THE DIABETES
MELLITUS
MANUAL

A PRIMARY CARE COMPANION TO
ELLENBERG AND RIFKIN'S

Edited by

SILVIO INZUCCHI, MD

Professor of Medicine
Section of Endocrinology
Director, Yale Diabetes Center
Yale University School of Medicine
New Haven, Connecticut

Daniel Porte, Jr, MD

Professor of Medicine
University of California, San Diego School of Medicine
San Diego, California
Emeritus Professor of Medicine
University of Washington School of Medicine
Seattle, Washington

Robert S. Sherwin, MD

C.N.H. Long Professor of Medicine
Director, General Clinical Research Center
Yale University School of Medicine
New Haven, Connecticut

Alain Baron, MD

Senior Vice President, Clinical Research
Amylin Pharmaceuticals, Inc.
San Diego, California
Professor of Medicine
Indiana University School of Medicine
Indianapolis, Indiana

McGraw-Hill
Medical Publishing Division

New York   Chicago   San Francisco   Lisbon   London   Madrid   Mexico City
Milan   New Delhi   San Juan   Seoul   Singapore   Sydney   Toronto

The Diabetes Mellitus Manual: A Primary Care Companion to Ellenberg & Rifkin's, Sixth Edition

Copyright © 2005 by The McGraw-Hill Companies, Inc. All rights reserved. Printed in the United States of America. Except as permitted under the United States Copyright Act of 1976, no part of this publication may be reproduced or distributed in any form or by any means, or stored in a data base or retrieval system, without the prior written permission of the publisher.

1234567890 DOC DOC 0987654

ISBN 0-07-143129-2

This book was set in Times Roman by PV&M Publishing Solutions.
The editors were James Shanahan, Michelle Watt, and Karen Davis.
The production supervisor was Sherri Souffrance.
The cover designer was Janice Bielawa.
The index was prepared by Robert Swanson.
RR Donnelley was printer and binder.

This book is printed on acid-free paper.

Library of Congress Cataloging-in-Publication Data

The diabetes mellitus manual : a primary care companion to Ellenberg and
    Rifkin's / edited by Silvio E. Inzucchi.
        p. cm.
    Includes bibliographical references and index.
    ISBN 0-07-143129-2
    1. Diabetes—Handbooks, manuals, etc.   I. Inzucchi, Silvio E.   II. Ellenberg,
Max.   III. Rifkin, Harold, 1916–
RC660.D5417 2004
616.4′062—dc22

                                                                2004052413

Contents

Contributors

Cameron M. Akbari, MD
Attending Vascular Surgeon and Director, Vascular Diagnostic Laboratory
Washington Hospital Center
Washington, DC
(Chapter 27)

K. George M.M. Alberti, DPhil, BM, Bch
Professor of Medicine
University of Newcastle Upon Tyne
Newcastle, England
(Chapter 15)

Stephanie A. Amiel, FRCP
Professor of Diabetic Medicine
Kings College School of Medicine
London, England
(Chapter 15)

Joyce P. Barnett, MS, RD, LD
Clinical Assistant Professor
Department of Clinical Nutrition
University of Texas Southwestern Medical Center
Dallas, Texas
(Chapter 7)

Peter H. Bennett, MB, FRCP
Senior Investigator
National Institute of Diabetes and Digestive and Kidney Diseases
Phoenix, Arizona
(Chapter 2)

Clifton Bogardus, MD
Chief, Clinical Diabetes and Nutrition Section
Chief, Phoenix Epidemiology and Clinical Research Branch
National Institute of Diabetes, Digestive, and Kidney Diseases
National Institutes of Health
Phoenix, Arizona
(Chapter 6)

Jennifer Bub, MD
Acting Instructor
Department of Medicine, Division of Dermatology
University of Washington School of Medicine
Seattle, Washington
(Chapter 29)

Joan I. Casey, MD, FRCPC
Professor of Medicine
Department of Internal Medicine
Albert Einstein College of Medicine
Bronx, New York
(Chapter 18)

Deborah A. Chyun, PhD, RN
Associate Professor
Yale University School of Nursing
New Haven, Connecticut
(Chapter 26)

William C. Coleman, DPM
Division of Podiatry
Division of Orthopedics
Ochsner Clinic Foundation
New Orleans, Louisiana
(Chapter 28)

C. Hamish Courtney, MD
Division of Endocrinology
University of California, San Diego School of Medicine
San Diego, California
(Chapter 5)

Brian P. Currie, MD
Associate Professor
Departments of Medicine and Epidemiology and Public Health
Albert Einstein College of Medicine
Bronx, New York
(Chapter 18)

Ralph A. DeFronzo, MD
Professor of Medicine and Chief, Diabetes Division
Department of Internal Medicine
University of Texas Health Sciences Center San Antonio
San Antonio, Texas
(Chapter 21)

Sharon L. Dooley, MD, MPH
Professor of Obstetrics and Gynecology
Northwestern University Feinberg School of Medicine
Chicago, Illinois
(Chapter 13)

Elizabeth Delionback Ennis, MD
Director, Internal Medicine and Transitional Year Residency Program
Baptist Health System
Birmingham, Alabama
(Chapter 16)

Tomris Erbas, MD
Department of Endocrinology and Metabolism
Hacettepe University
Hacettepe Medical School
Ankara, Turkey
(Chapter 22)

Eva L. Feldman, MD, PhD
Professor of Neurology
Director, JDRF Center for the Study of Complications
  in Diabetes
University of Michigan School of Medicine
Ann Arbor, Michigan
(Chapter 22)

Abhimanyu Garg, MD
Chief, Division of Nutrition and Metabolic Diseases
University of Texas Southwestern Medical Center
Dallas, Texas
(Chapter 7)

Robert R. Henry, MD
Professor of Medicine
University of California, San Diego Medical Center
Chief, Diabetes/Metabolism Section
VA San Diego Healthcare System
San Diego, California
(Chapter 12)

Silvio E. Inzucchi, MD
Professor of Medicine
Section of Endocrinology
Director, Yale Diabetes Center
Yale University School of Medicine
New Haven, Connecticut
(Chapter 1)

Steven E. Kahn, MB, ChB
Professor of Medicine
Division of Metabolism, Endocrinology, and Nutrition
University of Washington
Seattle Washington
(Chapter 4)

Norman M. Kaplan, MD
Clinical Professor of Internal Medicine
University of Texas Southwestern Medical Center
Dallas, Texas
(Chapter 25)

Ronald Klein, MD, MPH
Professor, Department of Ophthalmology and Visual Sciences
The University of Wisconsin-Madison Medical School
Madison, Wisconsin
(Chapter 20)

William C. Knowler, MD
Chief, Diabetes and Arthritis Epidemiology Section
National Institute of Diabetes and Digestive and Kidney Diseases
Phoenix, Arizona
(Chapter 2)

Robert A. Kreisberg, MD
Dean, Vice President of Medical Affairs
University of South Alabama College of Medicine
Mobile, Alabama
(Chapter 16)

Yolanta T. Kruszynska, MD, PhD
Associate Professor of Medicine
University of California, San Diego School of Medicine
San Diego, California
(Chapter 5)

Pierre Lefèvre, MD, PhD, FRCP
Emeritus Professor of Medicine
Division of Diabetes, Nutrition, and Metabolic Disorders
University of Liege, Medical School
Liege, Belgium
(Chapter 11)

Åke Lernmark, PhD
Robert H. Williams Professor of Medicine
Department of Medicine
Adjunct Professor of Immunology
University of Washington
Seattle, Washington
(Chapter 3)

Frank W. LoGerfo, MD
William V. McDermott Professor of Surgery
Harvard Medical School
Boston, Massachusetts
(Chapter 27)

Robert Matz, MD
Professor of Medicine
Division of Endocrinology and Metabolism
Mt. Sinai School of Medicine
New York, New York
(Chapter 17)

Boyd E. Metzger, MD
Division of Endocrinology, Metabolism & Molecular Medicine
Northwestern University Feinberg School of Medicine
Attending Physician
Northwestern Memorial Hospital
Chicago, Illinois
(Chapter 13, 14)

Sunder Mudaliar, MD
Staff Physician, Diabetes/Metabolism Section
VA San Diego Healthcare System
Assistant Clinical Professor of Medicine
University of California, San Diego
San Diego, California
(Chapter 12)

Ramachandra G. Naik, MD
Consultant Endocrinologist
Mumbai Hospital and Medical Research Center
Mumbai, India
(Chapter 3)

David M. Nathan, MD
Professor of Medicine
Harvard Medical School
Director, Diabetes Center and General Clinical Research Center
Massachusetts General Hospital
Boston, Massachusetts
(Chapter 10)

Edward S. Ogata, MD
Professor of Obstetrics and Gynecology
Northwestern University Feinberg School of Medicine
Chicago, Illinois
(Chapter 14)

Jerrold M. Olefsky MD
Professor of Medicine
Division of Endocrinology
University of California, San Diego
VA Medical Center
San Diego, California
(Chapter 5)

John Olerud, MD
Professor of Medicine
Head, Division of Dermatology
University of Washington Medical Center
Seattle, Washington
(Chapter 29)

Jerry P. Palmer, MD
Director, Diabetes Endocrinology Research Center
and Diabetes Care Center
Professor of Medicine
University of Washington School of Medicine
Seattle, Washington
(Chapter 3)

Amanda Peltier, MD
Department of Neurology
University of Michigan School of Medicine
Ann Arbor, Michigan
(Chapter 23)

Michael A. Pfeifer, MD
Medical Product Leader, Lantus
Avenits Pharmaceuticals
Bridgewater, New Jersey
(Chapter 22)

Richard L. Phelps, MD
Assistant Professor of Clinical Medicine
Northwestern University Feinberg School of Medicine
Chicago, Illinois
(Chapter 13)

Daniel Porte, Jr., MD
Professor of Medicine
University of California, San Diego School of Medicine
San Diego, California
Emeritus Professor of Medicine
University of Washington School of Medicine
Seattle, Washington
(Chapter 4)

Philip Raskin, MD
Professor of Internal Medicine
University of Texas Southwestern Medical Center
Medical Director, University Diabetes Treatment Center
Parkland Memorial Hospital
Dallas, Texas
(Chapter 9)

Marian J. Rewers, MD, PhD, MPH
Professor, Pediatrics and Preventive Medicine
Clinical Director, The Barbara Davis Center for Childhood Diabetes
University of Colorado Health Sciences Center
Denver, Colorado
(Chapter 2)

James W. Russell, MD
Associate Professor of Neurology
University of Michigan School of Medicine
Ann Arbor, Michigan
(Chapter 22, 23)

Lester B. Salans, MD
Clinical Professor of Medicine
Department of Medicine
Division of Endocrinology
Mt. Sinai School of Medicine
New York, New York
(Chapter 30)

André J. Scheen, MD, PhD
Professor of Internal Medicine
Department of Medicine
Head, Division of Diabetes, Nutrition, and Metabolic Disorders
Head, Division of Clinical Pharmacology
University Hospital
Liege, Belgium
(Chapter 11)

Clay F. Semenkovich, MD
Professor of Medicine
Professor of Cell Biology and Physiology
Washington University School of Medicine
St. Louis, Missouri
(Chapter 24)

Bernard L. Silverman, MD
Director, Therapeutics and Safety
Alkermes, Inc.
Cambridge, Massachusetts
(Chapter 14)

Jay S. Skyler, MD
Professor of Medicine, Pediatrics, and Psychology
University of Miami School of Medicine
Miami, Florida
(Chapter 19)

Geralyn R. Spollett, MSN, C-ANP, CDE
Adult Nurse Practitioner
Yale Diabetes Center
Yale School of Medicine
New Haven, Connecticut
(Chapter 8)

Martin J. Stevens, MD
Associate Professor of Internal Medicine
Associate Director, JDRF Center for the Study of Complications
    in Diabetes
University of Michigan School of Medicine
Ann Arbor, Michigan
(Chapter 22)

Suzanne M. Strowig, MSN, RN
Faculty Associate
Department of Internal Medicine
University of Texas Southwestern Medical Center
Dallas, Texas
(Chapter 9)

P. Antonio Tataranni, MD
Head, Obesity, Diabetes, and Energy Metabolism Unit
Director, Clinical Research Unit
Clinical Diabetes & Nutrition Section
National Institutes of Health
Phoenix, Arizona
(Chapter 6)

Aaron I. Vinik, MD
Director, The Strelitz Diabetes Research Institutes
Professor of Medicine
Eastern Virginia Medical School
Norfolk, Virginia
(Chapter 22)

Lawrence H. Young, MD
Professor of Internal Medicine
Section of Cardiovascular Medicine
Yale University School of Medicine
Attending Physician
Yale-New Haven Hospital
New Haven, Connecticut
(Chapter 26)

Preface

This is the companion Manual to the sixth edition of *Ellenberg & Rifkin's Diabetes Mellitus*. The chapters in the Manual were prepared by the authors of the corresponding chapters in the larger text and reflect recent developments of significance to all clinicians in the management of diabetes and its complications. In addition, there is a new chapter on the basics of diabetes education, not found in the larger text. The Manual was designed to provide a concise, portable reference source on diabetes mellitus for clinicians, trainees, and students who cannot always access the larger textbooks. However, it is not intended to replace the more detailed reference sources for diabetes mellitus.

Silvio E. Inzucchi
September 2004

TABLE 1-1 Etiologic Classification of Diabetes Mellitus

Type 1 (formerly insulin-dependent diabetes, IDDM)
β-cell destruction, resulting in absolute insulin deficiency
  Autoimmune
  Idiopathic
Type 2 (formerly non-insulin-dependent diabetes, NIDDM)
Variable disorder ranging from predominately insulin resistance with relative
  insulin deficiency to a predominately insulin secretory defect with or
  without insulin resistance
Other specific types (secondary diabetes)
  Genetic defects of β-cell function
    (i.e., maturity-onset diabetes of the young, MODY)
  Genetic defects of insulin action
  Diseases of the exocrine pancreas
  Other endocrinopathies
  Drug- or chemical-induced
  Infections
  Uncommon forms of immune-mediated diabetes
  Other congenital syndromes associated with diabetes
Gestational diabetes
  Diabetes diagnosed during pregnancy, with usual resolution postpartum

Source: Adapted with permission from Alberti KG, Zimmet PZ: *Diabet Med* 1998;
15:535.

patient at increased susceptibility to β-cell injury, through the interaction of one or several environmental factors. The presence of islet cell injury in patients with T1DM is reflected in certain circulating antibodies, such as islet cell antibodies (ICAs), insulin autoantibodies (IAAs), and antibodies to glutamic acid decarboxylase (GAD) and ICA512 (or IA2). Type 1A diabetes refers to the form that is associated with such immune markers, although it should be noted that as permanent islet cell destruction is established, antibody titers may dissipate or disappear entirely. A less common second subtype, type 1B, is idiopathic in origin, and may not have an immune-mediated etiology.

Although the islet autoimmunity can precede clinical manifestations of disease by years or even decades, the presentation of T1DM is often abrupt and severe because of the eventuation of a loss of a critical mass of insulin-producing cells. The clinical onset of T1DM is marked by hyperglycemia developing over several days to weeks, usually associated with weight loss, fatigue, polyuria, polydipsia, blurring of vision, and evidence of volume contraction. The presence of ketoacidosis indicates the severe deficiency of insulin, which leads to both the hyperglycemia as well as unrestrained lipolysis. T1DM is usually diagnosed prior to the age of 30–40 years, most commonly in childhood or in adolescence. However, T1DM occurs throughout life and is often misdiagnosed as T2DM when it appears after the age of 40 years. Individuals with T1DM are typically lean, although the presence of obesity certainly does not preclude the diagnosis. Despite the genetic predisposition for T1DM, most affected patients, in contrast to type 2 diabetes, have no family history of diabetes.

1 | Classification and Diagnosis of Diabetes Mellitus

Silvio E. Inzucchi

Diabetes mellitus is characterized by increased circulating glucose conc trations associated with abnormalities in carbohydrate, fat, and protein me olism, and a variety of microvascular and macrovascular complications. diabetic states result from an inadequate supply of insulin or an inadeq tissue response to its actions. The former occurs in, for example, type 1 betes, which culminates from the autoimmune destruction of the inst producing β-cells within the pancreatic islets. The latter occurs when insulin receptor is defective, or, more commonly, when genetic an acquired defects in postreceptor intracellular signaling pathways attenuate subsequent physiologic response. Such is the case with the more wic prevalent type 2 diabetes, a complex disorder resulting from periph insulin resistance, combined with relative insulin deficiency.

ETIOLOGIC CLASSIFICATION OF DIABETES

Diabetes is not a single disease, but a heterogenous group of disorders rel to each other only because of their primary manifestations: hyperglyce and resultant vascular complications. In the past, when the understandin underlying pathophysiologic mechanisms was less mature, its classifica was based on either the age groups affected or on conventional treatment adigms. For instance, the currently designated type 1 diabetes mellitus referred to as "juvenile-onset diabetes mellitus (JODM)" or "insulin-depen diabetes mellitus (IDDM)," while type 2 diabetes mellitus was labeled "ac onset diabetes mellitus (AODM)" or "non-insulin dependent diabetes m tus (NIDDM)." As knowledge regarding the underlying cellular and r molecular underpinnings of diabetes has matured, a more pathophysiol cally based nomenclature has developed (Table 1-1).

TYPE 1 DIABETES MELLITUS

Type 1 diabetes mellitus (T1DM) is responsible for approximately 5–10% c cases of diabetes in the Western world. It is characterized by severe insulin c ciency resulting from β-cell destruction. Ultimately, circulating insulin centrations are negligible or completely absent. When the disease is f expressed (and in the absence of insulin therapy), patients with T1DM exl not only hyperglycemia but are also ketosis-prone. Thus, these individual: "dependent" on insulin for survival. β-Cell destruction in T1DM is aut(mune in nature. Islet inflammation ("insulitis") may be seen in pathol pancreatic specimens from individuals prior to the development of diabe

As with most autoimmune diseases, T1DM is associated with genes w the major histocompatibility complex (MHC). The prevalence of certain tocompatibility locus antigens (HLAs) is either increased (DR3, DQ2 or E DQ8) or decreased (DR2, DQ6). One or several immune response or c genes are likely to enhance the effect of these HLA antigens, rendering

Type 2 Diabetes Mellitus

In many ways, type 2 diabetes mellitus (T2DM) is an entirely separate disorder from T1DM. It is a much more common condition, responsible for more than 90% of cases of diabetes worldwide. The autoimmune markers of type 1 diabetes are typically absent. While relative β-cell insufficiency is, by definition, present in all individuals with T2DM, the disorder in most is characterized by insulin resistance detected at the level of skeletal muscle, adipose tissue, and the liver. Insulin resistance at the former site results in decreased peripheral glucose disposal, while at the latter, in increased hepatic glucose production. Unlike T1DM, a family history is common, although the inheritance pattern of this disease is complex and suspected to be polygenic.

In many individuals, the natural history of T2DM begins with a period of insulin resistance with preserved, indeed augmented, pancreatic insulin secretion, as the insensitivity to insulin action in peripheral tissues is overcome by hyperinsulinemia. As a result, plasma glucose concentrations remain relatively normal. As the disease progresses, however, pancreatic islet cell function falters and is no longer able to meet peripheral demands. As a result, insulin levels fail to keep up with requirements, and hyperglycemia ensues. This may be first manifested in the postprandial setting, while fasting glucose is preserved early in the disease course. Even in those with late-stage T2DM, insulin secretion persists to an extent required to suppress lipolysis in most patients, so that ketoacidosis rarely occurs. Ketosis can develop, however, when an intervening medical illness poses a severe metabolic stress, further heightening insulin resistance and impairing the insulin secretory response. Because of renal glucose clearance, plasma glucose concentrations in T2DM typically plateau in the 250–350-mg/dL range. However, in the presence of any superimposed deterioration in renal function or marked dehydration, further elevations may occur. Hyperosmolar, hyperglycemic syndrome (HHS) may result and can be life-threatening.

Compared to patients with T1DM, those with T2DM are typically older, usually over 40 years, and are commonly overweight, if not frankly obese. Over the past decade, however, a frightening increase in the prevalence of T2DM has been noted in younger age groups, even in children. This is felt to result from increasing rates of obesity and inactivity in populations from certain ethnic groups predisposed to T2DM, including Native, African, and Hispanic Americans, and Pacific Islanders.

In patients with or at risk for T2DM, a group of other clinical and biochemical characteristics is frequently encountered. These include central obesity, hypertension, dyslipidemia (elevated triglycerides, decreased HDL-cholesterol, and increased small dense LDL-cholesterol), a procoagulant state, endothelial dysfunction, and an increased risk for premature cardiovascular morbidity. This constellation of findings is often referred to as the "metabolic syndrome" (formerly, syndrome X). Insulin resistance is felt by many to be the root cause of this complex, and, thus, many refer to it as the "insulin resistance syndrome." The striking predisposition of patients with T2DM to cardiovascular disease, even prior to their development of significant hyperglycemia, may result from the combined effects of the manifestations of the metabolic syndrome on the vasculature.

While patients with T2DM can use insulin for blood glucose control, they rarely require it to avoid the life-threatening complications of ketoacidosis. Importantly, however, when insulin is required for optimal blood glucose control, the designation of disease type is not changed. It should also be noted that some adult individuals with diabetes mellitus, usually between the ages of 20 and 40 years, share features of both type 1 and type 2 disease and, as a result, escape easy categorization, These individuals are often leaner and more insulin-deficient than those with classical T2DM. Frequently, immune markers of T1DM are present, and their hyperglycemia appears to represent a slowly progressive form of autoimmune diabetes. Furthermore, it has recently been discovered that as many as 10% of elderly patients classified as T2DM may also have measurable titers of autoantibodies associated with T1DM. Similarly, these patients may also have a slowly evolving form of T1DM, which is now referred to as "latent autoimmune diabetes of adulthood (LADA)"

Other Forms of Diabetes Mellitus (Secondary Diabetes)

Several forms of diabetes result from or are related to another specific disease process or genetic disorder. These conditions are considered neither T1DM nor T2DM and are grouped together under "other specific types," sometimes referred to as "secondary diabetes." This category represents a variety of conditions that are included because of (1) a recognized comprehension of the underlying pathogenensis; (2) the molecular defects governing the hyperglycemia are well defined; or (3) a clear association between the diabetes and an otherwise precisely defined clinical syndrome.

Genetic Defects in β-Cell Function

Maturity-onset diabetes of the young (MODY) is a clinically heterogeneous group of hyperglycemic disorders with an autosomal dominant mode of inheritance that may account for 1–5% of diabetes cases in the United States. Patients with MODY are usually not obese and may be mildly hyperglycemic. They are generally not predisposed to ketoacidosis. The onset of disease is typically before age 25 years, usually in childhood or adolescence, although the mild nature of the disorder may mask clinical detection for many years. There is a strong family history of diabetes in multiple generations. Primary defects in β-cell function, which are becoming well defined, appear to be responsible for all cases of MODY. To date, six separate genetic mutations have been characterized and numbered, MODY 1 through MODY 6. Each of the mutated genes is expressed in islets, and their mutations result in abnormal glucorecognition by the β-cell, or in insulin secretory dysfunction, or both.

Genetic Defects in Insulin Action

Abnormalities of the insulin molecule or its receptor can lead to diabetes, but these are extraordinarily rare conditions that are manifested in infancy. Leprechaunism, which results from an inactivating mutation in the insulin receptor, for example, is characterized by severe insulin resistance, dysmorphic features, intrauterine growth retardation, and acanthosis nigricans. Other forms of diabetes in this category include type A insulin resistance with acanthosis nigricans, Rabson-Mendenhall syndrome (dental dysplasia, dystrophic nails, precocious puberty), and lipodystrophic diabetes. More recently, genetic mutations in the nuclear transcription factor known as PPAR-γ (peroxisome proliferator-activated receptor-γ) has been associated with severe insulin resistance and diabetes.

Exocrine Pancreatic Diseases

Diseases of the nonislet pancreas are also frequently associated with abnormalities of glucose tolerance. Hyperglycemia can be a sequela of both acute and chronic pancreatitis, as well as other diseases that involve the pancreatic parenchyma, such as hemochromatosis and cystic fibrosis. In the tropics, malnutrition-related fibrocalculous pancreatitis has been linked to diabetes. Hyperglycemia is also commonly encountered in patients with carcinoma of the pancreas.

Other Endocrinopathies

Other hormonal disorders are frequently associated with glucose intolerance and, sometimes, frank diabetes. Most of these involve the secretion of counterregulatory factors, leading to a state of decreased insulin sensitivity. These include acromegaly (excess growth hormone), Cushing's syndrome (cortisol), and pheochromocytoma (catecholamines). Diabetes may also occasionally be encountered in patients with hyperthyroidism, presumably due to augmentation of β-adrenergic activity, and primary hyperaldosteronism, possibly related to decreased insulin release from hypokalemia. Finally, several neuroendocrine tumors of the pancreas are also associated with diabetes, including those elaborating primarily glucagon, vasoactive intestinal peptide, and somatostatin. Glucagonoma is rare, but carries the strongest association with diabetes. This tumor is associated with normocytic anemia and a pathognomonic rash involving the groin, genital, and perineal regions, known as necrolytic migratory erythema.

Drug- and Chemical-Induced Diabetes

A number of medications have been implicated in the development of diabetes. In most situations, the use of the drug may simply unmask an underlying tendency toward glucose intolerance. Such drugs include those that contribute to insulin resistance, most notably glucocorticoids, but also growth hormone, levothyroxine (in excess), and niacin. Atypical antipsychotics, especially clozapine and olanzapine, are associated with diabetes, at times manifested by severe hyperglycemia or even ketoacidosis. These drugs frequently lead to weight gain but also may directly alter insulin sensitivity. Other diabetogenic medications or chemical agents decrease insulin secretion (β-adrenergic antagonists; calcium channel antagonists; diuretics, especially thiazides; diazoxide; dilantin; and octreotide) or lead to β-cell destruction (pentamidine and the rodenticide Vacor). Certain chemotherapeutic agents or immunomodulators, such as mithramycin, L-asparaginase, and α-interferon, have also been associated with new cases of diabetes, although the precise mechanisms involved are not completely understood.

Infections

Certain viral agents have been implicated as the "environmental" factor that triggers the immune response in T1DM, including rubella, CMV, Coxsackie, mumps, and adenovirus. No specific virus appears to be responsible, however, for most cases.

Uncommon Forms of Immune-Mediated Diabetes

Rarely, patients may present with hyperglycemia and/or hypoglycemia due to anti-insulin or anti-insulin receptor antibodies. Stiff-man syndrome is an autoimmune neurologic affliction associated with increased circulating titers of anti-GAD antibodies and diabetes.

Other Genetic Syndromes

Diabetes or impaired glucose tolerance is also found with increased frequency in a number of congenital disorders such as Down's syndrome, Turner's syndrome, myotonic dystrophy, Klinefelter's syndrome, Prader-Willi syndrome, Huntington's chorea, Wolfram's syndrome, Werner's syndrome, Alstrom's syndrome, Friedrich's ataxia, porphyria, and the Laurence-Moon-Biedl syndrome. In most cases, the diabetes is non-insulin-requiring.

Gestational Diabetes Mellitus

Diabetes diagnosed during pregnancy is referred to as gestational diabetes mellitus (GDM), a category that necessarily includes both diabetes first appearing and first being recognized during pregnancy. (See Chapter 13).

DIAGNOSTIC CRITERIA AND THE SPECTRUM OF ABNORMALITIES IN GLUCOSE HOMEOSTASIS

Diabetes is characterized by progressive elevations in circulating glucose concentrations. In T2DM, these elevations occur over years to decades. As they pass from the normal into the diabetic range, glucose levels transition through an intermediate and less well categorized phase referred to as impaired glucose tolerance (IGT). While the hyperglycemia of diabetes is clearly associated with an increased risk of microvascular and macrovascular complications, as well as increased mortality, there has been less agreement on the implications of these earlier and more mild glucose elevations. Over the past decade, however, the risk associated with IGT has become clear, with affected individuals at increased risk not only for progression to diabetes, but also for increased cardiovascular morbidity. IGT, widely recognized to occur in patients destined to develop T2DM, may also be seen in individuals prior to the development of T1DM.

Report of the Expert Committee on the Diagnosis and Classification of Diabetes Mellitus, 1997

Until 1997, the ADA had endorsed the 1979 criteria of the National Diabetes Data Group (NDDG). The NDDG had denoted 140 mg/dL as the plasma glucose (PG) cutpoint for the diagnosis of diabetes by fasting criteria. Alternatively, the diagnosis could also be made if sustained elevation of PG during a 2-hour, 75-g oral glucose tolerance test (OGTT) was documented. In 1995, however, an international expert committee was invited by the ADA to review the scientific literature since 1979 and to decide if changes to the classification of and diagnostic criteria for diabetes were required. The committee published its findings in 1997, and these continue to be endorsed by the ADA. The most notable changes recommended by the committee included the following:

1. The previous terms (used by the NDDG) "insulin-dependent" and "non-insulin-dependent," as applied to diabetes, should be abandoned, as they were felt to be both confusing and imprecise. Instead, the main subclasses of diabetes would be, simply, "type 1" and "type 2."

TABLE 1-2 Diabetes Mellitus: 1997 ADA Diagnostic Criteria*

1. Symptoms of diabetes plus casual plasma glucose concentration ≥ 200 mg/dL (11.1 mmol/L). Casual is defined as any time of day without regard to time since last meal. The classic symptoms of diabetes include polyuria, polydipsia, and unexplained weight loss.

or

2. FPG ≥ 126 mg/dL (7.0 mmol/L). Fasting is defined as no caloric intake for at least 8 hours.

or

3. A 2-hour PG ≥ 200 mg/dL (11.1 mmol/L) during an OGTT. The test should be performed as described by WHO, using a glucose load containing the equivalent of 75 g of anhydrous glucose dissolved in water.

*In the absence of unequivocal hyperglycemia with acute metabolic decompensation these criteria should be confirmed by repeat testing on a different day. The third measure (OGTT) is not recommended for routine clinical use.

Source: Reprinted with permission from American Diabetes Association: *Diabetes Care* 2004; 27(Suppl 1):S9.

2. The fasting plasma glucose (FPG) threshold for the diagnosis of diabetes should be lowered from 140 to 126 mg/dL (Table 1-2).
3. Normal FPG should be <110 mg/dL; those individuals with FPGs between 110 and 125 mg/dL should be newly categorized as "impaired fasting glucose (IFG)," intended to be the fasting equivalent of IGT.
4. Although the older criteria, using both random (now called "casual," i.e., without regard to meals) and post-OGTT glucose concentrations, were not changed, FPG was recommended as the preferred screening and diagnostic test due to its wide availability, simplicity, and convenience over OGTT. (See Table 1-3 for the ADA recommended screening guidelines.)

This decision to reduce the diagnostic threshold for FPG was based on epidemiologic data that emerged after the NDDG criteria were developed. It was recognized that only one in four individuals without a prior diagnosis of diabetes but with a 2-hour PG ≥ 200 mg/dL during OGTT also had an FPG ≥ 140 mg/dL. The committee also had a practical concern. Many individuals who would have a 2-hour PG ≥ 200 mg/dL during an OGTT would not necessarily undergo such testing, either because they were asymptomatic or because the diagnosis of diabetes had already been confirmed on the basis of an FPG ≥ 140 mg/dL. Since the OGTT identifies more individuals with diabetes than does the FPG, routine use of the OGTT would be necessary for optimal case finding. Yet, in routine practice, the more expensive and inconvenient OGTT was rarely performed. Several studies had also shown that the actual FPG level equivalent to the 2-hour PG cutpoint of 200 mg/dL ranged between 120 and 126 mg/dL. In addition, and perhaps more importantly, the committee reviewed three studies relating plasma glucose levels to the prevalence of retinopathy. In each of these, the FPG threshold distinguishing those subjects at increased risk for microvascular disease was observed at approximately 120–130 mg/dL (with the 2-hour PG threshold remaining at approximately 200 mg/dL) (Fig. 1-1). Thus, the committee felt that it was mandatory that the fasting diagnostic criteria for diabetes be revised so that the discrepancy in diagnostic power between the FPG and 2-hour PG would be diminished and in order to facilitate and encourage the use of a simpler test, namely, FPG. The cutpoint of 126 mg/dL was chosen.

TABLE 1-3 Criteria for Testing for Diabetes in Asymptomatic, Undiagnosed Individuals

Testing for diabetes should be considered in all individuals at age 45 years and above and, if normal, it should be repeated at 3-year intervals.
Testing should be considered at a younger age or be carried out more frequently in individuals who:

- Are habitually inactive.
- Are obese (≥ 120% desirable body weight or a BMI ≥ 27 kg/m²).
- Have a first-degree relative with diabetes.
- Are members of a high-risk ethnic population (e.g., African-American, Hispanic American, Native American, Asian American, Pacific Islander).
- Have delivered a baby weighing > 9 lb or have been diagnosed with gestational diabetes mellitus (GDM)
- Are hypertensive (140/90 mmHg).
- Have an HDL cholesterol level ≤ 35 mg/dL (0.90 mmol/L) and/or a triglyceride level ≥ 250 mg/dL (2.82 mmol/L).
- Have polycystic ovary syndrome.
- On previous testing, had impaired glucose tolerance (IGT) or impaired fasting glycemia (IFG).
- Have other clinical conditions associated with insulin resistance (e.g., acanthosis nigricans).
- Have a history of vascular disease.

Source: Reprinted with permission from American Diabetes Association: *Diabetes Care* 2004; 27(Suppl 1):S17.

On the basis of epidemiologic estimates, the committee expected only slightly fewer individuals would be identified as having diabetes using the new FPG criteria, as compared to the WHO cutpoints using both FPG and 2-hour PG. In the Cardiovascular Health Study, however, Wahl and coworkers reported a significant difference in the prevalence of diabetes as identified by these two sets of criteria. The prevalence of untreated diabetes was found to be 14.8% using the WHO criteria and only 7.7% using the new ADA fasting criteria. Similar conclusions were made by Gabir and colleagues in Pima Indians and by Resnick and colleagues, using NHANES III data.

Overall, however, in clinical practice, because of low utilization of OGTTs, the change in the ADA criteria has effectively led to an increase in the number of patients identified as having diabetes. It has been estimated, for example, that the change has resulted in the diagnosis of patients an average of 7 years earlier as compared to the older fasting criteria.

In keeping with the new criteria of the ADA, in 1999, the WHO similarly reduced their cutpoint for venous FPG to 126 mg/dL and affirmed the new category of IFG (impaired fasting glycemia) for those with FPGs between 110 and 125 mg/dL. If an OGTT had been performed, however, and if the 2-hour PG reached or exceeded 140 mg/dL, the IGT diagnosis would predominate. The diagnostic glucose ranges for IGT were not changed from the WHO 1985 report, and remained identical to those accepted by the ADA. In contrast to the ADA criteria, however, the WHO continued to recommend use of the OGTT for purposes of clinical research. For clinical practice, unless the FPG was already in the diabetic range, the WHO also recommended an OGTT if a random glucose level was in the "uncertain" range [i.e., between the levels that "establish" (200 mg/dL) or "exclude" (100 mg/dL) diabetes]. It was also emphasized that IGT and IFG were not diagnostic classes by themselves, but instead stages in the natural history of abnormal carbohydrate metabolism.

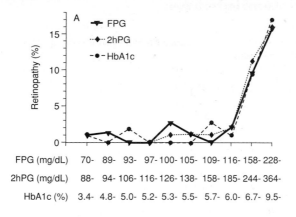

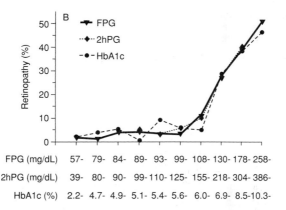

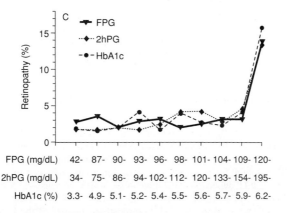

FIG. 1-1 Prevalence of retinopathy by deciles of the distribution of FPG, 2-h PG, and HbA1c. (Reprinted with permission from American Diabetes Association: *Diabetes Care* 2002; 25(Suppl 1):S13.)

In 2004, the ADA further reduced the glucose threshold for the diagnosis of IFG to 100 mg/dL.

Comparison of Current ADA and WHO Criteria

Since the release of the 1997 ADA diagnostic criteria, several studies have compared their performance with those of the WHO. Gabir and colleagues compared these two criteria and their relation to the development of microvascular complications, finding no difference in their predictive value. Others have also affirmed that, although OGTT-driven diagnostic algorithm will find more individuals with diabetes, the current ADA fasting criteria are adequate to identify those persons at risk for microvascular disease resulting from their hyperglycemia.

The DECODE Study Group evaluated the impact of using FPG versus OGTT criteria on the identification of individuals at risk for macrovascular disease. Existing baseline data on glucose concentrations in the fasting state and 2 hours after a 75-g glucose load from 10 prospective European cohort studies including more than 15,000 men and 7000 women were analyzed. Hazard ratios for all-cause mortality and cardiovascular disease endpoints were estimated. The investigators concluded that use of 2-hour PG enhanced the predictive value of FPG alone, whereas the converse was not true. Therefore, while both FPG and 2-hour PG appear to perform equivalently in the identification of microvascular risk, FPG alone may fail to sufficiently identify those at increased macrovascular risk, and the 2-hour glucose during an OGTT may provide additional prognostic information. Barzilay and coworkers performed a similar analysis on a separate data set. Not unexpectedly, there was a higher prevalence of cardiovascular disease among individuals with IGT or newly diagnosed diabetes by both ADA and WHO criteria than among those with normal glucose levels. However, since fewer subjects were classified as abnormal by the fasting ADA criteria than by the WHO criteria, the number of cases of cardiovascular disease attributable to abnormal glucose status by ADA criteria was one-third of that attributable by WHO criteria. Conversely, those classified as normal by the ADA fasting criteria had more cardiovascular events during the follow-up period than did those deemed normal by the WHO criteria. Thus, the current fasting ADA criteria may be less predictive than those of the WHO for the burden of cardiovascular disease associated with abnormal glucose metabolism in the elderly.

Comparison of Two Stages of Abnormal Glucose Homeostasis: IGT and IFG

Although IFG was devised to be the fasting equivalent of IGT, studies performed since 1997 demonstrate that these two categories of early abnormal glucose homeostasis are not necessarily interchangeable diagnoses. Based on NHANES III data, for example, 14.9% of Americans between the ages of 40 and 74 have IGT, whereas 8.3% have IFG, and 3.9% carry both diagnoses. That is, only a minority of patients with either IFG or IGT meet criteria for the other diagnosis. Moreover, while almost one-quarter of the U.S. population in this age group has either IFG or IGT, less than 1 in 25 has both conditions simultaneously.

Patients with IFG and those with IGT also appear to have distinct metabolic abnormalities. Investigators studied a large group of Pima Indians using hyperinsulinemic euglycemic clamps, glucose isotope infusions, and intravenous glucose tolerance tests (IVGTTs) to assess insulin sensitivity, insulin secretion, and endogenous glucose production. Subjects with isolated IFG (i.e., IFG, but not IGT) and those with isolated IGT (i.e., IGT, but not IFG) demonstrated equally reduced insulin sensitivity. IFG subjects had worse insulin secretory responses to IVGTTs and increased endogenous glucose production, compared to IGT subjects. Individuals with both IFG and IGT had the most severe abnormalities in all metabolic parameters. Thus, Pima Indians with isolated IFG and isolated IGT show similar impairments in insulin action, but those with isolated IFG have a relatively more pronounced defect in early insulin secretion and greater augmentation of endogenous glucose production. The most severe abnormalities are exhibited by those with combined IFG and IGT. The risk of progressing to T2DM appears to be equivalent between those with isolated IFG and isolated IGT, and those who carry both diagnoses progress at the highest rate. From the DECODE study, individuals with IGT seem to have the greater risk for developing cardiovascular disease, which may indicate a greater influence on vascular disease from postprandial hyperglycemia.

COMMON TESTS USED TO EVALUATE GLUCOSE HOMEOSTASIS

Type and Source of Body Fluid

Venous plasma or *serum* is considered the standard body fluid for the determination of glucose concentration, being representative of the extracellular glucose content. Serum and plasma glucose values are essentially identical. The latter is measured by most laboratories and has been historically used in most clinical research studies. *Whole blood* determinations are typically 15% lower than plasma or serum and may also be influenced by the hematocrit. Ideally, phlebotomized blood should be collected in test tubes containing sodium fluoride, which will inhibit red blood cell glycolysis. Alternatively, the blood can be chilled immediately, with the plasma or serum expeditiously separated from cellular contents. *Arterial blood* has a glucose content approximately 7% higher than that of venous blood. In the fasting state, this difference is less than in the postprandial setting. *Capillary blood* glucose is similar to that of arterial blood.

The easy availability of capillary blood is taken advantage of by home glucose meters, which are hand-held monitoring devices that provide the patient the ability to test his or her own blood glucose at any time of the day. Home glucose monitoring has become an integral part of the management of patients with diabetes. A large variety of meters are currently on the market, with many different features, including interfaces with computer software, allowing for intricate forms of data analysis. Many of the newer meters automatically adjust their results to be displayed as standardized to plasma glucose. While extremely useful for the monitoring of established patients, personal glucose monitors are neither accurate nor precise enough for diagnostic purposes.

Urine glucose is a poorly sensitive marker of diabetes, since the renal glucose threshold in most individuals is not reached until the extracellular glucose concentration exceeds 180 mg/dL. In addition, the urine glucose result is in part dependent on the dilutional effects of recent fluid intake. Prior to the availability of home capillary blood glucose meters, urine testing was an acceptable means for the rough assessment of glycemic control. Except for unusual circumstances where capillary glucose monitoring is impractical, urine glucose testing is no longer considered appropriate for either diagnostic or monitoring purposes.

Oral Glucose Tolerance Test

The homeostatic mechanisms serving to maintain normal glucose concentrations can be assessed using the physiologic "stress" of providing the patient a rapidly absorbed carbohydrate load: the oral glucose tolerance test (OGTT). As noted previously, more individuals will be diagnosed with various degrees of abnormal glucose homeostasis on the basis of their performance on OGTT than by the simpler measurement of fasting glucose alone. It is currently recommended by the WHO for use when blood glucose levels are otherwise equivocal, in epidemiologic settings to assess for diabetes and impaired glucose tolerance, and during pregnancy to screen for and diagnose gestational diabetes. Given its relatively cumbersome and time-consuming nature, the ADA recommends that, outside of pregnancy, FPG be used as the routine screening and diagnostic test. However, there is a recent move to expand utilization of the OGTT to detect earlier forms of abnormal carbohydrate metabolism. This has resulted both from recent evidence that the progression from IGT to DM is indeed preventable, with lifestyle change and/or pharmcotherapy, and because of emerging evidence that postchallenge blood glucose is a better prognosticator of cardiovascular morbidity than FPG. In clinical practice, the OGTT is also used in the rare patient who presents with microvascular complications suggesting diabetes (i.e., retinopathy, nephropathy, or neuropathy) but in whom initial glucodiagnostic studies show no abnormalities.

In the standard test, 75 g of anhydrous glucose is dissolved in 250–300 mL of water and administered over 5 minutes. (In children the glucose load should calculate to 1.75 g/kg body weight, up to a maximum of 75 g.) A base line glucose level is obtained prior to glucose ingestion, and subsequently every 30 minutes for 2 hours. (The WHO standard is for blood to be obtained fasting and then again only at 2 hours.) Variations of the standard OGTT include the 1-hour test using 50 g glucose for GDM screening and the 3-hour 100-g glucose test for formal testing for GDM. The 5-hour OGTT has recently fallen out of favor, having been used in the past for the evaluation of reactive hypoglycemia. The concurrent measurement of plasma insulin concentrations (as a surrogate marker of insulin sensitivity) is used occasionally for the inferential diagnosis of insulin resistance.

Glycosylated Hemoglobin, Hemoglobin A1c (HbA1c)

Due to wide fluctuations in circulating glucose concentrations in patients with diabetes, random glucose measurements are often not reflective of overall glycemic control. Even fasting determinations, which tend to be more stable, do not provide a complete picture. Like many proteins, erythrocyte hemoglobin is nonezymatically glycosylated at amine residues in the presence of glucose, which passes freely across red blood cell membranes. The percentage of hemoglobin molecules undergoing this reaction is proportional to the average ambient glucose concentrations during the preceding 60–90 days. "Glycohemoglobin" and "hemoglobin A1c" (HbA1c) are, therefore, commonly used laboratory tests for assessing long-term diabetic control. HbA1c, with a normal range of approximately 4–6% in most laboratories, refers to the percentage of hemoglobin molecules with glucose moieties attached to N-terminal valines of each of the two β-chains. Glycohemoglobin (normal range, approximately 6–8%) includes HbA1c, but also other forms of hemoglobin where glycosylation has occurred at other amino acids. HbA1c is more popular and is used primarily in the ongoing follow-up of diabetic patients. A highly specific test for diabetes, HbA1c is not sensitive enough to be used for screening purposes. That is, patients with mild hyperglycemia, clearly within the diabetic range by FPG or 2-hour PG, may have HbA1c in the high-normal range. This is particularly the case since the lower diagnostic criteria of the ADA have been used. For instance, in one analysis of two large data sets including NHANES III, 87% of individuals with IFG and 61% of those with FPGs in the diabetic range had normal HbA1c. In contrast, when the older criteria, FPG ≥ 140 mg/dL, were used, only 19% of diabetic patients had normal HbA1c. Hemoglobinopathies and states of rapid red cell turnover may make glycohemoglobin and HbA1c values difficult to interpret.

Emerging Technologies

Interstitial sensors are currently available for use in diabetic patients for continuous monitoring of extracellular glucose concentrations. Interstitial glucose approximates plasma glucose, particularly when determining glycemic trends. A current commercially available model is used for a 72-hour period, with the interstitial probe inserted subcutaneously and attached to a computerized unit that can be worn on the belt. The readings are downloaded at the end of the recording period for computerized analysis at the practitioner's office. Several companies are actively pursuing refined versions of sensors that can provide a live display to the patient. Recently, a wristwatch-like sensor device was approved by the U.S. Food and Drug Administration (FDA). This unit uses a process known as reverse iontophoresis (applying a gentle electrical current to the skin to express minute amounts of interstitial fluid, which can be analyzed for glucose content) and can measure glucose levels every 20 minutes. The results are provided to the patient on the device's display. Twice-daily calibration with the readings from routine capillary blood glucose monitoring is still required.

ADDITIONAL READINGS

Alberti KG, Zimmet PZ: Definition, diagnosis and classification of diabetes mellitus and its complications. Part 1: Diagnosis and classification of diabetes mellitus. Provisional Report of a WHO Consultation. *Diabet Med* 1998;15:535.

American Diabetes Association. Diagnosis and classification of diabetes mellitus. *Diabetes Care* 2004;27(Suppl 1):S5.

American Diabetes Association: Report of the Expert Committee on the Diagnosis and Classification of Diabetes Mellitus. *Diabetes Care* 1997;20:1183.

DECODE Study Group/European Diabetes Epidemiology Group: Glucose tolerance and mortality:comparison of WHO and American Diabetes Association diagnostic criteria. *Lancet* 1999;354:617.

Fajans SS, Bell GI, Polonsky KS. Molecular mechanisms and clinical pathophysiology of maturity-onset diabetes of the young. *N Engl J Med* 2001;345:971.

Ferrannini E: Insulin resistance versus insulin deficiency in non-insulin-dependent diabetes mellitus: problems and prospects. *Endocrine Rev* 1998;19:477.

World Health Organization:Definition, diagnosis and classification of diabetes mellitus and its complications. *Part 1: Report of a WHO Consultation: Diagnosis and Classification of Diabetes Mellitus.* Geneva: World Health Organization; 1999.

For a more detailed discussion of this topic and a bibliography, please see Porte *et al: Ellenberg & Rifkin's Diabetes Mellitus,* 6th ed., Chapter 18.

2 | Epidemiology of Diabetes Mellitus

Peter H. Bennett   Marian J. Rewers
William C. Knowler

TYPE 1 DIABETES MELLITUS

According to the current classification of diabetes mellitus, type 1 diabetes (T1DM; previously called insulin-dependent or juvenile diabetes) is caused by β-cell destruction, often immune-mediated, which leads to loss of insulin secretion and absolute insulin deficiency. Type 1a (autoimmune form) diabetes (T1aDM) is preceded by a subclinical period of T-cell-mediated autoimmune destruction of β-cells, marked by the presence of autoantibodies of variable duration. This is the most common form of diabetes among children and adolescents of European origin. In children, the disease is usually characterized by a rapid onset with acute symptoms and dependence on exogenous insulin for survival. T1aDM is nearly as frequent in adults, but often, less dramatic onset may lead to misclassification as type 2 (T2DM) and delayed insulin treatment. In most patients, the etiology of the autoimmune process and β-cell destruction is not known. T1DM also includes cases that are thought not to be immune-mediated, but are characterized by absolute insulin deficiency (T1bDM).

T1DM accounts for 5–10% of all diagnosed diabetes. About 40% of persons with T1DM are younger than 20 years of age at onset, thus making diabetes one of the most common severe chronic diseases of childhood, affecting 0.3% of the general population by the age of 20 years and 0.5–1% during the life span. The incidence of the disease appears to be increasing by 3–5% per year. It is estimated that approximately 1.4 million people in the United States, and perhaps 10–20 million people globally, suffer from the disease. The high incidence, associated severe morbidity, mortality, and enormous health care expenditures make T1DM a prime target for prevention.

NATURAL HISTORY OF TYPE 1a DIABETES

The natural history of T1aDM includes four distinct stages that can be observed in a vast majority of patients: (1) preclinical β-cell autoimmunity with progressive defect of insulin secretion, (2) onset of clinical diabetes, (3) transient remission, and (4) established diabetes associated with acute and chronic complications and premature death. At each stage, a spectrum of clinical manifestations and laboratory measurements helps to define the etiology, severity, prognosis, and prevention goals (Table 2-1).

PRECLINICAL β-CELL AUTOIMMUNITY

T1aDM results from a chronic autoimmune destruction of the pancreatic islet β-cells, probably initiated by exposure of a genetically susceptible host to an environmental agent. While the candidate genetic and environmental factors appear to be quite prevalent, β-cell autoimmunity develops in less than 5% and progresses to diabetes in less than 1% of the general population.

Table 2-1 Natural History of Type 1 Diabetes

	Preclinical autoimmunity	Clinical onset	Remission	Long-standing diabetes
Clinical	—	Polyuria, polydipsia Weight loss DKA in 20–40%	Insulin independence partial in 20–70% Total in 10–30%	Acute complications: DKA, hypoglycemia, infections Chronic complications: retinopathy, nephropathy, neuropathy, hypertension, atherosclerosis, growth impairment Premature mortality
Laboratory				
Genetic markers	Initiation: ? Progression: HLA-DR,DQ	IDDM1 (HLA-DR,DQ,DP) IDDM2 IDDM3-IDDM17?	?	ACE/ApoH—hypertension? Apo E, Apo A-IV—CHD? Others?
Autoantibodies to insulin GAD_{65}, ICA512 (IA-2)	Prevalence 85–100%	Prevalence 85–100%	Prevalence 40–60%	Prevalence ↓ 20–40%
Autoreactive cells	CD4, CD5, CD8	CD4, CD5, CD8	CD4, CD8	Mostly CD8 (?), CD4
Insulin secretion	Normal → low AIR	Low	Partially restored	Progressively lost
Blood glucose	Normal	>200 mg/dL (random)	Mostly <200 mg/dL	Depends on treatment
HbA1c	Normal (<6%)	Usually >11%	<7.5%	Depends on treatment
Prevention				
Primary	Of autoimmunity	Of diabetes onset	—	—
Secondary	Of diabetes	Remission induction	Remission extension	—
Tertiary	—	Of onset mortality	Of acute complications	Of complications, mortality

DKA, diabetic ketoacidosis

16

The autoimmune process is mediated by macrophages and T-lymphocytes with circulating autoantibodies to various β-cell antigens. Epidemiologic studies have defined autoimmunity as the presence of autoantibodies because, in contrast to cellular markers, their measurement is reliable and standardized across laboratories. A combination of assays for antibodies against insulin (IAA), glutamic acid decarboxylase (GAD), or ICA512 (IA-2) is quite sensitive and predictive in relatives of T1DM patients and in the general population.

Prevalence and Incidence

The prevalence of β-cell autoimmunity in school children from various countries is roughly proportional to the incidence of T1DM in the populations. In contrast, the prevalence of β-cell autoimmunity in first-degree relatives of T1DM persons does not differ as dramatically between high- and low-T1DM-risk countries.

In siblings of T1DM children, the incidence of combined β-cell autoimmunity or T1DM is up to 1.4% per year. Reliable estimates of the incidence of β-cell autoimmunity in the general population are expected from cohort studies underway in the United States (DAISY) and Finland (DIPP).

Among relatives of T1DM patients screened for the DPT-1 trial, lower prevalence of β-cell autoimmunity was observed in Asian-Americans (2.6%) and in Hispanics (2.7%), compared with African-Americans (3.3%) or non-Hispanic whites (3.9%).

Genetic Factors

In contrast to the wealth of data concerning genetic markers associated with clinical diabetes, little is known about the genetic determinants of β-cell autoimmunity. No particular HLA type seems to be associated with β-cell autoimmunity, although inconsistent associations between IAA or GAD HLA-DR,DQ phenotypes have been reported. The HLA-DR2, DQB1*0602 haplotype, which almost completely protects from T1DM, is found in about 15% of GAD- and IAA-positive young relatives of T1DM patients. However, over 90% of persons strongly and/or persistently islet autoantibody-positive are HLA-DR3 or 4, similar to T1DM patients. This may suggest that HLA genes are not involved in the initiation of β-cell autoimmunity, but rather determine progression to diabetes. More subjects with β-cell autoimmunity need to be genotyped to precisely determine the role of HLA and additional T1DM candidate genes in the initiation of autoimmunity and progression to diabetes.

Environmental Factors

Viruses

Viral infections appear to initiate autoimmunity rather than precipitate diabetes in subjects with autoimmunity. Islet autoantibodies have been detected after enteroviral, rotavirus, mumps, rubella, measles, and chickenpox infections. Newborns and infants are particularly likely to develop a persistent infection, and 70% patients with congenital rubella syndrome develop islet autoantibodies. The HLA-DR3,DQB1*0201 haplotype is associated with viral persistence. It remains to be established which additional genetic variants interact with infectious agents to promote β-cell autoimmunity in humans.

The evidence is strongest for enteroviruses, yet it is still inconclusive. Prospective studies of nondiabetic relatives and general-population children found an association between enteroviral infections, defined by polymerase chain reaction (PCR), and development of islet autoantibodies in Finland, but not in the United States or Germany.

Dietary Factors

Exposures to cereal or cow's milk prior to gut cellular tight junction closure or during gastroenteritis when the intestinal barrier is compromised are alternative causes of β-cell autoimmunity. Cereal or cow's milk introduced at weaning triggers insulitis and diabetes in animal models. Human data appear to support the role of cereals, but not cow's milk. The postulated autoimmune response to dietary proteins is likely amplified by the host's age and genetic background.

Chemical compounds, dietary nitrates, and nitrosamines can induce β-cell autoimmunity. Multiple hits of dietary β-cell toxins may render genetically resistant individuals susceptible to diabetogenic viruses, leading to T1DM.

Primary Prevention of β-Cell Autoimmunity

In mice, it is possible to prevent virus-induced diabetes by immunization with a nondiabetogenic variant of the virus. Alternative approaches to vaccination that would provide optimal antigenic stimulus providing long-term protection against diabetogenic viral variants include antiviral agents.

If too early or too late exposure to cereal or cow's milk triggers β-cell autoimmunity in humans, a logical primary prevention would be optimal timing of the introduction of these foods, especially in those with T1DM-associated genotypes. Such interventions are been carried out in newborn relatives of T1DM patients.

Progression from β-Cell Autoimmunity to Clinical Diabetes

Preclinical β cell autoimmunity precedes the diagnosis of diabetes by up to 9–13 years. In most persons with persistent autoantibodies, there is an early loss of spontaneous pulsatile insulin secretion and progressive reduction in the acute insulin response to intravenous glucose load, followed by decreased response to other β-cell secretagogues, impaired oral glucose tolerance, and fasting hyperglycemia. However, a nonprogressive β-cell defect can exist for many years.

Studies in first-degree relatives of T1DM patients and in school children with no family history of T1DM have reported ICA "remission" rates of 10–78%. It is unclear whether such remissions really occur or are an artifact of low specificity of autoantibody assays.

The cumulative β-cell damage and increases in insulin resistance with obesity and physical inactivity may eventually cause diabetes at a later age. Those persons in whom the disease process is slow may present with T1DM as adults, develop diabetes that does not immediately require insulin treatment, or may even fail to develop diabetes altogether. Markers of autoimmunity can be detected in 14–33% of diabetes patients classified on clinical grounds as "type 2" and are associated with early failure of oral hypoglycemic drug therapy and insulin dependence. The term *latent autoimmune diabetes of adults* (LADA) has been coined for this slowly progressing form of T1DM.

Primary Prevention of T1DM in Persons with β-Cell Autoimmunity

ICA-positive relatives of T1DM patients have become the primary target of clinical trials to prevent T1DM. Unfortunately, oral nicotinamide and parenteral or oral insulin have not been effective in preventing or delaying diabetes onset in large randomized clinical trails (ENDIT and DPT-1).

CLINICAL ONSET OF T1DM

In industrialized countries, 20–40% of T1DM patients younger than 20 years present in diabetic ketoacidosis (DKA). Younger age, female gender, HLA-DR4 allele, lower socioeconomic status, and lack of family history of diabetes have been associated with more severe presentation. Severe presentation in younger children may result from greater β-cell destruction at diagnosis; an average of 80% of the islets are damaged at diagnosis in children younger than 7 years, 60% in those 7–14 years old, and 40% in those older than 14. Case fatality in industrialized countries ranges between 0.4% and 0.9%.

Both DKA and onset death are largely preventable, because most of the patients have typical symptoms of polyuria, polydipsia, and weight loss 2–4 weeks prior to diagnosis. The diagnosis is straightforward in almost all cases and can be based on the symptoms, random blood glucose over 200 mg/dL, and/or HbA1c higher than 7%.

Prevalence and Incidence of T1DM

T1DM is one of the most common chronic childhood illnesses, affecting worldwide an estimated 50,000 new cases annually and, in Caucasian populations, 1–4 per 1000 children by the age of 20 years. The prevalence of T1DM in the age group 0–15 years ranges from 0.05% to 0.3% in most European and North American populations. Incidence, the rate at which new cases of T1DM appear in the population, varies by geographic location, ethnicity, age, gender, and time period.

Geographic Variation

One of the most striking characteristics of T1DM is the large geographic variability in the incidence. Scandinavia and Sardinia have the highest incidence rates in the world, and Asian populations have the lowest. This geographic and ethnic variation may reflect different pools of susceptibility genes, different prevalence of causative environmental factors, or both.

Race and Ethnicity

Racial differences in T1DM risk within the same population are striking, although not of the same magnitude as the geographic differences. U.S. non-Hispanic whites are about one-and-a-half times as likely to develop T1DM as African-Americans or Hispanics.

Age and Sex

T1DM incidence peaks at the ages of 2, 4–6, and 10–14 years, perhaps due to alterations in the pattern of infections or increases in insulin resistance. The age distribution of T1DM onset is similar across geographic areas and ethnic groups. The incidence decreases in the third decade of life, only to increase again in the fifth to seventh decades of life. It is not known whether there are etiologic differences between child- and adult-onset T1DM. Over 30% of those aged 25–34 are positive for islet autoantibodies, but the prevalence decreases with age, to less than 10% in those aged 55–65. The presence of the autoantibodies and age of presentation of diabetes were strongly associated with the presence of the HLA-DRB1*03/DRB1*04-DQB1*0302 genotype.

In general, males and females have similar risk of T1DM, with the pubertal peak of incidence in females preceding that in males by 1–2 years. In lower-risk populations, such as Japanese or U.S. blacks, there is a female preponderance, whereas in high-risk groups there is slight male excess. T1DM in adulthood is more commonly diagnosed in men.

Time

There is evidence for marked variations in the incidence of T1DM over time, both seasonally and annually. In both the Northern and Southern Hemispheres, the incidence declines during the warm summer months, implicating a climatic factor. This seasonal pattern appears to occur only in older children, suggesting that factors triggering diabetes may be related to school attendance, but they also differ by HLA-DR type.

Most population-based registries have shown increasing T1DM incidence over time, with periodic outbreaks superimposed on a steady secular increase in incidence.

Genetic Factors

Family History of T1DM

In moderate-T1DM-risk areas, such as the United States, the risk of T1DM by the age of 15 years is approximately 1/400. The risk is increased to about 1/40 in offspring of type 1 diabetic fathers and to 1/66 in offspring of type 1 diabetic mothers. The risk to siblings ranges from 1/12–1/35 and is further increased, to 1/4, in HLA-identical siblings. It is estimated that by the age of 60 years, approximately 10% of the relatives develop T1DM, due to a combination of genes and environmental exposures shared by family members.

"Familial" cases represent about 10% of T1DM and do not appear to be etiologically different from "sporadic" cases in HLA gene frequencies, seasonality of onset, or prevalence of immune markers. Familial cases tend to have lower glycated hemoglobin and higher C-peptide levels than sporadic cases, because relatives recognize diabetes symptoms earlier; however, these differences disappear soon after diagnosis.

Candidate Genes

The primary loci of genetic susceptibility to T1DM have been mapped to the HLA-DR and DQ regions, and new candidate genes outside the HLA region are being identified. While 50% of non-Hispanic whites in the United States have the HLA-DR3 or DR4 allele, at least one of these alleles is present in 95% of patients with T1DM. The estimated risk to HLA-DR3/4 children in the general population ranges from 1/35 to 1/90. The risk is further increased in those with HLA-DR3/4, DQB1*0302 genotype (about 2.2% of the general population versus 30–40% of T1DM patients).

Environmental Factors

Seasonality, increasing incidence, and epidemics of T1DM, as well as numerous ecologic, cross-sectional, and retrospective studies, suggest that certain viruses and components of early childhood diet may cause T1DM.

Viruses

Herpesviruses, mumps, rubella, and retroviruses have been implicated. While congenital rubella syndrome is responsible for a minute proportion of T1DM and postnatal rubella infection or vaccination does not cause T1DM, congenital rubella syndrome provides an example of viral persistence leading to T1DM after an incubation period of 5–20 years.

Enteroviruses have been most strongly linked to human T1DM, but convincing proof of causality remains elusive. At least 90% of T1DM patients demonstrate a prolonged period of β-cell autoimmunity that is hardly compatible with an acute cytolytic enteroviral infection being a major cause. Enteroviral infection could, however, initiate β-cell autoimmunity through a molecular mimicry or a persistent β-cell infection with impairment of insulin secretion and expression of self-antigens. Alternatively, acinar cell infection and limited capacity of β-cells to neutralize free radicals released in this process could initiate cell autoimmunity. Studies from Finland and Sweden have suggested that *in utero* enteroviral infections can lead to T1DM in a significant proportion of cases. Additional perinatal factors and season of birth have been associated with T1DM. In animal models, viral infection may protect the host from developing T1DM; however, evidence for such a protective effect in humans is speculative.

Susceptibility to diabetogenic enteroviruses in humans appears to be genetically restricted by HLA-DR and DQ alleles. Elevated antiviral IgM levels in subjects with T1DM appear to be driven by specific HLA phenotypes and may reflect a greater ability to mount an immune response or a higher susceptibility to infection, rather than a causal relationship to T1DM.

None of the routine childhood immunizations has been shown to increase the risk of diabetes or prediabetic autoimmunity.

Dietary Factors

Ecologic and case-control studies have suggested a relationship between the duration of breastfeeding and age at introduction of cow's milk and T1DM. Breastfeeding may be viewed as a surrogate for the delay in the introduction of diabetogenic substances present in formula or early childhood diet. More recent cohort studies failed to find an association between infant diet exposures and β-cell autoimmunity. Despite these limitations, a dietary intervention trial to prevent T1DM by a short-term elimination of cow's milk from infant diet (TRIGR) is underway. Circumstantial evidence suggests a connection between T1DM and consumption of foods and water containing nitrates, nitrites, or nitrosamines.

REMISSION ("HONEYMOON PERIOD")

Shortly after clinical onset, most T1DM patients experience a transient fall in insulin requirement due to an improved β-cell function. Total and partial remissions have been reported in 2–12% and 18–62%, respectively, of young T1DM patients. Older age and less severe initial presentation and low or absent autoantibodies have been consistently associated with longer remission. Most studies agree that preserved β-cell function is associated with better glycemic control (lower HbA1c) and preserved α-cell glucagon response to hypoglycemia.

The natural remission is always temporary, ending with a gradual or abrupt increase in exogenous insulin requirements. Destruction of β-cells is complete within 3 years of diagnosis in most young children, especially those with the HLA-DR3/4 phenotype. It is much slower and often only partial in older patients, 15% of whom have still some β-cell function preserved 10 years after diagnosis.

Secondary Prevention in New-Onset T1DM Patients

A number of placebo-controlled randomized trials using azathioprine, cyclosporin A, nicotinamide, prednisone, and other immunosupressive agents attempted to increase the rate and the duration of T1DM remission. Only cyclosporin A treatment has been shown to be partially effective, inducing total remission in 25–40% of patients and sustaining it for 1 year in 18–24% of newly diagnosed patients, compared with 0–10% in the placebo group. However, the drug is nephrotoxic, of little value in children, and effective for only as long as it is administered, rendering this approach to secondary prevention of T1DM unacceptable. Trials using intensive insulin treatment or immunomodulation have been even less successful.

ESTABLISHED DIABETES

Complications

Acute complications of T1DM (diabetic ketoacidosis, hypoglycemia, and infections) are described in detail elsewhere. The risk of hospital admission for acute complication is 30/100 patient years in the first year of the disease and 20/100 in the subsequent 3 years. An estimated 26% of patients have at least one episode of severe hypoglycemia within the initial 4 years of diagnosis, with little relation to demographic or socioeconomic factors. The incidence of severe hypoglycemic episodes varies between 6 and 20/100 patient-years, depending on age, geographic location, and intensity of insulin treatment.

Diabetes is the leading cause of end-stage renal disease, blindness, and amputation, and a major cause of cardiovascular disease and premature death in the general population. In the United States, the disease results in over $25 billion in medical care expenditures per year, with costs for patients being over 10 times those for nondiabetic persons.

Mortality

Insulin treatment dramatically prolongs survival, but it does not cure diabetes. Although the absolute mortality at onset and within the first 20 years of T1DM is low (3–6%), it is 5 times higher for diabetic males and 12 times higher for diabetic females, compared with the general population. This excess mortality is lowest in Scandinavia, intermediate in the United States, and highest in countries where T1DM is rare, due to a combination of the quality of care and access. Even in Finland, at least half of the deaths are due to currently preventable causes such as acute complications, infections, and suicide. On the other hand, 40% of patients survive over 40 years, and half of these have no major complications. Survival and avoidance of complications have been related to better metabolic control; however, genetic factors also are involved.

TYPE 2 DIABETES MELLITUS

Type 2 diabetes mellitus (T2DM), formerly known as non-insulin-dependent diabetes, is the most frequent form of diabetes mellitus in all parts of world. The prevalence of the disease is increasing globally. It is estimated that in 2000 there were approximately 150 million individuals with the disease and that this number is likely to double by 2025. In most countries, including those with a high level of medical care, there is typically one undiagnosed case of T2DM for each that is known. Thus, studies that ascertain only previously diagnosed cases are subject to limited interpretation.

As T2DM may remain undetected for many years, investigations of its development, natural history, and complications are compromised when cases are identified only by routine clinical diagnosis. As undiagnosed diabetes represents an important fraction of the population with the disease, most epidemiologic studies are performed by testing all subjects in the population of interest. Without systematic testing, an incomplete and potentially misleading picture of the frequency or distribution of the disease is obtained. Furthermore, because of the differences in criteria, comparisons of rates from recent and earlier studies must be made with caution.

Prevalence

The prevalence of T2DM varies enormously in different countries and among different racial and ethnic groups (Fig. 2-1). The prevalence and incidence of T2DM have increased dramatically during the past 50 years in many countries. Countries such as Japan and India that used to have low prevalences now have rates that exceed those found in the United States and Europe. In the United States, the rates have increased considerably in the past 30 years and have continued to do so over the past decade. The majority of cases of T2DM in the future will occur in developing countries, with India and China having the highest number of cases in the world.

T2DM in developed countries most often occurs in the middle to older age groups. In developing countries, because of the younger age distribution of the population, many cases occur in young to middle-aged adults. The disease, however, can develop in childhood or adolescence and its occurrence in these age ranges appears to be increasing rapidly, especially in populations that already have a high overall prevalence of T2DM. In Caucasian populations, in the United States and Europe the prevalence of T2DM increases with age at least into the seventies.

Data from health examination surveys (NHANES III) conducted between 1988 and 1994 showed that 5.1% of U.S. adults age 20 years and over already carried a diagnosis of diabetes. The prevalence of undiagnosed diabetes, based on fasting plasma glucose levels of 126 mg/dL or higher, was 2.7%, or, based on glucose tolerance tests and the 1985 WHO criteria, was 6.3%. The total prevalence was 7.8% based on diagnosed diabetes and fasting plasma glucose levels only, or 11.4% when based on the 1985 WHO criteria, rates appreciably higher than were seen in earlier surveys.

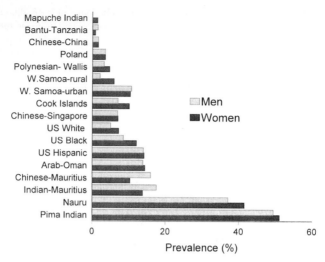

FIG. 2-1 Prevalence of diabetes according to 1980 WHO criteria in men and women aged 30–64 years in different countries and various ethnic groups. (*Adapted from King H, Rewers M: Global estimates for prevalence of diabetes mellitus and impaired glucose tolerance in adults. WHO Ad Hoc Diabetes Reporting Group.* Diabet Care *1993; 16:157–177.*)

Incidence

Incidence is the rate of development of new cases of disease. Only a few studies of the incidence of T2DM using standardized and comparable methods have been reported. Incidence studies using standardized glucose tolerance tests have been performed in the Pima Indians of Arizona and among Micronesians on the central Pacific island of Nauru. Both groups have very high incidence rates. Among Pima Indians, the age-specific incidence rates of diabetes have increased over the course of two decades, whereas in Nauru the incidence may now be falling.

Mortality

T2DM is associated with excess mortality, mainly attributable to the vascular complications of the disease. In Caucasian populations, much of the excess mortality is attributable to cardiovascular disease, especially ischemic heart disease, but in others, such as Asian and Native American populations, renal disease contributes to a considerable extent. In developing nations, an important component of the excess is due to infections. Age-adjusted mortality rates among persons with diabetes are 1.5–2.5 times higher than in the general population, but the excess is greater in younger age groups and diminishes at older ages.

The increased mortality in patients with T2DM is seen mainly among those with complications. Risk factors include proteinuria, retinal disease, and the classic risk factors for heart disease. Hyperlipidemia, hypertension, and smoking contribute disproportionately to death rates among those with T2DM. Mortality rates also increase with increasing duration of the disease.

Risk Factors

Familial Aggregation

The empiric risk of having T2DM is increased two- to sixfold if a parent or sibling has the disease. Consequently, a positive family history is a practical, albeit crude, way of estimating if an individual is likely to have inherited susceptibility to the disease, although familial aggregation alone is not definitive evidence of genetic determinants.

Genetic Factors

Genes that specifically confer risk for the development of T2DM have been identified only to a limited extent. Genes have been identified that determine susceptibility to several rare forms of monogenic diabetes, such as maturity-onset diabetes of the young (MODY), that were formerly classified as non-insulin-dependent diabetes. Many patients with such forms of diabetes may still be inaccurately diagnosed as T2DM unless specific attempts are made to identify them. These monogenic forms of diabetes, now classified as other specific types of diabetes.

Genomic scans have identified several regions in the genome where putative susceptibility genes are located. These observations suggest that the common forms of T2DM are multigenic and that the relative importance and frequency of the genes determining susceptibility varies from population to population.

Age and Sex

The prevalence and incidence of T2DM vary to some extent between the sexes from one population to another, but these differences are relatively small and appear to be accounted for by differences in other risk factors, such as obesity and physical activity. The prevalence of T2DM increases with age, although these patterns of incidence vary considerably. In populations with high frequencies of the disease, the incidence may be high and the prevalence may increase markedly in the younger adult years; in others, the incidence and prevalence increase mainly in older individuals. In most populations, a decrease in prevalence is seen in the oldest age groups (e.g., at least 75 years) because of higher mortality rates in those with T2DM.

Obesity

Obesity is a frequent concomitant of T2DM. In many longitudinal studies, it has been shown to be a powerful predictor of its development. In nonobese individuals, the incidence of T2DM is low, even in populations such as Pima Indians, whose overall risk of the disease is very high. The relationship of incidence of T2DM to obesity also varies with other risk factors. For example, in Pima Indians, the incidence rises much more steeply with body mass index (BMI) in those whose parents have diabetes than in those who do not. This relationship indicates an interaction between risk factors.

Obesity has increased rapidly in many populations in recent years. This increase has been accompanied by an increasing prevalence of T2DM. As obesity is such a strong predictor of diabetes incidence, the rapid increases in the prevalence of T2DM seen in many populations in recent decades are almost certainly related to increasing obesity. Furthermore, interventions directed to reducing obesity reduce the incidence of T2DM in obese individuals with impaired glucose tolerance (*vide infra*).

Physical Inactivity

Many studies indicate the important role of physical inactivity in the development of T2DM. Nevertheless, its relative importance may be underestimated in most studies because of imprecision in measurement. Several studies do provide evidence of a causal role of physical inactivity in T2DM. Intervention studies that have included increased physical activity to prevent diabetes among subjects with impaired glucose tolerance (*vide infra*) demonstrate a reduced incidence of T2DM, but the dose-response relationship of physical activity to diabetes incidence and the extent that the relationship is mediated by concomitant weight loss remain unclear.

Other Risk Factors

Genes, obesity, and physical inactivity appear to be the most important risk factors for T2DM. There are, however, others that influence the risk of developing T2DM, but their importance on a population level is much less than those of obesity and physical inactivity. These include low birth weight, exposure to a diabetic intrauterine environment, and other metabolic and environmental exposures.

T2DM Prevention

As important lifestyle factors have been identified and groups of persons at high risk are identifiable, several recent randomized controlled clinical trials have examined whether lifestyle intervention or pharmacologic interventions can reduce the incidence of T2DM.

Studies in DaQing, China, among 530 persons with IGT were the first to show that lifestyle interventions could reduce the rate of progression to diabetes. The effects of diet alone, exercise alone, and both diet and exercise together reduced the incidence of diabetes by about 30% over a 6-year period compared with a control group who received only general lifestyle-change recommendations. There was no significant difference among the three intervention groups.

A study from Finland also demonstrated that lifestyle changes reduced the incidence of T2DM among overweight individuals with IGT. Specific dietary goals were given and a target of at least 30 minutes of exercise per day was set. Compared with the control group, who lost 0.8 kg over a 2-year period, the intervention group lost 3.5 kg. After an average of 3.2 years, the incidence of diabetes in the lifestyle-intervention group was 58% lower than in the control groups.

A much larger multicenter study, the Diabetes Prevention Program (DPP), was conducted in the United States among 3234 subjects with IGT and BMI of at least 24 kg/m^2. This study showed a 58% reduction in the incidence of T2DM over a 3-year period in the lifestyle-intervention group (Fig. 2-2) One-third of the subjects were randomized to metformin treatment. This therapy resulted in a 31% lower incidence of T2DM, significantly less than in the placebo group, but the lifestyle intervention was significantly more effective overall than the metformin intervention.

Another multicenter study (STOP NIDDM), also among subjects with IGT, examined whether an α-glucosidase inhibitor, acarbose, delayed (or prevented)

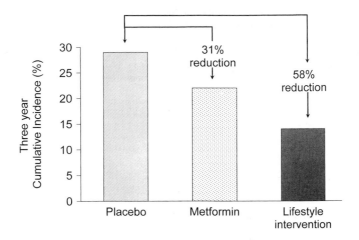

FIG. 2-2 Results of the Diabetes Prevention Program. Diabetes incidence was reduced in persons with impaired glucose tolerance randomized to lifestyle intervention. *(Adapted from The Diabetes Prevention Program Research Group: Reduction in the incidence of type 2 diabetes with lifestyle intervention or metformin. N Engl J Med 2002; 346:393–403.)*

the onset of T2DM. This study reported a 25% reduction in the incidence of T2DM over a 3-year period.

Yet another intervention study (TRIPOD, Troglitazone in the Prevention of Diabetes) examined the effect of a thiazolidinedione, troglitazone, on the development of T2DM in women with previous gestational diabetes. Although this trial was stopped prematurely because of the withdrawal of troglitazone from the market, a 50% reduction in the incidence of T2DM was seen compared with the placebo treatment. This trial, therefore, suggests that other thiazolidinedione drugs might also be effective in delaying or preventing the onset of T2DM. Such trials have recently been initiated.

Other pharmacologic agents may also reduce the incidence of T2DM. Secondary analyses of the WOSCOPS (West of Scotland Cardiovascular Disease Prevention Study) and HOPE (Heart Outcomes Prevention Evaluations) studies suggest that the incidence of T2DM may be lower in patients receiving a statin, pravistatin, or ramipril, an angiotensin-converting enzyme inhibitor, than among those receiving placebo. Further trials are required to determine if this is indeed true.

ADDITIONAL READINGS

Atkinson MA, Eisenbarth GS: Type 1 diabetes: New perspectives on disease pathogenesis and treatment. *Lancet* 2001;358:221–229.

The Diabetes Prevention Program Research Group: Reduction in the incidence of type 2 diabetes with lifestyle intervention or metformin. *New Engl J Med* 2002; 346: 393–403.

Knowler WC, Pettitt DJ, Saad MF, *et al*: Diabetes mellitus in the Pima Indians: Incidence, risk factors and pathogenesis. *Diabetes Metabolism Rev* 1990;61:1–27.

Redondo MJ, Eisenbarth GS. Genetic control of autoimmunity in type I diabetes and associated disorders. *Diabetologia* 2002;45:605–622.

Wild S, Roglic G, Green A, et al: Global prevalence of diabetes: Estimates for the year 2000 and projections for 2030. *Diabetes Care* 2004;27:1047–1053.

For a more detailed discussion of this topic and a bibliography, please see Porte *et al: Ellenberg & Rifkin's Diabetes Mellitus,* 6th ed., Chapter 19.

3 | The Pathophysiology and Genetics of Type 1 (Insulin-Dependent) Diabetes

Ramachandra G. Naik   Åke Lernmark
Jerry P. Palmer

The term *diabetes* does not denote a single disease entity, but rather a clinical syndrome. Fundamental to all types of diabetes is impairment of insulin secretion by the pancreatic β-cells. The etiologic classification currently accepted by the American Diabetes Association (ADA) and the World Health Organization (WHO) recognizes two major forms of diabetes, type 1 diabetes mellitus (earlier known as insulin-dependent diabetes mellitus, IDDM) and type 2 diabetes (earlier known as non-insulin-dependent diabetes mellitus, NIDDM). Type 1 diabetes encompasses the vast majority of patients with pancreatic islet β-cell destruction and proneness to ketoacidosis. This form includes those patients in whom β-cell destruction is currently ascribable to an autoimmune process and those for whom an etiology is unknown. It does not include those forms of β-cell destruction or failure for which non-autoimmune-specific causes can be assigned (e.g., cystic fibrosis). While most type 1 diabetes is characterized by the presence of autoantibodies that identify the autoimmune process that leads to β-cell destruction, in some subjects no evidence of autoimmunity is present; these cases are classified as type 1 idiopathic. Type 2 diabetes is the most prevalent form of diabetes and results from insulin resistance with an insulin secretory defect. Although the exact causes of the insulin resistance and the insulin secretory defect are not fully known, both are strongly genetically determined and the β-cell defect does not have an autoimmune etiology.

Epidemiologic studies have suggested that the incidence rate of type 1 diabetes peaks twice, once close to the puberty and again around 40 years of age. It has also been suggested that the overall incidence rate of type 1 diabetes is approximately equivalent above and below the age of 20. Many of these older patients, especially early in the course of their diabetes, are clinically similar to classical type 2 diabetes patients. This relatively high incidence rate of type 1 diabetes in adults is often not appreciated, probably because of the over 10-fold greater frequency of type 2 diabetes in this age group. Furthermore, the finding of antibodies characteristic of type 1 diabetes such as islet cell antibodies (ICA) and glutamic acid decarboxylase antibodies (GADAb) in 10–30% of type 2 diabetes patients suggests that in older individuals the type 1 disease process may result in a similar clinical phenotype as the type 2 disease process. This subset has been variously described as latent autoimmune diabetes in adults (LADA), slowly progressive IDDM, late-onset type 1 diabetes, and type 1½ diabetes.

NATURAL HISTORY

Based on data mainly from prospective studies of nondiabetic relatives of patients with type 1 diabetes, the natural history of type 1 diabetes includes the following major concepts. First, there is a long preclinical period. During this time antibodies and T-cells reactive with β-cell antigens can be detected, perhaps due to an immunologic attack on the β-cells. Loss of β-cell function has been observed years prior to the onset of clinical type 1 diabetes. Second, at least 80–90% of the functional capacity of the β-cells must be lost before hyperglycemia occurs. It was believed for a long time that β-cell destruction was the primary mechanism responsible for the loss of insulin secretory capacity during the preclinical period of type 1 diabetes. We now recognize that at least some of the impairment in insulin secretion may be functional and due to inhibition of insulin secretion by cytokines and possibly other factors. Third, as implied by the insulitis and the presence of antibodies and T-cells directed against islet antigens, the β-cell lesion is autoimmune in nature. And fourth, this autoimmune destructive process occurs specifically in genetically susceptible individuals.

Type 1 diabetes is not a disease of unbridled destruction. The autoimmune attack on pancreatic β-cells has two distinct stages—insulitis and diabetes—and progression of the former to the latter appears to be regulated. A major question pertaining to the natural history of type 1 diabetes centers around whether the diabetogenic process, once initiated, is relentlessly progressive and always culminates in clinical type 1 diabetes. The alternative is that the process is more variable, waxing and waning, and sometimes remitting without eventual progression to overt type 1 diabetes (Fig. 3-1). It is now recognized that insulitis can occur in animals that will not develop clinical type 1 diabetes and changes in immune markers may not always be reflective of changes in the immune attack on the β-cells. ICA, and even other antibodies

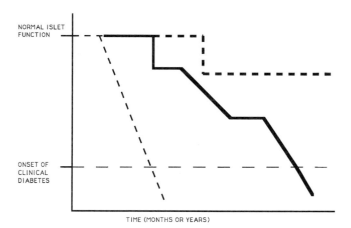

FIG. 3-1 Hypothetical courses of pancreatic function after islet insult. Inexorable linear decline in function after islet insult leading to rapid onset of clinical disease (-----). Multiple islet insults leading to eventual clinical disease (——). Islet insult and recovery, without development of clinical disease.(------). *(Reproduced with permission from Greenbaum CJ, Brooks-Worrell BM, Palmer JP, Lernmark A: Autoimmunity and prediction of insulin dependent diabetes mellitus. In: Marshall SM, Home PD, eds.* The Diabetes Annual/8. *Elsevier. 1994:21.)*

such as insulin autoantibodies (IAA), GADAb, and insulinoma-associated protein-2 (IA-2) antibodies, show fluctuations in their levels over time. In nondiabetic individuals with autoantibodies directed against islet antigens, impaired β-cell function is very common. A combination of immune markers with impaired β-cell function is associated with a greater risk of subsequent clinical type 1 diabetes than immune markers in combination with normal β-cell function. But impaired β-cell function is also common in ICA-negative relatives of type 1 diabetes patients. Because less than 20% of these individuals would be expected to progress to clinical type 1 diabetes, these observations suggest that in many of these individuals the β-cell destructive process has remitted.

The temporal development of autoantibodies was studied in offspring of parents with type 1 diabetes in the German BABYDIAB study. By 2 years of age, autoantibodies appeared in 11% of offspring, 3.5% having more than one autoantibody. Cumulative risk for disease by 5 years of age was 1.8%, and it was 50% for offspring with more than one autoantibody in this 2-year sample. It was concluded that autoimmunity associated with childhood diabetes is an early event and a dynamic process, presence of IAAs is a consistent feature of this autoimmunity, and IAA detection can identify children at risk. The Childhood Diabetes in Finland Study Group showed that positivity for multiple diabetes-related autoantibodies is associated with accelerated β-cell destruction and an increased requirement for exogenous insulin over the second year of clinical disease, indicating that multiple autoantibodies reflect a more aggressive progression of β-cell destruction. Patients testing negative for diabetes-associated autoantibodies at diagnosis seemed to have a milder degree of β-cell destruction, but their metabolic decompensation was similar to that seen in other affected children, suggesting that they do represent classical type 1 diabetes.

In the LADA group mentioned earlier, it is believed that the autoimmune β-cell destructive process proceeds more slowly, or the destruction stops at a "moderate" stage. A prospective observation on the natural history of the ICA-positive type 2 diabetes patients in Japan disclosed characteristic findings which included a late onset, a family history of type 2 diabetes, a slow progression of β-cell failure over several years with persistently positive low-titer ICA, and incomplete β-cell loss. Similar presentations have been described in various other countries. The typical patient, however, is generally younger than 35 years (age at onset 30–50 years) and nonobese (lower body mass index); the diabetes is often controlled with diet, but within a short period (months to years), metabolic control by oral agents fails, and progression to insulin dependency is more rapid than in antibody-negative, obese type 2 diabetics. The eventual clinical features of these patients include weight loss, ketosis proneness, unstable blood glucose levels, and an extremely diminished C-peptide reserve; in retrospect, these subjects possess additional classical features of type 1 diabetes, including increased frequency of HLA-DR3 and -DR4, and islet cell antibody positivity . Various studies have shown that patients positive for GADAb and/or ICA have a more rapid decline in C-peptide, fail oral agents, and require insulin treatment earlier. Another study showed that the positive rate for GADAb was as high as 23.8% in the nonobese and insulin-deficient patients with sulfonylurea failure, suggesting that autoimmune mechanisms may play an important role in the pathogenesis of secondary failure of sulphonylurea therapy. Thus, loss of β-cell function in approximately two-thirds of phenotypic type 2 diabetes subjects can be predicted by GADAb and ICA. However, as a result of lower cost and relative ease of performance, and the availability of several simple and robust assays for GADAb, GAD antibodies may provide a practical alternative to ICA assay, particularly in population screening. Early detection of these immune markers of β-cell damage creates the future potential for immune modulation to limit such damage. The associations between clinical type 1 diabetes and HLA genotype appear in part to be determined by age of diagnosis. It appears that the type 1 diabetes disease process is more aggressive resulting in clinical presentation at a younger age in individuals with more susceptibility genes and less protective genes; and the reverse: the disease process is less aggressive resulting in clinical presentation at older ages in individuals with less susceptibility genes and/or more protective genes.

GENETIC ASPECTS

Association with Human Leukocyte Antigens (HLA)

The association between HLA and type 1 diabetes (see Table 3-1 for definitions) was first demonstrated for HLA-B8 and/or B15. Recent technologies have allowed rapid detection of new alleles now explained by gene sequencing. The HLA molecules have structural similarities to an array of related molecules (Fig. 3-2). The marked polymorphism is one distinct feature of the HLA complex. Another feature of the HLA class I and II molecule genes encoded on the short arm of chromosome 6 is the phenomenon of linkage disequilibrium. This means that certain alleles in a haplotype tend to be inherited together, because the recombination frequency at certain parts of the HLA complex is markedly reduced compared to other parts of the human genome. The phenomenon of linkage disequilibrium is important when an association between HLA and a disease such as type I diabetes is analyzed. The alternative approach is to estimate susceptibility by genetic linkage. Analysis of linkage is used when investigating sib pairs, which is necessary in studying type 1 diabetes because of the rarity of large, multigeneration families. It is critical to the understanding of type 1 diabetes etiology that the majority of new patients do not have a first-degree relative with the disease. It has therefore been extremely complicated to determine the mode of inheritance of type 1 diabetes.

TABLE 3-1 Nomenclature and Abbreviations for HLA Molecules

MHC	Major histocompatibility complex
MHC molecules	Proteins encoded on the short arm of chromosome 6; these proteins are involved in various functions of the human immune response
Class I molecules	The heavy chain (M, 43,000) is encoded in the HLA-A, -B, and -C loci; the light chain is β_2-microglobulin, coded for on chromosome 9
Class II molecules	A dimer composed of two transmembrane polypeptide chains (α and β) with M, 34,000 and 29,000, respectively
Class III molecules	Plasma proteins such as C2 or C4, or cytokines such as tumor necrosis factor (TNF)-α and -β

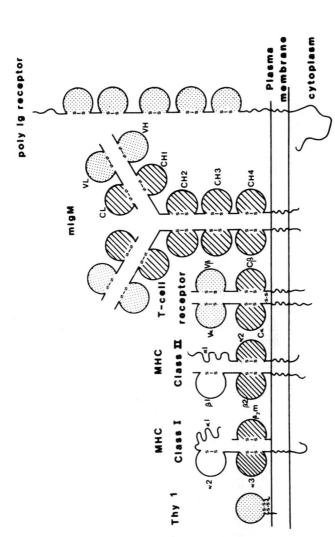

FIG. 3-2 Schematic structures of proteins in the "immunoglobulin superfamily." (Adapted with permission from Kaufman JF, Auffray C, Korman AJ, et al: The class II molecules of the human and murine major histocompatibility complex. Cell 1984;28:891.)

33

TABLE 3-2 Lifetime Recurrence Risk of Type 1 Diabetes

| | Age at onset of proband | |
Age corrected empirical risk of type 1 diabetes	< 25 years	≥ 25 years
A. Parents	2.2 ± 0.6%	4.9 ± 1.4%
Siblings	6.9 ± 1.3%	5.6 ± 1.8%
Children	5.6 ± 2.8%	4.3 ± 2.2%
B. HLA-identical siblings	15.5%	ND
HLA-haploidentical siblings	4.9%	ND
HLA-nonidentical siblings	1.2%	ND
C. Identical twins	25–50%	ND

ND. not determined.

Lifetime risks for type 1 diabetes (Table 3-2) in first-degree relatives of an individual with type 1 diabetes have been calculated to be about 3% for parents, 7% for siblings, and 5% for children. A recent study including patients at an older age at onset and a longer follow-up than in previous studies indicated that 25% of type 1 diabetes patients had at least one affected sibling. The lifetime recurrence risk for siblings from time of birth up to 30 years of age was 6%, which increased to 10% at 60 years of age. Studies of families with multiple affected members have shown that the occurrence of type 1 diabetes is 16% if the parent or sibling shares both HLA markers with the proband (HLA identical), 5% for one HLA marker (HLA haploidentical), and 1% or less for HLA nonidentical. Certain HLA-DR specificities, such as DR2 or HLA haplotypes such as DQB1*0602-DQA1*0102 (DQ6.2), are rarely found among young type 1 diabetes patients, although the frequency of the haplotype among patients increases with age of diagnosis of diabetes. The association with the disease is negative, which is interpreted as protection from type 1 diabetes.

Statistical analyses demonstrate that type 1 diabetes patients with HLA-B8 more often are HLA-DR3-positive than are healthy HLA-B8 positive controls. These analyses suggest that the DR locus is indeed closer to a putative risk gene for type 1 diabetes than the locus coding for the HLA-B specificities. In children or young adults, the overall findings were that more than 90% of type 1 diabetes patients were positive for DR3, DR4, or both, compared with 60% of the controls. It was also found that among Caucasians as many as 35–40% of type 1 diabetes patients were DR3/4 (heterozygotes). Monozygotic twins concordant for type 1 diabetes showed an increased frequency of DR 3/4 heterozygocity.

The HLA class II molecules are central to the human immune response because they present peptide antigens to T-helper (CD4-positive) cells. It is therefore a reasonable hypothesis that HLA class II molecules associated or linked to type 1 diabetes may present peptides that are diabetogenic. Recent advances in molecular genetics have allowed detailed studies of the genes that code for the HLA class II molecules, including their precise chromosomal location, nucleotide sequences, and transcriptional regulation. In fact, the entire HLA class II region has been sequenced, and bioinformatics details are available at http://www.anthonynolan.org.uk/HIG/index.html. Knowledge of the nucleotide sequence permits a derivation of the expected amino acid sequence of the individual class II molecules. A schematic map of the HLA-D region of human chromosome 6 is shown in Fig. 3-3. The size of the HLA-D region has been estimated to be as large as 1.1×10^6 base pairs. The DQ and DR subre-

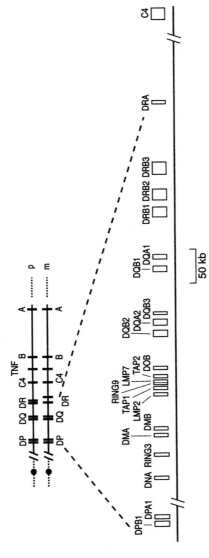

FIG. 3-3 Schematic map of the HLA region of chromosome 6. The major loci are shown for a paternal (p) and maternal (m) chromosome. The loci between DP and DR are amplified to indicate the location of currently known genetic factors in the HLA class II region.

gions are harbored within 450×10^3 base pairs. The current order of known genes from the centromere toward the telomere is illustrated in Fig. 3-3. Genomic HLA typing by PCR analyses (Table 3-3) made it possible to test the hypothesis that genetic determinants other than DR explained the association between HLA and type 1 diabetes. Evidence that DQ is closer to type 1 diabetes than DR was first obtained by RFLP analysis, followed by direct cDNA sequence analysis, and confirmed in numerous investigations by allele-specific PCR analyses.

As indicated previously, DR4 is a broad serologic specificity now explained by several DRB1 alleles such as DRB1*0401, DRBI*0402, and DRBI*0403. While DRB1*0401 and DRB1*0405 were strongly associated with type 1 diabetes, DRB1*0403 was found to be protective. It is therefore possible that antigen presentation by different HLA-DR or DQ molecules may make variable contributions to type 1 diabetes risk. Taken together, current available data suggest that certain DQ alleles are more closely associated with type 1 diabetes than the associated DR alleles. The data by several investigators suggest that among DR4-positive individuals the DQ8 specificity confers the highest risk for type 1 diabetes. This risk may be modulated, however, by different DRB1*04 subtypes.

Large population-based investigations provide sufficient statistical power for the association between HLA and type 1 diabetes to be critically analyzed. A genetic factor in the HLA region that totally controlled the development of diabetes would be expected to be present among all (100%) patients. The frequency of this factor in the healthy control population would be expected to be significantly lower, but not necessarily to the level of disease prevalence itself. Studies in identical twins and in families suggest that the genetic factors may account for only 30–40% of disease susceptibility, the rest probably

TABLE 3-3 Caucasian HLA Haplotypes

DQB1	DQA1	DRB
0201 (DQ2)	0501	3
0201 (DQ2)	0201	7
0301 (DQ7)	0301	4
0301 (DQ7)	0501	5
0302 (DQ8)	0301	4
0303 (DQ9)	0201	7
0303 (DQ9)	0301	9
0402 (DQ4)	0401	8
0501 (DQ5)	0101	1
0502 (DQ5)	0102	2
0503 (DQ5)	0101	6
0601 (DQ6)	0103	2
0602 (DQ6)	0102	2
0603 (DQ6)	0103	6
0604 (DQ6)	0102	6

TABLE 3-4 Genotypes and Haplotypes Associated with Insulin-Dependent Diabetes Mellitus (IDDM)

	Association with IDDM	
	Positive	Negative
■ GENOTYPES		
DR	DR4	DR2
	DR3	
DQA1	0301	0102
DQB1	0302	0602
	0501	
■ HETEROZYGOSITY	DQ-DR heterozygotes	
Positive association	DQ 2/8 > DQ 8/8>DQ8/DQB1*0604-DQA1*0102	
Negative association	DQ 6/6 > DQ 6/8 > DQ6/2	
■ HAPLOTYPES	DQ-DR haplotype	
Positive association	DQB1*0302-DQA1*0301(DQ8)-DR4	
	DQB1*0201-DQA1*0501(DQ2)-DR3	
Negative association	DQB1*0602-DQA1*0102(DQ6)-DR2	
	DQB*0301-DQA1*0301(DQ7)-DR4	

being the environment. Among the genetic factors, linkage analysis suggests that HLA contributes only 60%. Individual alleles may be considered, such as DQB1*0302, which is positively associated with type 1 diabetes, or DQB1*0602, which is negatively associated with type 1 diabetes (Table 3-4). The association between HLA and type 1 diabetes with the DQB1 alleles therefore would take into account one-half of the HLA-DQ class II molecule (Fig. 3-2), and a functional consequence that controls type 1 diabetes development needs to be identified. The same reasoning is applicable to the many different known alleles of DQA1. Therefore, type 1 diabetes susceptibility and protection is most likely controlled by the expression and function of HLA-DQ class II molecules (Fig. 3-4). The mechanism would be specific peptide binding to the groove and selective initiation of an immune response, perhaps to a type 1 diabetes-associated autoantigen such as GAD65, insulin, or IA-2.

The particular proneness to develop type 1 diabetes among HLA-DR3/4 DQ 2/8-positive individuals remains to be explained. It has been speculated that the formation of transcomplementation HLA class II molecules explains the markedly increased risk of DR3-DQ2 and DR4-DQ8 together (Fig. 3-5). Transcomplementation HLA-DQ molecules have been demonstrated in DR3/4-positive IDDM patients. The role of such class II molecules in cell-cell interaction, antigen processing, and presentation is currently not known. The specific amino acid sequence of the α- and β-chains may determine in part their ability to form such heterodimers.

One possible mechanism to explain cell-specific autoimmunity would be if the target cell were able express HLA class II molecules. It is conceivable that cell-specific self-antigens could be presented by the target cell itself and thereby induce an immune response by activating appropriate T-lymphocytes. Class II molecules are rarely expressed on nonlymphoid cells. The first evidence of aberrant expression was obtained in skin cells in mice with graft-versus-host disease. In organ-specific autoimmunity, thyroid cells may express class II molecules in thyroiditis-affected glands. *In vitro* studies indicated that it was possible to induce class II expression by mitogens or

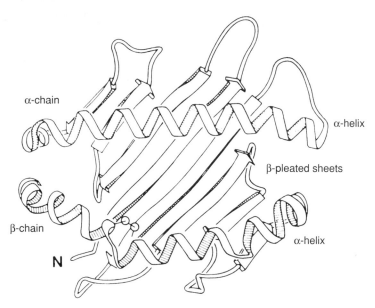

FIG. 3-4   Hypothetical structure of the HLA class II molecule foreign antigen binding site. *(Reproduced with permission from Bjorkman PJ, Saper MA, Samraou B. Structure of the human class I histocompatibility antigen. HLA A2. Nature 1987;329:506.)*

cytokines such as IL-1, IL-2, INF-γ, or TNF in both thyroid and islet cells. Studies in the NOD mouse and the BB rat failed to reveal class II expression on β-cells, but did on endothelial cells and on infiltrating mononuclear cells. The detection of class II-positive β-cells in a newly diagnosed patient evaluated by immunocytochemistry could not be confirmed in other patients.

Association with Other Genes on Chromosome 6

The genes for TNF-α and TNF-β are also located in the MHC region (see Fig. 3-4). Both genes have polymorphisms associated with type 1 diabetes. Although TNF-β alleles differ between HLA-DR-matched Caucasian type 1 diabetes patients and controls, this was not found in North Indian Asians, suggesting that TNF-β does not directly predispose to type 1 diabetes. The genes for heat-shock protein (HSP) are also located in the MHC region. The increased frequency of a HSP70-2 9.5-kb Pst fragment among type 1 diabetes patients compared with controls was explained by linkage disequilibrium with DR3. Consistent with this conclusion is the observation that Japanese type 1 diabetes patients do not show an association with HSP70.

Association and Linkage with Chromosome 11

Sequence analysis of the human insulin gene revealed the presence of upstream (5'-flanking) variable-number tandem repeat (VNTR) sequences.

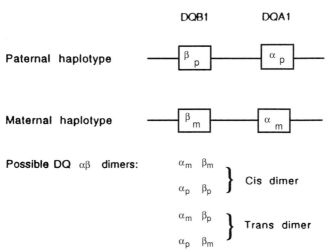

FIG. 3-5   The location of DQB1 and DQA1 genes on paternal (p) and maternal (m) chromosomes. Possible HLA-DQ class II molecules that may be formed in *cis* and *trans*-complementaton are indicated. *(Reproduced with permission from Kockum I, Wassmuth R, Holmberg E, et al: HLA-DQ primarily confers protection and HLA-DR susceptibility in type I (insulin-dependent) diabetes studied in population-based affected families and controls. Am J Human Gent 1993;53:150.)*

Although an association with type 2 diabetes was eventually excluded, the type 1 diabetes association was reproducible in several ethnic groups. Polymorphisms in the 5'-flaking region of the insulin gene were not found to be directly associated with type 1 diabetes because these markers were present on haplotypes that were either associated or not with type 1 diabetes. It was suggested that the size variation of the VNTR at the 5' end of the insulin gene could have a direct effect on the insulin gene regulation. The short class I VNTR alleles (26–63 repeats) predispose to type 1 diabetes, while class III alleles (140–210 repeats) have a dominant protective effect. When expression of insulin in human fetal thymus was examined, it was found that class III VNTR alleles were associated with two- to threefold higher proinsulin mRNA levels than class I. It was suggested that higher levels of thymic insulin expression may facilitate immune tolerance induction as a mechanism for the dominant protective effect of class III alleles.

Association with Other Genetic Markers from Genome Scanning

Other genetic markers for type 1 diabetes (Table 3-5) have been obtained by recent human genome scanning studies to support the previous observation that other genetic factors may contribute to the risk for type 1 diabetes. DNA collection available to investigators throughout the world through the Human Biological Data Interchange (HBDI) and from the British Diabetic Association (BDA) made it possible to identify several type 1 diabetes risk loci. There may be as many as 14–18 such risk loci, although it is controversial as to how many of them are reproducible in all populations.

TABLE 3-5 Candidate Type 1 Diabetes Susceptibility Loci Identified by Linkage Analysis

Locus	Chromosome	Candidate genes or microsatellites
IDDM1	6p21.3	HLA (DQA1, DQB1, DRB1)
IDDM2	11p15.5	INS-VNTR, TH
IDDM3	15q26	D15S107
IDDM4	11q13.3	FGF3, D11S1917, MDU1, ZFM1, RT6, ICE, CD3, etc.
IDDM5	6q25	ESR, a046Xa9, MnSOD
IDDM6	18q12-q21	D18S487, D18S64, JK (Kidd locus)
IDDM7	2q31-33	D2S152, D2S326, GAD1
IDDM8	6q25-27	D6S281, D6S264, D6S446
IDDM9	3q21-25	D3S1303
IDDM10	10p11-q11	D10S193, D10S208, GAD2
IDDM11	14q24.3-q31	D14S67
IDDM12	2q33	CTLA-4, CD28
IDDM13	2q34	D2S137, D2S164, IGFBP2, IGFBP5
IDDM14	Not assigned	Not assigned
IDDM15	6q21	D6S283, D6S434, D6S1580

HLA and insulin VNTR are estimated to contribute about 40% and 10%, respectively, of familial clustering of type 1 diabetes. Other contributing genes are therefore expected. A strong contributing gene reproduced in several ethnic groups is CTLA-4 on chromosome 2. Polymorphisms in the coding as well as in the noncoding regions of the CTLA-4 gene are associated with autoimmune diseases such as Graves' disease as well as type 1 diabetes. The association between CTLA-4 and type 1 diabetes in a case-control study indicated that long (AT)n repeats at the 3' end of the gene are associated with type 1 diabetes. One possible mechanism is that the CTLA-4 polymorphism affects the survival of autoreactive T-cells. While HLA seems necessary, it is clearly not sufficient for appearance of type 1 diabetes. However, HLA in combination with one or several contributing genes may affect the pathogenetic process, thereby affecting age at onset. It cannot be excluded, however, that other genetic factors important to β-cell function may contribute to type 1 diabetes risk.

IMMUNE ASPECTS

Autoantibodies

Autoantibodies that are reactive with antigens in pancreatic islet cells are common in type 1 diabetes (Table 3-6). Most of these antibodies occur with high prevalence in newly diagnosed type 1 diabetes subjects and before clinical appearance of type 1 diabetes. Their presence is useful in detecting β-cell autoimmunity and in assessing risk of subsequent clinical type 1 diabetes in genetically susceptible individuals. However, the relationship between the various islet-cell autoantibodies, β-cell autoimmunity, and eventual clinical type 1 diabetes is very complex and is still not fully characterized or understood. Of all the autoantibodies described in type 1 diabetes, four are clinically most useful: ICA, IAA, GADAb, and IA-2 Ab.

When ICAs were first discovered in 1974, it was felt that all individuals with ICAs would eventually develop clinical type 1 diabetes. This is not the

TABLE 3-6 Islet Cell Autoantigens of Insulin-Dependent Diabetes Mellitus

Autoantigen	Characteristics
Sialogylcolipid	Target of ICA in humans, GM2-1, non-beta-cell specific
Glutamate decarboxylase	Target of 64-kd antigen/GAD antibody in humans and animal models of IDD, two forms (GAD65 and 67), cellular immune antigen, synaptic like microvesicle protein, disease-modifying antigen
Insulin	Target of IAA in humans and non-obese diabetic (NOD) mice, cellular immune antigen, disease-modifying antigen
Insulin receptor	Target of autoantibodies in humans determined by bioassay
38 kd	Target of 38-kd antigen in humans, induced by cytomegalovirus, localized to insulin secretory granules, cellular immune antigen, multiple antigens of this molecular mass?
Bovine serum albumin	Target of BSA antibody, antigen in humans and animal models of IDD, contains ABBOS peptide, has molecular mimic in beta cell p69 protein (PM-1), disease-modifying antigen
Glucose transporter	Target of autoantibodies in humans, inhibits glucose stimulation, Glut-2 directed?
hsp 65	Target of autoantibodies and cellular immunity in NOD mice, disease-modifying antigen, contains p277 peptide.
Carboxypeptidase H	Target of autoantibodies in humans, identified by immunoscreening of islet cDNA, insulin secretory granule protein
52 kd	Target of autoantibodies in humans and NOD mice, molecular mimic with rubella virus
ICA12/ICA512	Target of autoantibodies in humans, identified by immunoscreening of islet cDNA, 5123 homology to CD45
150 kd	Target of autoantibodies in humans, beta-cell specific, membrane associated
RIN polar	Target of autoantibodies in humans and NOD mice, present on insulinoma cells

Source: Reprinted with permission from Atkinson MA, Maclaren NK: Islet cell autoantigens in insulin-dependent diabetes. *J Clin Invest* 1993; 92:1608–1616.

case, and recent extensive investigation in this area has revealed considerable complexity. When ICAs are detected in nondiabetic individuals identified because of other autoimmune diseases besides diabetes, the risk of subsequent clinical type 1 diabetes is less than when ICAs occur in relatives of type 1 diabetes patients. Similarly, ICA-positive individuals from the general population without a family history of type 1 diabetes have a much lower risk of type 1 diabetes than ICA-positive relatives of type 1 diabetes patients. In fact, ICAs can occur in people with protective HLA haplotypes, and in these individuals subsequent clinical type 1 diabetes is unusual. Insulin autoantibodies have become equally complex. In relatives of type 1 diabetes patients, the presence of IAAs in addition to ICAs greatly increases the risk of subsequent clinical type 1 diabetes compared to ICAs alone, but relatives with IAAs without ICAs have only a minimally increased risk of clinical type 1 diabetes.

In 1990, Baekkeskov and colleagues reported that the 64K autoantigen recognized by antibodies from type 1 diabetes patients was glutamic acid decarboxylase (GAD). GAD exists in at least two major isoforms, GAD65 and GAD67. Their respective distribution in β-cells and neural tissue varies between species, and although antibodies to both isoforms can occur, antibodies to GAD65 are predominantly associated with type 1 diabetes in humans. GAD autoantibodies are very common in a rare neurologic disorder, stiff-man syndrome, and only a small percentage of these patients develop type 1 diabetes. Furthermore, the GAD autoantibodies in type 1 diabetes and stiff-man syndrome appear to differ in ability to inhibit GAD enzymatic activity and in recognizing antigen in Western blot assays. It is now shown that recognition of GAD epitopes by GAD65Ab in type 1 diabetes is different from that in non-type 1 diabetes, GAD65Ab-positive individuals. Falorni *et al*, in their studies in the LADA subjects, demonstrated that antibodies to the COOH terminus of GAD (GADAb-C) have a diagnostic specificity for predicting insulin dependency as high as 99.4% (compared with 96.6% for GADAb measured in the traditional radiobinding assay), suggesting that epitope-specific assays can improve the diagnostic specificity of GADAb for insulin requirement.

In very elegant experiments, Christie *et al* demonstrated antibodies in type 1 diabetes to a 64K islet protein distinct from known isoforms of heat-shock protein or GAD. Antibodies recognizing a 37-kDa tryptic fragment of this non-GAD 64K antigen were more predictive of type 1 diabetes than GAD autoantibodies. These autoantibodies are now known as ICA512 or IA-2 (directed to the neuroendocrine protein insulinoma-associated protein 2, a member of the protein tyrosine phosphatase family). IA-2 autoantibodies were detected in 65–70% of patients with new-onset type 1 diabetes and 60–65% of prediabetic relatives of patients with type 1 diabetes. With sophisticated studies, it is now demonstrated that a major unique epitope for IA-2 autoantibodies is localized to amino acids 762-887.

Further studies looking at the relationships between genetic markers and disease-associated autoantibodies demonstrated that a combination of the genetic markers and autoantibodies increased the positive predictive values of all autoantibodies substantially, which may have clinical implications when evaluating the risk of developing type 1 diabetes at the individual level or when recruiting high-risk individuals for intervention trials. Increased prevalence of all the antibodies was closely associated with HLA identity to the index case, the DR4 and DQB1*0302 alleles, the DR3/4 phenotype, and the DQB1*02/0302 genotype. GADA were also associated with the DR3 and DQB1*02 alleles, and siblings carrying the protective DR2 and DQB1*0602-3 alleles were characterized by lower frequencies of ICAs, IA-2A, and GADA. However, because such combinations also resulted in reduced sensitivity, autoantibodies alone rather than in combination with genetic markers are recommended as the first-line screening in siblings.

To summarize, subjects develop autoantibodies to increasing number of islet antigens during the preclinical period, and multiple islet autoantibodies are much more predictive of future type 1 diabetes than a single antibody. Although autoantibodies could damage β-cells by antibody-dependent complement cytotoxicity or by targeting natural killer cells to β-cell antigens, transfer of type 1 diabetes in the animal models requires T-cells, and consequently a major direct role for antibodies in causing the β-cell damage of type 1 diabetes is unlikely.

Cellular Immune Response and Cytokines

Type 1 diabetes is thought to result from a T-cell-mediated destruction of the pancreatic β-cells. Antigen-specific T-cell activation requires two signals. One is imparted by interaction of the T-cell receptor (TcR)/CD3 complex with the antigen:MHC class II protein complex expressed by antigen-presenting cells (APCs). The second signal is provided by cell-bound and secreted co-stimulatory molecules, which, while not imparting any antigenic specificity, synergizes with TcR/CD3 signals in augmenting T-cell activation. Several signal transduction pathways operate as a result of T-cell activation.

As part of the insulitis process, a number of cytokines (soluble polypeptide mediators) are released from the immune cells infiltrating the islet. In addition to their immunologic function to modulate, amplify, and direct the immune response, several of the cytokines have been found to have direct effects on the pancreatic β-cells. The direct effects potentially involved in the pathogenesis of type 1 diabetes include inhibition of insulin release, cytotoxicity, and altered antigen expression. The cytokines IL-1, TNF, and IFN have been the most intensively studied. In general, the above-mentioned cytokines, especially when administered in combination, are cytotoxic to pancreatic β-cells. In addition to the impairment in insulin secretion resulting from this cytotoxicity, inhibition of insulin secretion, independent of cytotoxicity, is also observed. This distinction is potentially very important because it raises the attractive possibility that, especially early in the preclinical period of type 1 diabetes, much of the loss of insulin secretory function may be functional in nature and therefore potentially reversible rather than due to irreversible β-cell destruction. Both *in vitro* and *in vivo* experimental data suggest that β-cells are indeed able to repair after damage.

Cytokines also cause alterations in the β-cell expression of many other proteins besides insulin. Some proteins are stimulated, whereas others are inhibited. IL-1 inhibits the expression of GAD and stimulates the expression of other islet proteins. We have proposed that some of these proteins, especially heat-shock protein 70, hemoxygenase, and superoxide dismutase, may be protective of the β-cell and/or aid in recovery of the β-cell from damage. Cytokines are recognized to be an important component of the immune mechanism determining whether the immune response of CD4+ T-cells to an antigen is primarily cellular (Th1) or humoral (Th2). T-helper cells differentiate into at least two major subtypes, Th1 and Th2, which are functionally distinct and distinguished by different cytokine secretion patterns. Th1 and Th2 responses are largely mutually inhibitory; Th2 cytokines suppress Th1 responses, and vice versa. A large number of factors, including antigen dose, antigen affinity, route of administration, genetics including HLA type, and type of antigen-presenting cell, control differentiation into Th1 versus Th2 responses. Considerable data suggest that Th1-type immune responses against islet antigens are associated with progression to clinical type 1 diabetes in animals. In contrast, a predominantly Th2-type immune response appears to confer protection against type 1 diabetes. The Th1/Th2 paradigm may not be as distinct in humans as in the mouse. For example, in humans both Th1 and Th2 clones produce IL-10. The observations that subjects develop autoantibodies to increasing number of islet antigens during the preclinical period, and that multiple islet autoantibodies are much more predictive of future type 1 diabetes than single antibody, further supports the Th1/Th2 paradigm in humans.

Parenteral insulin therapy has been shown to protect against type 1 diabetes in the animal models, and in pilot studies in humans. Several observations support an immunologic effect of insulin as mediating, at least in part, the protection in the NOD mouse. If parenteral insulin prevents clinical type 1 diabetes and if this were mediated by an immunologic response to insulin, the mechanism would likely be a shift in the immune response toward a Th2-type pattern. Th2-type immune responses are preferentially generated by antigen presentation via the gut and consequently "oral tolerance" and resultant protection against autoimmune disease is in some ways analogous to the Th1/Th2 paradigm. *Oral tolerance* is a term used to describe the tolerance that can be induced by the exogenous administration of antigen to the peripheral immune system via the gut. It is a form of antigen-driven peripheral immune tolerance, and appears to involve two main mechanisms that are in part dependent on the antigen dose. The tolerance induced by lower doses of orally administered antigen appears to be mediated predominantly by active suppression, whereas higher doses tend to induce clonal anergy and/or deletion. The active suppression by low doses of oral antigen appears to be mediated by the oral antigen-generating regulatory T-cells that migrate to lymphoid and target organs expressing the antigen administered orally, and confer suppression via the secretion of downregulatory cytokines including IL-4, IL-10, and TGF-β. Unfortunately, the Diabetes Prevention Trial-Type 1 (DPT-1) did not confirm the beneficial effect of either parenteral or oral insulin on the type 1 diabetes disease process in humans. The divergent findings could be explained by any of several variables, including disease severity at the time of recruitment to the study (established diabetes versus high-risk subjects), age, disease subtype (LADA or classical type 1 diabetes), and ethnic background (Japanese or North American). It is important not to overinterpret these negative findings, since they apply only to high-risk subjects, as defined by the DPT-1, and to insulin at the doses and by the routes tested.

ENVIRONMENTAL FACTORS

Epidemiology

Various environmental triggers, such as certain viruses and dietary factors, may initiate the autoimmune process, leading to the destruction of the pancreatic β-cells and consequent type 1 diabetes. Several epidemiologic observations such as the age of onset, seasonality, and marked geographic differences in incidence and prevalence provide circumstantial evidence in support of environmental factors being involved in type 1 diabetes. Initial studies in monozygotic twins had shown that fewer than 50% of such twins are concordant for type 1 diabetes. Concordance can be the result of genetic and/or environmental similarity, but discordance, especially of this degree, suggests that type 1 diabetes, at least in part, is due to nongenetic factors. More recent longitudinal twin studies, with up to 39 years of follow-up from the onset of diabetes in index twins, have shown that identical twins may develop diabetes after a prolonged period of discordance and approximately two-thirds of long-term discordant twins have evidence of persistent β-cell autoimmunity and/or β-cell damage. This presence of discordance of age of disease presentation also supports the role of environmental factors. The diagnosis of type 1 diabetes follows a seasonal pattern, with incidence peaks in autumn and winter and a nadir in late spring/early summer. This seasonality has suggested a viral connection, but a single virus is unlikely to be responsible, because in children the autumn peak is primarily enteroviral infections and the winter peak is respiratory viruses. Furthermore, because infection usually results in immunity to subsequent infection by similar viruses for several years, most viruses pass through a given community with cycles of 2 or more years. Consequently, if the seasonality were due to viral infections, a number of different viruses would have to be involved to be consistent with the remarkably stable seasonal and yearly incidence of type 1 diabetes. The age pattern of onset of type 1 diabetes is in part compatible with an infectious etiology. Type 1 diabetes is rare in the first 9 months of life, has an increase at about 5–6 years of age, peaks at approximately 12 years of age, and has a less well defined peak at ages 20–35. No known infectious agent has an incidence pattern similar to this.

Another epidemiologic observation supporting a pathogenetic role for environmental factors is the marked geographic variation in incidence of type 1 diabetes. Earlier studies had reported the age-adjusted incidence rates for type 1 diabetes to have a 30-fold difference between the population extremes; the highest incidence rate, 29.5 per 100,000 person-years, was noted from Finland and the lowest, 1.6 per 100.000 person-years, from Hokkaido, Japan. The EURODIAB collaborative group prospectively analyzed geographically defined registers of new cases diagnosed under the age of 15 years in several centers representing most European countries with population coverage of about 28 million children, and reported standardized average annual incidence rates ranging from 3.2 cases per 100,000 per year in the former Yugoslav republic of Macedonia to 40.2 cases per 100,000 per year in two regions of Finland. The Diabetes Mondiale (DiaMond) Project Group has reported that the overall age-adjusted incidence of type 1 diabetes varied from 0.1/100,000 per year in China and Venezuela to 36.8/100,000 per year in Sardinia and 36.5/100,000 per year in Finland. This represents a >350-fold variation in incidence worldwide. This marked difference in incidence is much greater than for most other chronic diseases.

Analytical epidemiologic studies have further indicated exposures that are associated with an increased risk for the disease. In early perinatal life the immune system is inducible, and exposures in this period may initiate autoimmunity. Findings from Sweden and Finland suggest that enterovirus exposure during fetal life may initiate autoimmunity leading to diabetes. In addition, food components such as nitrosamine components, cow's milk protein, and gliadin have been proposed to initiate the autoimmunity of type 1 diabetes. A prospective natural history cohort study (the German BABYDIAB study) showed that food supplementation with gluten-containing foods before age 3 months was associated with significantly increased islet autoantibody risk (adjusted hazard ratio, 4.0) versus children who received only breast milk until age 3 months. Another birth cohort study from Denver showed that children initially exposed to cereals between ages 0 and 3 months (hazard ratio 4.32) and those who were exposed at 7 months or older (hazard ratio 5.36) had increased hazard of islet autoimmunity compared with those who were exposed during the fourth through sixth month, after adjustment for HLA genotype, family history of type 1 DM, ethnicity, and maternal age; there may be a window of exposure to cereals in infancy outside which initial exposure increases islet autoimmunity risk in suscepti-ble children. The diversity of determinants that are associated with type 1 diabetes risk points to a complex interaction between the genome and envi-ronment, and multivariate analyses have disclosed different risk profiles in different age groups. Evidence has been accumulating indicating that peri-natal exposures may be important for the initiation of β-cell destruction. Such risk factors may be the targets for primary prevention strategies of type 1 diabetes. As discussed earlier, considerable evidence supports the concept that a neonatal wave of β-cell apoptosis precedes insulitis in spon-taneous, induced, and accelerated models of autoimmune diabetes, and the wave of apoptosis provides the antigens necessary for priming the β-cell-specific T-cells.

The precise mechanisms whereby environmental factors contribute to the pathogenesis of human type 1 diabetes are not known. Some of the major possibilities include: (1) the agents may be directly toxic to the β-cells; (2) the agents, by an effect on the β-cells, may trigger an autoimmune response directed against the β-cells; (3) the agents, by providing specific peptides that share antigenic epitopes with host-cell protein ("molecular mimicry"), may trigger an immune response against β-cells; (4) the agents may cause insulin resistance; and (5) the agents may alter the β-cells in a way that increases their susceptibility to damage by other mechanisms (Table 3-7). These mech-anisms are not mutually exclusive. Even a protective rather than offensive role has also been suggested for specific viral and bacterial antigens. It is of interest to note also that a pathogen-free environment increases diabetes in BB rats and NOD mice, and in NOD mice nonspecific immune stimulation is usually protective. As we live in a "cleaner environment," the decreasing chances of natural infection in the general population may contribute to the induction of autoimmunity because the developing immune system is not exposed to stimulation that may be necessary to generate regulatory cells involved in the modulation and prevention of autoimmunity.

Drugs

Potential environmental factors fall into three main groups: specific drugs or chemicals, nutritional constituents consumed in the diet, and viruses. Specific drugs or chemicals include alloxan, streptozocin, pentamidine, and Vacor. The major mechanism underlying the diabetes in these patients appears to be direct β-cell toxicity, but these patients also provide evidence that primary β-cell damage can result in secondary autoimmunity, as islet-cell antibodies have been found in some of these patients.

Recently, attention has been paid to the long-term adverse effects of highly active antiretroviral therapy (HAART). Nucleoside and nucleotide reverse transcriptase inhibitors induce mitochondrial toxicity (inhibition of mito-chondrial DNA polymerase-γ), and this is the most likely cause of the adverse

TABLE 3-7 Possible Environmental Mechanisms in Type 1 Diabetes

1. Directly toxic to β-cells
2. Trigger an autoimmune reaction directed against the β-cells
3. Trigger an immune response by "molecular mimicry"
4. Induce increased insulin need that cannot be met by damaged β-cells
5. Alter β-cells to increase susceptibility to damage

effects associated with these drugs. Patients treated with human immunodeficiency virus-1 protease inhibitors often develop impaired glucose tolerance or diabetes, most likely due to an induction of insulin resistance; the protease inhibitor, indinavir has been shown to alter insulin signaling.

It is unlikely, except in rare cases, that drugs or chemicals in the external environment are common and/or major etiologic factors in human type 1 diabetes. The observations cited are primarily important because they document that β-cells are uniquely sensitive and can be selectively destroyed by certain chemicals, and that primary β-cell damage can elicit an immune response directed against the β-cells. The latter view is also supported by studies in transgenic mice expressing lymphocytic choriomeningitis virus (LCMV) in their β-cells. Animals are tolerant to the transgene and remain nondiabetic until infected with the virus exogenously. They then develop an immune response to LCMV, severe insulitis, and type 1 diabetes.

Dietary Factors

Among the environmental triggers, exposure to cows' milk in early neonatal life and development of type 1 diabetes has received considerable attention. The hypothesis was developed more than a decade ago, and the issue is still not settled. Literature review shows that as many as 19 groups from different parts of the world have implicated exposure to cows' milk protein in early neonatal life in the development of type 1 diabetes, whereas six other groups have found no such relationship. The major reasons for this discrepancy could be problems with case-control studies (maternal recall bias of early infant feeding history), problems with population controls, and use of smaller odds ratios (OR)/relative risk (RR < 2).

Epidemiologic and experimental evidence suggested that denial of dietary cows' milk protein early in life protects genetically susceptible children and animals from type 1 diabetes. Elimination of intact cows' milk proteins from the diet significantly reduced the incidence of type 1 diabetes in the spontaneously diabetic BB rat, the elimination being most effective when it occurred during the preweaning period. Bovine serum albumin (BSA) was proposed as a candidate milk-borne mimicry antigen responsible for the diabetogenic cows' milk effect. Elevated anti-BSA antibodies have been observed in patients and diabetic rodents. The anti-BSA antibodies cross-react with a β-cell membrane protein of Mr 69,000 (known as p69 or ICA 69), and precipitate p69 from islet-cell lysates. BSA-specific T-cells have recently been detected in culture system, and this response is mapped to a 17-amino acid sequence of BSA, known as ABBOS peptide (pre-BSA position 152-169), previously identified as a possible mimicry epitope.

A multicenter trial is being conducted in the United States, Canada, Europe, and Australia to test whether avoidance of dietary cows' milk protein for at least the first 6 months of life in genetically at-risk infants prevents the subsequent development of type 1 diabetes during the first 10 years of life. This "Trial to Reduce IDDM in Genetically at Risk" (TRIGR) project is a randomized, prospective trial and involves newborn infants with first-degree relatives with type 1 diabetes. Those genetically determined to be at high risk are randomized to receive a baby formula free of cows' milk (the formula containing a nonantigenic protein hydrolysate) or a conventional cows' milk-based formula. The intervention period is for a 6-month period, with a follow-up of 10 years. This would be a "true" primary prevention strategy.

Viruses

Viral infections can cause diabetes in a variety of animal species, frequently with important similarities to human type 1 diabetes. Although it is clear that, in certain animal species, viruses can cause diabetes and that sometimes the diabetogenic process is in part immune-mediated, the situation in humans is far more controversial.

Among the many viruses potentially involved in the etiology of human type 1 diabetes, three have received the greatest attention: mumps, coxsackie, and rubella. Numerous investigators have noted temporal associations between type 1 diabetes and mumps infections, although the proposed time interval between the reported viral infection and type 1 diabetes has ranged from several years to weeks or months. However, available data about mumps and type 1 diabetes are incomplete and difficult to interpret. Recent evidence from animal studies has raised the possibility that immunization by vaccines can influence the pathogenesis of type 1 diabetes mellitus. The possibility that widespread vaccination against mumps might offer protection against type 1 diabetes has also been investigated. A decline in mumps antibodies in type 1 diabetes patients and a plateau in the rising incidence of type 1 diabetes after introduction of mumps vaccine has been reported from Finland. However, there is no evidence that mumps-measles-rubella (MMR) mass vaccination programs have changed the incidence of diabetes mellitus in any population.

Several studies have indicated that enterovirus infections, coxsackievirus B (CVB) infections especially, are frequent at the diagnosis of clinical type 1 diabetes or may play a role in the initiation of the β-cell-damaging process. Prospective studies have suggested that enterovirus infections can also initiate the process several years before clinical type 1 diabetes. A temporal relationship between enterovirus infections and the induction of autoimmunity was demonstrated by Lonnrot *et al* in the Finnish Diabetes Prediction and Prevention Study. Three other observations support a potential role for coxsackie B in the etiology of type 1 diabetes. First, human β-cells are susceptible to coxsackie B viral infection and second, this infection results in decreased insulin production. Third, coxsackie B viral infection of diabetes-susceptible mice results in increased β-cell expression of GAD, and GAD antibodies. Finally, a portion of the GAD molecule shares homology to coxsackie B4, and this portion of the GAD molecule appears to contain an immune dominant epitope stimulatory to T-cells from human type 1 diabetes patients. However, only some strains of coxsackie B virus are diabetogenic, and exposure of mice to the more common nondiabetic strains probably confers protection against infection with the diabetic strains.

"Molecular mimicry" is one mechanism by which infectious agents (or other exogenous substances) may trigger an immune response against autoantigens (Tables 3-8 and 3-9). Structural similarity (molecular mimicry)

TABLE 3-8 Potential Viral Mechanisms in IDDM

1. Direct β-cell destruction
2. Increased insulin resistance and β-cell destruction
3. "Molecular mimicry"
4. Protection from diabetogenic strain by prior infection with nondiabetogenic strain
5. Stimulation of regulatory T-cells
6. Stimulation of effector T-cells

TABLE 3-9 Examples of "Molecular Mimicry" Potentially Related to Type 1 Diabetes

Pancreatic antigen	Foreign antigen
Insulin (IAA)	p73 protein of mouse endogenous retrovirus
GAD	PC2 protein of coxsackievirus
ICA69	ABBOS peptide of bovine serum albumin
38K	Cytomegalovirus
52K	Rubella virus

between viral epitopes and self-peptides can lead to the induction of auto-aggressive T-cell responses. It has been proposed that a self-peptide could replace a viral epitope for T-cell recognition and therefore participate in pathophysiological processes in which T-cells are involved. The tolerance to autoantigens breaks down and the pathogen-specific immune response that is generated cross-reacts with host structures to cause tissue damage and disease. Mimicry related to viral infection has been proposed on the basis of sequence homology between GAD65 and coxsackievirus P2-C, an enzyme involved in the replication of coxsackievirus B. However, a search of data bases identified 17 viruses with some homology to various fragments of GAD65, indicating that cross-reactivity between GAD65 and coxsackie-viruses is not unique. To conclude, the currently available information supports the assumption that the role of enterovirus infections may be more important than previously estimated. Enterovirus infections are associated with increased risk of type 1 diabetes, but whether this association reflects a causal relationship remains to be determined.

The incidence of diabetes in the congenital rubella syndrome is approximately 10–20%. Most important, the diabetes induced by rubella is similar genetically and immunologically to the type 1 diabetes occurring spontaneously in the absence of rubella. These similarities suggest that the diabetes associated with congenital rubella is not etiologically distinct, but that rubella virus triggers at least some of the same mechanisms that are operative in most spontaneous cases of type 1 diabetes. Rubella virus has also been demonstrated to infect human β-cells and to result in impaired insulin production, and there is antigen homology between a rubella virus capsid protein and an epitope in an unidentified 52-kDa islet protein. The similarity between these findings and those previously summarized for coxsackievirus make it tempting to speculate that molecular mimicry may be applicable to both viruses.

Recently, data have also been reported regarding an association of rotavirus infection and type 1 diabetes. Rotavirus, the most common cause of childhood gastroenteritis, contains peptide sequences highly similar to T-cell epitopes in the islet autoantigens GAD and tyrosine phosphatase IA-2 (IA-2), suggesting that rotavirus could also trigger islet autoimmunity by molecular mimicry. It appears that rotavirus infection may trigger or exacerbate islet autoimmunity in genetically susceptible children.

SUMMARY

Dramatic advances have been made in recent years in our understanding of the pathogenesis of type 1 diabetes. Using this information plus genetic and immunologic measurements, nondiabetic individuals can now be identified at high risk of subsequent clinical type 1 diabetes. In turn, this ability to identify high-risk subjects and to predict subsequent clinical type 1 diabetes plus knowledge of pathogenic mechanisms set the stage for large-scale intervention trials to test whether type 1 diabetes can be prevented (recently completed DPT-1, Diabetes Prevention Trial-Type 1, and ENDIT, European Nicotinamide Diabetes Intervention Trial; and ongoing trials that include DIPP, Finnish Diabetes Type 1 Prediction and Prevention Project; and TRIGR, Trial to Reduce IDDM in Genetically at Risk). The long-term goal of researchers working in this field may soon be realized; the type 1 diabetes disease process may be susceptible to interruption, and some people may be prevented from developing clinical type 1 diabetes.

ACKNOWLEDGMENTS

This work was supported in part by grants from the Medical Research Service of the Department of Veterans Affairs and from the National Institutes of Health (P30DK17047, RO1HD42444, and UO1DK46639).

ADDITIONAL READINGS

Akerblom HK, Knip M: Putative environmental factors in Type 1 diabetes. *Diabetes Metab Rev* 1995;14:31–67.
Diabetes Prevention Trial—Type 1 Diabetes Study Group: Effects of insulin in relatives of patients with type 1 diabetes mellitus. *N Engl J Med* 2002;346:1685–1691.
Naik RG, Palmer JP. Latent autoimmune diabetes in adults (LADA). *Rev Endocr Metab Disorders* 2003;4:233–241.
Palmer JP, Hirsch IB: What's in a name?: Latent autoimmune diabetes in adults, type 1.5, adult-onset, and type 1 diabetes. *Diabetes Care* 2003;26:536–538.
Von Herrath MG: Selective immunotherapy of IDDM: a discussion based on new findings from RIP-LCMV model for autoimmune diabetes. *Transplant Proc* 1998; 30(8):4115–4121.

For a more detailed discussion of this topic and a bibliography, please see Porte *et al: Ellenberg & Rifkin's Diabetes Mellitus,* 6th ed., Chapter 20.

4 | The Pathophysiology and Genetics of Type 2 Diabetes Mellitus

Steven E. Kahn   Daniel Porte, Jr.

Both fasting hyperglycemia and excessive increases in glucose concentration following oral glucose loading are criteria for the diagnosis of type 2 diabetes mellitus (T2DM). In both the postabsorptive and fed states, three important defects have been demonstrated in subjects with T2DM: (1) impaired basal and stimulated insulin secretion, (2) an increased rate of endogenous hepatic glucose release, and (3) inefficient peripheral tissue glucose use. In this chapter we will review the closed feedback loop comprising the pancreatic islet, liver, and peripheral tissues, which together are responsible for the regulation of plasma glucose. Then we will describe the nature of the three major defects observed in T2DM and how they interact in the pathophysiology of hyperglycemia. We will use this same feedback loop to provide a perspective of how the different therapeutic interventions act to alter the steady-state glucose level. Finally, we will discuss studies of the genetic basis for hyperglycemic syndromes including T2DM, maturity-onset diabetes of the young (MODY), and other rare genetic forms of T2DM.

NORMAL PHYSIOLOGY OF GLUCOSE REGULATION

The maintenance of a stable fasting plasma glucose level is dependent on a closed-feedback-loop relationship among the liver, peripheral tissues, and the pancreatic islet (Fig. 4-1). After an overnight fast, glucose is produced largely in the liver by glycogen breakdown and gluconeogenesis, with the rate of production being dependent on the availability of hepatic glycogen and gluconeogenic precursors. About 70–80% of the glucose released by the liver is metabolized independent of insulin by the brain and other insulin-insensitive tissues, such as the gut and red blood cells. Insulin-sensitive tissues, such as muscle and fat, use only small quantities. A number of neural and hormonal influences regulate hepatic glucose production, and in the presence of adequate amounts of insulin, the glucose level itself can regulate hepatic glucose release. Short-term hormonal regulators of physiologic importance include insulin, glucagon, and the catecholamines; a more long-term influence on hepatic glucose production is provided by growth hormone, thyroid hormone, and glucocorticoids.

The liver is exquisitely sensitive to changes in insulin and glucagon levels, which, due to the fact that these hormones drain directly into the liver, are ideally suited to regulate moment-to-moment changes in hepatic glucose output. An impairment in β-cell function reduces insulin levels and removes its inhibitory effect on the liver, which permits a slow rise in hepatic glucose production and the development of hyperglycemia. This impairment also raises glucagon output, which would increase glucose production by the liver and be associated with a concomitant rise in plasma glucose level. The elevated glucose level will stabilize if the feedback loop is intact, because of the effect

51

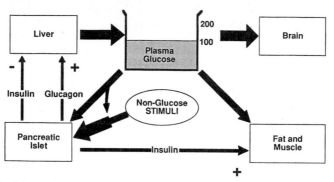

FIG. 4-1 A model for the normal steady-state regulation of plasma glucose level. Plasma glucose has direct effects on the pancreas to modulate insulin and glucagon secretion as well as interacting with nonglucose stimuli to modify α- and β-cell responses to these stimuli. During hyperglycemia, insulin secretion is increased and glucagon secretion reduced. When hypoglycemia prevails, glucagon secretion is enhanced and insulin secretion is diminished. Glucagon stimulates hepatic glucose production. Insulin inhibits glucose release by the liver and stimulates glucose use in insulin-sensitive tissues. Glucose uptake by the brain is insulin-independent, but in the periphery glucose uptake by fat and muscle is enhanced by insulin. Any change in hormone or substrate concentration or glucose use will be modulated by the loop in order that glucose use and production remain balanced. The plasma glucose level at which this occurs is determined by the efficiency with which the peripheral tissues take up glucose, the rate of hepatic glucose production, and islet α- and β-cell responsiveness to glucose. *(Adapted with permission from Porte D Jr: β-cells in type II diabetes mellitus.* Diabetes *1991; 40:166–180.)*

of the glucose feedback and the stimulation of pancreatic insulin and inhibition of glucagon secretion.

In situations in which peripheral insulin sensitivity changes, this would also tend to cause a change in plasma glucose level. For example, if insulin-mediated peripheral glucose uptake or utilization were to decrease, a rise in the fasting plasma glucose level would occur. If the pancreatic islet is normal, it will appropriately modify its secretion by reducing glucagon output by the α-cell and increasing β-cell insulin secretion. These secretory changes will reduce the rate of hepatic glucose output so that the glucose level will tend to be minimally disturbed. In instances in which peripheral glucose utilization rises, the opposite will occur, so that hepatic glucose production will increase and glucose level will once again return toward normal. It is important to realize that complete islet adaptation cannot occur; otherwise no stimulus for the changes in insulin and glucagon secretion would be present. Thus, when tissue insulin sensitivity changes, a new steady-state glucose level results, at a value somewhere between that expected for the change in insulin action and that expected for the change in pancreatic hormone secretion, with the exact level depending on islet α- and β-cell responsiveness and sensitivity to glucose and insulin.

Following food ingestion, plasma glucose excursions are minimized by the islet. This is accomplished by a reduction in hepatic glucose production and an increase in peripheral glucose uptake. These changes in glucose metabolism arise as a result of alterations in insulin and glucagon secretion, which are regulated on a minute-to-minute basis by an interaction among glucose, amino acids, the autonomic nervous system, and the gut hormones. Among these, glucose is the key islet regulator because it not only regulates insulin and glucagon secretion directly, it also modulates responses to the other substrates as well as gut hormones and neural factors released during nutrient ingestion.

From this description it is clear that when the feedback loop is functional, interpretation of any isolated aspect of this homeostatic mechanism cannot be meaningfully performed without taking into account all of the participating variables. Thus it is vitally important that comparisons of islet secretory function, hepatic glucose output, or peripheral tissue glucose uptake among different groups of individuals be performed at similar hormonal and substrate levels or that differences in these levels be taken into account. Failure to do so could lead to a gross misinterpretation of the status of these various components of the feedback loop.

PATHOPHYSIOLOGY OF ISLET DYSFUNCTION IN T2DM

Basal Insulin Secretion

Fasting plasma insulin levels in patients with T2DM, as compared with nondiabetic controls, have been reported as low, normal, and elevated. However, when type 2 diabetic patients are adiposity-matched and have their insulin levels evaluated at matched plasma glucose concentrations the resulting steady-state insulin levels in diabetic patients are lower than those of weight-matched and presumably insulin sensitivity-matched controls. Thus, regardless of the absolute levels, there is always a deficiency of basal insulin secretion in patients with T2DM. In T2DM there is a fundamental decrease in β-cell responsiveness to the prevailing plasma glucose level, but the effect of the resultant hyperglycemia is to stimulate basal insulin output to the point where the insulin levels will often appear normal or, if insulin resistance is present, will be higher than those of normal, insulin-sensitive lean subjects.

Insulin release is not simply a continuous process, but rather it has both pulsatile and oscillatory characteristics. The 10- to 15-minute pulses occur on a background of longer oscillations with cycles approximately every 120 minutes. Examination of these patterns reveals both to be abnormal in subjects with T2DM and in individuals at high risk for developing the disease.

Comparisons of basal insulin secretion in type 2 diabetic subjects and normal individuals may also be confounded by the fact that proinsulin cross-reacts in many conventional insulin radioimmunoassays. Using a radioimmunoassay specific for insulin, it has been shown that proinsulin and proinsulin intermediates contribute an average of twice as much to basal insulin immunoreactivity (approximately 30%) in subjects with T2DM as in healthy subjects (approximately 15%). Thus the true insulin levels in these patients are lower than those measured as immunoreactive insulin.

Glucose-Stimulated Insulin Secretion

Although measurement of plasma glucose levels during the oral glucose tolerance test provides the standard method for the diagnosis of T2DM, the use of this test as a means of assessing β-cell function in patients with this disorder is difficult and imprecise. This is because it is difficult to control factors such as gastric emptying time, gut hormone secretion rates, and the differences in glucose levels, which are important variables during the test. Thus, although some patients with T2DM will demonstrate an exaggerated insulin response late in the oral test, this seems to be the result of an early deficient response leading to markedly increased glucose levels that provide both a prolonged and exaggerated stimulus to the β-cell. Nevertheless, the magnitude of the insulin response over the first 30 minutes following oral glucose administration is reduced in both T2DM and impaired glucose tolerance. In fact, in subjects with reduced glucose tolerance, small changes in the magnitude of this response are associated with progressive reductions in glucose tolerance.

Use of an intravenous glucose challenge avoids many of the complicating variables associated with oral glucose tolerance testing as a means to assess β-cell function. With this test, T2DM has been shown to be characterized by total absence of the acute or first-phase insulin response measured during the first 10 minutes following intravenous glucose administration (Fig. 4-2). Loss of this response can in fact be documented at a fasting plasma glucose level above 115 mg/dL (6.4 mmol/L), now considered impaired fasting glucose. The insulin response after the first 10 minutes is called the second phase. Like the fasting insulin level, it is a function of the prestimulus glucose level. Thus, second-phase insulin responses may appear normal or even increased in patients with obesity and insulin resistance whose fasting plasma glucose levels are less than 200 mg/dL (11.1 mmol/L) (Fig. 4-2). However, when comparisons are made to adiposity- or insulin sensitivity-matched normal subjects at matched plasma glucose levels, it is apparent that second-phase insulin secretion is decreased in type 2 diabetic patients. When plasma glucose levels rise above 200–250 mg/dL (11.1–13.9 mmol/L), glycosuria ensues, thus preventing a sufficient rise in glucose level to compensate for the impaired insulin secretion. Therefore, patients with fasting plasma glu-

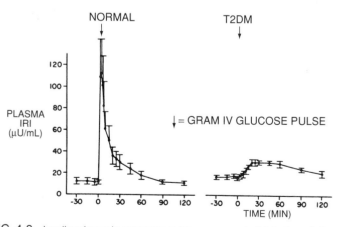

FIG. 4-2 Insulin release in response to intravenous administration of glucose in normal (n = 9) and T2DM (n = 9) subjects. Mean fasting plasma glucose concentrations: normal subjects, 85 ± 3 mg/dL (4.7 ± 0.2 mmol/L); diabetic subjects, 160 ± 10 mg/dL (5.9 ± 0.6 mmol/L). IRI, immunoreactive insulin; ↕ ± SEM. Note the relative preservation of the second-phase insulin response in T2DM subjects. *(Reprinted with permission from Pfeifer MA, Halter JB, Porte D Jr: Insulin secretion in diabetes mellitus.* Am J Med *1981;70:579.)*

cose levels above 250 mg/dL (13.9 mmol/L) are usually absolutely insulin-deficient, and their second-phase responses are characterized by absolute reductions in insulin release. These individuals have been termed as having *decompensated* T2DM.

Non-Glucose-Stimulated Insulin Secretion

Administration of one of a variety of nonglucose secretagogues, such as the amino acid arginine, the gastrointestinal hormones secretin or glucagon-like peptide 1 (GLP-1), the β-adrenergic agent isoproterenol, or the sulfonlyurea tolbutamide, is also followed by an acute insulin response. In T2DM patients with a fasting plasma glucose level less than 200 mg/dL (11.1 mmol/L), the acute insulin response to any of these secretagogues is of normal magnitude when subjects are matched for body adiposity or sensitivity. However, as is the case for basal and second-phase insulin secretion, the elevated plasma glucose level appears to be responsible for the maintenance of these apparently normal insulin responses to nonglucose stimuli. When plasma glucose levels are matched by either a glucose infusion in normal subjects or an insulin infusion in type 2 diabetic subjects, the acute insulin response to a nonglucose stimulus is also found to be reduced in weight-matched diabetic subjects (Fig. 4-3). This regulatory effect of glucose, termed *glucose potentiation,* can be expressed as the slope of the line relating the acute insulin response to a nonglucose secretagogue as a function of plasma glucose level between 100 and 250 mg/dL (5.6 and 13.9 mmol/L). Type 2 diabetic subjects with fasting hyperglycemia have been shown to have a much flatter slope of potentiation than normal individuals.

At a glucose level above 450 mg/dL (25.0 mmol/L), both normal and diabetic subjects reach their maximal acute insulin responses, termed *AIRmax* (Fig. 4-3). The observed reduction in maximal responsiveness in diabetic subjects denotes a decrease in insulin secretory capacity. The similarity of the glucose level giving a half-maximal response (PG50) in both diabetic and healthy individuals indicates an equivalent β-cell sensitivity to glucose. However, AIRmax has a curvilinear negative relationship to the fasting plasma glucose level (Fig. 4-4), with a reduction of 50–75% in secretory capacity by the time the diagnostic fasting level of diabetes mellitus is reached (126 mg/dl, 7.0 mM).

Basal and Stimulated Glucagon Secretion

Abnormalities of glucagon secretion have also been demonstrated in T2DM. The normal regulation of glucagon release is not entirely understood but appears to be dependent on inhibition of the α-cell by glucose or insulin alone or by insulin and glucose together. Bearing this in mind, T2DM patients with plasma glucose levels below 250 mg/dL (13.9 mmol/L) have been shown to have apparently normal basal plasma glucagon levels. Though matching of plasma glucose levels does not provide evidence as to whether glucose or insulin regulation of the α-cell is impaired, it has demonstrated that these normal glucagon levels are inappropriately elevated for the prevailing hyperglycemia.

The glucagon response to an intravenous glucose challenge is also abnormal in T2DM patients. Bolus administration of intravenous glucose normally results in suppression of glucagon release, but suppression is a slow phe-

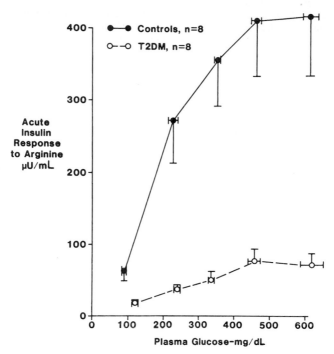

FIG. 4-3 A comparison of acute insulin responses to 5 g IV arginine (mean 2- to 5-minute insulin increment) at five matched plasma glucose levels in eight patients with T2DM and in eight controls of similar age and body weight. The slope of potentiation is the linear portion of the relation between plasma glucose (100–250 mg/dL, 5.5-13.9 mmol/L) and the acute insulin response. It is much flatter in the diabetic group. The maximal insulin response, a measure of β-cell secretory capacity, is the response at a glucose concentration greater than 450 mg/dL (25 mmol/L). It is also much lower in the diabetic group. The half-maximal glucose level, a measure of glucose sensitivity of the β-cell, is between 150 mg/dL (8.3 mmol/L) and 200 mg/dL (11.1 mmol/L) and is unchanged in the diabetic group. *(Reprinted with permission from Ward WK, Bolgiano DC, McKnight B, Halter JB, Porte D Jr: Diminished β-cell secretory capacity in patients with non-insulin-dependent diabetes mellitus. J Clin Invest 1984; 74: 1318–1328.)*

nomenon. In T2DM, insulin levels are similar because glucose disposal rates are lower and therefore a higher glucose level prevails, leading to what appears to be a normal suppressive response. However, when glucose levels in T2DM subjects are matched to controls, then glucagon levels are higher. In addition, the magnitude of the acute glucagon response to amino acid stimulation is greater at matched glucose levels in type 2 diabetic subjects. Therefore, there is also an abnormality in regulation of α-cell secretory function related to glucose.

Assessment of α-cell secretory function by oral glucose tolerance testing is, as in β-cell evaluation, confounded by the inability to control the plasma glucose level, the rate of gastric emptying, and gut peptide secretion. Despite these caveats, when oral testing is performed, defects in α-cell function are often apparent. Thus, carbohydrate ingestion in T2DM may not be followed by suppression of glucagon and may even demonstrate a paradoxical increase rather than the usual suppression observed with hyperglycemia. In addition, ingestion of a pure protein meal produces an exaggerated glucagon response in type 2 diabetic patients regardless of whether their fasting glucose levels are normal or elevated.

Thus it appears that an abnormality in α-cell function is present in most patients with T2DM. At the present time, however, it is unclear whether this abnormality results from reduced insulin regulation of the α-cell, diminished glucose sensing, or a combination of factors.

Nature of the Islet Lesion in T2DM

Although it is clear that islet dysfunction is present in T2DM, it is still not certain whether the defects in insulin secretion are the result of a reduction of β-cell mass, dysfunction of a normal number of β-cells, or some combination. In addition, as the normal physiologic regulation of glucagon secretion is

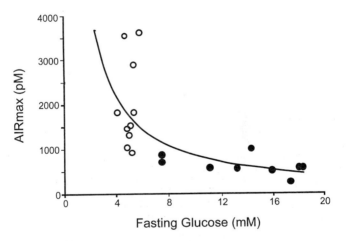

FIG. 4-4   Curvilinear relationship between β-cell secretory capacity (AIRmax) and fasting plasma glucose in nine subjects with T2DM (●) and nine subjects with normal glucose tolerance (○). There is a broad range of β-cell secretory capacity in the healthy subjects due to large differences in insulin sensitivity, whereas in the subjects with T2DM the range is narrower, a manifestation of the impaired islet function. The nonlinear relationship between these two parameters ($r = -0.76$; $p < 0.0001$) demonstrates that the degree of β-cell function is a determinant of the fasting glucose level. This relation predicts that a relatively large initial loss of β-cell function should result in only a small increase of fasting plasma glucose level. However, further small declines in β-cell function would lead to much larger increases of glucose level. *(Adapted from Røder ME, Porte D Jr, Kahn SE: Disproportionately elevated proinsulin levels reflect the degree of impaired β-cell secretory capacity in patients with non-insulin dependent diabetes mellitus.* J Clin Endocrinol Metab *1988; 83:604–608.)*

incompletely understood, the contribution of the β-cell defect to α-cell dysfunction is also not entirely clear.

From studies of all of these possibilities it is apparent that although many different perturbations can reproduce some features of the β-cell secretory abnormalities observed in T2DM, no single experimental approach has been able to fully replicate the findings of this disorder in humans. This suggests the possibility that the abnormalities of islet function characteristic of T2DM are the result of a combination of a variety of lesions and supports the concept that considerable heterogeneity is probably involved in the pathogenesis of the β-cell defects of this disorder.

PATHOPHYSIOLOGY OF INSULIN RESISTANCE AND GLUCOSE RESISTANCE IN T2DM

Tissue resistance to insulin is an important component of the glucose intolerance of T2DM . The etiology of defects in insulin action observed in the liver and peripheral tissues of the common forms of T2DM is not clear. However, it does appear that a major component of this abnormality may be related to obesity, with central fat distribution, particularly intra-abdominal fat, being important. Glucose-mediated glucose disposal independent of insulin is also important to glucose tolerance and requires that its role in the pathophysiology of T2DM also be recognized.

Hepatic Insulin Resistance

Basal rates of hepatic glucose production in patients with T2DM have been documented as normal or increased. As with measurements of insulin secretion, it is important that these production rates be evaluated in the context of the glucose concentration at which they were measured. When this is done, it is apparent that even if "normal," the values are inappropriately elevated for the ambient glucose level. In most studies, the degree of the abnormality in hepatic glucose output is positively correlated with the degree of fasting hyperglycemia, indicating that the rate of hepatic glucose production is an important determinant of the fasting plasma glucose level (Fig. 4-5).

The increased rate of hepatic glucose production results from an impairment of the effects of insulin and glucose to normally suppress glucose release by the hepatocyte. A shift to the right in the insulin dose-response curve with no reduction in the maximal suppressive response at supraphysiologic insulin levels has been demonstrated in diabetic subjects studied at euglycemia. This type of change is compatible with a reduction in hepatic sensitivity to insulin produced by a decrease in insulin receptor number. However, when similar studies are performed in T2DM subjects at basal hyperglycemia, maximal suppression of hepatic glucose production occurs at lower insulin levels, but the dose-response relation still demonstrates a defect in insulin action when compared to control subjects studied at normoglycemia. Thus, hyperglycemia appears capable of exerting a suppressive effect on hepatic glucose output independent of insulin, but is unable to fully compensate for the reduction in insulin sensitivity found in T2DM. This suggests that a defect in the ability of glucose to inhibit its own release from the liver is also contributing to the observed glucose overproduction in the basal state. Glucagon, of major importance to the maintenance of postabsorptive hepatic glucose release, appears to be responsible for more than half of the hepatic glu-

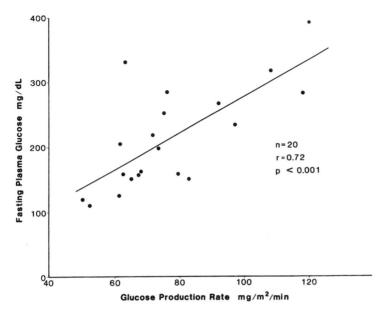

FIG. 4-5 Correlation between fasting plasma glucose levels and glucose production rate in 20 patients with untreated T2DM. Despite the suppressive effect of hyperglycemia on glucose production, those patients with the highest glucose levels had the highest production rates. *(Reprinted with permission from Best JD, Judzewitsch RG, Pfeifer MA, Beard JC, Halter JB, Porte D Jr: The effect of chronic sulfonylurea therapy on hepatic glucose production in non-insulin-dependent diabetes. Diabetes 1982; 31:333–338.)*

cose production observed in T2DM. As a result, the abnormal regulation of glucagon secretion in these subjects may help explain the observed hepatic resistance of T2DM to the suppressive effects of both insulin and glucose.

During oral caloric intake the liver plays a critical role in the maintenance of glucose homeostasis. The meal-induced alterations in the concentrations of glucose, insulin, and glucagon entering the liver through the portal circulation contribute to the liver changing from its status in the fasted state as an organ responsible solely for glucose production to one that, during refeeding, restores its glycogen content by increasing its uptake and/or synthesis of glucose. Therefore, considering the defects in hepatic sensitivity to glucose and insulin, it is not surprising that following an oral glucose load a delayed reduction in hepatic glucose production can be demonstrated in T2DM. This failure of the liver to adequately suppress its glucose production accounts for a considerable proportion of the observed rise in plasma glucose concentrations following meal ingestion. Although a large proportion of this defect in suppression of hepatic glucose release may result from the deficient insulin response, neither the contribution of the increased glucagon response during meals nor the potential for variability in hepatic sensitivity to other neurohormonal responses following oral intake has yet been defined.

Peripheral Insulin Resistance

Using the euglycemic insulin clamp technique, it has been conclusively demonstrated that a major reduction in the mean glucose disposal rate exists in subjects with T2DM. Further analysis of the *in vivo* dose-response relation suggests that this reduction in insulin responsiveness is the result of two abnormalities. First, the rightward shift in the curve is compatible with a reduction in cellular insulin receptor number. A decrease in receptor number has been reported in *in vitro* studies using monocytes, erythrocytes, and adipocytes. Despite the presence of spare or unoccupied receptors, the marked decrease in the maximal rate of glucose disposal indicates the existence of a postbinding (intracellular) defect as well. Insulin-binding studies on isolated adipocytes from individuals with T2DM have shown that the predominant determinant of the severity of the peripheral insulin resistance in untreated patients is this reduction in postreceptor insulin action. Initial analysis suggested that part of this defect in intracellular insulin action resulted from a reduction in the number of glucose transporters. However, it appears that the total amount of GLUT-4 mRNA and protein is normal, although the function or the intracellular movement to the cell membrane of this insulin-dependent glucose transporter is diminished. Assessments of a number of the key molecules involved in intracellular transmission of the insulin signal following insulin binding to its receptor (e.g., insulin receptor substrate-1 [IRS-1] and phosphotidylinositol-3-kinase [PI3 kinase]) have demonstrated defects in the activity or amounts of these molecules, but these changes are not distinct from those observed in obesity.

These preceding observations of reduced insulin effectiveness were all made under euglycemic conditions and thus do not take into account the ability of glucose, by virtue of mass action, to augment its own disposal into the peripheral tissues independent of a change in insulin. When incremental insulin dose-response studies are performed at the basal level of hyperglycemia in T2DM subjects, insulin's effect on peripheral glucose disposal is essentially identical to that observed in matched control subjects studied at euglycemia. These findings suggest that in the presence of hyperglycemia, any impairment of peripheral insulin action is overcome by a mass action increase of glucose uptake. Therefore, as glucose levels rise due to the increase in hepatic glucose production, peripheral glucose uptake increases by mass action so that a new steady state is created in which the increased glucose levels are associated with increased glucose use despite the impairment of insulin action.

The efficiency of glucose uptake following oral glucose ingestion is also defective in T2DM subjects. In the peripheral tissues, ingested glucose normally undergoes oxidative and nonoxidative metabolism, with the rate of these processes being controlled by the enzymes pyruvate dehydrogenase and glycogen synthase, respectively. At low insulin concentrations the major route of peripheral glucose disposal is via glucose oxidation, while at higher levels disposal occurs predominantly by glycogen synthesis. In T2DM, the efficiency of glucose uptake by both processes is reduced, with the predominant abnormality being a defect in nonoxidative glucose storage. As glycogen synthase activity is stimulated by insulin, the diminished insulin sensitivity compounded by the reduced insulin secretory response to meals leads to a failure to stimulate normal enzyme activity.

Glucose Resistance

Besides insulin resistance and islet dysfunction as causes of decreased glucose tolerance, insulin-independent glucose uptake or glucose-mediated glucose uptake is an important factor determining glucose use. In fact, about 80% of tissue glucose uptake in the fasting state occurs by insulin-independent mechanisms, primarily into the brain. However, insulin-independent glucose uptake also takes place in muscle, fat, and other tissues. During intravenous glucose tolerance testing, insulin-independent glucose-mediated glucose uptake, also known as glucose effectiveness, is important in determining the rate of glucose disappearance.

Glucose-mediated glucose uptake has been quantified using a number of methods, and has been shown to be regulated in normal subjects and abnormal in patients with T2DM. As suggested in the foregoing discussions of hepatic and peripheral insulin resistance, glucose-mediated glucose disposal is important in decreasing glucose production by the liver and increasing glucose uptake in muscle. Thus, it could be envisaged that in T2DM, glucose resistance would result in a reduced ability of the liver to suppress glucose production and/or a decrease in the effectiveness of peripheral tissues to take up glucose by mass action, thereby contributing to hyperglycemia.

The cellular processes underlying alterations in glucose effectiveness have not been fully elucidated. This function could be dependent on glucose transporter number and/or activity as well as processes involving glucose metabolism after its entry into the cell. These posttransport processes could include regulation of enzymes responsible for glucose use, as well as others that may regulate glucose transporter function such as the enzyme glucosamine fructose amino transferase (GFAT), which metabolizes glucose through a shunt from the glycolytic breakdown process. Although glucose effectiveness is independent of a sudden change in insulin level, this process can apparently be regulated by changes in circulating insulin over time. Up until now, all conditions in which glucose effectiveness has been shown to be reduced have been associated with impaired islet function and therefore associated with reduced circulating basal and stimulated insulin levels. This finding suggests that improvements in insulin secretion may be associated with an increase in glucose effectiveness, a hypothesis that has yet to be tested.

Role of Obesity, Counterregulatory Hormone Secretion, and Insulin Deficiency

It has long been recognized that obesity is associated with insulin resistance. In the absence of carbohydrate intolerance, dramatic compensatory hyperinsulinemia is present. Though this adaptive response effectively maintains normoglycemia in more than 85% of obese individuals, these elevated plasma insulin levels may contribute to the alterations in insulin action that are a feature of obesity. With mild degrees of obesity, the predominant change is a reduction in tissue insulin binding. As body weight and fat cell size increase further, a proportional increase in basal insulin secretion occurs. These changes are associated with the development of a postreceptor defect, the severity of which is related to the change in body weight and plasma insulin concentration. Because central adiposity rather than lower-body adiposity is the major determinant of the insulin resistance of obesity, and intra-abdominal fat appears to be particularly critical, there are difficulties in estimating the role of obesity in the insulin resistance of any particular type 2 diabetic person.

Secretion of counterregulatory hormones has been shown to be altered in some patients with T2DM. Marked hyperglycemia by inducing glycosuria and resultant volume depletion leads to baroreceptor stimulation and increased sympathetic nervous system activation, which can explain increased levels of catecholamines observed in out-of-control T2DM subjects. This effect is more marked as hyperglycemia becomes more severe due to greater urinary glucose losses. Thus, hyperglycemia acts as a stimulus for a neuroendocrine stress response, which leads to counterregulatory hormone secretion. This excessive catecholamine release in turn impairs islet function, reducing both insulin-mediated and glucose-mediated glucose disposal producing more hyperglycemia. Since counterregulatory hormones are all capable of producing insulin resistance, it appears that even a mild increase in plasma concentrations of such hormones observed in T2DM patients could contribute to their insulin resistance. With severe hyperglycemia it is likely that the more pronounced neuroendocrine abnormalities contribute to the greater degrees of insulin and glucose resistance observed with poorer glycemic control.

A variety of studies suggest that insulin deficiency, or the metabolic derangements arising from it, is involved in the development of insulin and glucose resistance. Animal studies in which insulin deficiency has been created using agents toxic to the β-cell, such as streptozocin, have demonstrated the existence of an abnormality in insulin action. Similarly, type 1 diabetic (T1DM) subjects who are totally insulin-deficient are insulin-resistant, and both type 1 and T2DM subjects increase their rates of glucose disposal with an amelioration of the postreceptor defect in insulin action when treated with insulin. In addition, states of glucose resistance have been associated with an absolute or relative reduction of β-cell function. From the foregoing discussion it is apparent that the simultaneous presence and interaction of obesity, excessive counterregulatory hormone effects, and the metabolic events related to hypoinsulinemia contribute significantly to the diminished insulin and glucose sensitivity of T2DM. The inability to control for all these factors makes it difficult to discern whether a primary alteration in insulin or glucose action also exists in this disease. However, by virtue of its relation with islet function, it is clear that insulin and glucose resistance are of major importance in determining the degree of the metabolic derangement present in T2DM.

THE INTERACTION BETWEEN INSULIN RESISTANCE AND INSULIN SECRETION IN T2DM

The feedback loop comprising the liver, pancreas, and peripheral tissues requires that islet function be an important determinant of the basal glucose level. If islet responsiveness to glucose is high, then changes in insulin action will not perturb the plasma glucose level very much. Thus, in the presence of normal islet function, isolated insulin resistance does not usually result in fasting hyperglycemia. A common condition that exemplifies this is obesity, in which the majority of subjects are insulin-resistant but do not have impaired glucose tolerance (IGT) or diabetes. This lack of change in fasting glycemia is because there is a reciprocal and proportionate increase in insulin secretion, representing an adaptive phenomenon by the normal β-cell to insulin resistance (Fig. 4-6). From percentile charts based on data comparing

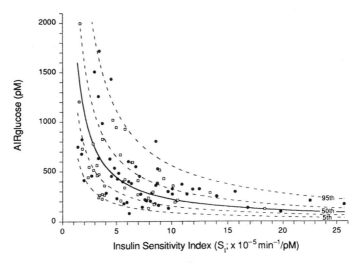

FIG. 4-6   Relationship between insulin sensitivity and the first-phase insulin response (AIRglucose) in 93 healthy subjects (55 males [•] and 38 females [□]). The best fit of the relationship is described by a hyperbolic function, that is, insulin sensitivity × first-phase insulin response is a constant. The 5th, 25th, 50th, 75th, and 95th percentiles for the relationship are illustrated. *(Reprinted with permission from Kahn SE, Prigeon RL, McCulloch DK, et al: Quantification of the relationship between insulin sensitivity and β-cell function in human subjects. Evidence for a hyperbolic function. Diabetes 1993; 42:1663–1672.)*

β-cell function and insulin sensitivity in healthy subjects, it is possible to determine the adequacy of insulin secretion (Fig. 4-7). When the relationship places an individual in a low percentile, this would be predicted to be associated with reduced glucose tolerance.

Although the exact mediator responsible for this alteration in α- and β-cell function has not been identified, evidence in normal subjects suggests that glucose may be responsible for this change. When healthy individuals are given glucose infusions for 2–3 hours, they demonstrate enhanced insulin secretory responses to a later intravenous glucose challenge despite the fact that glucose levels under both the basal and postinfusion conditions are similar at the time of the test. When studies of islet secretory function are performed following a 20-hour glucose infusion, consistent increases in the slope of glucose potentiation provide evidence of β-cell adaptation, while consistent decreases in the acute glucagon responses suggest adaptation of α-cell function. Thus it appears that the normal pancreatic islets possess an adaptive capability involving both the α- and β-cells, and that this adaptation, which may be mediated by changes in glucose level, prevents the development of marked hyperglycemia in individuals with insulin resistance and normal islet function. However, when β-cell dysfunction is present, the degree of glycemia needed to compensate will be greater. When insulin sensitivity is normal, it is unclear what degree of β-cell mass reduction is necessary before fasting hyperglycemia occurs. Some individuals do not develop diabetes mellitus after 70–90% pancreatectomies. Whether this or lesser degrees of β-cell

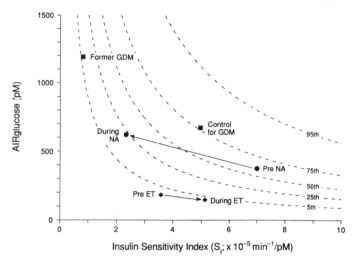

FIG. 4-7 Percentile lines for the relationship between insulin sensitivity and the first-phase insulin response (AIRglucose). Data from three studies are plotted. Individual data for a former gestational diabetic (former GDM) and a control individual (control for GDM) demonstrate that although β-cell function may be greater in absolute terms, when evaluated relative to the degree of insulin sensitivity, the response is inappropriately low in the former GDM, compatible with β-cell dysfunction. Mean data show that exercise training (ET) in older males does not alter the relationship between insulin sensitivity and the first-phase insulin response and thus glucose tolerance does not change. In contrast, nicotinic acid (NA)-induced insulin resistance in young males results in a change in the relationship between insulin sensitivity and the first-phase insulin response, which is associated with a reduction in glucose tolerance. *(Reprinted with permission from Kahn SE, Prigeon RL, McCulloch DK, et al: Quantification of the relationship between insulin sensitivity and β-cell function in human subjects. Evidence for a hyperbolic function. Diabetes 1993; 42: 1663–1672.)*

loss are associated with clinically significant hyperglycemia if insulin resistance develops is as yet undetermined. Because this question cannot be easily addressed in humans, mathematical modeling has been utilized to predict the various degrees of β-cell loss and insulin resistance required to produce fasting hyperglycemia. Such modeling predicts that in the presence of marked insulin resistance a 50% decrease in β-cell function would result in significant hyperglycemia. From this type of analysis it is predicted that tissue insensitivity to insulin will become a more important determinant of plasma glucose concentration as the loss of β-cell function becomes greater. Observations in T2DM are consistent with this prediction. Thus, a decrease in insulin sensitivity such as that induced by the development of adiposity will cause only a small change in glucose level in a person with a normal pancreas, but a much larger rise in glucose concentration will be observed in a patient with reduced islet function (Fig. 4-8). This is due to the curvilinear relation between islet β-cell function and plasma glucose level shown in Fig. 4-8. It requires more than a 75% loss of islet function for plasma glucose to

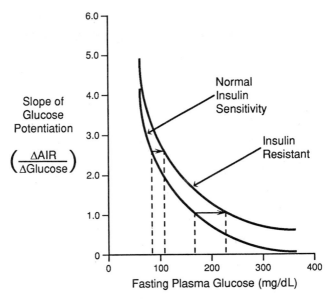

FIG. 4-8   Relationship of β-cell function to plasma glucose concentration and the impact of insulin resistance. The curvilinear relationship between β-cell function and fasting plasma glucose concentration dictates that in an individual with normal insulin sensitivity, the fasting glucose concentration will only reach the diagnostic level for T2DM (126 mg/dL; 7.0 mmol/L) when approximately 75% of β-cell function has been lost. When insulin resistance coexists in an individual with intact islet function and normal fasting plasma glucose, the compensatory enhancement in insulin output will prevent a marked change in plasma glucose concentration. Alternatively, in an individual with islet dysfunction sufficient to produce an elevation in the fasting glucose concentration, the additive effect of insulin resistance will produce a large increase in fasting glucose. A therapeutic intervention that reduces insulin resistance will reverse this change, resulting in a reduction in the glucose concentration. *(Reproduced with permission from Porte D Jr: β-Cells in type II diabetes mellitus. Diabetes 1991; 40:166–180.)*

rise above 126 mg/dL (7.0 mmol/L), but there is an increasingly greater glucose rise as islet function deteriorates. Insulin resistance shifts the curve to the right, amplifying this effect. When tissue insulin sensitivity is improved by weight loss, again only small changes in fasting plasma glucose levels will be observed in subjects with normal α- and β-cell function, but a marked lowering of the glucose concentration will occur in the hyperglycemic obese individual with impaired islet β-cell function.

A PATHOPHYSIOLOGIC MODEL OF T2DM

Figure 4-9 illustrates how the basal glucose concentration is regulated by a feedback loop in which the pancreatic islet acts as a glucose sensor to balance hepatic glucose delivery to the rate of insulin-dependent and insulin-independent glucose use. The occurrence of any change in glucose production

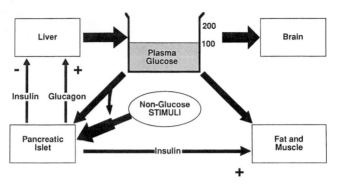

FIG. 4-9 Model for the development of hyperglycemia in T2DM: normal basal glucose regulation. Insulin and glucagon, through their effects on the liver, fat, and muscle, modulate the plasma glucose level. Plasma glucose, by its direct interaction with the endocrine pancreas and by its modulation of the secretory response to nonglucose stimuli, feeds back to the islet to regulate insulin and glucagon output. *(Reproduced with permission from Porte D Jr: β-Cells in type II diabetes mellitus.* Diabetes *1991; 40:166–180.)*

by the liver or glucose use by the peripheral tissues leads to a change in glucose levels. This, in turn, is sensed by the islet, leading to changes in insulin and glucagon secretion to minimize the overall change in glucose levels at a new, minimally changed steady state. While this new steady state returns the glucose concentration toward normal, complete compensation cannot occur because this would result in the loss of the stimulus responsible for the adaptive change. The β-cell lesion in T2DM would, if uncompensated, lead to reduced plasma insulin levels. Because glucagon secretion is either wholly or partially regulated by the neighboring β-cell, an abnormal rise in α-cell release of glucagon would also occur (Fig. 4-10). This reduction in insulin and increase in glucagon draining into the liver would be expected to produce an increase in hepatic glucose production. Further, the reduced peripheral insulin level would impair glucose use by both fat and muscle, while glucose use in the non-insulin-dependent tissues proceeds normally. Because of the reduction in insulin secretion, insulin-mediated glucose uptake cannot increase sufficiently to compensate for the increased rate of hepatic glucose release, and the fasting glucose level tends to rise. This situation is only transient, because the elevation in the fasting plasma glucose level would lead to increased β-cell stimulation, thereby producing a more "normal" plasma insulin level, as depicted in Fig. 4-11. In addition, the increase in glucose and insulin concentrations results in a reduction in glucagon secretion, but at the new steady state the glucagon level is not appropriately reduced for the degree of glycemia. Concurrent with these changes in islet hormone secretion, glucose production and use are moderated. However, at the new steady state, the rate of hepatic glucose release will remain elevated, glucose levels will be elevated, and therefore total glucose uptake will be increased due to the hyperglycemia. When hepatic and peripheral insulin resistance develops, the impairment of glucose uptake leads to a further increase in plasma glucose. This additional hyperglycemia leads to further stimulation of the β-cell with resultant normal or even supranormal insulin levels as well as further

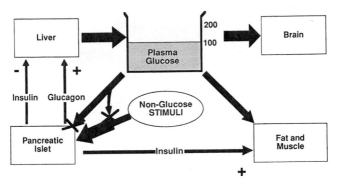

FIG. 4-10 Model for the development of hyperglycemia in T2DM: hypothetical initial islet lesion of T2DM. The impairment of islet function would be expected to reduce insulin and increase glucagon output, which would result in overproduction of glucose by the liver and underuse of glucose in the periphery, with a resultant increase in the glucose level. *(Reproduced with permission from Porte D Jr: β-Cells in type II diabetes mellitus. Diabetes 1991; 40:166–180.)*

increase in hepatic glucose delivery and peripheral glucose uptake (Fig. 4-12). Although a further reduction in the glucagon level occurs, the resultant level is still inappropriately elevated for the degree of hyperglycemia.

From this model it is apparent that islet dysfunction may be present regardless of whether basal insulin and glucagon levels are normal, high, or low in T2DM. Hyperglycemia is a compensatory mechanism that occurs in an attempt to overcome the islet secretory defect and insulin resistance. These

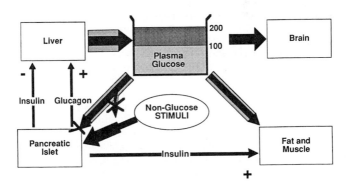

FIG. 4-11 Model for the development of hyperglycemia in T2DM: hyperglycemia's effect to compensate for the islet lesion of T2DM. The increased glucose concentration that develops as a result of the deficient insulin and enhanced glucagon secretion in turn modulates the islet by increasing insulin secretion and decreasing glucagon release. As a result of these secretory changes, glucose production and use return toward normal but still remain elevated. *(Reproduced with permission from Porte D Jr: β-Cells in type II diabetes mellitus. Diabetes 1991; 40:166–180.)*

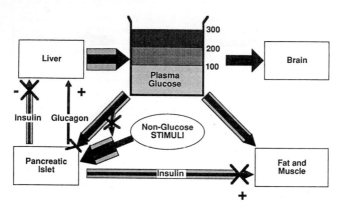

FIG. 4-12 Model for the development of hyperglycemia in T2DM: interaction of islet dysfunction and insulin resistance on basal glucose regulation in T2DM. The impairment of insulin action in the liver and peripheral tissues requires a marked additional increase in glucose concentration in order that, in the presence of an impaired islet, a new steady state is achieved. Under these conditions, the islet may secrete "normal" or even "supranormal" quantities of insulin while secreting "normal" or "subnormal" amounts of glucagon, despite the presence of islet α- and β-cell dysfunction. The net result is a further increase in glucose production by the liver and glucose use by the peripheral tissues, until the renal threshold is exceeded when decompensation occurs. *(Reproduced with permission from Porte D Jr: β-Cells in type II diabetes mellitus.* Diabetes *1991; 40:166–180.)*

adaptive changes result in a reregulated steady-state hyperglycemia, but complete compensation can occur only at glucose levels below the renal threshold. Once the renal threshold is exceeded, glycosuria occurs and the plasma glucose level cannot rise sufficiently to compensate. This then results in the development of a state of absolute insulin deficiency and glucagon excess with metabolic decompensation.

TREATMENT OF T2DM

At the present time, three major therapeutic modalities are used in T2DM subjects: diet, oral agents, and insulin administration. These interventions produce alterations in hepatic glucose production, insulin sensitivity, and/or insulin secretion, and, as is apparent from the previously described closed feedback loop, any change in these variables should result in a reregulated steady state at a new level of glycemia.

Body Weight Reduction

Body-weight reduction comprises two distinct phases: a period of weight loss, during which time there is a marked reduction in caloric intake, and later weight maintenance at a new lower level, during which time more calories are being consumed, albeit less than the quantity taken before the initiation of weight loss. Although a decline in glucose level occurs during both these phases, the mechanism by which glucose decreases is different. For an individual to lose weight, a reduction in caloric intake is required so that a state of negative caloric balance exists. Although it has been claimed that caloric restriction is associated with an improvement in insulin sensitivity, this does not occur during the period of weight loss. In fact, during periods of caloric restriction, the opposite is true and a state of insulin resistance exists. Therefore, the initial decrease in fasting plasma glucose level that is observed during caloric restriction results from a reduction in hepatic glycogen stores, a resultant decline in glycogenolysis, and a reduced rate of hepatic glucose release. As glycogen stores become progressively depleted, the liver tends to produce glucose predominantly by gluconeogenesis, with the rate of hepatic glucose production remaining low as the body attempts to maintain energy stores and minimize the protein losses. Thus, after a period of fasting as short as 3 days, T2DM patients will demonstrate a significant reduction in their glucose levels, but these levels, while approximating those of healthy unfasted individuals, never reach the same low levels as normal subjects during a similar fast. However, as soon as caloric intake increases and weight maintenance is achieved, hepatic glycogen is replaced, glucose release is enhanced, and glucose levels tend to rise once again. Thus, although improved insulin action is not a factor in the lowering of glucose levels during a hypocaloric diet, once body adiposity is reduced and weight is stabilized at a new lower level, any lowering of plasma glucose is now due to improved hepatic and peripheral insulin sensitivity. The magnitude of the glucose level reduction will in large part be related to this enhancement of insulin sensitivity and is of most benefit to those individuals with poor islet function and marked hyperglycemia, in whom even a small improvement in insulin action can lower glucose concentrations (see Fig.4-8). This improvement in peripheral insulin sensitivity is due largely to an enhancement of postreceptor insulin action, with some increase in insulin receptor number also occurring. Some of these improvements in hepatic and peripheral glucose metabolism may also be the result of an increase in insulin secretion. Enhanced insulin release has been demonstrated in some T2DM patients given an oral glucose challenge following marked weight reduction and in a group of severely hyperglycemic subjects in whom the plasma gluscose level was halved to approximately 150 mg/dL (8.3 mmol/L) following 4–12 weeks of severe caloric restriction, with a resultant increase of about 65% in the insulin response to tolbutamide.

Oral Agents

A number of oral agents are now available that are capable of stimulating insulin secretion, but this effect is dependent on the presence of a responsive endocrine pancreas. Long-term administration of sulfonylureas is associated with reduced plasma glucose levels, but basal and stimulated insulin levels are often unchanged. The similarity of insulin levels is misleading, however, because when glucose is administered to match the glucose levels to those present prior to initiation of treatment, marked increases in basal and stimulated insulin levels are apparent. Sulfonylureas are also capable of reducing basal hepatic glucose production, and this reduction has been maintained for periods of up to 18 months. The magnitude of this reduction appears to be a major determinant of the hypoglycemic effectiveness of those compounds. This decrease in the rate of hepatic glucose output is related to the change in basal insulin secretion. This relation between hepatic glucose release and basal insulin secretion, coupled with a marked enhancement of β-cell responsiveness to glucose, clearly links a major proportion of the decline in hepatic glucose production and the resultant glucose-lowering effect of these agents to the improved insulin secretion. In many patients, sulfonylurea administration does appear to improve peripheral insulin sensitivity measured *in vivo*, resulting in an increase in insulin binding and an enhancement of postreceptor function, the latter being the predominant improvement. This ability of sulfonylureas to improve peripheral insulin sensitivity also appears to be a function of their capacity to enhance insulin secretion. This is suggested by the fact that type 1 diabetic subjects who are insulin resistant and incapable of enhancing their insulin output do not exhibit an improvement of insulin sensitivity when treated with these agents. Therefore, we conclude that sulfonylureas result in a steady-state reregulation of plasma glucose at a lower level largely due to their direct and persistent effects on the pancreatic islet. More recently, two new classes of β-cell secretagogues have been developed and introduced into clinical practice. The first is the meglitinide repaglinide and the second the D-phenylalanine analogue nateglinide. As with the sulfonylureas, they appear to bind to the ATP-sensitive potassium channel. However, due to the fact that these newer classes of agents have a more rapid onset of action and a shorter half-life, they tend to have a greater effect on early postprandial insulin release compared to basal insulin, thereby being more efficient in suppressing meal-related hepatic glucose production.

The biguanide metformin's predominant effect appears to be on the liver, where it primarily reduces basal hepatic glucose production. This effect may be mediated by an enhancement of the action of insulin in the liver or perhaps by an alteration in substrate flow, primarily from the splanchnic bed. It has been postulated that a portion of the effect of this agent to improve glucose metabolism may also be mediated by an improvement in peripheral insulin sensitivity. However, this effect does not appear to be consistent, although it is clear that the major beneficial effect is mediated through the liver.

The PPAR-γ-agonist thiazolidinediones work primarily by enhancing insulin sensitivity in the peripheral insulin-sensitive tissues, namely, the muscle and adipose tissue, while having a much smaller effect on the liver. The effect of these agents to enhance insulin action may be mediated in part by a change in free fatty acid flux from the adipocyte. In small studies it has been demonstated that administration of these compounds has been associated with a redistribution of central adiposity from the intra-abdominal to the subcutaneous fat depot. It also appears that these agents may improve β-cell function as the relationship between insulin sensitivity and insulin levels is improved and disproportionate proinsulinemia is partially ameliorated. The recent suggestion that PPAR-γ-receptors may be present on islets raises the interesting possibility that this effect of thiazolidinediones to improve β-cell function may be in part occurring via a direct effect on the β cell.

Insulin Therapy

Exogenous insulin serves to substitute for the β-cell defect of type 2 diabetes, and if sufficient insulin is administered, normoglycemia can be achieved. This reduction in glucose level is a function of glucose's ability to suppress hepatic glucose release and enhance peripheral glucose uptake. Intensive insulin treatment is capable of reducing hepatic glucose production so that after only

3 weeks of therapy, the rate of glucose output approximates that observed in normal subjects. Improved glucose utilization has been demonstrated for periods of up to 2 weeks following withdrawal of insulin therapy. Although this lower plasma glucose level may provide less stimulation to the β cell, resulting in reduced basal insulin secretion, it has been demonstrated that intensive glucose control may improve the insulin response to glucose and nonglucose stimuli. Although the first-phase insulin response to glucose, long considered a marker of T2DM, does not improve, the second-phase insulin response is enhanced. However, once intensive insulin therapy is discontinued, the subsequent rise in glucose levels is again associated with steadily deteriorating β-cell function. Even though β-cell function may improve when glucose levels decline as a result of insulin treatment, islet stimulation is reduced, and usually the endocrine pancreas is suppressed. Therefore, the total insulin requirement will need to be met by exogenous insulin administration and the treatment program for an insulin-treated T2DM subject becomes very similar to the regimen of a T1DM patient. Thus the treatment program will require well-spaced meals and multiple doses of insulin. When complete replacement is required, the amount of insulin needed is not related to the degree of hyperglycemia, but rather relates to body adiposity and other factors that determine insulin resistance. Thus in lean individuals a daily dose of 40–50 U may suffice, while in grossly obese subjects the requirement may be as great as 150–200 U/d.

GENETIC FACTORS IN T2DM

Two groups of patients with T2DM and identified gene defects associated with β-cell dysfunction have been described. The first group consists of the maternally inherited mitochondrial syndromes with diabetes, originally described as being associated with various neuromuscular disorders but recently found to present at any age independent of or prior to neuromuscular disease with glucose intolerance or T2DM. The second group also presents as glucose intolerance or T2DM but with a different inheritance pattern and has been called maturity-onset diabetes of the young (MODY), since it was first described clinically on the basis of its presentation under age 40 with a dominant inheritance pattern. Similarly, molecular studies have found relatively rare defects associated with insulin resistance that are associated with T2DM and mutations in the insulin receptor gene.

These known β-cell and insulin receptor genetic syndromes and the high concordance of T2DM in identical twins compared with fraternal twins have stimulated a major search for predisposing gene defects in the more typical older-onset T2DM patients, but the likely heterogeneity of defects has made their identification difficult, and despite many promising associations between gene polymorphisms and hyperglycemia, there is no genetic defect that has yet been unequivocally identified to cause the disease more commonly affecting T2DM patients.

Genetic Studies of T2DM

A variety of metabolic studies have demonstrated impaired β–cell function and insulin resistance in family members of subjects with T2DM and in identical twins of T2DM patients with normal glucose tolerance who have a high likelihood of developing the syndrome. It is still not clear in any individual patient which of these two disorders began first, how much is related to the environment and to genetic dysfunction, and how much of the full-blown syndrome is secondary to the hyperglycemia. There is evidence that both β-cell function and insulin sensitivity are familial traits in certain populations, and abnormalities of insulin secretion and sensitivity have been reported to predate the onset of glucose intolerance. Nevertheless, there remain many uncertainties regarding progression from normal to IGT and eventually to fasting hyperglycemia and clinical T2DM.

GENETIC STUDIES OF RARER FORMS OF ALTERED GLUCOSE METABOLISM ASSOCIATED WITH DEFECTS IN β-CELL GENES

Mitochondrial Diabetes

Maternally Inherited Diabetes and Deafness (MIDD)

Van den Ouweland and colleagues described a pedigree with maternally inherited diabetes and deafness with a heteroplasmic A → G mutation at 3243 in the tRNA$^{leu(UUR)}$ portion of the mitochondrial genome. The clinical diagnosis of diabetes usually, but not always, precedes the detection of clinical sensorineural hearing loss, but the age of presentation in a rather large Japanese population has varied from 11 to 68 years. The identical clinical picture has also been associated with several other, less common mitochondrial mutations. The most common of these, the tRNA$^{(lys)}$ 8296 A → G mutation, was estimated to explain 1% of Japanese T2DM cases, and the 3271 T → C tRNA$^{leu(UUR)}$ mutation to explain one-tenth as many.

Other Mitochondrial Syndromes

Several neuromuscular mitochondrial syndromes are also associated with diabetes. The most common one is the MELAS syndrome, and it is usually also associated with the same 3243 A → G mutation that can lead to MIDD. Other mutations have been reported to be associated with this syndrome. Another rare mitochondrial syndrome is the Kearns-Sayre syndrome (KS syndrome), which is usually associated with a mitochondrial DNA deletion on muscle biopsy and is frequently associated with diabetes mellitus.

Maturity-Onset Diabetes of the Young (MODY)

In the great majority of patients with T2DM, a diagnosis is made in middle age. However, a subclass of this syndrome includes families in whom diabetes can be recognized in children, adolescents, and young adults, and has been clinically termed MODY. Autosomal dominant inheritance has been established in these families, and at least five specific mutations have been described. However, this does not include all of the families in whom a dominant genetic pattern with young family members has been observed, so more mutations are yet to be discovered. At times these patients have been confused with T1DM patients because they are young, some variants lead to relatively severe forms of insulin-deficient diabetes, and by and large most patients with this syndrome are lean. However, most of the patients are ketosis-resistant, and even those who need insulin for control of glycemia are not usually ketosis-prone. Since the more common variety of T2DM can also be present among these families, it is possible for an individual family member to have both syndromes, and therefore relative insulin deficiency may become more evident in the presence of insulin resistance and obesity and during periods of stress, infection, or trauma. The true prevalence of MODY is unknown, but estimates have varied from 2–5% of patients with T2DM to 10–20% of families with T2DM in multiple family members. Studies of the insulin secretory defects early in the course of the disease can distinguish among the various genetic mutations.

MODY-1 (Hepatocyte Nuclear Factor-4α [HNF-4α])

In 1996, mutations in the HNF-4α gene were shown to be the cause of MODY-1. In this early large pedigree, there was a C → T substitution in codon 130 leading to a threonine-to-isoleucine substitution and a C → T substitution in codon 268 which generated a nonsense mutation CAG (Gln) → TAG (AM) (Q268X). Both the isoleucine 130 and the amber mutation at codon 268 were present on the same allele.

Approximately one-third of affected individuals will require insulin treatment, and patients with this form of diabetes may have microvascular complications.

MODY-2 (Glucokinase)

The first candidate gene linkage in the MODY syndrome was described from a study of 16 French families with three or more generations of IGT or T2DM, and was found to link to glucokinase on chromosomal 7. By 2002, a large number of families with more than 130 different mutations involving all 10 exons in populations distributed worldwide of all racial types (Caucasian, black, and Asian) were described. Twenty-eight of these mutations alter the protein sequence by changing one amino acid; six transform the sequence at the site of RNA splicing of an intron-exon or exon-intron junction, resulting in the expression of an abnormal species of messenger RNA; and eight are responsible for the synthesis of a truncated protein by creating a premature termination codon by point mutation or deletion. Most are only present in single families.

Glucokinase is present at critical levels in the liver and the pancreas, playing an important role in hepatic glucose storage by phosphorylation of glucose after absorption and in the endocrine pancreas by coupling the first step of glucose metabolism to insulin secretion through the generation of ATP and regulation of β-cell potassium conductance and calcium levels. The degree of hyperglycemia is relatively mild, although it can be usually detected in children. Long-term complications are relatively unusual with this form of diabetes. Hyperglycemia remains stable for many years whether treated or not and progresses very little, in contrast to typical T2DM. Treatment with oral agents is usually satisfactory, and can lead to reasonable control for many years.

MODY-3 (Hepatocyte Nuclear Factor-1α [HNF-1α])

In 1996, Yamagata and associates showed that MODY-3 was the gene encoding HNF-1α, a transcription factor involved in tissue-specific regulation of liver genes which is also expressed in pancreatic islets and other tissues. More than 120 different mutations have now been identified in MODY-3 families of various populations. This type of MODY resembles late-onset T2DM in its natural history, with patients progressing rapidly from IGT to overt hyperglycemia with severe deterioration of insulin secretion. Thus, it is frequently treated with oral hypoglycemic agents for a time, but often later requires insulin therapy. Complications, such as proliferative retinopathy, have been observed frequently and at rates comparable to those seen in late-onset T2DM patients. However, there is a low prevalence of obesity, dyslipidemia, and arterial hypertension, and unlike MODY-2, clinical disease with hyperglycemia usually develops after puberty.

MODY-4 (Insulin Promoter Factor-1 [IPF-1])

One family with a mutation in the IPF-1 gene has been reported. IPF-1, also known as IDX-1, STF-1, and PDX-1, regulates both early pancreatic development and the expression of key endocrine β-cell-specific genes, most notably insulin.

MODY-5 (Hepatocyte Nuclear Factor-1β [HNF-1β])

One family with a nonsense mutation in codon 177 (R177X) of HNF-1β was found, which in this family was associated with diabetes. This MODY family has diabetes in three generations with renal dysfunction consisting of renal cysts, proteinuria, and/or elevated creatinine. Additional families screened for MODY or renal disease in the UK uncovered additional mutations segregating with hyperglycemia and renal disease.

More MODY mutants presumably will be found, as only 60% of clinically dominant families with T2DM had an identified defect in 2002.

GENETIC STUDIES OF RARER FORMS OF ALTERED GLUCOSE METABOLISM ASSOCIATED WITH MUTATIONS IN THE INSULIN RECEPTOR GENE

Two clinical features commonly observed in these syndromes are acanthosis nigricans and hyperandrogenism (in female patients). However, each set of defects is defined by the presence or absence of specific clinical features.

Leprechaunism

Leprechaunism is the most severe clinical syndrome caused by mutations in the insulin receptor gene. These patients have glucose intolerance despite having extremely high insulin levels (100-fold above the normal range). In addition to insulin resistance, patients have multiple abnormalities (e.g., intrauterine growth restriction and fasting hypoglycemia) and usually die within the first year of life. These patients have inactivating mutations in both alleles of the insulin receptor gene. In inbred pedigrees, the patients are usually homozygous for a single mutant allele. In the absence of consanguinity, they are usually compound heterozygotes with two different mutant alleles.

Type A Insulin Resistance

Most patients with type A insulin resistance are heterozygous for a single mutant allele, most often a mutation in the tyrosine kinase domain of the receptor. It is defined by the triad of insulin resistance, acanthosis nigricans, and hyperandrogenism in the absence of obesity or lipoatrophy. Although some heterozygotes have abnormal glucose tolerance, most do not exhibit fasting hyperglycemia. These patients are usually less insulin-resistant than patients with two mutant alleles. Patients with type A insulin resistance with two mutant alleles of the insulin receptor gene can develop overt diabetes with fasting hyperglycemia during childhood or adolescence, but usually do not have fasting hyperglycemia as infants.

Rabson-Mendenhall Syndrome

The Rabson-Mendenhall syndrome is defined by the presence of several clinical features, including extreme insulin resistance, acanthosis nigricans, short stature due to growth retardation, abnormalities of teeth and nails, and pineal hyperplasia. As in leprechaunism, patients with the Rabson-Mendenhall syndrome have inactivating mutations in both alleles of the insulin receptor gene.

Specific Mutations

Many different mutations have been identified in the insulin receptor. However, there are insufficient data to provide a reliable estimate of the prevalence of mutations in the insulin receptor gene, although currently available data are consistent with estimates that about 1% of patients with T2DM may have such mutations in their receptor gene. In several instances the same mutation has been identified in two apparently unrelated patients. However, most of the published mutations have only been identified in single kindreds.

ACKNOWLEDGMENTS

This work was supported in part by National Institutes of Health grants DK-02654, DK-17047, DK-50703, and RR-37, and grants from the Medical Research Service of the Department of Veterans Affairs, and the American Diabetes Association.

ADDITIONAL READINGS

Bell GI, Polonsky KS: Diabetes mellitus and genetically programmed defects in beta-cell function. *Nature* 414:778–791, 2001.

DeFronzo RA: Pathogenesis of type 2 diabetes mellitus. *Med Clin North Am* 88: 787–835, 2004.

Kahn SE: The relative contributions of insulin resistance and beta-cell dysfunctin to the pathophysiology of type 2 diabetes. *Diabetologia* 46:3–19, 2003.

Kahn SE, Porte D, Jr: β-cell dysfunction in type 2 diabetes: pathophysiologic and genetic bases. In *The Metabolic and Molecular Bases of Inherited Disease*, 8th ed. Scriver CR, Beaudet AL, Sly WS, et al, eds. New York, McGraw-Hill, 2001, pp. 1401–1431.

Porte D, Jr: β-cells in type II diabetes mellitus. *Diabetes* 40:166–180, 1991.

For a more detailed discussion of this topic and a bibliography, please see Porte *et al: Ellenberg & Rifkin's Diabetes Mellitus,* 6th ed., Chapter 21.

5	Insulin Resistance
	C. Hamish Courtney Yolanta T. Kruszynska
	Jerrold M. Olefsky

GENERAL CONSIDERATIONS

Insulin resistance is the state in which a given concentration of insulin produces a less than normal biologic response. Because one of insulin's major effects is to promote overall glucose metabolism, abnormalities of this action of insulin may lead to a number of important clinical and pathophysiologic states. As insulin travels from the β-cell through the circulation to the target tissue, events at any one of these loci can influence the ultimate action of the hormone. Insulin resistance may be categorized according to known etiologic mechanisms (Table 5-1).

The Metabolic Syndrome

The term *syndrome X* or *metabolic syndrome* has been coined to refer to subjects exhibiting features of insulin resistance, and this has been further defined by the National Cholesterol Education Program (NCEP) (Table 5-2). Besides insulin resistance, associated manifestations of the syndrome include hypertension, dyslipidemia, and obesity. This cluster of abnormalities reflects the diverse actions of insulin, so that resistance to the action of insulin is not simply limited to disruption of glucose homeostasis.

Clinically, the association of many features of metabolic syndrome with premature atherosclerosis and subsequent cardiovascular disease means that it represents a condition of considerable importance.

CAUSES OF INSULIN RESISTANCE

Abnormal β-Cell Secretory Product

Rare patients have been described who secrete a structurally abnormal insulin molecule, either because of an insulin gene mutation or as a result of defective processing of proinsulin within the β-cell. These syndromes do not, however, represent insulin-resistant states in the most common usage of the term.

Circulating Insulin Antagonists

Circulating antagonists may be hormonal or nonhormonal.

Hormonal Antagonists

All of the known counterregulatory hormones, such as cortisol, growth hormone, glucagon, and catecholamines, antagonize insulin action. Well-known clinical syndromes exist (Cushing's disease, acromegaly, glucagonoma, pheochromocytoma) in which elevated levels of these hormones can induce insulin resistance. However, in the usual case of obesity or type 2 diabetes

TABLE 5-1 Causes of Insulin Resistance

Abnormal β-cell secretory product
   Abnormal insulin molecule
   Incomplete conversion of proinsulin to insulin
Circulating insulin antagonists
   Elevated levels of counterregulatory hormones,
      (e.g., growth hormone, cortisol, glucagon, or catecholamines)
   Elevated free fatty acid levels
   Anti-insulin antibodies
   Anti-insulin receptor antibodies
   Resistin
   Cytokines (TNF-α, interleukin-6)
Target tissue defects
   Insulin receptor defects
   Postreceptor defects

mellitus (T2DM), excessive levels of counterregulatory hormones are not an important contributory factor to insulin resistance.

Nonhormonal Antagonists

Free fatty acids: Fasting plasma free fatty acid (FFA) levels tend to be higher in T2DM patients than in lean subjects, and postprandial FFA suppression is impaired. Randle and coworkers, many years ago, showed that FFAs could compete with glucose for oxidative metabolism in skeletal muscle. They hypothesized that elevated circulating levels of FFAs could impair peripheral glucose use.

Glucose clamp studies have confirmed that elevated FFAs can induce mild insulin resistance. The mechanism may differ from that originally proposed. According to Randle's hypothesis, FFA oversupply inhibits glucose oxidation and glycolysis, leading to increased intracellular glucose-6-phosphate levels, in turn inhibiting phosphorylation of incoming glucose and hence glucose uptake. It now appears that additional direct effects of FFAs on insulin-stimulated glucose transport occur, as muscle glucose-6-phosphate levels have been shown to decrease, rather than increase, in response to FFA elevation. Recent data implicate activation of the inflammatory cascade by lipid oversupply with subsequent impairment of the insulin-signaling pathway.

TABLE 5-2 NCEP Definition of Metabolic Syndrome

At least three of the following:
- Fasting plasma glucose ≥ 110 mg/dL
- Abdominal obesity [waist girth > 102 cm (men), > 88 cm (women)]
- Serum triglycerides ≥ 150 mg/dL
- Serum HDL cholesterol < 40 mg/dL (men), < 50 mg/dL (women)
- Blood pressure ≥ 130/85 mmHg (or medication)

Source: Expert Panel on Detection, Evaluation, and Treatment of High Blood Cholesterol in Adults: *JAMA* 2001; 285:2486–2497.
Executive Summary of the Third Report of the National Cholesterol Education Program (NCEP) Expert Panel on Detection, Evaluation, and Treatment of High Blood Cholesterol in Adults (Adult Treatment Panel III).

Increased circulating FFA levels might be expected to promote the accumulation of triglycerides within muscle, if their supply exceeds immediate energy needs. Intramyocellular triglyceride (IMTG) levels in nondiabetic subjects correlate inversely with whole-body insulin sensitivity. IMTG levels are increased in T2DM patients and in the insulin-resistant offspring of T2DM patients relative to insulin-sensitive offspring matched for age, body mass index, physical activity, and percentage of body fat. It is likely that increased IMTG content may not in itself impair insulin signaling, but act as a marker of increased intracellular long-chain fatty acyl coenzyme A and lipid intermediates which may mediate the deleterious effects of lipid accumulation.

FFAs also play an important role in the regulation of hepatic glucose output and may contribute to hepatic insulin resistance in obesity and T2DM (see later).

Anti-insulin antibodies: In the past, patients receiving animal-derived insulin developed anti-insulin antibodies, which although not usually resulting in clinically significant insulin resistance, did alter insulin pharmacokinetics. In recent years, highly purified insulins have been available and these have proven to be much less antigenic, making development of anti-insulin antibodies much less of a problem than in the past.

Anti-insulin receptor antibodies: In rare cases, circulating endogenous immunoglobulins directed against the insulin receptor have been described.

Other Insulin Antagonists

Resistin is a circulating protein secreted by adipocytes, which in some studies in mice has been shown to antagonize the metabolic actions of insulin. Its role in humans is as yet unclear.

Tumor necrosis factor-α (TNF-α) produced by adipocytes is elevated in several genetic forms of obesity in animal models. *In vitro* studies have shown that TNF-α can impair insulin signaling. Furthermore, neutralization of TNF-α by *in vivo* administration of soluble TNF-α receptors or TNF-α antibodies ameliorates insulin resistance in obese animals. However, in obese T2DM patients, intravenous infusion of an antibody neutralizing TNF-α had no effect on insulin resistance. Thus, if excess adipocyte production of TNF-α contributes to insulin resistance, it may not do so in an endocrine fashion, but in a local autocrine or paracrine fashion.

Interleukin-6 (IL-6) has been suggested to play a role in the insulin resistance. It is produced by adipocytes and immune cells, with circulating levels increased in obesity and T2DM. IL-6 appears to stimulate the hypothalamic-pituitary-adrenal axis and also elevate FFA levels, both of which may contribute to insulin resistance.

IN VIVO INSULIN RESISTANCE IN T2DM AND OBESITY

Type 2 Diabetes Mellitus

Pathogenesis and Etiology

Metabolic abnormalities in T2DM: Figure 5-1 summarizes the physiologic abnormalities commonly seen. Target tissues are insulin-resistant, a feature characteristic of this disease and seen in essentially all population groups studied.

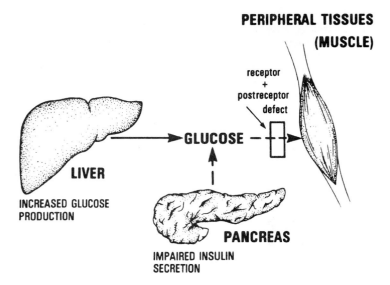

FIG. 5-1   Summary of the metabolic abnormalities in T2DM that contribute to hyperglycemia. Increased hepatic glucose production, impaired insulin secretion, and insulin resistance due to receptor and postreceptor defects all combine to generate the hyperglycemic state. NIDDM, non-insulin-dependent diabetes mellitus.

- Liver: Increased basal hepatic glucose production is characteristic of essentially all T2DM patients with fasting hyperglycemia.
- Skeletal muscle: Depicted as the prototypical peripheral insulin target tissue, as in the *in vivo* insulin-stimulated state, 70–80% of all glucose uptake is into skeletal muscle.
- Pancreas: Abnormal islet cell function with decreased insulin and increased glucagon secretion plays a central role in the eventual development of hyperglycemia in T2DM.

Progressive development of T2DM: Figure 5-1 represents a pathophysiological view at a single time point after overt diabetes has developed. This does not provide insight into the natural history of the disease, which is progressive (Fig. 5-2).

Whether the insulin resistance of T2DM is a primary or a secondary phenomenon has been the subject of intense study. To answer this question, various prediabetic populations have been examined prospectively. In these studies, insulin resistance has been shown in the prediabetic state, many years before T2DM supervenes. At this stage, insulin secretion in response to intravenous glucose is often increased. Thus, while acquired factors, such as obesity and a sedentary lifestyle, may be additive, insulin resistance is likely to be a primary inherited component of the disease in most patients.

In the presence of primary insulin resistance, if β-cell function is normal, hyperinsulinemia ensues with maintenance of relatively normal glucose homeostasis. Impaired glucose tolerance (IGT) eventually develops in a subpopulation of individuals with compensated insulin resistance. Those with IGT also typically have fasting and postprandial hyperinsulinemia, but this is insufficient to compensate fully for insulin resistance. This may be because of a more profound degree of insulin resistance or because of a limited ability to augment insulin secretion rates. Although some subjects with IGT may revert to normal glucose tolerance, many will progress to overt T2DM. The latter display a marked decline in insulin secretion. This may result from pre-programmed genetic abnormalities and/or from acquired insults such as those caused by the chronic effects of mild hyperglycemia or elevated FFA levels, commonly referred to as glucotoxicity and lipotoxicity, respectively.

The contribution of genetics to the etiology of T2DM is well accepted, and is demonstrated by studies showing a greater than 90% concordance rate for T2DM in identical twins. In addition, the incidence of T2DM is much higher in individuals with first-degree relatives with the disease. Given this strong

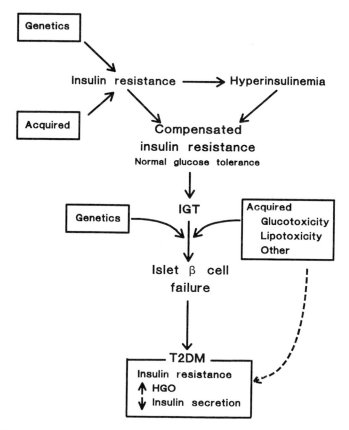

FIG. 5-2 Proposed etiology for the development of T2DM. HGO, hepatic glucose output.

genetic component to T2DM and that insulin resistance predates the development of T2DM in most populations, it is likely that insulin resistance is an inherited initial lesion in most patients.

Many reports also indicate that the magnitude of the insulin resistance is greater in T2DM than it is in the prediabetic IGT state. It appears that once T2DM develops, some factor creates a secondary component of insulin resistance that is additive to that which existed in the prediabetic state. There is strong evidence that hyperglycemia *per se* plays such a role. Other factors associated with the poorly controlled hyperglycemic state, such as elevated FFA levels, may also play a role. Obesity is associated with insulin resistance. Since most T2DM patients are overweight, obesity-induced insulin resistance is thought to be a contributing factor in these patients. However, obesity does not account for all of the insulin resistance in T2DM, since the insulin resistance exceeds that caused by obesity alone, and nonobese T2DM patients are also insulin-resistant.

In vivo Assessment of Insulin Sensitivity

Several methods are used to measure insulin sensitivity.

Homeostasis model assessment of insulin resistance (HOMA-IR): The HOMA model uses fasting blood glucose and insulin to give a measure of insulin sensitivity, calculated using the formula

$$\text{HOMA-IR} = [\text{insulin (mU/L)} \times \text{glucose (mmol/L)}]/22.5$$

It is based on the principle that for a given level of glucose, insulin levels reflect overall insulin sensitivity. This test is easy to perform, making it useful for epidemiologic research, although other methods are preferred for a more precise assessment of insulin sensitivity.

Steady-state plasma glucose and insulin: In this method, insulin and glucose are infused at fixed rates with endogenous insulin secretion inhibited by either a combination of epinephrine and propranolol or by somatostatin. The resulting steady-state plasma glucose level reflects the action of the concomitantly infused insulin, with higher steady-state plasma glucose levels associated with a greater degree of insulin resistance.

Minimal model method: In this method, the plasma glucose and insulin levels following an intravenous glucose bolus are fed into a mathematical model to generate an index of insulin sensitivity (*Si*). The test has been adapted for T2DM patients with poor insulin secretion by giving an injection of insulin 20 minutess after the glucose bolus.

Glucose clamp: In this method, insulin is infused at a constant rate to maintain a steady-state plasma insulin level with the blood glucose "clamped" at a predetermined level by the titration of a variable-rate glucose infusion. If a radioactive or stable isotope of glucose is also infused, the rate of hepatic glucose output during the clamp can be quantified. At steady state, the isotopically measured rate of glucose disposal provides an excellent quantitative assessment of the biologic effect of a particular steady-state insulin concentration.

The steady-state glucose disposal data from such a glucose clamp study, in which a submaximally stimulating insulin infusion rate was used in normal, nonobese IGT subjects and obese and nonobese T2DM subjects, are shown in Fig. 5-3. Steady-state insulin levels were comparable in all subjects, but the glu-

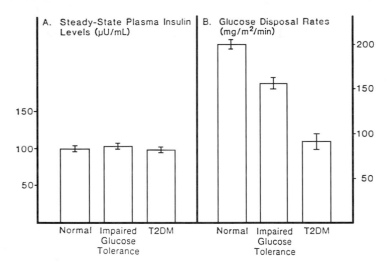

FIG. 5-3 Mean steady-state glucose disposal rates *(right panel)* and plasma insulin levels *(left panel)* for control subjects, nonobese subjects with impaired glucose tolerance, and T2DM patients during euglycemic glucose clamp studies performed at an insulin infusion rate of 40 mU/m²/min. Results are plotted as means ± SEM.

cose disposal rates were decreased in the patient groups and the magnitude of this defect was greatest in the patients with the worst carbohydrate intolerance.

Hepatic Glucose Metabolism

The liver is capable of extracting glucose from the blood delivered via the portal vein and hepatic artery as well as releasing glucose derived from glycogenolysis or gluconeogenesis into the hepatic vein.

Hepatic glucose production: *Normal physiology:* After an overnight fast, about 90% of the glucose released into the circulation comes from the liver. After carbohydrate ingestion, hepatic glucose output (HGO) falls to limit the rise in plasma glucose levels. As intestinal delivery of glucose wanes, basal HGO rates must be restored to prevent hypoglycemia. These changes in HGO are largely mediated by changes in insulin and other hormones that oppose insulin's effects on hepatic gluconeogenesis and glycogenolysis through alterations in the supply of gluconeogenic substrate, and by the effects of the hepatic plasma glucose concentration per se.

Abnormal physiology in T2DM: The basal rate of HGO is increased in diabetes, but is normal in subjects with IGT (Fig. 5-4A). Figure 5-4B illustrates the close correlation between HGO and the fasting plasma glucose level, indicating that it is the rate of glucose production by the liver that appears to be most directly responsible for the level of fasting hyperglycemia in T2DM. Gluconeogenesis is increased in T2DM, and this appears to be the cause of the increased basal HGO. The exact mechanism remains unclear, but is likely to include factors such as elevated glucagon levels.

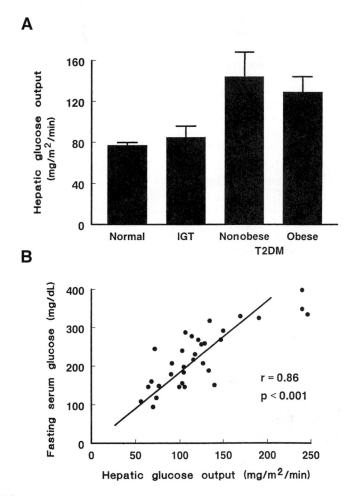

FIG. 5-4 *A.* Rates of hepatic glucose output (HGO) in the basal state (7–9 AM following an overnight fast) in normal subjects, subjects with IGT, and obese or nonobese subjects with type 2 diabetes. HGO is normal in patients with IGT but is increased in type 2 diabetes. *B.* Relationship between hepatic glucose production rates and fasting serum glucose levels in type 2 diabetic subjects.

HGO can be completely suppressed by high physiologic or supraphysiologic insulin levels in T2DM, but there is resistance to suppression of HGO at lower insulin concentrations. This hepatic insulin resistance also likely contributes to exaggerated glucose production rates in diabetes. Because insulin's effect on HGO may in part be indirect, mediated by suppression of adipose tissue lipolysis and plasma FFA levels, it is possible that the defect of HGO suppression in T2DM may be secondary to impaired suppression of plasma FFA levels by insulin. However, resistance to insulin's direct effects on HGO is also present in T2DM. Additionally, increased flux of the gluconeogenic precursors lactate, alanine, and glycerol from peripheral tissues to the liver may participate in the maintenance of the increased rate of HGO in T2DM.

Hepatic glucose uptake: Insulin does not directly stimulate postprandial hepatic glucose uptake, although it does play a permissive role. An increase in the portal venous glucose concentration and the establishment of a positive portal-arterial glucose gradient is a prerequisite for net hepatic glucose uptake and under these circumstances insulin will augment the net uptake of glucose by the liver. In T2DM, uptake of glucose by the liver after glucose ingestion (newly absorbed and recirculating) is impaired.

Insulin-Mediated versus Non-Insulin-Mediated Glucose Uptake and the Pathogenesis of Hyperglycemia

In the *basal state,* insulin-mediated glucose uptake (IMGU) accounts for only ~30% of overall glucose disposal, whereas non-insulin-mediated glucose disposal (NIMGU), primarily in the central nervous system (CNS), compromises ~70%. Therefore, impairment in IMGU due to insulin resistance will have little effect on overall basal glucose disposal or fasting glucose levels. As the fasting glucose level reflects the balance between HGO and glucose disposal, it follows that if reduced glucose disposal does not contribute to significant fasting hyperglycemia, then increased glucose entry into the circulation (increased HGO) is the factor most directly responsible for fasting hyperglycemia.

In the *postprandial state,* IMGU normally predominates, and the limited ability of T2DM subjects to increase this allows marked postprandial glucose excursions. Postprandial hyperglycemia is thus primarily due to glucose underutilization by peripheral tissues (primarily muscle).

Obesity

Whole-Body Insulin Sensitivity

Insulin resistance has been widely described in obesity. Using the glucose clamp, a rightward shift in the dose-response curve for insulin-stimulated glucose disposal is a consistent finding. The response to a maximally stimulating insulin concentration, however, is quite variable, covering the whole spectrum from normal to markedly reduced, indicating a continuum of insulin resistance in human obesity.

Hepatic Insulin Sensitivity

Basal HGO is similar in control and obese subjects; however, the dose-response curve for HGO suppression by insulin is shifted to the right in obese subjects, indicating hepatic insulin resistance.

Fat Distribution

Obese subjects with a predominantly central (abdominal/truncal) distribution of body fat are more insulin-resistant than those with peripheral obesity, independent of the overall degree of obesity. In contrast, total body fat content rather than its distribution is an important determinant of insulin sensitivity in mildly obese subjects. Once an individual exceeds 25–30% of ideal body weight (body mass index, BMI > 27 kg/m^2), further increases in total fat mass

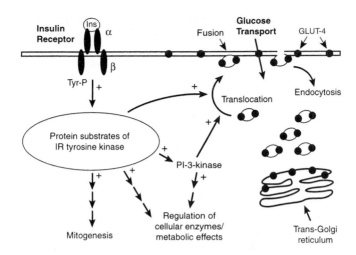

FIG. 5-5 Model of insulin action. Abnormalities can occur at the prereceptor phase, involving biosynthesis and secretion of abnormal β-cell products; at the receptor binding phase, involving decreased insulin binding to receptors due to decreased receptor number or affinity; or at the postreceptor phase, involving any defect in the insulin action cascade distal to the initial binding event.

have relatively little additional influence on insulin sensitivity, and the distribution of fat assumes greater importance as a determinant of insulin action.

The adverse metabolic effects associated with central obesity are likely due to the accumulation of visceral fat, which is lipolytically more active. FFAs released directly into the portal vein may impair hepatocyte insulin receptor function, resulting in decreased hepatic insulin clearance. High circulating insulin levels may desensitize target tissues at several steps in the insulin action sequence, causing a decrease in maximal insulin responsiveness.

CELLULAR DEFECTS IN INSULIN ACTION

Normal Insulin Action

Insulin first binds to the insulin receptor, resulting in autophosphorylation of the β-subunit of the receptor. Receptor activation then initiates a signaling cascade by which the insulin signal is transmitted downstream to the various insulin-regulated enzymes, transporters, and insulin-responsive genes, culminating in the metabolic and growth effects of insulin (Fig. 5-5). Clearly, because insulin action involves a cascade of events, abnormalities anywhere along this sequence can lead to insulin resistance.

Insulin Binding

Insulin binding to a variety of tissues is decreased in T2DM patients relative to controls, and in most studies of obese subjects. Since the first step in insulin action involves binding to the receptor, it is apparent that a decrease in cellular insulin receptors could lead to insulin resistance. However, this potential relationship is not as clear as it might seem, because insulin target tissues possess "spare" receptors.

Insulin-Stimulated Autophosphorylation

Insulin receptor autophosphorylation is decreased in insulin-responsive tissues in subjects with T2DM. This, however, appears to be the result of glucotoxicity rather than a primary inherited cause of insulin resistance, as it is not observed in nondiabetic obese subjects with insulin resistance and has also been shown to normalize in obese T2DM patients who lose weight and thus improve their hyperglycemia.

Postreceptor/Glucose Transport Defects

Postreceptor defects may account for a large portion of insulin resistance in T2DM.

In vitro Glucose Transport

Experiments performed in adipocytes demonstrate a rightward shift in the glucose transport dose-response curve with no change in the maximal response in patients with IGT. This is explained largely by decreased number of insulin receptors. In T2DM patients, however, decreased glucose transport is seen at all insulin concentrations (Fig. 5-6).This *in vitro* reduction in glucose transport correlates with the decrease in glucose rates seen *in vivo.*

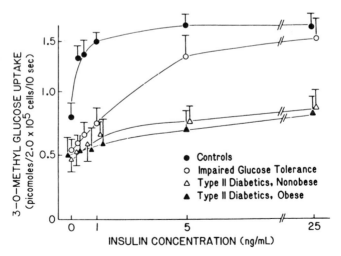

FIG. 5-6   Dose–response curve for insulin's ability to stimulate glucose transport (3-O-methylglucose uptake) in isolated adipocytes prepared from normal subjects, subjects with IGT, and obese or nonobese subjects with type 2 diabetes. The functional form of these dose–response curves is quite comparable to the shape of the dose–response curves for *in vivo* insulin-stimulated overall glucose disposal.

Glucose Transport as Rate-Limiting Step

Available evidence indicates that glucose transport is rate-determining for glucose metabolism *in vivo*. For example, if intracellular metabolism, rather that transport, were limiting the rate of glucose disposal, one would expect an accumulation of free intracellular glucose. However, a buildup of intracellular glucose is not observed in skeletal muscle. Additionally, apparent K_m values reported for *in vivo* glucose disposal are similar to measured values of muscle glucose transport *in vitro*, consistent with the view that transport governs glucose disposal. Cline and colleagues, using nuclear magnetic resonance spectroscopy, measured skeletal muscle glucose-6-phosphate levels and intracellular free glucose levels during a hyperinsulinemic, hyperglycemic clamp and produced evidence that glucose transport is also the rate-controlling step in insulin-stimulated muscle glucose uptake in T2DM. They found that the reduction in muscle glucose uptake and glycogen synthesis was associated with lower steady-state muscle glucose-6-phosphate levels and very low intracellular free glucose levels, implying a defect at the level of glucose transport.

GLUT-4

One potential cellular locus for a postreceptor defect is the glucose transport effector system. Insulin stimulates glucose transport primarily by causing translocation of GLUT-4 proteins from an intracellular vesicular compartment to the plasma membrane, thus initiating glucose uptake. Insulin stimulation of glucose transport in target tissues thus reflects GLUT-4 activity.

GLUT-4 mRNA and protein levels, however, are normal in skeletal muscle in T2DM. An explanation for decreased glucose transport activity may therefore be either decreased insulin-mediated translocation of GLUT-4 to the plasma membrane or decreased GLUT-4 intrinsic activity or both. Evidence points to impaired insulin-stimulated translocation of GLUT-4 in skeletal muscle of obese and T2DM patients, associated with a marked impairment of insulin-stimulated muscle glucose transport.

Decreased GLUT-4 intrinsic activity resulting from alteration in the GLUT-4 primary structure due to genetic variation in the GLUT-4 gene appears less likely. One mutation in the GLUT-4 gene has been identified, but larger-scale molecular scanning studies have found this mutation in only a small percentage of T2DM, and it also exists in low frequency in nondiabetic subjects. Since no other mutations in the GLUT-4 gene have been identified, it appears that abnormalities in the GLUT-4 gene are rare.

Translocation of GLUT-4 involves a complex system, and an expanding list of proteins involved in GLUT-4 vesicle trafficking, regulation of membrane fusion, and endocytotic events are being identified. Thus it is possible that decreased GLUT-4 translocation could be due to altered expression or a functional defect of one or more of the GLUT-4 vesicle-trafficking proteins. An impairment of insulin signaling downstream of the receptor is also a likely cause of decreased insulin-stimulated GLUT-4 translocation.

Insulin Receptor Substrate-1 (IRS-1)

After insulin receptor autophosphorylation, a number of endogenous protein substrates, including IRS-1, are phosphorylated on tyrosine residues by the insulin receptor kinase. The ability of insulin to stimulate IRS-1 phosphorylation is decreased in both adipocytes and skeletal muscle in T2DM. The IRS-1 protein content of adipose tissue is reduced in T2DM patients, potentially contributing to decreased IRS-1 phosphorylation observed in adipocytes. However, this is not a factor in muscle, as skeletal muscle IRS-1 levels are similar in T2DM patients and in lean and obese normal subjects. The insulin dose-response curves for stimulation of tyrosine phosphorylation of IRS-1 and of the insulin receptor β-subunit are almost identical in adipocytes from control, obese, and T2DM subjects, with the ability of phosphorylated insulin receptors to phosphorylate IRS-1 also normal. It is therefore likely that the reduction in IRS-1 phosphorylation in T2DM is essentially secondary to the insulin receptor kinase defect.

PI-3-Kinase

PI-3-kinase is essential for insulin's effects on GLUT-4 translocation and glycogen synthase activation. It is activated by the binding of its regulatory subunit to tyrosine phosphorylated IRS-1 and IRS-2. Several studies have shown that association of the p85 regulatory subunit of PI-3-kinase with IRS-1 and IRS-2 in response to insulin is impaired in muscle of T2DM patients, with a corresponding defect of PI-3-kinase activation. Some but not all studies have found that activation of muscle PI-3-kinase by insulin is also impaired in obese nondiabetic subjects.

Glycogen Synthesis

Glycogen synthase, the rate-controlling enzyme of glycogen synthesis, is another potential locus for insulin resistance in T2DM. Diminished activation of glycogen synthase, decreased insulin-stimulated muscle glycogen deposition, impaired insulin-mediated glucose disposal, and defective nonoxidative glucose disposal all exist in T2DM.

The reduction in glycogen synthase activity in T2DM persists even when glucose uptake rates are normalized, indicating that the effect of insulin on glycogen synthesis is separate from its effect on glucose transport and that the defect in glycogen synthase activity is not due simply to a decline in glucose flux into the cell.

FUNCTIONAL ASPECTS OF INSULIN RESISTANCE

Kinetic Defects in Insulin Action

While most quantitative assessments of *in vivo* insulin resistance report impaired insulin action based on steady-state measurements, kinetic defects in insulin action in obesity have also been demonstrated. In these reports the rate of activation of insulin's effect to stimulate glucose disposal is decreased and the rate of deactivation of insulin's effect is increased. The abnormal kinetics of insulin action in obesity may therefore represent a functionally important manifestation of the insulin resistance. It is possible that in obesity, insulin's effects never reach steady state in the physiologic situation, and that the decrease in the rate of onset of insulin action and rapid deactivation serve to minimize the biologic effects of the insulin secreted after oral glucose or meals, in spite the fact that obese subjects are hyperinsulinemic.

Functional studies of adipocyte glucose transport in obesity indicate that the kinetic abnormalities observed *in vivo* are most likely related to cellular defects in insulin action. Decreased *in vitro* rate of activation of glucose transport correlates with slower rates of activation of glucose disposal *in vivo*.

Glucose Mass Action in Obesity

If hyperinsulinemia does not fully compensate for insulin resistance in obesity, what does? From analysis of the oral glucose tolerance profile, it is clear that obese subjects, while not glucose-intolerant, are somewhat hyperglycemic compared to controls. It is this hyperglycemia, by virtue of mass action, that helps compensate for the insulin resistance to restore glucose disposal to normal during meals. Thus, following a meal, insulin-resistant obese subjects achieve relatively normal rates of glucose disposal (and therefore can accommodate an incoming glucose load), but only at the expense of hyperinsulinemia and relative hyperglycemia.

Kinetic Defects in Insulin Action in T2DM

Comparable kinetic defects in insulin action have been reported in T2DM, with the magnitude of the kinetic defects generally greater in T2DM than in simple obesity. The presence of insulin resistance in T2DM, coupled with the impaired insulin secretion, explains the marked postprandial hyperglycemia in this condition. With this formulation it is evident that hyperglycemia is the major factor driving glucose disposal in T2DM, allowing these subjects eventually to dispose of an incoming meal or glucose load. These concepts may have implications regarding the treatment of T2DM patients. For example, intensive insulin therapy relies on algorithms for insulin delivery that were developed largely in T1DM patients. Clearly, such algorithms do not account for the kinetic defects present in insulin-resistant T2DM subjects. As such, these kinetic defects provide part of the explanation of why such large daily doses of insulin are needed to achieve ideal control in T2DM patients.

TYPE 1 DIABETES MELLITUS

When applied to the patient with type 1 diabetes mellitus (T1DM), the term *insulin resistance* is more difficult to evaluate. It usually denotes a patient who requires a large amount of insulin (> 100 U/day) to maintain an acceptable level of glycemia. These patients are unusual and may have high titers of anti-insulin antibodies. It is unclear whether the typical T1DM patient responds normally to insulin. One reason for this is that insulin sensitivity in T1DM is at least partially dependent on the degree of diabetic control. Subjects in poor control are more hyperglycemic, with hyperglycemia *per se* able to induce a secondary state of insulin resistance as already discussed. In addition to hyperglycemia, increases in $[H^+]$, counterregulatory hormones, and FFA concentrations can all impair insulin action. It has been reported, however, that insulin sensitivity may be normal if a T1DM patient is maintained in euglycemic control.

In conclusion, it is clear that insulin resistance is both a prominent feature of obesity and also fundamental to the pathogenesis of T2DM. It is thus an important cause of morbidity and mortality in the Western and developed world. A more complete understanding of the pathophysiological mechanisms underlying insulin resistance is of great interest, as it will potentially allow development of appropriate therapies.

ADDITIONAL READINGS

Bergman RN, Finegood DT, Ader M: Assessment of insulin sensitivity *in vivo. Endocr Rev* 1985;1:45.

Cline GW, Petersen KF, Krssak M, et al: Impaired glucose transport as a cause of decreased insulin-stimulated muscle glycogen synthesis in type 2 diabetes. *N Engl J Med* 1999;341:240.

Kolterman OG, Gray RE, Griffin J, et al: Receptor and post-receptor defects contribute to the insulin resistance in non-insulin dependent diabetes mellitus. *J Clin Invest* 1981;68:957.

Reaven GM: Role of insulin resistance in human disease. *Diabetes* 1988;37:1595.

Roden M, Price TB, Perseghin G, et al: Mechanism of free fatty acid induced insulin resistance in humans. *J Clin Invest* 1996;97:2859.

For a more detailed discussion of this topic and a bibliography, please see Porte *et al: Ellenberg & Rifkin's Diabetes Mellitus,* 6th ed., Chapter 22.

6 Obesity and Diabetes Mellitus

P. Antonio Tataranni   Clifton Bogardus

OBESITY

Obesity is clinically defined as a body mass index (BMI) of ≥ 30 kg/m^2, which represents an overweight of approximately 30 lb (14 kg) for any given height. In the United States during the late 1990s, one of two adults was overweight and one of four was obese. More alarming, the prevalence of obesity has been rising drastically among children, and The World Health Organization (WHO) has identified obesity as one of the major emerging chronic disease throughout the world. Obesity increases the risk for a number of noncommunicable diseases (i.e., type 2 diabetes, hypertension, dyslipidemias) and reduces life expectancy.

The exact cause of obesity in the majority of humans is not known. It is widely accepted, however, that it results from a chronic imbalance between energy intake and energy expenditure. While the impact of the environment is thought to be substantial, several studies indicate that obesity is a heritable disease caused primarily by the effect of multiple susceptibility genes on eating behavior. Thus, a greater knowledge of its pathophysiology will ultimately come from the current efforts to isolate all these genes. Genome-wide scans continue to be completed in human populations, and major loci linked to obesity have been found on several chromosomes. These areas of the genome are currently under intense investigation, as they may lead to the cloning of obesity-susceptibility genes.

OBESITY AND TYPE 2 DIABETES

Individuals with type 2 diabetes are so commonly obese that Sims coined the term *diabesity* to describe this increasingly occurring syndrome. In addition to being more obese than nondiabetic people, people with type 2 diabetes have a more central distribution of body fat.

Longitudinal data in a group of Pima Indians followed for 5 years indicated that the transition from normal glucose tolerance to impaired glucose tolerance (IGT) was associated with increased body weight, a reduction in peripheral insulin action (i.e., increased insulin resistance), and a decline in insulin secretion, but no changes in hepatic glucose production. Further increase in body weight and further decrease in both insulin action and insulin secretion, but an increase in hepatic glucose production, characterized progression from IGT to diabetes. By comparison, in Pimas who maintained normal glucose tolerance over the same period of time, a twofold smaller increase in body weight was associated with a decline in insulin action and an increase in insulin secretion. These data are consistent with a pathogenic role of obesity and its duration in the progressive impairment of insulin action and insulin secretion that lead to diabetes.

Despite the overwhelming evidence showing the association between obesity and diabetes, however, obesity is neither necessary nor sufficient for the development of type 2 diabetes. In all populations, a vast majority of the individuals who are obese do not have type 2 diabetes. Although more than 50% of individuals in the United States are overweight, less than 10% of the population has type 2 diabetes. Finally, the association between obesity and diabetes is strongly influenced by the parental history of diabetes, suggesting that obesity may be more harmful in subjects who are genetically predisposed to develop type 2 diabetes. The reason(s) why obesity causes diabetes in some but not all people will remain unclear until the exact molecular mechanisms linking excessive adiposity to insulin resistance and insulin secretory dysfunction are unequivocally identified.

OBESITY AND INSULIN RESISTANCE

Weight gain causes hypeinsulinemia and insulin resistance in animals and humans, but a convincing explanation of how excess adiposity and/or its metabolic/hormonal consequences impair glucose uptake and storage in the muscle remains elusive.

Possible Role of Free Fatty Acids (FFAs)

An acute elevation of plasma FFA levels, such as can be generated by intralipid/heparin infusion, results in insulin resistance. Conversely, acute and chronic lowering of FFA improve insulin sensitivity. Obesity is characterized by chronically elevated circulating FFA, and there is increasing evidence for an accumulation of fat within muscle and liver in insulin-resistance states in humans. However, the causal links between tissue accumulation of fat and reduced glucose uptake remain to be established. Proposed mechanisms include inhibition of carbohydrate metabolism at the mitochondrial level by competition for the same oxidative pathways, direct or indirect inhibition of the activity of glycogen synthase, and activation of the glucosamine pathway.

Possible Role of Adipocyte-Secreted Hormones

The adipose tissue is now recognized as an endocrine and paracrine organ from which a number of signals emanate. These include leptin, tumor necrosis factor-α (TNF-α), interleukin-6 (IL-6), complement C3 and its cleavage product acylation-stimulating protein (ASP), enzymes of lipoprotein metabolism (LPL, CETP, and Apo-E), growth factors (TGF-β and IGF-1), angiotensinogen, PAI-1, adiponectin, resistin, and a number of other adipokines. It has been proposed that the role of adipose tissue in regulating glucose metabolism may in part be explained through a direct or indirect action of these adipocyte-secreted hormones to impair insulin signaling in peripheral tissues (Fig. 6-1).

Possible Role of Obesity-Induced Changes in Skeletal Muscle

Obesity is associated with an increase in both fat mass and fat-free mass. With an increase in fat-free mass, muscle cells are hypertrophied and capillaries in the muscle are more widely spaced. It has been proposed that the association between obesity-induced changes in skeletal muscle morphology and insulin action may be explained by the fact that lower capillary density results in reduced access of insulin to muscle of obese subjects.

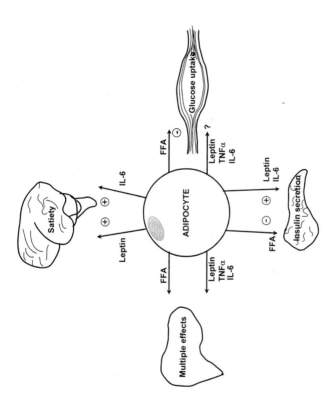

FIG. 6-1 The adipose tissue is an endocrine organ. Several signals (endocrine, paracrine, and metabolic) emanate from adipocytes and are believed to affect several organs, including brain, liver, skeletal muscle, and pancreas. The strength and direction of the effect of the signals emanating from the adipose tissue to other organs is the object of intense investigation.

OBESITY AND INSULIN SECRETION

The links between obesity and the abnormal insulin secretory function that precipitates an insulin-resistant state into frank diabetes are even less well understood. Recent studies indicate that chronic exposure of the pancreas to excessive FFA concentration may have deleterious effects on the β-cell. An attractive hypothesis is that tissue accumulation of fat plays a role in inducing both muscle insulin resistance and pancreatic glucose hyporesponsiveness. Possible mechanisms underlying the "lipotoxic" effects of FFA on the β-cell include overproduction of NO, interleukin-1β, and/or ceramide, the latter possibly being responsible for the accelerated apoptosis observed in fat-laden β-cells.

Parasympathetic, sympathetic, and sensory nerves richly innervate the pancreatic islets. Experimental evidence indicates that insulin secretion is stimulated by parasympathetic nerves and their neurotransmitters and inhibited by sympathetic nerves and their neurotransmitters. Because defects of both parasympathetic and sympathetic nervous system activity have been reported in obese individuals, it is possible that they contribute to an abnormal adaptation of the pancreatic islets to insulin resistance, with possible implications for the development of type 2 diabetes.

OBESITY AND TYPE 2 DIABETES IN CHILDREN AND ADOLESCENTS

One of the most troubling aspects of the current epidemic of obesity is the increasing prevalence of type 2 diabetes among children and adolescents. Until recently, immune-mediated type 1 diabetes was the only type of diabetes considered prevalent among children. Recent reports indicate that 8–45% of children with newly diagnosed diabetes have non-immune-mediated diabetes. While percentages vary greatly depending on ethnicity and sampling strategies, the majority of these children have type 2 diabetes. Obesity is the hallmark of type 2 diabetes in youth, with up to 85% of affected children being either overweight or obese at diagnosis.

Studies in Pima Indians indicate that offspring of women who had diabetes during pregnancy are especially at risk of early-onset obesity and type 2 diabetes. Exposure to the diabetic intrauterine environment was responsible for about 40% of the type 2 diabetes in 5–19-year-old children between 1987 and 1994, approximately twice the attributable risk found between 1967 and 1976. It remains to be seen whether gestational diabetes is a factor in the alarming rise of obesity and type 2 diabetes in youth nationally.

SUMMARY AND CONCLUSION

Obesity is a chronic disease, which is quickly reaching epidemic proportions, and which increases the risk for other noncommunicable diseases, thus reducing life expectancy. Obesity is heritable and results from a chronic imbalance between energy intake and energy expenditure. However, its exact etiology is unknown.

While obesity is often observed in association with type 2 diabetes, it is neither necessary nor sufficient to cause type 2 diabetes. In some predisposed individuals/populations, obesity substantially increases the risk of developing type 2 diabetes by worsening insulin resistance, and possibly by causing insulin-secretory dysfunction. The mechanistic links between obesity and type 2 diabetes have yet to be unequivocally identified. Thus, further research is needed to understand the etiology of obesity and how obesity precipitates the development of type 2 diabetes in predisposed individuals.

ADDITIONAL READINGS

Dabelea D, Knowler WC, Pettitt DJ. Effect of diabetes in pregnancy on offspring: Follow up research in the Pima Indians. *J Matern Fetal Med* 2000;9:83–88.

Rajala MW, Scherer PE. Mini Review: The adipocyte—at the cross-road of energy homeostasis, inflammation, and atherosclerosis. *Endocrinology* 2003;144:3765–73.

Snyder EE, Walts B, Perusse L, et al. The human obesity gene map: The 2003 update. *Obes Res* 2004;12:369–439.

Weyer C, Bogardus C, Mott DM, Pratley RE. The natural history of insulin secretory dysfunction and insulin resistance in the pathogenen's of type 2 diabetes mellitus. *J Clin Invest* 1999;104:787–794.

WHO Report: Obesity, preventing and managing the global epidemic. WHO/NUT/NCD/98.1. WHO, 1997.

For a more detailed discussion of this topic and a bibliography, please see Porte *et al: Ellenberg & Rifkin's Diabetes Mellitus,* 6th ed., Chapter 23.

7 | Nutritional Management of the Person with Diabetes

Abhimanyu Garg   Joyce P. Barnett

INTRODUCTION

Revised nutritional guidelines of the American Diabetes Association (ADA) address the importance of optimizing plasma glucose and lipid levels. Specific goals of therapy are outlined in Table 7-1. Greater emphasis on nutritional management, or medical nutrition therapy, should help achieve improved metabolic control and prevent diabetic complications. To achieve the goals of therapy, a coordinated team approach is optimal. The ADA guidelines emphasize the importance of individualizing the nutrition prescription to meet specific goals of therapy and allow more variation in the proportion of energy from carbohydrate and fat with limited variation in protein intake. The focus for carbohydrate intake has shifted away from restriction of sugar, or sucrose, to the total amount of carbohydrate in the diet. The purpose of this chapter is to review the scientific rationale for nutritional management and provide practical insight on its implementation.

NUTRITION RECOMMENDATIONS

Energy Needs

The most important decision for diabetes nutritional management involves deciding the appropriate total energy intake for each patient (Tables 7-2 and 7-3). Total energy intake should be appropriately increased for growing children and for pregnant and lactating women. Obesity is a major predisposing factor for type 2 diabetes mellitus (T2DM); thus reduced energy intake is an important aspect of management for these patients as well as for prevention of T2DM in susceptible individuals. Even those patients with T2DM who do not appear obese may have truncal obesity and could benefit from small amounts of weight loss (5–10%). After achieving reasonable body weight, energy intake can be adjusted to maintain body weight and prevent future weight gain. Instances where patients with T2DM may need increased energy intake beyond maintenance levels include:

- Following significant weight loss at diagnosis
- During chronic infections
- During severe illness
- During a postoperative period

Such patients lose not only body fat but also lean body mass that needs to be recovered.

While controversy exists over whether high-carbohydrate or high-fat diets are more effective in causing weight loss, studies show that if reduction of total energy intake is similar, the diets cause equal weight loss. Emphasis should be on reduction of total energy intake, not necessarily the source of the energy.

TABLE 7-1 Goals of Medical Nutrition Therapy (MNT)

Attain and maintain optimal metabolic outcomes to prevent or reduce risks of
complications of diabetes:
    Normal or near-normal blood glucose levels
    Optimal lipid and lipoprotein profile
    Optimal blood pressure control
Prevent and treat chronic complications of diabetes by modification of:
    Nutrient intake
    Lifestyle
Improve health through optimal food choices and physical activity
Address individual nutritional needs with consideration for personal, cultural,
and lifestyle preferences

Source: Modified with permission from the American Diabetes Association.
American Diabetes Association Position Statement: Evidence-based nutrition
principles and recommendations for the treatment and prevention of diabetes
and related complications. *Diabetes Care* 2002; 25:202.

Two approaches may be considered for reduction of total energy intake:
very-low-calorie diet (VLCD, less than 800 kcal or 3350 kJ per day) or low-
calorie diet (LCD, 800–1500 kcal or 3350–6300 kJ per day). The VLCD
promotes rapid weight loss and leads to reduction of blood pressure, serum
glucose, and lipid levels. To safely implement the VLCD, close medical supervision is required. Care must be taken to include adequate protein (1.0–1.4 g/kg
of ideal body weight per day), vitamins, electrolytes, and fluids.

TABLE 7-2 Estimating Energy Requirements for Adults

Basal energy requirements:	20–25 kcal/kg (80–100 kJ/kg) of desirable body weight
*Additional energy required for activity level:	
Sedentary	30% of estimated basal energy requirements
Moderate	50% of estimated basal energy requirements
Strenuous	100% of estimated basal energy requirements
*Adjustments:	
During pregnancy:	
Second trimester	Add 340 kcal (1420 kJ) per day
Third trimester	Add 450 kcal (1880 kJ) per day
During lactation:	
First 6 months postpartum	Add 330 kcal (1380 kJ) per day
6–12 months postpartum	Add 400 kcal (1675 kJ) per day
For weight gain (0.5 kg/wk)	Add 500 kcal (2100 kJ) per day
For weight loss (0.5 kg/wk)	Subtract 500 kcal (2100 kJ) per day

*Adjustments are approximate: weight changes should be monitored and energy
intake adjusted as indicated to achieve desired body weight.

TABLE 7-3 Estimating Energy Requirements for Children and Adolescents

Age in Years	kcal(kJ)/kg body weight*
≤3	~100 (~400)
4–6	90 (375)
7–10	70 (300)
11–14 Males	55 (230)
15–18 Males	45 (190)
11–14 Females	47 (200)
15–18 Females	40 (165)

*Adjustments may be needed for activity level and other individual variations.
Source: Recommended Dietary Allowances, 10th ed., Washington, D.C.: National Academy Press, 1989.

Significant side effects of VLCDs include:

- Rapid loss of lean body mass
- Electrolyte imbalances
- Cardiac arrhythmias
- Gout
- Gallstones

VLCDs should not be used for mildly overweight individuals (BMI less than 30 kg/m^2) and may lead to binge eating in some people. Even though short-term weight loss is greater on VLCDs, the long-term results are no more effective than a LCD.

The preferred approach to energy reduction is the LCD, a reduction of 500–1000 kcal (2100–4200 kJ) per day to produce weight loss of 0.5–1 kg per week. However, reduction in energy intake of 1000 kcal (4200 kJ) per day can be difficult to sustain. An alternative approach which is more likely to be successful is to reduce energy intake gradually by 250–500 kcal (1050–2100 kJ) per day for weight loss of 0.25–0.5 kg per week.

Some people claim that high-protein, low-carbohydrate diets promote weight loss. They suggest that carbohydrate intake, by stimulating insulin secretion, contributes to insulin resistance, obesity, and other metabolic abnormalities, and therefore should be reduced. Clinical investigation of these diets is limited, especially in the long-term. A recent meta-analysis suggested that weight loss on such diets is the simple result of decreased calorie intake. Proposed benefits of low-carbohydrate diets are initial rapid weight loss and short-term improvements in serum lipids. The low-carbohydrate level in some of these diets leads to ketosis. Studies of ketogenic diets for seizure control have reported adverse effects:

- Increased risk of kidney stones
- Constipation
- Dehydration
- Hyperlipidemia
- Osteoporosis
- Optic neuropathy

Very-low-energy ketogenic diets have also been reported to have a negative effect on cognitive function. High protein intake can contribute to kidney stone formation, gout, and possible reduction in bone density. Most individuals can tolerate unlimited intake of high-protein, high-fat foods for only a short time, leading to decreased total energy intake, weight loss, and decreased vitamin and mineral intake.

Macronutrients

Dietary Carbohydrates

Equal energy intake from complex carbohydrates such as starch or naturally occurring simple carbohydrates causes similar increases in plasma glucose concentrations. Fructose causes a reduced glycemic excursion compared to sucrose. However, sucrose or fructose intake may increase serum triglyceride and cholesterol concentrations compared to starch intake. Therefore, while small amounts of simple sugars can be ingested as part of a healthful diet, overall intake should be limited. Other nutritive sweeteners have no advantage or disadvantage over sucrose.

The amount of carbohydrate in the meal plan should be based on individualized assessment of current intake. Patients using oral antidiabetes agents or insulin need to maintain day-to-day and meal-to-meal consistency in the amount of carbohydrate consumed. Experts advise dietary carbohydrate-based calculation of insulin dose in patients with type 1 diabetes mellitus (T1DM). Complex carbohydrates should be encouraged, and simple sugars from fruits and vegetables are preferred because of their higher nutrient content.

The glycemic index is a ranking of foods based on their immediate effect on blood glucose levels. Molecular and physical characteristics of the carbohydrates, as well as processing and cooking methods, can affect glycemic index. Long-term intake of low-glycemic-index foods has not shown consistent improvement in plasma glucose or lipid concentrations in patients with diabetes. Many experts, including the ADA, do not recommend the use of the glycemic index in diabetes management.

Sweeteners

Sugar alcohols (or polyols), such as sorbitol, provide 2–3 kcal (8–12 kJ) per gram. Polyols can cause significant gastrointestinal distress if consumed in large amounts (20–50 g). Children may be particularly susceptible to developing diarrhea from ingestion of as little as 0.5 g/kg body weight of polyols. Polyols should not be used to treat hypoglycemia.

Non-nutritive sweeteners include saccharin, aspartame, acesulfame K, and sucralose. Because saccharin crosses the placenta, its use in pregnancy is questionable, even though it has been removed from the list of potential carcinogens. Although aspartame contains 4 kcal (17 kJ) per gram, it is consumed in very small amounts, contributing negligible energy. People with phenylketonuria should not use aspartame because its metabolism yields phenylalanine.

Protein

Adequate protein intake is necessary for maintenance of lean body mass in adults. Children have higher protein needs to support growth. Protein needs are also increased during pregnancy and lactation, catabolic illness or stress, and vigorous exercise.

The recommended dietary allowance (RDA) for protein is approximately 10% of total energy (0.8 g/kg). Protein intake of 10–20% of total energy is recommended by the ADA, and will meet protein needs in most situations.

Reduction of protein intake to 0.8 g/kg is recommended for patients with chronic renal insufficiency and diabetic renal disease; however, protein malnutrition can occur on lower intakes. Although studies suggest that decreasing protein intake in people with T1DM may delay the progression of nephropathy, it is not clear whether all patients with diabetes would benefit from reduced protein intake.

Because meat, poultry, and dairy products can be major sources of saturated fat and cholesterol, lower-fat selections should be made. Consumption of 500 mL (2 cups) of milk and 140–170 g of meat, poultry, or fish per day can provide approximately 20% of total daily energy requirements from protein in adults. In contrast, lacto-ovo vegetarian diets provide about 12–14% of energy from protein, while vegan diets provide about 10–12%.

Dietary Fats

Dietary fats, or triglycerides, usually contain a mixture of saturated, monounsaturated, and polyunsaturated fatty acids. Mono- and polyunsaturated fatty acids can be further classified as *cis* or *trans,* depending on the geometric configuration of the double bonds. Two-thirds of the saturated fat in the diet comes from animal fats, emphasizing the need to limit the quantity of animal products eaten. The importance of reducing cholesterol-raising fatty acids (mainly the saturated and *trans* variety) in the diet to achieve maximum reduction in serum low-density lipoprotein (LDL)-cholesterol is well established. The goals for serum lipid and glycemic control can provide the basis for individualizing the amount of dietary fat.

Saturated fatty acids: Saturated fatty acids should be limited to <10% and preferably <7% of total energy. Saturated fatty acids with the most potent serum cholesterol-raising effect are

- Lauric (C12:0, twelve carbon chain length with no double bond)
- Myristic (C14:0)
- Palmitic (C16:0).

Stearic acid (C18:0) does not raise serum LDL-cholesterol. Studies have found that the medium-chain fatty acids caprylic (C8:0) and capric (C10:0) acids, as well as the long-chain fatty acid behenic acid (C22:0), also raise serum LDL-cholesterol.

Polyunsaturated fatty acids: Polyunsaturated fatty acids should also be limited to ≤ 10% of total energy intake. Polyunsaturated fatty acids are classified as *n*-6 (ω-6) or *n*-3 (ω-3). Consumption of approximately 2–3% of total energy intake from *n*-6 polyunsaturated fatty acids supplies adequate amounts of essential fatty acids. The essential fatty acids are linoleic acid (*n*-6, C18:2) and α-linolenic acid (*n*-3, C18:3). Arachidonic and γ-linolenic acids can be formed from linoleic acid. Linoleic acid, when substituted for saturated fatty acids, lowers LDL-cholesterol, but does not decrease triglycerides. Large intakes of linoleic acid, however, may decrease high-density lipoprotein (HDL)-cholesterol concentrations.

Omega-3 (*n*-3) fatty acids, eicosapentaenoic acid (C20:5) and docosahexaenoic acid (C22:6), reduce serum triglycerides by competitively inhibiting hepatic triglyceride synthesis. Exacerbation of hyperglycemia can occur with high fish oil intake (up to 5–10 g of *n*-3 fatty acids per day) but not with small doses. Reduced risk of acute myocardial infarction as a result of decreased platelet aggregation could be a potential benefit of *n*-3 fatty acids. The increase in consumption of *n*-3 fatty acids should be via increased intake of fish, except for patients with hypertriglyceridemia, who require concentrated fish oil supplements.

cis-*Monounsaturated fatty acids:* When oleic acid (C18:1) is substituted for saturated fatty acids, serum LDL-cholesterol declines just as much as with polyunsaturated fatty acids. A recent meta-analysis of several randomized crossover studies in patients with T2DM reported that, in comparison to high-carbohydrate diets, diets high in *cis*-monounsaturated fatty acids reduce plasma triglycerides and very-low-density-lipoprotein (VLDL)-cholesterol levels by 19% and 22%, respectively. The diets high in *cis*-monounsaturated fatty acids also raised HDL-cholesterol by 4% and led to a modest increase in apolipoprotein A-I concentrations. No significant changes were reported in plasma total cholesterol, LDL-cholesterol, and apolipoprotein B. The high-*cis*-monounsaturated-fat diet also lowered plasma glucose and insulin concentrations.

Diets rich in *cis*-monounsaturated fatty acids may increase compliance for some individuals used to a high-fat diet. Good sources of *cis*-monounsaturated fatty acids are shown in Table 7-4.

trans-*Fatty acids:* Dietary *trans*-fatty acids should be limited as much as possible because they raise serum LDL-cholesterol and may lower serum HDL-cholesterol. Intake of *trans*-fatty acids is associated with higher risk of coronary heart disease. In Western countries, approximately 0.5–3% of the total daily energy is provided by *trans*-fatty acids.

TABLE 7.4 Various *cis*-Monounsaturated Fatty Acids and Their Dietary Sources

Common name	Notation	Sources
Lauroleic	C12:1	Fish oils
Myristoleic	C14:1	Fish oils, beef fat
Palmitoleic	C16:1	Fish oils, beef and pork fat
Oleic	C18:1	Oils: olive; canola; ground nut (peanuts); high-oleic safflower and sunflower; avocado; aceituno; shea nut; rice bran; sesame; *Jessenia bataua;* tea seed
		Nuts: filberts, almonds, pistachios, pecans, macadamias, cashews
		Others: mowrah butter; illipe butter; fat of cattle*, pigs, goats, chicken, and sheep; cocoa butter*
Gadoleic	C20:1	Fish oils (such as herring, sardines, mackerel), jojoba oil
Erucic	C22:1	Mustard seed oil, rape seed oil, nasturtium seed oil

*Although a source of oleic acid, these fats should be used sparingly because they are high in cholesterol-raising saturated fatty acids.
Source: Padley FB, Gunstone FD, Harwood JL, in Gunstone FD, Harwood JL, Padley FB (eds): *The Lipid Handbook,* 2nd ed, London: Chapman & Hall, 1994, pp 49–183.

TABLE 7-5 Fiber Content of Some Foods Particularly Rich in Soluble Fiber

Food item	Amount	Weight (g)	Total dietary fiber (g)	Insoluble fiber (g)	Soluble fiber (g)
Legumes and Grains (cooked)					
Lima beans	1 cup	188	13.2	6.2	7.0
Navy beans	1 cup	182	11.7	7.3	4.4
Oatmeal	1 cup	234	4.0	2.1	1.9
Fruits (fresh)					
Grapefruit	½ medium	128	1.4	0.2	1.2
Mango	1 medium	207	3.7	2.2	1.5
Nectarine	1 medium	136	2.2	1.4	0.8
Orange	1 medium	131	3.1	1.3	1.8
Papaya	1 cup	140	2.5	1.3	1.2
Peach	1 medium	98	2.0	1.2	0.8
Plums	1 cup	165	2.5	1.2	1.3
Vegetables (cooked)					
Artichokes	1 cup	168	9.1	2.5	6.6
Broccoli	1 cup	184	5.5	2.8	2.7
Cabbage	1 cup	150	3.4	1.9	1.5
Kohlrabi	1 cup	165	1.8	0.6	1.2
Okra	1 cup	184	5.1	3.1	2.0
Squash, winter	1 cup	240	6.7	2.9	3.8
Sweet potatoes	1 cup	255	7.6	4.8	2.8
Zucchini	1 cup	180	2.5	1.4	1.1

Source: Schakel SF, Pettit, Himes JH. Dietary fiber values for common foods. In Spiller GA (ed.): *CRC Handbook of Dietary Fiber in Human Nutrition*, 3rd ed. Boca Raton, Florida: CRC Press Inc., 2001:615.

Fat Replacers

Reduced-fat products are of questionable benefit in weight management because many have only slightly reduced energy compared to the regular product. Lower satiety value of reduced-fat products may lead to increased overall intake. Carbohydrate-based fat replacers can contribute a significant amount of carbohydrate to the diet.

Dietary Cholesterol

Both serum LDL- and total cholesterol are increased by high intake of dietary cholesterol. Limiting dietary cholesterol to 300 mg or less per day is recommended, and reduction to 200 mg or less may be necessary to achieve maximal lowering of LDL-cholesterol. Animal products are the sole sources of dietary cholesterol, and their intake should be limited.

Dietary Fiber

The recommended intake for total dietary fiber, including both soluble and insoluble types, for patients with diabetes is 20–35 g/day, a significant increase over the usual intake of 16–22 g/day. Soluble, but not insoluble fibers, reduce serum cholesterol by approximately 5%. A recent study in subjects with T2DM, using a diet high in total fiber (50 g total, 25 g soluble) reported improvement in glycemic control and lipid levels. Selection of fruits, vegetables, and grains with a high proportion of soluble to insoluble fiber is recommended (Table 7-5).

Alcohol

The ADA recommends the same guidelines for alcohol consumption for patients with diabetes as for the general population. Additional concerns about alcohol use exist in the following conditions:

• Pregnancy
• History of alcohol abuse
• Pancreatitis and gastritis

In large amounts, alcohol causes peripheral insulin resistance, and may lead to hyperglycemia, hypertriglyceridemia, and hypertension. Alcohol may also contribute to development of truncal obesity and fatty liver. Because alcohol ingestion may enhance glucose-stimulated insulin secretion and reduce gluconeogenesis, binge drinking and/or failing to consume food with alcohol increases the likelihood of hypoglycemic events. To reduce the risk of hypoglycemia when insulin is required, food should never be omitted to compensate for the alcohol consumed. With good glycemic control, moderate ingestion of alcohol (two drinks for men and one for women) has limited acute effect on blood glucose levels. Alcohol provides 7 kcal (30 kJ) per gram and in T2DM, where weight management is a concern, energy from alcohol should be substituted for fat energy.

Micronutrients: Vitamins and Minerals

There is little need for vitamin and mineral supplementation in patients who eat a variety of foods and consume adequate energy to maintain body weight. Unless the diet is deficient in chromium, its supplementation does not improve glucose tolerance. Patients with diabetes tend to have low blood magnesium levels, most likely due to urinary loss of magnesium associated with chronic glycosuria. Repletion with oral magnesium chloride is recommended only for those who have documented hypomagnesemia.

Reduction of sodium intake has been found to be effective in lowering blood pressure in subjects with hypertension. Older individuals, especially those with diabetes, appear to be more sensitive to sodium than others. For individuals with hypertension, moderate restriction of sodium (2400 mg/day) is recommended. Patients with diabetic nephropathy should limit intake of sodium to 2000 mg/day. A diet based primarily on fresh rather than processed foods is essential to reduce sodium intake.

Phytochemicals and Supplements

Plant sterols or stanols lower serum LDL-cholesterol by 10–15% in mildly hypercholesterolemic subjects by competitive inhibition of gastrointestinal absorption of cholesterol. It may be a useful dietary adjunct for patients with diabetes.

Clinical evidence to support the efficacy and safety of many botanical (herbal) supplements is limited. Because of the potential for harmful effects and possible interaction with prescription medications, patients should be asked about their use of supplements.

Meal Frequency and Timing

For patients with T1DM, consistency in timing of meals and amount of carbohydrate is important to prevent fluctuations in blood glucose levels. Adjustments should be made in the timing of insulin injections to match peak glucose excursion. Multiple daily injections or use of an insulin pump provides greater flexibility in meal times. Patients taking oral antidiabetes agents should be advised to avoid skipping meals, to prevent hypoglycemia. Multiple small meals (compared to a pattern of less frequent meals) have been shown to have a positive effect on metabolic control and weight loss efforts.

SPECIAL ISSUES

Type 1 Diabetes Mellitus

Infants and Children

Providing adequate nutrition for normal growth and development and prevention of hypoglycemic events are two major goals in management of diabetes in infants and children. Important factors in diabetes management in this group include:

- Monitor growth every 3–6 months
- Use higher preprandial blood glucose target goals
  - — 120–220 mg/dL for infants and toddlers
  - — 100–200 mg/dL for preschool children
  - — 70–150 mg/dL for school-age children
- Monitor blood glucose levels frequently
- Adjust insulin to match carbohydrate consumed

Adolescents

Rapid growth and hormonal changes in the adolescent years influence insulin needs. Extra energy intake may be needed for catch-up growth if the child has lost weight or has experienced poor growth. Intensive glycemic control may induce excessive weight gain. Children with T1DM are typically thin or even underweight at the time of diagnosis, but with the increased prevalence of obesity, approximately 25% of children diagnosed with T1DM are now obese. When a child participates in vigorous physical activity, periodic guidance by a dietitian is recommended to facilitate appropriate adjustments in the child's meal plan.

Type 2 Diabetes Mellitus

Adults

Focus on improved metabolic control, rather than weight loss, provides greater incentive for long-term change in T2DM. Long-term maintenance of reduced weight is problematic for many individuals. Key factors for maintaining reduced body weight are

- Continued self-monitoring (food and weight records)
- Increased physical activity

Many chronic illnesses and physical conditions limit patients' physical activity. Some medications can also adversely affect weight loss efforts, including glucocorticoids, thiazolidinediones, antipsychotics, tricyclic antidepressants, antiepileptics, and antihistamines (increased appetite), nonsteroidal anti-inflammatory drugs (increased intake due to gastritis), and β-blockers (decreased metabolic rate).

Children and Adolescents

The prevalence of obesity and T2DM is increasing among children. The goal for children is to maintain weight while providing adequate energy for continued linear growth. Modest energy restriction and increased physical activity to promote weight loss in adolescents who are past the growth spurt is appropriate. Encouraging decreased sedentary time can also promote a healthy weight.

Pregnancy and Lactation

Nutritional planning should begin 3–6 months prior to conception, to achieve near-normal glycemic control before pregnancy. Increased energy should be provided during pregnancy and lactation. Recommended weight gain for women with diabetes is the same as for nondiabetic women. Some changes occurring in pregnancy include:

- Lower fasting blood glucose levels
- Increased likelihood of hypoglycemia with morning sickness
- Increasing insulin resistance as pregnancy progresses

Approximately 4% of women develop gestational diabetes. They are often overweight and are at increased risk for developing T2DM. Energy restriction during pregnancy is controversial, but energy consumption of 1600–1800 kcal (6700–7500 kJ) per day can improve hyperglycemia without causing ketosis. Severe energy restriction can result in ketosis and adversely affect the fetus.

Recommendations for diet during pregnancy include:

- Energy intake based on present pregnant weight of:
  — 30 kcal/kg if normal-weight
  — 24 kcal/kg if overweight
  — 12 kcal/kg if morbidly obese
- Carbohydrate limited to 40% of total energy intake
- Food intake distributed into six small meals
- Adequate protein (additional 25 g/day)
- Weight loss postpartum

Breastfeeding should be encouraged for any new mother. Lactation does tend to lower blood glucose. Breastfeeding can promote gradual weight loss in overweight women with T2DM. Nutritional recommendations during lactation include:

- Extra energy [~330 (first 6 months) to 400 (second 6 months) kcal or 1390–1680 kJ per day]
- Adequate protein (additional 25 g/day)

- Moderate weight loss (0.5–1.0 kg/month)
- Additional snacks, especially at night
- Insulin adjustments to maintain blood glucose levels

Eating Disorders

The prevalence of eating disorders among people with diabetes is at least as great as in the general population. Eating disorders, particularly prevalent in young females, can significantly complicate diabetes management.

Acute and Chronic Illnesses

Sick-Day Guidelines

Nutritional management during acute illnesses requires maintenance of appropriate fluid and electrolyte balance and intake of ≥ 150 g of carbohydrates to avoid ketosis. The nutritional goal during periods of stress is to avoid over- and underfeeding. Overfeeding exaggerates the hyperglycemia caused by metabolic stress. Maintenance of blood glucose levels between 100 and 200 mg/dL is recommended. Impaired wound healing has been observed when blood glucose exceeds 200 mg/dL.

Enteral and Parenteral Nutrition Support

The indications for nutritional support for patients with diabetes are similar to those without diabetes. Energy and protein needs should be determined based on thorough nutrition assessment. Monitoring of blood glucose and urine ketones is recommended every 6 hours during enteral nutrition and every 4 hours during parenteral nutrition. Reduced fluid intake and high-carbohydrate formulas may increase risk of hyperosmolar nonketotic coma. Excess administration of glucose (0.5 mg/kg body weight/min) may cause hyperglycemia and require a higher dose of insulin for glycemic control.

Other Complications

Diabetic Nephropathy

In chronic renal insufficiency and nephrotic syndrome, a reduction in dietary protein to 0.8 g/kg is recommended. Dextrose in the dialysate used for peritoneal dialysis can be absorbed and contribute to hyperglycemia. Supplementation of certain vitamins and minerals may be needed due to the metabolic alterations of renal failure as well as poor dietary intake.

Autonomic Neuropathy

Gastroparesis: Gastroparesis is a complication of diabetes with significant nutritional management implications. Decreased intake and weight loss can result from the early satiety and gastrointestinal symptoms. The patient may experience postprandial hypoglycemia and fluctuating plasma glucose levels. Optimal glycemic control is important because hyperglycemia slows gastric emptying. Nutritional management recommendations include:

- Low-fat, low-fiber diet
- Small, frequent meals

- Replace solid foods with liquid meals
- Eat solid foods in the morning, then switch to liquids
- Sit up during and after meals
- Use a jejunostomy feeding route if enteral feeding is required

Diarrhea and constipation: Diabetic diarrhea occurs in approximately 10–20% of patients with poorly controlled diabetes. Adjustments in diet have not been very effective in management of diarrhea or constipation that results from diabetic autonomic neuropathy; therefore, good glycemic control for prevention of neuropathy is essential.

OVERCOMING BARRIERS TO CHANGE

Medical nutrition therapy is effective in improving metabolic control in diabetes. Numerous barriers to dietary compliance have been identified. Factors that facilitate compliance are

- Simplified, individualized meal plans
- Time-management skills
- Physician referral for medical nutrition therapy

Lack of physician referral is often the reason cited for not consulting a dietitian. Patients with diabetes of long duration, with poor metabolic control, and with major obstacles to lifestyle changes, are most likely to benefit from intensive nutrition therapy.

SUMMARY

The goals of nutritional management for diabetes mellitus can be achieved in a number of ways. Provision of adequate energy intake to meet needs during periods of growth and development, pregnancy and lactation, and times of stress, injury, or illness are of primary importance. For patients with T2DM, reduction of total energy intake and an increase in physical activity consistent with the patient's physical capabilities should be recommended in order to reduce body fat, decrease insulin resistance, and improve glycemic and lipid control. Either a high-carbohydrate diet or a diet rich in *cis*-monounsaturated fats can be used as long as intake of dietary cholesterol and cholesterol-raising fats is limited. Intake of added sugars should be limited, and carbo-hydrates rich in soluble fiber should be preferentially consumed. Recommendations for protein, vitamins, minerals, and fluids are similar to those for people without diabetes. Emphasis should be on a healthy lifestyle with a wholesome diet rich in whole grains, fresh fruits, and vegetables. Referral to a qualified dietitian to assist the patient in establishing an individualized, realistic meal plan is essential. Because changing dietary habits is difficult, frequent follow-up will increase the likelihood of long-term positive outcomes and prevention of complications.

ADDITIONAL READINGS

American Diabetes Association Position Statement: Evidence-based nutrition principles and recommendations for the treatment and prevention of diabetes and related complications. *Diabetes Care* 2002;25:202.

Chandalia M, Garg A, Lutjohann D, et al: Beneficial effects of high dietary fiber intake in patients with type 2 diabetes mellitus. *N Engl J Med* 2000;342:1392.

Franz MJ, Monk A, Barry B, et al: Effectiveness of medical nutrition therapy provided by dietitians in the management of non-insulin-dependent diabetes mellitus: A randomized, controlled clinical trial. *J Am Diet Assoc* 1995;95:1009.

Franz MJ, Bantle JP, Beebe CA, et al: Evidence-based nutrition principles and recommendations for the treatment and prevention of diabetes and related complications, Technical Review. *Diabetes Care* 2002;25:148.

Garg A: High-monounsaturated-fat diets for patients with diabetes mellitus: A meta-analysis. *Am J Clin Nutr* 1998;67(suppl):577S.

For a more detailed discussion of this topic and a bibliography, please see Porte *et al: Ellenberg & Rifkin's Diabetes Mellitus,* 6th ed., Chapter 26.

8 | Basics of Diabetes Education

Geralyn R. Spollett

Self-management education is a critical part of the medical plan for people with diabetes, such that medical treatment without systematic self-management education cannot be regarded as acceptable care. Patients with chronic illness must be educated in a way which assists them in self-managing their illness successfully. It is not enough merely to impart information. The health care provider joins in partnership with the patient to provide education, guidance, and support in the management of diabetes. Within the framework of the care visit, patients have the opportunity to rethink decisions made in the home setting and strategize changes in therapy that can help them achieve health care goals. Self-management education focuses on those skills and techniques integral to attaining competency in all aspects of diabetes self-care. Ultimately, the patient is responsible for the day-to-day decision making concerning dietary intake, medication adjustment, and the amount and frequency of exercise. Therefore, self-management education is the cornerstone of all diabetes therapies.

Historically, diabetes self-management education was divided into two categories: (1) survival skills and (2) lifestyle management issues. Survival skills encompassed those skills and techniques every person with diabetes should know to safely manage in the home setting (Table 8-1). The lifestyle management issues focused on the educational topics that, while important, were not integral to the daily management of the disease—for example, travel, sick-day rules, skin care, and stress management.

While it is essential for patients to understand the rudiments of diabetes self-care, the way in which this educational process is conducted has changed to allow for more input and information selection by the patient.

The components of diabetes self-management education (DSME) as defined by the American Diabetes Association (ADA) in the consensus statement, "National Standards for Diabetes Self-Management Education," include an individualized assessment of the patient's learning needs, development of an educational plan, and periodic reassessment and evaluation to direct the selection of appropriate educational materials and interventions. In DSME, the emphasis is on the individualization of self-management education and the formation of mutually set health care goals.

The curriculum for a diabetes education program should include a solid core of information (Table 8-2) designed to give the participant the knowledge and skills necessary to begin to make informed choices regarding the management of his or her disease. Incorporating behavioral change strategies (Table 8-3) and using the patient's past experiences strengthens the knowledge base and reinforces the practical application of the curriculum content. The goal of the educational process is for the participant to apply the principles learned, thereby enhancing decision making within the context of disease self-management.

Self-monitoring of blood glucose (SMBG) gives the patient the necessary feedback on changes made in therapy toward achieving health care goals in diabetes management.

109

TABLE 8-1 Survival Skills

How to take prescribed medication
Timing, action of medication, technique for administration (insulin)
How to test blood glucose
Meter usage, schedule for testing
Warning signs of hypo/hyperglycemia
Respective causes and treatments
Basic nutrition guidelines
Food types, timing of meal, balancing content and quantity

All patients with diabetes need to learn to self-monitor and be able to relate the results to medication, dietary, or activity changes. Acquiring this ability to analyze glucose results takes both time and experience but is a critical step in the process of self-management of diabetes (Table 8-4). In portraying the glucose results as information to guide therapy rather than a report card of the patient's failures and successes, the health care provider reinforces the importance of SMBG as a tool that assists patients in the decision-making process. The number of glucose meters on the market can make selection of a meter seem difficult. However, most meters are very simple to operate, requiring a two- or three-step procedure. A diabetes educator can guide the patient in the selection of a meter and instruct the patient in its use.

The health care provider will need to work with the patient to establish glucose target ranges for the various testing times recommended. The ADA has defined glycemic targets, but these should be considered a starting point (Table 8-5). These target goals are individualized to the patient and take into consideration age, health status, duration of disease, and complications secondary to diabetes such as hypoglycemic unawareness.

Another method for assisting patients in evaluating self-care is the glycated hemoglobin test (HbA$_{1c}$). By giving a retrospective picture of glucose control over a 2–3-month time frame, HbA$_{1c}$ provides a broader view of glucose control and can assist the patient and provider in making the necessary therapeutic changes for improvement. Patients should know their HbA$_{1c}$ level and understand its meaning in the process of achieving glucose control. As with SMBG, goals for HbA$_{1c}$ must be established by patient and provider. When target goals are not met, the ADA recommends a change in therapy.

Addressing changes in lifestyle—diet and activity level—is usually the best starting point.

Medical nutrition therapy (MNT) is a central component of all diabetes care. A registered dietitian, in a series of visits that allow for assessment, indi-

TABLE 8-2 Content Areas for DSME

Diabetes disease process and treatment options
Nutritional management
Physical activity
Utilizing medications for therapeutic effectiveness
Monitoring blood glucose and utilizing results to improve control
Acute complications—their prevention, detection, and treatment
Chronic complications—their prevention, detection, and treatment
Goal setting and problem solving
Psychosocial adjustment
Preconception care, management during pregnancy, and gestational
diabetes management

TABLE 8-3 Behavioral Change Strategies

1. Patient sets an attainable goal
2. Identifies steps necessary to achieve goal
3. Assesses resources needed or available for meeting goal
   (includes support system, financial resources, equipment, etc.)
4. Creates a timeline for meeting initial steps toward goal
5. Performs a self-evaluation and readjusts plan to meet goal

Example:
   1. "I will increase my physical activity with a walking program. I would like to walk 3 miles per week by the end of November."
   2. "I will begin by walking 15 minutes 3 days per week during my lunch hour for the next 2 weeks."
   3. "I will buy good walking shoes, ask a friend to walk with me for encouragement, and plan to bring my lunch on the days I walk to save time."
   4. "I will block out the time on my calendar to walk on Monday, Tuesday, and Friday for the next 2 weeks."
   5. "I was able to walk on Monday and Tuesday, but Friday was too hectic. I need to change to another day. I need to increase my time to 20 minutes and to buy a pedometer to measure miles walked."

vidualized meal planning, and a follow-up evaluation visit, is the best resource for this self-management education. When a dietitian is not available, the best strategy is to make simple changes in the patient's current eating pattern that will modify or reduce carbohydrate and fat in the diet. Simple suggestions, such as limiting the use of sugared beverages, or switching to 2% milk rather than cream in coffee, can have an impact on glucose and saturated fat levels. At the very least, the health care provider should ask what the patient normally eats—portion size, nutrient balance, and timing of the meals—to gain an insight into areas that need to be considered when choosing medication therapy. Highlighting these problem areas in a referral to a dietitian helps to individualize education and counseling.

Sedentary patients who are encouraged to increase their physical activity need to understand the vital role activity plays in reducing insulin resistance, maintaining weight loss, and improving cardiovascular function. The concept of continuous daily exercise, that is, short, 10-minute periods of exercise done three or four times a day, can improve their diabetes dramatically. Building these increments of activity into the day—using stairs rather than elevators, walking to the store rather than driving the short distance—makes exercise

TABLE 8-4 Blood Glucose Monitoring Guidelines

Have the patient demonstrate meter usage during an office visit.
Assess for:
   Correct coding/calibrating of meter
   Lancet device usage
   Strip expiration and proper storage of open strip vials
   Adequate blood sampling
   Meter memory access
   Use of control solution
   Battery replacement
Discuss record-keeping methods (handwritten log, computer download).
Identify most useful testing times given the patient's therapy.
Establish glycemic goals and adjustments in therapy to achieve goals.

TABLE 8-5 Glycemic Control for Nonpregnant Individuals with Diabetes

	Normal	Goal	Additional action suggested
Plasma values			
Average preprandial glucose (mg/dL)	<110	90–130	<90 or >150
Average bedtime glucose (mg/dL)	<120	110–150	<110 or >180
Whole blood values			
Average preprandial glucose (mg/dL)	<100	80–120	<80 or >140
Average bedtime glucose (mg/dL)	<110	100–140	<100 or >160
A1c (%)	<6	<7	>8

Source: ADA Clinical Practice Recommendation, Diabetes Care 2002 (suppl 1); 25:S37.

"doable." For those patients over age 40 starting a more strenuous exercise program, cardiac evaluation and an exercise tolerancy test is recommended by the American Diabetes Association.

When glucose targets are not achieved through changes in exercise and diet, the initiation of drug therapy, or adjustment in a preexisting pharmacologic regimen, is the next step. Importantly, patients benefit by knowing how to take the medication (timing, amount or dosage, with or without food), any adverse effects, and even a rudimentary knowledge of how a specific drug works (i.e., sulfonylureas by increasing pancreatic insulin output, thiazolidinediones by increasing the body's response to insulin, etc.).

The transition to insulin from oral medications can be difficult for both patient and provider. Addressing the patient's fears and helping him or her to see insulin as a safe, effective therapy is an important first step to patient acceptance. The basic components of initiating insulin therapy are outlined in Table 8-6. The health care provider may need to enlist the help of a visiting nurse or family member to supervise the first at-home injection.

Once the patient has mastered the rudimentary skills of insulin administration, whether by pen device or syringe, the next step is to assist the patient in making adjustments in insulin therapy to meet target goals for glucose control. "Fix fasting first" is an easy alliterative rule that helps the patient to understand the importance of starting the day within the target glycemic range. Adjustments made to any of the basal insulins (NPH, Lente, or glargine)

TABLE 8-6 Initiation of Insulin

1. Select easiest method for patient to use, taking into account visual acuity, dexterity, etc.
2. Have the patient inject prior to learning drawing technique.
3. Teach pen or syringe usage. (Make sure patient is able to demonstrate both preparation and injection before leaving the office).
4. Give a sample of the insulin product or pen device when possible.
5. Write down number units of insulin to be given and the time of the injection.
6. Give patient contact information—next appointment, phone or e-mail contact time
7. Anticipate possible changes due to insulin therapy, such as blurry vision, less nocturia, and hypoglycemic symptoms, and discuss with patient.

TABLE 8-7 Insulin Adjustment Rules

Establish target blood glucose goals.
In general, change only one insulin dosage at a time.
Strive for meal consistency, especially carbohydrate intake, when making
    insulin adjustments.
Determine insulin doses by looking at glucose patterns.
Use postmeal glucose levels to assist in adjusting premeal insulin dosage.

should result in an improvement in the fasting level. While the approach must be individualized for each patient, a good starting place is to increase insulin by 2 units every third day until goal ranges are reached. Entrusting the patient to make these minor adjustments empowers the patient and establishes a partnership between the patient and provider. Table 8-7 lists general rules for teaching insulin adjustment.

Adjustments in preprandial or meal insulin doses require the ability to synthesize information and make decisions based on the result. There are four questions the patient can ask himself prior to making this dosage decision: (1) What is my current glucose level? (2) Do I plan to eat a larger or smaller meal than usual? (3) Will I be more or less active in the next few hours than usual? (4) What has happened under these circumstances previously? These questions help the patient to focus on the factors that influence the amount of insulin necessary for the meal.

When a patient is ill, blood glucose levels rise and the usual adjustments will not be adequate in treating the hyperglycemia. Sick-day rules (Table 8-8) encourage the patient to take at least his usual dose of insulin and to supplement this with fast or rapid-acting insulin every 4 hours until glucose levels are within target ranges. All patients with diabetes must be taught the sick-day guidelines. Familiarity with them can make the critical difference in being able to manage at home or being admitted to the hospital.

Similarly, all patients using secretagogues or insulin must be taught to recognize the signs and symptoms of hypoglycemia and its treatment

TABLE 8-8 Sick-Day Rules

Increase hydration—at least 8 oz/hour.
    If unable to eat, use caloric beverages such as ginger ale, apple juice,
    or broth.
Try to maintain usual diet—do not skip or reduce meals to lower glucose
    levels.
    Adjust food types as necessary to maintain nutrition.
Check blood glucose every 4 hours and record.
    For glucose readings >250 mg/dL, check urine ketones.
Notify health care provider if fever, vomiting, or diarrhea persist for
    > 24 hours or if symptoms are severe.
Rest; do not use exercise to try to lower glucose levels.
Do not withhold usual insulin dose.
    Insulin supplements using lispro, aspart, or regular insulin may be
    needed to reduce high glucose levels caused by illness.
Take oral medications as directed.
    May need to withhold metformin if dehydration, vomiting, diarrhea
    present.

TABLE 8-9 Hypoglycemia Treatment Guidelines

Increase awareness of hypoglycemia symptoms:
 Shakiness, sweating, heart palpitations, hunger
 Change in visual acuity, headache, tremors, irritability
Treat symptoms promptly with 15–20 g of carbohydrate:
 4 oz fruit juice, 8 oz skim milk, 2 tsp sugar or honey, 3–6 glucose tablets
 1 small box of raisins, 5–7 Lifesavers
Wait 15–20 minutes for symptoms to subside.
Test glucose level and retreat if necessary.
Follow treatment with a small snack (1 starch serving, 1 protein serving) if
 next meal time is longer than 45–60 minutes away.
Administer glucagon by IM injection if the patient is unable to swallow safely.

(Table 8-9). The health care provider should emphasize to the patient that quick action is necessary to treat hypoglycemia. In the aftermath of a hypoglycemic event, the patient can examine the factors that may have brought it about—lack of food, inappropriate amount of medication, or increased physical activity without adequate food—and make the necessary changes to avoid future episodes.

In the case of those patients who have had severe hypoglycemic episodes characterized by an inability to take nourishment or loss of conscientiousness, a family member or significant other must be taught to give glucagon by injection to stimulate hepatic glucose release.

A frequent cause of hypoglycemia is unplanned exercise or increased physical activity. An important part of hypoglycemia prevention is educating patients in the need for "extra food for extra activity." When possible, the patient should try to plan for exercise by adjusting food and/or medication (Table 8-10).

Good planning and preparation can help the diabetic patient avoid problems when traveling that place health at risk (Table 8-11). Whether the travel is for work or pleasure, certain preventive measures need to be taken to

TABLE 8-10 Exercise Tips

Always warm up before and cool down after exercise.
Wear appropriate protective equipment and foot wear.
Test blood glucose before and after exercise.
 If exercising longer than 1 hour, check glucose during exercise period
 as well.
Do not exercise if glucose levels are below 100 mg/dL or above 300 mg/dL.
 Bring glucose levels to a safe range before initiating exercise.
Exercise with a buddy when possible.
Carry an appropriate treatment for hypoglycemia and treat at the first
 symptom.
When exercising for longer than 30 minutes, snack to maintain glucose
 levels.
During prolonged exercise, 2 hours or more, adjustments in both food and
 medication may be necessary.
Strenuous exercise during the day may result in hypoglycemia up to 24
 hours later. Increasing the evening snack may prevent exercise-related
 nocturnal hypoglycemia.
Review glucose results from past exercise episodes and try to learn from
 both the positive and negative aspects of the experience.

TABLE 8-11 Travel Guidelines

Pack sufficient medical supplies for the entire trip. Carry them with you.
Bring two glucose monitors with strips, lancets, and extra batteries. Pack them in two separate bags.
Carry simple carbohydrate sources such as glucose tablets, gel, candy, or juice packs to treat hypoglycemia.
Wear a medical identification bracelet or necklace. Also have a letter from your health care provider verifying your need for the medical supplies to treat diabetes adequately.
Pack portable food sources such as snack mix, peanut butter crackers, granola bars, or fruit for nourishment when meals are missed or delayed.
Keep a traveler's emergency kit with medication for nausea, vomiting, diarrhea, and fever. Include bandages, antibiotic ointment, sterile gauze, and adhesive tape.
Pack all prescription medications in their original, labeled vials.
In advance, know what medical coverage is available to you as you travel. Have appropriate phone numbers and insurance cards with you.
If using a pump: carry not only sufficient pump supplies for the entire trip but also backup intermediate/long-acting insulin and syringes in case of pump malfunction.

Source: Adapted from Chandran M, Edelman SV: *Clin Diabetes* (2003); 21:82–85.

ensure safety. Individualized counseling regarding insulin adjustment takes into consideration types of insulin used and timing of dosages for air flights that cross two or more time zones.

Practicing good foot care is important for all persons with diabetes and can be easily accomplished by most patients (Table 8-12). Fifty percent of all non-traumatic amputations each year occur in the diabetic population. Prevention of foot trauma and routine foot evaluations are key to reducing the disabilities and economic burden associated with amputations. Patients with peripheral neuropathy and/or poor circulation are at highest risk. The importance of foot care cannot be overemphasized in this patient group.

TABLE 8-12 Foot Care Guidelines

Wash and dry feet well every day.
Wear well-fitting shoes and clean, dry, cotton socks.
Never walk barefoot.
Follow the contour of the toe when trimming toenails.
    To prevent ingrown nails, do not cut into the corners
Apply moisturizing lotion daily.
    Avoid using lotions that are perfumed or that contain alcohol.
See a podiatrist regularly for removal of corns, warts, and calluses.
    A yearly foot evaluation is recommended.
Buy shoes mid-day, when feet are at their largest. Break in new shoes gradually.
    Leather shoes will stretch and mold to the foot and provide less pressure areas.
Notify your health care provider within 24 hours if your foot becomes infected or injured.
    Keep the area clean, dry and covered. Apply antibiotic ointment and gauze wrap as needed. Try to stay off the foot as much as possible until it is evaluated.

Table 8-13 Complications Screening

Diabetic retinopathy screening—yearly*
Macular edema, glaucoma, and cataract screening included
Urine microalbumin screening—yearly*
Comprehensive foot exam—yearly
Visual inspection at every office visit
Cardiac risk assessment—yearly
Lipid evaluation
Exercise stress test
Smoking cessation
BP evaluation
Evaluation for aspirin therapy

*For type 1 diabetic patients with ≥ 5 years' duration and for all type 2 diabetic patients, starting at diagnosis.

Source: American Diabetes Association: *Clinical Recommendations 2003— Standards of Medical Care for Patients with Diabetes Mellitus.* 2003: s33–s50.

The prevention of long-term complications in persons with diabetes is a pivotal issue in self-care. Most, if not all, of the patient education and self-management in diabetes is aimed at promoting a healthy, long life in the presence of chronic disease. Therefore, screening for complications, both macrovascular and microvascular, is a critical element in the preservation of health. All patients with diabetes need to know the importance of renal and eye screening and cardiovascular risk analysis (Table 8-13).

Diabetes education plays a critical role in comprehensive diabetes care. It is important for all practitioners caring for patients with diabetes to understand the basic tenets of diabetes education. Moreover, it is important for these caregivers to help their patients take advantage of resources (nutritionists, diabetes educators, etc.) available to them to help manage this challenging chronic disease.

ADDITIONAL READINGS

American Association of Diabetes Educators: Individuation of diabetes-self-management education. *Diabetes Educ* 2002;28:741.

American Diabetes Association: National Standards for Diabetes Self-Managment Education. *Diabetes Care* 2004;27 (suppl 1):S143.

American Diabetes Association: Standards of Medical Care in Diabetes. *Diabetes Care* 2004;27 (suppl 1):S15.

Franz MJ: 2002 diabetes nutrition recommendations: Grading the evidence. *Diabetes Educ* 2002;28:756,762,766.

Polonsky WH, Earles J, Smith S, et al: Integrating medical management with diabetes self-management training: A randomized control trial of the Diabetes Outpatient Intensive Treatment Program. *Diabetes Care* 2003;26:3048.

9 | Intensive Management of Type 1 Diabetes Mellitus

Suzanne M. Strowig   Philip Raskin

INTRODUCTION

The Diabetes Control and Complications Trial (DCCT) and the Epidemiology of Diabetes Interventions and Complications (EDIC) trial demonstrated the benefit of near-normal glycemic control in the prevention of diabetic complications. These results led to the recommendation that intensive therapy should be implemented as early as is safely possible, and that such therapy be maintained for as long as possible.

Although intensive diabetes treatment techniques are recommended to achieve near-normal glycemic control, some individuals with type 1 diabetes mellitus (T1DM) may not be candidates for intensive diabetes treatment or may not be willing to accept the personal commitment inherent in such treatment. Any improvement in glycemic control, however, will be of benefit to the patient.

Patients for whom the risk–benefit ratio of intensive therapy may be less favorable include those with repeated episodes of severe hypoglycemia or hypoglycemia unawareness, children under 13 years of age, the elderly, patients with coronary artery disease who may be at higher risk for severe sequelae from hypoglycemia, patients with proliferative or severe nonproliferative retinopathy who may experience a transient acceleration of their retinopathy, and patients with advanced complications. These individuals may not be good candidates for intensive diabetes treatment, or may require higher glycemic goals.

FEATURES OF INTENSIVE DIABETES TREATMENT

Treatment Plan

- Multiple daily insulin injections or continuous subcutaneous insulin infusion pump therapy
- Blood glucose monitoring 4–8 times daily
- Meal planning based on a systematic approach to quantifying food and matching insulin to food intake

Treatment Goals

- Individualized based on capabilities and risk factors
- Ideal glycemic goals:
  Blood glucose: Before meals: 70–120 mg/dL
  After meals: <150 mg/dL
  Bedtime: 100–130 mg/dL
  3:00 A.M.: >70 mg/dL
- Glycated hemoglobin level: nondiabetic range for the assay performed

117

Characteristics

- Integrates insulin and food preferences into lifestyle practices
- Basic prescription that can be adjusted by the patient
- Liberal, flexible, adapts to changing circumstances, and allows for patient choice

Patient Education

- Basic education initially; teach what is necessary to implement the treatment plan, i.e., insulin administration, blood glucose self-monitoring, meal planning, management of hypoglycemia and hyperglycemia
- Ongoing education integrated into each office visit; focuses on self-care behaviors and relevant issues within the context of lifestyle practices and experiences
- Emphasizes patient problem solving and decision making
- Emphasizes a systematic approach to matching insulin, food, and exercise rather than a fixed regimen

Interventions

- Nursing, nutrition, behavioral, and medical interventions are provided at each office visit.
- Once the treatment plan is prescribed, taught, and implemented, interventions become more behavioral, directed at assisting patients to overcome obstacles to implementing treatment recommendations.

Team Collaboration

- Team consists of patient, nurse, dietitian, physician, and mental health professional.
- Each member contributes equally and is part of the ongoing care of the patient; communication is open and ongoing.
- Decisions are made jointly; a unified message is delivered to the patient.

INSULIN REGIMENS

In general, insulin injection regimens consist of a combination of basal insulin [intermediate-acting insulin such as NPH or Lente, or long-acting insulin such as Ultralente or insulin glargine (Lantus insulin)] and short-acting (regular) or rapid-acting insulin such as insulin lispro (Humalog™ insulin) or insulin aspart (Novolog insulin). Short- or rapid-acting insulin is used before meals to control postprandial blood glucose levels.

CONVENTIONAL INSULIN TREATMENT REGIMENS

Twice-Daily Insulin Injections

Premixed Insulin Preparations

70/30 insulin (premixed 70% NPH and 30% regular insulin)
Novolog 70/30 insulin (70% insulin aspart protamine suspension and 30% insulin aspart)

Humalog mix 75/25 insulin (premixed 75% insulin lispro protamine suspension and 25% insulin lispro)

Timing of Injections

- 70/30 insulin: 30 minutes before breakfast and supper
- Novolog mix 70/30 or Humalog mix 75/25 insulin: 5–15 minutes before breakfast and supper

Insulin Action

- Peak insulin action before breakfast from supper NPH insulin, insulin aspart protamine, or insulin lispro protamine component
- Peak insulin action after breakfast and before lunch from breakfast regular insulin, insulin aspart, or insulin lispro component (see Fig. 9-1)
- Peak insulin action before supper from breakfast NPH insulin, insulin aspart protamine, or insulin lispro protamine component
- Peak insulin action after supper and before bedtime from supper regular insulin, insulin aspart, or insulin lispro component

Advantages

- Simple and easy to use; draw a single dose of a combination of insulin in one syringe.
- Minimum insulin dosing that provides 24-hour insulin coverage.
- Humalog mix 75/25 insulin or Novolog mix 70/30 insulin can be taken 5–15 minutes before a meal.

Disadvantages

- 70/30 insulin: should wait 30 minutes after insulin injection before eating the meal.

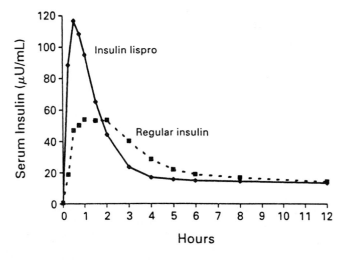

FIG. 9-1   Effects of subcutaneous administration of insulin lispro and regular insulin on serum insulin concentrations. *(Reproduced with permission from Holleman F, Hoekstra JBL: Insulin lispro.* N Engl J Med *1997;337:176.)*

- Fixed ratio of intermediate and short or rapid-acting insulin may not control blood glucose levels.
- Cannot adjust intermediate-acting insulin component without adjusting the short or rapid-acting insulin component.
- Cannot adjust regular insulin, insulin aspart, or insulin lispro for variations in food intake, blood glucose level, or exercise.
- Must take insulin and eat meals about the same time every day (± 1 hour); must eat a consistent amount of carbohydrate at each meal from day to day.
- Least flexible of all regimens.

Indications
- Patients with limited capabilities
- Patients who are unwilling to intensify regimen
- Initial regimen after diagnosis to learn and adapt to injections
- Type 2 diabetes

Starting Dose
- ⅔ total daily dose before breakfast, ⅓ total daily dose before supper
- 0.5–1.0 U/kg/day

NPH and Short-Acting (Regular) Insulin or NPH and Rapid-Acting Insulin (Insulin Lispro or Insulin Aspart)

Timing of Injections
- NPH and short-acting (regular) insulin 30 minutes before breakfast and supper or NPH and rapid-acting insulin 5–15 minutes before breakfast and supper

Insulin Action
- NPH and short-acting (regular) insulin as for 70/30 insulin (see Fig. 9-2)
- NPII and rapid-acting insulin as for Humalog mix 75/25 or Novolog mix 70/30 insulin

Advantages
- Relatively simple regimen
- Can adjust short-acting or rapid-acting insulin before breakfast and supper for variations in food intake, blood glucose reading, and activity
- Can adjust NPH and short-acting or rapid-acting insulin independently from each other

Disadvantages
- Must take insulin and eat meals about the same time every day (± 1 hour); limited flexibility.
- NPH insulin may peak too early, i.e., mid- to late afternoon and/or in the middle of the night, leading to hypoglycemia between meals and/or during the night, and hyperglycemia before breakfast and/or supper.

Indications
- Patients with a consistent schedule
- Patients with limited capabilities or who are unwilling to intensify therapy

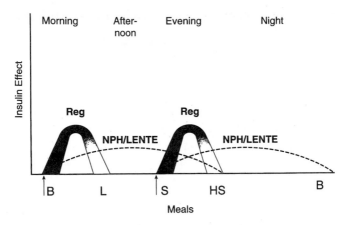

FIG. 9-2   Representation of idealized periods of insulin effect for a split-and-mixed insulin regimen, consisting of two daily doses of short-acting (regular) and intermediate-acting insulin. Symbols: **B**, breakfast; **L**, lunch; **S**, supper; **HS**, bedtime; **arrows,** time of insulin injection 30 minutes before meal; **Reg**, regular or short-acting insulin effect; **NPH/LENTE**, intermediate-acting insulin effect. *(Reproduced with permission from Hirsch IB, Farkas-Hirsch R, Skyler JS: Intensive insulin therapy for treatment of type I diabetes.* Diabetes Care *1990;13:1265.)*

Starting Dose
- ⅔ total daily dose before breakfast; ⅓ total daily dose before supper.
- Each injection should consist of ⅔ NPH insulin and ⅓ short or rapid-acting insulin.
- 0.5–1.0 U/kg/day.
- Adjust short or rapid-acting insulin based on patient's sensitivity (approximately 0.5–2.0 U/15 g carbohydrate; 0.5–2.0 U/50 mg/dL blood glucose level; must be individualized to patient).

INTENSIVE INSULIN REGIMENS

Three Daily Insulin Injections

NPH and Short-Acting (Regular) Insulin or NPH and Rapid-Acting Insulin (Insulin Lispro or Insulin Aspart)

Timing of Injections
- NPH and short-acting insulin 30 minutes before breakfast or NPH and rapid-acting insulin 5–15 minutes before breakfast
- Short-acting insulin 30 minutes before supper or rapid-acting insulin 5–15 minutes before supper
- NPH insulin at bedtime (short or rapid-acting insulin at bedtime if needed)

Insulin Action
- Peak insulin action before breakfast from bedtime NPH insulin

- Peak insulin action after breakfast and before lunch from breakfast short or rapid-acting insulin
- Peak insulin action before supper from breakfast NPH insulin
- Peak insulin action before bedtime from supper short or rapid-acting insulin (see Fig. 9-3)

Advantages

- Reduces risk for nocturnal hypoglycemia that can result from taking NPH insulin before supper
- Can adjust short or rapid-acting insulin before breakfast and supper for variations in food intake, blood glucose reading, and activity
- Can adjust NPH and short or rapid-acting insulin independently from each other

Disadvantages

- Preferable to take insulin and eat meals about the same time every day (± 1 hour)
- Third injection required

Indications

- Nocturnal hypoglycemia, often experienced when supper dose of NPH insulin is increased in an effort to improve fasting blood glucose levels.
- Patients do not want to take a fourth injection of short or rapid-acting insulin before lunch.
- Reasonably consistent schedule.

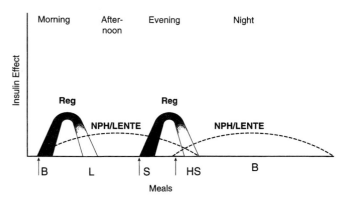

FIG. 9-3 Representation of idealized periods of insulin effect for a three-injection-a-day regimen in which split-and-mixed dose is given in the morning, short-acting (regular) insulin before supper, and intermediate-acting insulin is delayed until bedtime. Symbols: **B**, breakfast; **L**, lunch; **S**, supper; **HS**, bedtime; **arrows**, time of insulin injection 30 minutes before meal; **Reg**, regular or short-acting insulin effect; **NPH/LENTE**, intermediate-acting insulin effect. *(Reproduced with permission from Hirsch IB, Farkas-Hirsch R, Skyler JS: Intensive insulin therapy for treatment of type I diabetes.* Diabetes Care *1990;13:1265.)*

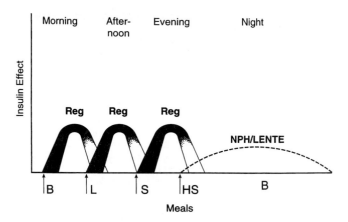

FIG. 9-4   Representation of idealized periods of insulin effect for a multiple-dosage regimen providing short-acting (regular) insulin before each meal and intermediate-acting insulin at bedtime. Symbols: **B**, breakfast; **L**, lunch; **S**, supper; **HS**, bedtime; **arrows**, time of insulin injection 30 minutes before meal; **Reg**, regular or short-acting insulin effect; **NPH/LENTE**, intermediate-acting insulin effect. *(Reproduced with permission from Hirsch IB, Farkas-Hirsch R, Skyler JS: Intensive insulin therapy for treatment of type I diabetes.* Diabetes Care *1990;13:1265.)*

- Patient is willing to check blood glucose levels at least three to four times daily before meals and at bedtime.

  Starting Dose

- Same as for twice-daily NPH and short or rapid-acting insulin except the evening dose of NPH insulin is taken at bedtime

Four Daily Insulin Injections

NPH and Short-Acting (Regular) Insulin or NPH and Rapid-Acting Insulin (Insulin Lispro or Insulin Aspart)

Timing of Injections

- NPH Insulin before breakfast and at bedtime or at bedtime only (if using rapid-acting insulin, patient will likely need NPH insulin twice daily at breakfast and bedtime)
- Short-acting insulin 30 minutes before or rapid-acting insulin 5–15 minutes before breakfast, lunch, and supper; use at bedtime if needed for bedtime snack or elevated bedtime blood glucose reading
- Should take short-acting insulin 4–6 hours apart to avoid overlap in insulin action

Insulin Action

- Peak insulin action before breakfast from bedtime NPH insulin
- Peak insulin action after breakfast and before lunch from breakfast short or rapid-acting insulin

TABLE 9-1 Clinical Considerations for the Use of Rapid-Acting Insulin versus Short-Acting Insulin

Regimens using rapid-acting insulin (insulin lispro or insulin aspart) will differ from those using short-acting insulin (regular insulin) as follows:

- Rapid-acting insulin is absorbed and eliminated faster than regular insulin, has a shorter duration of action of insulin, and reaches a peak serum insulin concentration that is two times higher and is achieved in half the time than regular insulin (see Fig. 9-1).
- The peak action of rapid-acting insulin is about 1 hour after injection, compared with 2–4 hours for regular insulin; the duration of action of rapid-acting insulin is about 3 hours after injection, compared with 4–6 hours for regular insulin.
- Regular insulin is ideally taken 30 minutes before a meal; rapid-acting insulin should be taken 5–15 minutes before a meal.
- The rapid onset and short duration of action of rapid-acting insulin may more adequately control postprandial blood glucose readings than will regular insulin, but may not have a long enough duration of action to control blood glucose levels before the subsequent meal as well as does regular insulin.
- The rapid onset and short duration of action of rapid-acting insulin makes it useful for correcting hyperglycemia or for those who take frequent injections because there is less concern about the overlap of insulin action, and the effect of the insulin can be observed sooner.
- Patients who switch from regular insulin to rapid-acting insulin may require less rapid-acting insulin and more intermediate-acting, long-acting, or basal insulin. A four-daily-injection regimen using NPH or ultralente insulin and rapid-acting insulin will generally require a morning and evening dose of NPH or ultralente insulin.
- Patients who eat between-meal snacks while using regular insulin may not be able to do so while using rapid-acting insulin. Patients may need to take an additional injection of rapid-acting insulin before the snack to maintain desired glycemic control.
- Patients should check blood glucose levels frequently during the first 2 weeks after switching to rapid-acting insulin to detect hypoglycemia or hyperglycemia, and to assist in making adjustments as needed.

- Peak insulin action after lunch and before supper from lunch short or rapid-acting insulin (and morning NPH insulin if used)
- Peak insulin action before bedtime from supper short or rapid-acting insulin (see Fig. 9-4, Table 9-1)

Advantages

- As for three daily injections but can also adjust insulin at lunch for variations in food intake, exercise, and blood glucose level, allowing for greater flexibility and increasing potential for improved blood glucose control.
- Using a single bedtime dose of NPH insulin avoids the problems associated with afternoon peak insulin activity from a morning dose of NPH insulin (a single dose of bedtime NPH insulin is not advisable when using rapid-acting insulin before meals).
- Can use a pen-like device to take frequent injections; device is portable and easy to use, especially when away from home; dial up desired dose and inject insulin with replaceable needles that are attached to the insulin pen.

Disadvantages

- Ideally, NPH insulin is taken about the same time every day (±1 hour).
- Short-acting insulin injections taken less than 4 hours or more than 6 hours apart can result in overlap or gaps in insulin action, leading to hypo- or hyperglycemia.
- Short duration of action of rapid-acting insulin taken before meals may not adequately control blood glucose levels before subsequent meals.
- Four injections per day are required.

Indications

- Inadequate glycemic control using three injections each day; morning NPH insulin does not adequately control before supper blood glucose levels.
- Patient requires more flexibility and is willing to assume the added responsibility associated with adjusting short or rapid-acting insulin for variations in blood glucose levels, food intake, and activity.
- Patient is willing to check blood glucose levels four times daily before meals and at bedtime.

Starting Dose

- NPH insulin should be 35–50% of total daily dose.
- If on morning and bedtime injections of NPH insulin, give 30–40% of total dose of NPH insulin before breakfast and the remainder at bedtime.
- Short or rapid-acting insulin can be given as a percentage of the total daily dose as follows: breakfast, 20–25%; lunch, 10–15%; supper, 15–20%; and bedtime (if needed) 3–5%, base on dietary intake according to patient's sensitivity (i.e., 0.5–2.0 U/15 g carbohydrate).
- Provide an algorithm for adjusting pre-meal short or rapid-acting insulin (i.e., increase insulin by 0.5–2 U for every 50 mg/dL greater than 150 mg/dL).

Ultralente and Short-Acting (Regular) Insulin or Ultralente and Rapid-Acting Insulin (Insulin Lispro or Insulin Aspart)

Timing of Injections

- Ultralente insulin is taken as a single dose before breakfast or divided so that half is given before breakfast and half before supper.
- Short-acting insulin is given 30 minutes before meals or rapid-acting insulin is given 5–15 minutes before meals (short or rapid-acting insulin can be given at bedtime if needed for bedtime snack or elevated blood glucose reading).

Insulin Action

- Ultralente insulin is considered a sustained, long-acting "peakless" insulin, but small peaks in its action can occur 15–24 hours after injection; peaks in insulin action are difficult to predict.
- Peak insulin action after breakfast and before lunch from breakfast short or rapid-acting insulin.
- Peak insulin action after lunch and before supper from lunch short or rapid-acting insulin.

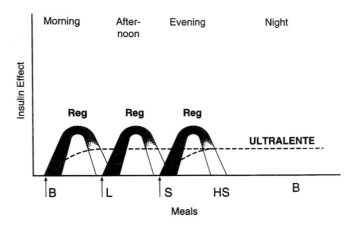

FIG. 9-5 Representation of idealized periods of insulin effect for a multiple-dosage regimen using pre-meal short-acting (regular) insulin and basal insulin as Ultralente. Symbols: **B**, breakfast; **L**, lunch; **S**, supper; **HS**, bedtime; **arrows**, time of insulin injection 30 minutes before meal; **Reg**, regular or short-acting insulin effect. *(Reproduced with permission from Hirsch IB, Farkas-Hirsch R, Skyler JS: Intensive insulin therapy for treatment of type I diabetes.* Diabetes Care *1990;13:1265.)*

- Peak insulin action after supper and before bedtime from supper short or rapid-acting insulin (see Fig. 9-5).

Advantages
- Flexibility in timing and dosing of insulin; can adjust for variations in food intake, exercise, and blood glucose level.
- Ultralente may allow for more flexibility in the timing of injections because of its sustained activity.

Disadvantages
- Four injections per day are required.
- Unpredictable peaks in action of ultralente insulin can occur.
- Taking short-acting insulin injections less than 4 hours or more than 6 hours apart can result in overlap or gaps in insulin action, leading to hypo- or hyperglycemia.
- Short duration of action of rapid-acting insulin may not adequately control blood glucose levels before subsequent meals.

Indications
- As for four daily injections using NPH and short or rapid-acting insulin, but prefer action profile of ultralente insulin over that of NPH insulin.
- NPH insulin does not adequately supply basal insulin needs or peak action of NPH insulin results in frequent hypoglycemia in the afternoon or during the night.

Starting Dose

- Ultralente insulin should be 35–50% of total daily dose; half can be given before breakfast and half before supper.
- Short or rapid-acting insulin before meals as for four daily injections using NPH and short or rapid-acting insulin.

Insulin Glargine (Lantus) and Short-Acting (Regular) Insulin or Insulin Glargine and Rapid-Acting Insulin (Insulin Lispro or Insulin Aspart)

Timing of Injections

- Single injection of insulin glargine at bedtime (single injection of insulin glargine can be given before breakfast if clinically indicated).
- Short-acting insulin 30 minutes before or rapid-acting insulin 5–15 minutes before breakfast, lunch, and supper; bedtime short or rapid-acting insulin can be given if needed.

Insulin Action

- Insulin glargine provides a sustained 24-hour duration of action without peaks.
- Peak insulin action after breakfast and before lunch from breakfast short or rapid-acting insulin.
- Peak insulin action after lunch and before supper from lunch short or rapid-acting insulin.

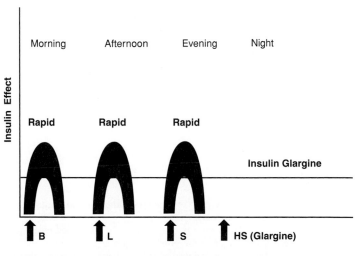

FIG. 9-6   Representation of idealized periods of insulin effect for a multiple-dosage regimen using pre-meal rapid-acting (insulin lispro or insulin aspart) insulin and basal insulin as insulin glargine (G). Symbols: **B**, breakfast; **L**, lunch; **S**, supper; **HS**, bedtime; **arrows**, time of insulin injection 5–15 minutes before meal.

- Peak insulin action after supper and before bedtime from supper short or rapid-acting insulin (see Fig. 9-6).

Advantages

- 24-hour basal insulin coverage with a single injection without peaks in activity.
- Less potential for hypoglycemia related to peak activity of intermediate-acting or ultralente insulin, especially during the night (if insulin glargine is administered at bedtime).
- Great degree of flexibility in timing of meals and injections.
- Adjustments can be made for short or rapid-acting insulin before each meal for variations in blood glucose level, food intake, and activity.

Disadvantages

- Insulin glargine cannot be mixed with any other insulin in the same syringe.
- Taking short-acting insulin injections less than 4 hours or more than 6 hours apart can result in overlap or gaps in insulin action, leading to hypo- or hyperglycemia.
- Short duration of action of rapid-acting insulin may not adequately control blood glucose levels before subsequent meals.

Indications

- As for four daily injections using NPH and short or rapid-acting insulin, but prefer action profile of insulin glargine over that of NPH or ultralente insulin
- Unable to achieve glycemic goals using NPH or ultralente insulin, or patient experiences frequent hypoglycemia in the afternoon or during the night

Starting Dose

- For patients on a single daily dose of NPH or ultralente insulin, give equivalent dose as a single injection of insulin glargine at bedtime or before breakfast.
- For patients on two daily doses of NPH or ultralente insulin, give 80% of the total daily dose of NPH or ultralente insulin as a single dose of insulin glargine at bedtime or before breakfast.
- Insulin glargine should constitute 35–50% of the patient's total daily insulin dose.

Subcutaneous Insulin Infusion Pump Therapy

Timing of Injections

- Use only buffered short-acting (regular) insulin or rapid-acting insulin (insulin lispro or insulin aspart).
- The insulin is drawn into a syringe or reservoir that is placed in the pump and connected to a catheter at the end of which is a 27-gauge needle or Teflon catheter; the catheter is inserted subcutaneously into the abdomen (can use the hip or thigh, but the abdomen is the preferred site), and is secured with an adhesive dressing or tape.
- 24-hour basal insulin is delivered automatically once programmed; can give multiple basal rates in 24 hours to adjust for variations in diurnal insulin needs (see Fig. 9-7).

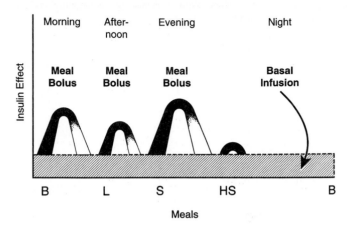

FIG. 9.7 Representation of insulin effect provided by continuous subcutaneous insulin infusion. A continuous infusion (basal rate) is delivered, with premeal boluses administered before meals. Only short- or rapid-acting insulin is used. Symbols: **B,** breakfast; **L,** lunch; **S,** supper; **HS,** bedtime. *(Reproduced with permission from Hirsch IB, Farkas-Hirsch R, Skyler JS: Intensive insulin therapy for treatment of type I diabetes.* Diabetes Care *1990;13:1265.)*

- Boluses of short or rapid-acting insulin are given before meals and snacks, or to lower elevated blood glucose levels.
- Boluses of short-acting insulin should be given 30 minutes before a meal, rapid-acting insulin should be given 5–15 minutes before a meal.

Insulin Action

- Basal insulin should maintain blood glucose levels in desired range overnight and in the absence of meals or change in activity; in general, the total daily basal rate should not exceed 60% of the total daily dose.
- Assess nighttime basal rates based on 3:00 A.M. and fasting blood glucose levels; assess daytime basal rates based on blood glucose levels when meals are skipped or delayed.
- Assess boluses based on 2-hour postprandial and subsequent pre-meal blood glucose levels.

Advantages

- Maximum flexibility; can adjust insulin for diurnal variations and changes in blood glucose levels, food intake, and exercise (see Fig. 7, Table 9-2).
- Meals can be skipped or delayed without loss of blood glucose control.
- No peak insulin activity from intermediate or long-acting insulin.
- More physiologic and more predictable insulin activity related to use of short or fast-acting insulin and mode of insulin delivery.
- Can vary timing of meals, sleep, activity, and work, and can travel across time zones without loss of blood glucose control and without having to adjust dose and timing of intermediate or long-acting insulin.
- Insulin infusion set needs to be inserted every 2–3 days instead of four daily injections.

TABLE 9-2 Features to Consider When Selecting an Insulin Infusion Device for Continuous Subcutaneous Insulin Delivery

- Size of pump
- Type and size of reservoir
- Type of infusion set
- Power source (type of batteries)
- Ease of wear
- Ease of programmability
- Safety features and alarm systems
- Special features
  - Number of programmable basal rates and basal rate patterns
  - Units of adjustment
  - Bolus delivery options such as square wave or extended boluses
  - Temporary basal rate options
  - Resistance to moisture
  - Display
  - Data storage and computer interface capability
  - Audio bolus delivery
  - Tamper-resistant blocks
  - Remote programmer
  - Built-in prompts
  - Communication with a blood glucose meter with automatic calculation of bolus
- Warranty
- Availability of 24-hour technical assistance and record of reliability

- Can remove or disconnect from insulin pump for short periods of time if desired for specific activities and substitute with multiple daily insulin injections.

Disadvantages

- Expensive.
- Must wear device 24 hours a day.
- Interruption of short or rapid-acting insulin can result in hyperglycemia and ketoacidosis within hours; do not suspend basal insulin delivery for more than 1 hour.
- Infection can occur at infusion site.
- Pump or infusion system malfunction (catheter occlusion, empty insulin reservoir, dead batteries, needle displacement, leakage of insulin from the catheter) can result in loss of blood glucose control or ketoacidosis in a few hours (pumps have alarms to warn of problems).

Indications

- Suboptimal glycemic control using multiple daily insulin injections.
- Cannot control overnight blood glucose levels using intermediate or long-acting insulin.
- Frequent and/or nocturnal hypoglycemia.
- Preconception/pregnancy.
- Gastroperesis.
- Patient's lifestyle requires flexibility in timing and dosing of insulin (travels, works different shifts, meal times are erratic and unpredictable).

- Motivated with necessary cognitive and physical capabilities to operate the pump safely and anticipate and evaluate adjustments made in insulin dosage for a variety of circumstances.
- Patient has financial resources.
- Patient has demonstrated willingness to check blood glucose levels at least four times daily and can quantify food intake.

Starting Dose

- Total daily basal dose should be 40–60% of total daily dose (divide by 24 to obtain hourly basal rate); usual range is 0.5–2.0 U/hour for type 1 diabetic individuals.
- May need to reduce prepump dose by 10–20% before calculating pump dosages.
- Total daily basal dose can be calculated by multiplying the patient's weight in kg by 0.3 (divide by 24 to obtain hourly basal rate).
- Usually one to three basal rates per 24-hour period are sufficient; i.e., lower basal rate at bedtime, higher basal rate during predawn hours (3:00–9:00 A.M.), and an intermediate basal rate during the day.
- Pre-meal boluses can be calculated as a percentage of the total daily dose as follows: breakfast, 20%; lunch, 10%; supper, 15%; bedtime (if needed for elevated blood glucose level or bedtime snack), 5%; base on dietary intake according to patient's sensitivity (i.e., 0.5–2.0 U/15 g carbohydrate).
- Provide an algorithm for adjusting pre-meal short-or rapid-acting insulin (see Table 9-3) (i.e., increase insulin by 0.5–2 U for every 50 mg/dL over desired blood glucose level).
- Adjust basal rates and boluses by 10–20% based on blood glucose readings before and after meals, at bedtime, and at 3:00 A.M.
- If pump malfunction occurs, or patient does not wish to wear pump for a brief period of time, administer usual dose of short or rapid-acting insulin before meals, and take intermediate or long-acting insulin at bedtime; if using rapid-acting and intermediate-acting insulin, take dose of intermediate-acting insulin in the morning, as well; recommended bedtime dose of intermediate or long-acting insulin should be about 70–80% of the patient's total daily basal insulin while on the insulin pump or 1.0–1.5 times the amount of basal insulin the patient would receive overnight while using the pump.

TABLE 9-3 Example of Variable Insulin Dosage Schedule for Insulin Infusion Pump Therapy (Short- or Rapid-Acting Insulin Only) (Basal Rate 0.8 U/hour)

Plasma glucose (mg/dL)	Pre-meal insulin dose (short- or rapid-acting insulin 1.0 U/15 g carbohydrate)
<80	Minus 1 U
80–120	Usual Dose
121–170	Add 1 U
171–220	Add 2 U
221–270	Add 3 U
271–300	Add 4 U
>300	Add 5 U

EXAMPLES OF HOW TO CALCULATE STARTING INSULIN DOSAGE BASED ON TWICE-DAILY INSULIN REGIMEN

Twice-Daily Insulin Injection Regimen

Breakfast: NPH 20 U, regular 10 U
Supper: NPH 10 U, regular 5 U
Total daily dose: 45 U

Conversion to Four Daily Insulin Injection Regimen

Single Bedtime Injection of NPH Insulin and Four Pre-meal Injections of Short-Acting (Regular) Insulin

Bedtime NPH insulin: 40% of 45 (0.40×45) = 18 U
Regular insulin*:
  Breakfast: 22% of 45 (0.22×45) = 10 U
  Lunch: 13% of 45 (0.13×45) = 6 U
  Supper: 20% of 45 (0.20×45) = 9 U
  Bedtime: none

NPH Insulin before Breakfast and at Bedtime and Pre-meal Rapid-Acting Insulin (Insulin Lispro or Insulin Aspart)

Total daily dose of NPH insulin: 50% of 45 (0.50×45) = 23 U
Morning NPH insulin: 35% of 23 (0.35×23) = 8 U
Bedtime NPH insulin: 23 − 8 = 15 U

Rapid-acting insulin*:
  Breakfast: 20% of 45 (0.20×45) = 9 U
  Lunch: 10% of 45 (0.10×45) = 5 U
  Supper: 15% of 45 (0.15×45) = 7 U
  Bedtime snack: 2% of 45 (0.02×45) = 1 unit

Insulin Glargine at Bedtime and Pre-meal Rapid-Acting Insulin (Insulin Lispro or Insulin Aspart)

Bedtime dose of insulin glargine = 80% of 30 U (total daily dose of NPH insulin on twice-daily injection regimen) (0.80×30) = 24 U

Rapid-acting insulin*:
  Breakfast: 20% of 45 (0.20×45) = 9 U
  Lunch: 10% of 45 (0.10×45) = 5 U
  Supper: 15% of 45 (0.15×45) = 7 U
  Bedtime snack: 2% of 45 (0.02×45) = 1 unit

Continuous Subcutaneous Insulin Infusion Pump Therapy Using Insulin Lispro

Reduce total daily dose by 10% ($0.10 \times 45 = 45 − 4.5 = 40.5$)
Basal rate: 50% of 40.5 (0.50×40.5) = 20.25 U/24 hours ÷ 24 = 0.80 U/hour**
Boluses*:
  Breakfast: 20% of 40.5 (0.20×40.5) = 8 U
  Lunch: 10% of 40.5 (0.10×40.5) = 4 U
  Supper: 15% of 40.5 (0.15×40.5) = 6 U
  Bedtime snack: 5% of 40.5 (0.05×40.5) = 2 U

If basal rate adjustment is needed for nocturnal hypoglycemia and fasting hyperglycemia:
  Basal rates:
  Midnight to 3:30 A.M.: 0.7 U/hour
  3:30 A.M. to 8:00 A.M.: 1.0 U/hour
  8:00 A.M. to 10:00 P.M.: 0.80 U/hour
  10:00 P.M. to midnight: 0.70 U/hour

*Starting dose must be individualized for each patient. Short- or rapid-acting insulin should be based on patient's dietary intake. These percentages represent typical distributions of pre-meal insulin doses. Once initiated, adjust insulin dose by 10–20% as needed based on blood glucose levels.

**Alternative way to calculate total daily basal rate is based on weight (0.3 U/kg); i.e., weight = 70 kg, 70 × 0.3 = 21 U − 10% = 19 ÷ 24 = 0.8 U/hour.

TEACHING PATIENTS TO ADJUST SHORT OR RAPID-ACTING INSULIN FOR VARIATIONS IN FOOD INTAKE

1. Teach patient how to quantify food using one of the following methods:
   • Count grams of carbohydrate.
   • Count starch, fruit, vegetable, and milk exchanges.
   • Use Healthy Food Choices (simplified version of exchange list) and count starch equivalents: one starch equivalent is comparable to one starch exchange, one fruit exchange, one milk exchange, and three vegetable exchanges; one starch equivalent is equal to approximately 15 g of carbohydrate.
2. Have patient keep food records for at least 3 days; dietary intake should reflect patient's usual eating habits, not some "ideal" food intake.
3. Design a meal plan based on patient's 3-day food records, reflecting patient's usual eating habits; no food, including sucrose-containing food, is prohibited; advocate healthy eating as appropriate based on patient's health status and readiness to change (i.e., low fat, high fiber, low sodium, low cholesterol, reduced calorie).
4. Initiate insulin regimen based on current total daily dose and meal plan; average dose of pre-meal short or rapid-acting insulin is 1 U per 15 g of carbohydrate (1 U per starch), but can range from 0.5 to 2.0 U per starch.
5. Have patient keep food records for 4–8 weeks until glycemic goals are achieved; food records are also useful for verifying patient's understanding of how to quantify food and are a good teaching tool.
6. Determine insulin/carbohydrate ratio for each meal based on amount of pre-meal short or rapid-acting insulin needed to achieve glycemic goals; i.e., patient needs 6 U of insulin lispro for a four-starch-equivalent lunch (60 g of carbohydrate); patient needs 1.5 U per starch equivalent or 1 U per 10 g of carbohydrate at lunch time.
7. When patient can quantify food intake competently, patient can simply estimate anticipated food intake and calculate insulin dose.
8. After estimating amount of insulin needed for anticipated food intake, patient can further adjust pre-meal short or rapid-acting insulin based on pre-meal blood glucose reading; i.e., patient can take additional 0.5–2.0 (average 1.0) U for every 50 mg/dL > 150 mg/dL.
9. Resume food records when needed to help patient achieve glycemic goals, to reeducate patient, or to identify and solve a self-management problem.

Adjusting Insulin for Exercise

General Guidelines

- Check blood glucose level prior to exercise.
- Before initiating any activity, correct hypoglycemia with 15–30 g of carbohydrate and repeat treatment until blood glucose reading is >100 mg/dL.
- Check blood glucose reading every 60–90 minutes while exercising, and at the end of the exercise period.
- Always carry source of carbohydrate while exercising, such as juice, regular soda, or glucose tablets.
- Drink fluids every hour, especially if exercising in warm temperatures.
- Avoid exercising when expect peak in insulin activity.
- Adjust insulin or food intake if needed to avoid delayed hypoglycemia that can occur many hours after exercise.
- Day-to-day activities such as housework, yard work, shopping, moving furniture, and unpacking boxes involve exercise that can result in low blood glucose levels if patient does not eat additional carbohydrate or does not take less insulin.
- A bedtime snack may be necessary if patient exercises in the evening.

Unplanned Exercise

- Ingest 15–30 g of carbohydrate for every 30–45 minutes of moderate exercise.
- Ingest one or two protein exchanges prior to a period of sustained exercise.

Planned Exercise

- Decrease short or rapid-acting insulin 25–50% prior to moderate level of planned activity.
- Additional carbohydrate may be needed (15–30 g of carbohydrate), depending on length and intensity of the activity.
- If the patient takes morning NPH insulin, reduce the dose of morning NPH insulin by 15–25% for afternoon or evening exercise.
- If the patient is on an insulin pump, temporarily lower the basal rate 20–40% for sustained periods of exercise; may need to lower the basal rate by 25% for a few hours postexercise; do not suspend the basal rate for more than 1 hour, if at all.

HYPOGLYCEMIA

Preventing Hypoglycemia

- Educate patient and family about causes, symptoms, and treatment of hypoglycemia, including administration of glucagon if patients cannot treat themselves.
- Teach patient a systematic approach to matching insulin to food intake and changes in routine.
- Patient should check blood glucose levels at least four times daily (before meals and at bedtime), weekly at 3:00 A.M., before and after exercise, every 2 hours during an illness, and anytime the patient deviates from usual routine.
- Patient should check blood glucose level prior to operating a motor vehicle and should restore blood glucose level to >80 mg/dL before driving.
- Patient should not take insulin prior to arriving at a restaurant; should take insulin only after food is ordered or served.

- Identify situations patient is likely to encounter that may lead to hypoglycemia; develop a plan to deal with the situation in order to avoid hypoglycemia.
- Have patient pay attention to symptoms when blood glucose level is <70 mg/dL; symptoms may become more vague as glycemic control improves.
- Patients should keep source of carbohydrate with them at all times (car, office, desk, locker, purse, briefcase, gym bag, at the bedside, while exercising, while traveling).
- Bedtime snacks consisting of protein and carbohydrate may be needed to avoid nocturnal hypoglycemia.
- Avoiding hypoglycemia may restore symptomatic perception of hypoglycemia.
- Alter glycemic goals for patients who have hypoglycemia unawareness.
- Review any episode of hypoglycemia to identify cause(s) so that a plan can be developed and patient can be educated to avoid the situation in the future.

Treating Hypoglycemia

- Ingest 15–30 g of rapidly absorbed carbohydrate such as juice, sweetened soft drinks, commercially prepared tablets or gels.
- Repeat treatment every 15–20 minutes until blood glucose level is >70 mg/dL.
- If prior to a meal, treat hypoglycemia and take pre-meal insulin when blood glucose level is restored to normal.
- Teach family member, friend, and/or coworker how to administer glucagon when patient is unable to treat himself (0.5–1.0 mg IM).

Blood Glucose Self-Monitoring

- Select a blood glucose meter suited to the patient's needs, abilities, resources, and personal preferences.
- Consider the meter's attributes:
  — Size
  — Display
  — Ease of use
  — Amount of blood required to do the test
  — Ability to use alternate blood testing sites
  — Strip size and method of strip insertion
  — Dependence on user technique
  — Type of batteries
  — Calibration procedure
  — Cost
  — Manufacturer support and warranty
  — Accuracy and precision
  — Storage capability for blood glucose results
  — Ability to interface with computer software
- Provide technical instruction
- Monitor the patient's technical competence; i.e., observe technical performance and check patient-obtained results against laboratory results performed simultaneously.
- Specify the frequency and circumstances under which blood glucose monitoring is to be performed.

- Specify desired blood glucose targets.
- Educate the patient on the meaning of blood glucose results; identify the relationship between blood glucose levels and self-care behaviors.
- Specify guidelines for dealing with blood glucose levels within and outside the desired range.
- Use a meter with storage capability and download data at each office visit to improve accuracy of records and increase potential for improved glycemic control.
- Provide feedback regularly.
- Sensors (Glucowatch, Cigna; others in development) that provide automatic frequent glucose testing with alarms for individually set high and low readings may be useful for some patients, especially those with hypoglycemia unawareness.

EDUCATION FOR INTENSIVE DIABETES TREATMENT

Initial Education

Three to four outpatient visits and a 3-day inpatient hospital stay, or three to four outpatient visits and a 3–7-day intensive outpatient course

- Blood glucose monitoring
- Insulin administration
- Meal planning and system for quantifying food
- Management of hypoglycemia and hyperglycemia

Education and Management Postinitiation of Intensive Therapy

Biweekly visits and weekly phone calls for 1–2 months

- Keep food and blood glucose records.
- Identify relationship between dietary intake and blood glucose readings.
- Confirm patient's ability to accurately quantify food and calculate needed short or rapid-acting insulin.
- Identify problem areas and revise meal plan as needed.
- Educate on how to deal with specific situations.
- Adjust insulin dosages as needed to achieve glycemic goals.

Ongoing Education and Follow-up

Monthly for 2–6 months, then every 2–3 months

- Teach patient to interpret blood glucose readings.
- Teach patient to adjust insulin for deviations in dietary intake and activity.
- Identify problems with implementation of the treatment plan.
- Identify strategies for dealing with obstacles that interfere with implementing the treatment plan.
- Adapt treatment recommendations for lifestyle situations.
- Anticipate problems and develop strategies to prevent potential problems from interfering with achieving treatment goals.

STRATEGIES THAT ENHANCE ADHERENCE TO TREATMENT

- Match the diet and other aspects of the regimen to the patient's current lifestyle, habits, and personal preferences.

- Design the insulin regimen to match the patient's dietary intake.
- Keep the treatment plan as simple as possible.
- Do not overwhelm the patient with too much information at one time; focus on the information the patient needs to implement the treatment plan.
- Integrate education into every office visit; teach concepts as issues arise and provide information when relevant to a specific situation or experience.
- Create an environment in which the patient feels comfortable to be honest:
  — Allow the patient to disagree with you.
  — Respect the patient's feelings.
  — Encourage the patient to express his or her own views.
  — Incorporate the patient's views into treatment recommendations.
  — Avoid interrupting the patient.
  — Avoid being critical or judgmental.
  — Avoid an authoritative tone.
- Allow the patient as much choice and as many options as possible; allow for flexibility.
- Encourage the patient to be the problem-solver and decision-maker; ask questions so the patient will identify the solution.
- Negotiate specific and realistic goals; establish goals that will lead to success.
- Assist the patient to change health care behaviors when the patient is ready; make changes one small step at a time; consider implementing components of an intensive treatment program in an incremental fashion.
- Provide frequent opportunities for positive feedback and encouragement.
- Help the patient to identify obstacles that can interfere with achieving treatment goals.
- Help the patient develop a plan to minimize obstacles.
- Use contracts to define measurable and realistic goals as well as reward contingencies.

ADDITIONAL READINGS

Klingensmith GJ, ed: *Intensive Diabetes Management*, 3rd ed. Alexandria, VA: American Diabetes Association;2003.

Lalli C, Ciofetta M, Del Sindaco P, et al: Long-term intensive treatment of type 1 diabetes with the short-acting insulin analog lispro in variable combination with NPH insulin at mealtime. *Diabetes Care* 1999;22:468.

Lepore M, Pampanelli S, Fanelli C, et al: Pharmacokinetics and pharmacodynamics of subcutaneous injection of long-acting human insulin analog glargine, NPH insulin, and ultralente human insulin and continuous subcutaneous infusion of insulin lispro. *Diabetes* 2000;49:2142.

Strowig SM: Initiation and management of insulin pump therapy. *Diabetes Educator* 1993;19:50.

Strowig SM, Rashkin P: Improved glycemic control in intensively treated diabetic patients using blood glucose meters with storage capability and computer-assisted analyses. *Diabetes Care* 1998;21:1694.

For a more detailed discussion of this topic and a bibliography, please see Porte *et al: Ellenberg & Rifkin's Diabetes Mellitus,* 6th ed., Chapter 29.

10 | Insulin Treatment of Type 2 Diabetes Mellitus

David M. Nathan

INTRODUCTION

The classification of diabetes mellitus into insulin-dependent or type I (IDDM) and non-insulin-dependent or type II diabetes mellitus (NIDDM), and other types, by the National Diabetes Data Group and the World Health Organization more than two decades ago provided a working model of different phenotypes of diabetes. The division of the diabetic population into IDDM and NIDDM was based on differences in their clinical characteristics, natural history, and presumed pathogenesis. The absolute dependence of IDDM patients on insulin therapy for survival was connoted by the "insulin-dependent" classification. Unfortunately, many clinicians continued to confuse insulin treatment with insulin dependence, and patients who clearly had phenotypic NIDDM, but who were treated with insulin, were often inaccurately described in medical records as having IDDM.

The most recent iteration of the classification of diabetes by the Expert Committee convened by the American Diabetes Association (ADA) refined the diagnostic plasma glucose criteria for diabetes, lowering the fasting plasma glucose threshold from 140 to 126 mg/dL. In addition, and in part to decrease the misclassification of patients using the old nomenclature, non-insulin-dependent diabetes mellitus was to be called type 2 diabetes (T2DM).

This chapter focuses on the insulin treatment of patients with T2DM. The population of insulin-treated T2DM patients in the United States is currently two to three times larger in number than the type 1 diabetic population and is growing at a rapid rate. The worldwide population of T2DM, already pandemic in nature, is projected to reach 300 million in the next 20 years. Although there have been numerous reviews of insulin therapy of type 1 diabetes, relatively few major reviews of insulin therapy of T2DM have appeared. This chapter reviews the magnitude of the problem, the pathophysiology of T2DM as it relates to insulin treatment, the goals of therapy including the role of intensive therapy, the relative attributes of insulin therapy compared with other available treatments, the spectrum of insulin regimens and new insulins that have been tested and their relative advantages and disadvantages, the use of combination therapy, and criteria for selecting T2DM patients for insulin therapy. The treatment of T2DM patients who require insulin transiently, such as during perioperative or other stress, is not discussed in this chapter.

BACKGROUND: THE SCOPE OF THE PROBLEM

Despite the remarkable increase in prevalence of T2DM in the twentieth century, it remained an underrecognized and underdiagnosed disease. The failure of patients to recognize and of clinicians to diagnose T2DM was and continues to be predicated on its subtle clinical presentation compared with type 1 diabetes. (Based on the relatively frequent appearance of long-term complications in "newly diagnosed" T2DM patients, it has been estimated that diabetes has been present for 4–7 years, on average, before it is diagnosed.) T2DM was probably relatively uncommon before the extension of life span and the increased obesity and sedentary lifestyle that have accompanied widespread industrialization in the latter part of the twentieth century.

The spread of T2DM is reaching pandemic proportions. It currently affects 7% of the adult population in the United States, including 12% of the adult population older than 45 and almost 20% of those older than 65. In developing countries in Asia and Africa, where T2DM has historically been relatively rare, the shift to more industrial economies with sedentary lifestyles and Westernized diets has resulted in a startling increase in T2DM.

Currently, at least 2 million T2DM patients in the United States (30% of all diagnosed patients) are treated with insulin, compared with an estimated 600,000 to 1.2 million patients with T1DM (Fig. 10-1). The increasing size of the T2DM population, the disappointing long-term results with diet therapy (the first choice in treating the majority of T2DM patients who are obese), and the relatively high primary and secondary failure rates of oral hypoglycemic therapy strongly suggest that the fraction of the T2DM population and the total number of T2DM patients treated with insulin will increase.

PATHOPHYSIOLOGY OF T2DM: IMPLICATIONS FOR THERAPY

The pathogenesis of T2DM is multifactorial and includes decreased sensitivity to insulin action (insulin resistance) secondary to obesity and genetic factors, and decreased insulin secretion. While insulin resistance may be the inherited defect that accompanies most cases of impaired glucose tolerance, progressive worsening of glucose tolerance with the development of fasting hyperglycemia and T2DM is usually preceded by decreased insulin secretion. Fasting hyperglycemia is primarily a consequence of increased hepatic glucose output in the setting of relatively low insulin levels. In addition, the development of hyperglycemia further compromises insulin secretion and increases resistance (Fig. 10-2). This effect of hyperglycemia, often termed glucotoxicity, is at least partially reversible if basal glycemia is restored to normal. The

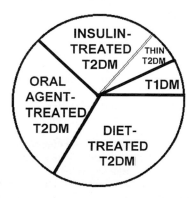

FIG. 10-1 Prevalence of different types of diabetes mellitus.

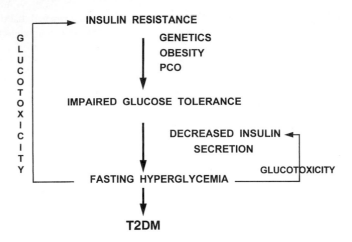

FIG. 10-2 Pathophysiology of type 2 diabetes mellitus.

beneficial effect of achieving normoglycemia in T2DM (lower glycemia begets further improvement in glycemia with restored endogenous insulin secretion) has been demonstrated with diet, sulfonylurea, and insulin therapy.

The implications of these studies with regard to therapy are the following:

1. By the time that T2DM is established, insulin secretion is relatively decreased and the absolute level may be very low.
2. With longer duration, metabolic control worsens with higher glycemic levels. This is largely attributable to progressive deterioration in insulin secretion.
3. Residual insulin secretion in T2DM, at least early in its course, provides a degree of stability to glucose levels not present in type 1 diabetes. Insulin regimens need not be as complex in the treatment of T2DM as in the treatment of type 1 diabetes.
4. Although T2DM patients may have severely impaired insulin secretion, they rarely become ketotic. There have been several populations identified, including an African-American population in Brooklyn, New York, that appear to be more vulnerable to the development of ketoacidosis. T2DM patients who are thin and/or ketonuric should probably be treated, at least initially, as if they have type 1 diabetes.
5. Correction of fasting hyperglycemia by any means has been demonstrated to result in improved insulin secretion and a modest improvement in resistance. Therapy with insulin early in the course of T2DM may result in remission for as long as several years with no need for hypoglycemic drugs and normal glycemia.
6. Ideally, suppression of increased overnight hepatic glucose output should normalize fasting blood glucose and improve endogenous insulin secretion in response to meals during the day. This effect is presumably mediated by ameliorating the toxic effects of hyperglycemia on the islets.
7. Insulin given in the morning will cover postprandial glucose excursions but may further suppress endogenous insulin secretion during the day.

METABOLIC GOALS OF THERAPY

The Diabetes Control and Complications Trial (DCCT) conclusively established blood glucose goals for type 1 diabetes. The similar clinical characteristics of the microvascular and neurologic complications in type 1 and type 2 diabetes, and the similar relationship between the occurrence of long-term complications and level of glycemia demonstrated in epidemiologic studies of type 1 and type 2 diabetes, support a similar benefit in T2DM as demonstrated in the DCCT. More importantly, the Kumamoto study and the United Kingdom Prospective Diabetes Study (UKPDS) have established the role of intensive therapy in type 2 diabetes mellitus.

The UKPDS compared an "active" treatment policy with either sulfonylurea or insulin (or metformin in the obese subjects) with a dietary policy. Over 10–12 years of average follow-up, the active policy, which decreased HbA_{1c} by approximately 1% compared with the dietary policy, was associated with a 12% decreased risk for aggregate diabetes complications. The major effect was mediated through a 25% decrease in microvascular complications.

These studies support the use of intensive therapy, with the goal of achieving near-normal glucose levels, in T2DM. Of note, the UKPDS demonstrated a seemingly inexorable worsening of metabolic control over time, which required the progressive addition of more hypoglycemic agents and insulin.

COMPARISON OF INSULIN WITH OTHER AVAILABLE THERAPIES FOR T2DM

Efficacy

Short-term randomized studies of glycemic response to insulin versus sulfonylurea, including one that was double-blind, have demonstrated only modest differences in glycemic control in the first weeks to months of therapy. The vast majority of studies that have examined and compared the metabolic benefits of diet, sulfonylurea, and insulin therapy have been short-term studies; longer-term controlled trials are few in number. Although the longest-term observational studies and controlled clinical trials, including the UGDP, the Kumamoto study, and the UKPDS, were 6–12 years in duration, they are relatively brief for a chronic disease such as T2DM. In concert, these studies demonstrate very limited long-term efficacy of diet therapy. The majority of the benefit with regard to weight loss and lowering of glycemia commonly noted in the first year is lost within 2–3 years with weight regain. In the UKPDS more than 50% of the patients with recent-onset T2DM assigned to diet therapy required subsequent reassignment to pharmacologic therapy in order to maintain even a modicum of glycemic control.

Similarly, the lowering of glycemic levels with sulfonylureas or biguanides is transient, with as many as 50% of sulfonylurea-treated patients failing therapy, either in the first 3 months of therapy (primary failure) or after a salutary initial response (secondary failure). Results with either sulfonylurea or biguanides are remarkably similar. In the UGDP and UKPDS, glycemic levels were lowered from baseline for the first several years of therapy, but drifted back to baseline by years 3–5 of therapy. In the UKPDS, worsening metabolic control in patients originally assigned to sulfonylurea or metformin occurred despite the addition or substitution of alternative therapies in as much as 30% of the patients originally assigned to the oral hypoglycemics as glycemic levels rose over time. There are no comparable long-term data available with thiazolidinediones or the meglitinides.

In contrast to sulfonylureas, biguanides, and thiazolidinediones, insulin has no upper dose limit and can be adjusted over time to achieve normal or near-normal glycemic levels. This attribute of insulin therapy has been demonstrated to provide lower levels of glycemia in oral agent failures or when intensive insulin therapy was compared with a conventional insulin regimen in the UGDP, Kumamoto, or Veterans Administration Cooperative Study of Diabetes Mellitus (VACSDM). In most studies of typically obese patients with T2DM, relatively large doses ranging from 50–200 U/day (usually 0.65 U/kg) are required to achieve near-normal glycemia (Table 10-1). Insulin doses had to be raised progressively from approximately 25 U/day at baseline to 90 U/day by 2 years in order to maintain near normal glycemia in the VACSDM.

Other Effects and Adverse Events

A comparison of diet, sulfonylureas, biguanides, and insulin with regard to effects other than glucose control is shown in Table 10-2. Diet therapy has the best benefit–risk ratio, with weight loss resulting in improved lipid levels, blood pressure, and other cardiovascular risk factors. Sulfonylureas and insulin share several metabolic benefits other than glycemic control, such as a reduction in free fatty acid levels. Insulin raises high-density lipoprotein (HDL)-cholesterol more than sulfonylurea therapy. The frequency of severe hypoglycemia, defined in the DCCT as any episode requiring assistance, is generally low; however, modest weight gain (2–5 kg) is relatively common with insulin or sulfonylurea therapy (Table 10-1). Hypoglycemia associated with sulfonylurea use can be more prolonged and dangerous than the usually self-limited hypoglycemia seen with insulin. Finally, drug-specific complications occur.

Metformin, a relatively old drug that was developed in 1959 but did not become available in the United States until 1995, provides several interesting benefits. When used as sole therapy, it has potency similar to that of sulfonylureas, but does not appear to promote weight gain or cause hypoglycemia. The gastrointestinal side effects of bloating and diarrhea that are seen with higher doses and rapid escalation of the dose are usually transient and can be largely eliminated if doses are titrated slowly. The risk of lactic acidosis with metformin is almost nil if patients with decreased renal function, liver disease, severe congestive heart failure, and binge alcohol drinking are excluded from treatment.

The thiazolidinediones are relatively new oral hypoglycemic agents that appear to act by binding to peroxisome proliferator activated receptor-γ (PPAR-γ) receptors and reducing insulin resistance. They appear to be more efficacious when used in combination with other hypoglycemic medications, including insulin. Owing to rare but severe idiosyncratic liver toxicity, the first approved thiazolidinedione, troglitazone, had to be withdrawn from the U.S. market. Pioglitazone and rosiglitazone do not appear to suffer from the same problem, although fluid retention can be problematic.

The meglitinides are nonsulfonylurea insulin secretagogues that have been introduced recently. With a shorter half-life than the sulfonylureas, they are probably less likely to cause hypoglycemia than sulfonylureas, but need to be administered before each meal.

TABLE 10-1 Insulin Treatment Regimens to Acheive Normoglycemia in Patients with Type 2 Diabetes

Duration (mo)	Subjects (#)	Regimen*	Dose (U/kg)	Glycemia achieved (HbA$_{1C}$ or HbA$_1$/ upper limit of normal)	Adverse events[†] (weight gain in kg/ % severe hypoglycemia)
9	15	AM NPH	0.66	7.1/6.4	3.8/0
4	12	Bedtime NPH	0.86	7.2/6.7	2.4/0
120	911	AM UL or NPH[‡]	0.42	7.1/6.2	6/2.3[‡]
6	21	BID NPH	0.63	9.5/7.4	4.7/0
4	10	BID NPH/REG	0.65	10.6/7.8	4.2/0
2	10	BID NPH/REG	NA	5.7/5.0	NA/0
6	14	BID NPH/REG	0.98	5.1/NA	8.7/0
3	29	BID NPH/REG	0.53	7.9/6.0	1.8/NA
6	34	BID 70:30	0.58	8.2/6.2	4.0/0
3	30	NPH + TID REG	0.55	8.0/6.0	2.9/NA
2	10	NPH + TID REG	NA	5.6/5.0	NA/0
27	75	1–3 Injections§	NA	7.2/6.1	NA/3.0
6	21	TID REG	0.55	9.7/7.0	3.3/0
4	10	CSII	0.58	9.2/7.8	4.5/0
1	12	CSII	0.81	NA	NA
1	12	CSII	0.61	NA	NA
12	51	IP Insulin by implantable pump	NA	7.1/6.1	NA/1.0
24	3	IV Insulin by implantable pump	0.75	6.2/6.3	9/0

*UL, ultralente insulin; REG, CZI insulin; NPH, neutral protamine Hagedorn insulin; CSII, continuous subcutaneous insulin infusion; NA, information not available.

[†]Defined as hypoglycemia requiring assistance for treatment and including coma, seizures, and/or treatment with glucagon or IV dextrose (episodes/100 patient-years).

[‡]Daily UL or NPH (+ regular if premeal BG >126 mg/dL). "Major" hypoglycemia in 2.3% of patients.

§Stepwise therapy with evening intermediate- or long-acting insulin proceeding to insulin plus sulfonylurea, to twice-per-day intermediate-acting insulin, and finally to multiple (≥ 3) daily injections.

TABLE 10-2 Comparison of Therapies for Type 2 Diabetes Currently Available in the United States When Used as Monotherapy

	Diet	Sulfonylurea	Biguanides	Glycosidase inhibitors	Thiazolidinediones	Insulin
Metabolic effects						
Improves resistance	+	+	++	+	+++	++
Secretion	+	++	+	+	+	+
Overnight HGO	+	+	++	+	+	+
Postprandial excursions	+	++	+	++	+	++
Glycosylated hemoglobin	+	++	++	+	+	+++
Lowers FFA	+	+	+	+	+	++
Weight gain	–	+	–	–	+	++
Hypoglycemia	–	+	–	–	–	++
Allergic phenonema	–	+	+	–	+	+
Other side effects						
Antabuse effect	–	+*	–	–	–	–
Hyponatremia	–	+*	–	–	–	–
Lactic acidosis†	–	–	+	–	–	–
Gastrointestinal	–	–	+	++	–	–
Hepatic dysfunction	–	–	–	–	+‡	–

*Very uncommon with second-generation sulfonylureas such as glyburide and glipizide. Most common with chlorpropamide.

†Very rary with metformin (<3/100,000 patients).

‡Severe idiosyncratic liver failure in approximately 1/35,000–50,000 patients treated with troglitazone (discontinued in March 2000). Rosiglitazone and pioglitazone thought to be less likely to cause hepatic dysfunction.

INSULIN THERAPY

Doses

As noted above, the dose of insulin required to normalize glycemia in T2DM is often more than 60 U/day. More obese, insulin-resistant patients invariably need more insulin. When calculated on the basis of body mass, most studies have required 0.6–1.0 U/kg. In general, insulin treatment is started with conservative doses, with empiric adjustment based on glucose levels. Since most T2DM patients are insulin-resistant, they can usually tolerate fairly high initial doses of insulin without hypoglycemia. On the other hand, hyperglycemia is very diet-responsive in T2DM, and if patients initiate their dietary efforts concurrently with beginning insulin, they can develop hypoglycemia with relatively small doses. For the reasons above, it is prudent to begin with 10–15 U of intermediate-acting insulin, at bed or before breakfast. Alternatively, a very long-acting insulin, such as insulin glargine, can be initiated in the evening. Adjustments can be made relatively quickly, guided by self-monitoring of blood glucose results.

As noted in Table 10-1, many studies attempting to normalize glycemia in T2DM have required large doses of insulin. However, when calculated on the basis of units per kilogram, these doses are only modestly higher than the range of doses used in the DCCT to treat adult type 1 diabetes mellitus (T1DM) intensively (0.66–0.73 U/kg). The largest doses are generally required in the most obese, most resistant T2DM patients.

The widespread availability of self-monitoring, which should be implemented in all insulin-treated patients, has made adjustment of insulin doses safer and easier. The results of insulin adjustments can be monitored by the patient and the rate and magnitude of further adjustments determined on the basis of self-monitoring. The decision when to split insulin from a single daily dose to two or more doses can also be guided by the results of self-monitoring. For those patients who cannot master self-monitoring, the relative stability of glycemia in T2DM makes possible monitoring of glycemia by visiting nurses or in the office setting to guide adjustment of doses. Timed glucose levels, fasting and/or before dinner, are most useful.

Regimens

Although many insulin treatment regimens have been tried (Table 10-3), most studies achieving glycemic control in the near-normal range, albeit for relatively brief periods of time, have done so with one or two daily insulin injections (Table 10-1). The UKPDS, which failed to maintain stable glycemia with its intensive regimen, perhaps owing to inadequate dosing, used a regimen based on a once-per-day Ultralente or NPH insulin supplemented with regular insulin as needed. The VACSDM employed increasingly complex regimens based on glycemia. In order to maintain stable glycemia over a 10-month follow-up, 64% of the subjects were advanced to two or three daily injections of insulin by study's end. Whether single injections of intermediate- or long-acting insulin in larger doses will perform as well as split doses has not been adequately studied, but is unlikely.

There are surprisingly few data available on the best timing of the injection. Conventionally, insulin therapy is initiated with morning intermediate-acting insulin, with or without rapid-acting insulin. Pre-dinner intermediate-acting insulin, again with or without rapid-acting insulin,

TABLE 10-3 Insulin Regimens for Type 2 Diabetes

Morning intermediate*
Bedtime intermediate or very long-acting
Morning intermediate + rapid†
Morning intermediate + rapid‡ with bedtime intermediate
Morning and predinner intermediate and rapid‡
Dinner and or morning long-acting (Ultralente) with rapid
Morning and bedtime intermediate and prebreakfast and predinner rapid (multiple daily injection—MDI)
Evening Ultralente with premeal rapid (MDI)
Continuous subcutaneous insulin infusion with an external pump (CSII)
Premeal inhaled insulin with bedtime intermediate
Bedtime intermediate with morning sulfonylurea, or daily metformin, thiazolidinedione, or α-glycosidase inhibitor (combination therapy)

*Intermediate-acting: NPH or lente.
†Rapid-acting: CZI (regular) or lispro (very-rapid acting).
‡May be administered as premixed (e.g., 70:30 NPH/regular insulin).

or prebedtime intermediate-acting insulin can be added as needed. As with intensive therapy in T1DM, the choice of doses of rapid-acting (Regular, CZI), or very-rapid-acting (lispro or aspart), insulin before meals is dictated by the results of self-monitoring of blood glucose. However, since blood glucose levels in T2DM are much less labile than in type 1 diabetes, probably mediated by endogenous insulin secretion, frequent adjustment of insulin is less necessary.

The use of nocturnal insulin has been championed on the basis of its ability to suppress overnight glucose output and not inhibit endogenous secretion in response to meals; however, there are few studies to recommend it over the more conventional morning regimens. Nevertheless, it is reasonable to initiate insulin therapy with intermediate-acting insulin at bedtime, adjusting the dose until fasting blood glucose levels are in the therapeutic range. This strategy can normalize fasting glucose levels and HbA_{1c} levels. If blood glucose levels during the day remain elevated, morning intermediate-acting insulin, with or without rapid- or very-rapid-acting insulin, can be added. Premixed insulins such as 70:30 or 50:50 mixtures of NPH and rapid-acting or 75:25 or 70:30 mixtures involving very-rapid-acting insulins are available. These mixtures are relatively stable, preserving the individual time action profiles of the components, and can be used in T2DM when day-to-day insulin doses remain relatively stable.

The use of long-acting insulin has also been espoused as a means of supplementing basal endogenous insulin without exogenous peaks which might suppress endogenous secretion. A new insulin analog, glargine, has a long half-life and no apparent peak. In clinical trials, it has been comparable with once- or twice-per-day NPH but may result in less nocturnal hypoglycemia.

Other more complicated regimens, including continuous subcutaneous insulin infusion (CSII) with an external pump, have been used. Whether they are ever necessary or advantageous compared with less complex regimens is unknown. A crossover study between premeal rapid-acting insulin and twice-per-day (before breakfast and dinner) intermediate-acting insulin revealed no significant benefit of the more frequent injection regimen. In contrast to intensive regimens in type 1 diabetes, which are accompanied by a relatively high risk of hypoglycemia (60–100 episodes/100 patient-years), intensive therapy of type 2 diabetes has much lower risk of hypoglycemia.

Intermittent, or short-term, intensive insulin therapy has been tested in clinical studies. The rationale behind this approach is to lower glycemia to the normal range and, by eliminating glucotoxicity, improve endogenous insulin secretion and decrease insulin resistance. After days to weeks of such therapy, insulin treatment is withdrawn. Glucose levels have been maintained at a near-normal range for as long as 2–3 years. These remissions have been demonstrated most reliably in relatively new-onset T2DM.

COMBINATION THERAPY

Insulin has been used in combination with virtually every other therapeutic modality. Conventionally, diet and exercise recommendations accompany insulin therapy. In addition, combination therapy with sulfonylurea (bedtime insulin daytime sulfonylurea, BIDS) has also been espoused. The rationale behind combination therapy is that nocturnal insulin therapy suppresses overnight glycemia and morning short-acting sulfonylurea stimulates endogenous insulin. The only potential benefit of combining insulin and sulfonylurea, which is more expensive than using insulin alone, is a modest reduction in insulin doses required to achieve a similar level of glycemia.

Other combination regimens, using drugs with different primary mechanisms of action than insulin, such as metformin or thiazolidinediones, have been examined. Most studies have not provided for aggressive adjustment of insulin in the insulin-only arm; thus, whether any benefits that occur when oral agents are added are unique to combination therapy, or whether similar results might be obtained merely by adjusting insulin, has not been conclusively established. The glycosidase inhibitor acarbose will lower HbA_{1c} levels achieved with insulin alone by 0.5%. The thiazolidinediones (with most data available using the troglitazone, which is no longer available) can lower HbA_{1c} when added to insulin or maintain HbA_{1c} with lower doses of insulin. Only rarely does thiazolidinedione therapy allow insulin-treated patients to stop their insulin therapy. The use of metformin with insulin has also been investigated. Although HbA_{1c} levels are only modestly lower with additional metformin, weight gain is less with this combination therapy. Whether the added expense, need for additional monitoring of renal and hepatic function (for metformin and thiazolidinediones), the potential for added toxicity and drug interactions, and decreased compliance associated with combination therapy are merited by the modest improvements in HbA_{1c}, and limited weight gain (with metformin) is not clear.

HOW TO SELECT T2DM PATIENTS FOR INSULIN THERAPY

Patients who have evidence of severe insulin deficiency and a catabolic state on the basis of ketonuria, profound weight loss, or dehydration, or who are thin, should be treated as if they have T1DM (Table 10-4). This will protect such patients from more profound metabolic decompensation if, in fact, they have type 1 diabetes, and will rapidly restore all of them to a safe metabolic state. Although criteria based on fasting and stimulated C-peptide levels have been proposed to help identify such patients, the majority of them can be identified on the basis of the clinical criteria listed above. In addition, patients who are symptomatic from hyperglycemia and have not responded initially, or have failed to respond after preliminary success with diet and/or sulfonylurea or metformin, should be treated with insulin. Finally, patients with very elevated triglyceride levels who are at risk for pancreatitis should be treated

TABLE 10-4 Indications for Insulin Therapy in Type 2 Diabetes Mellitus

Presence of ketonuria in unstressed state
Nonobese with persistently elevated glucose levels
Uncontrolled weight loss and hyperglycemia
Dehydration secondary to glycosuria and unresponsive to diet and/or oral
    agents
Severe hypertiglyceridemia
Diet or oral agent failure with or without symptomatic hyperglycemia
Hyperglycemia with aim of obtaining near-normal glycemia and/or inducing
    remission

with insulin and diet, rather than with an oral hypoglycemic agent, as the most effective way to rapidly lower the abnormal lipid levels.

The implications of the UKPDS and Kumamoto studies are that insulin should be started in T2DM patients whose level of glycemia is not in the near-normal range with diet and/or oral agents, regardless of the presence of symptoms. In the past, clinicians have generally implemented stepped intervention of T2DM in a relatively unaggressive fashion, reserving insulin as a last resort, and often after patients had diabetes for many years and had established complications. The now demonstrated beneficial effects of tight control of T2DM and the recognition that dietary and oral agent interventions are, in many cases, temporizing at best, with progressive worsening of metabolic control over time, suggest that insulin treatment should be implemented earlier and aggressively in the course of T2DM. Moreover, reports of "remissions" of T2DM with early and intensive insulin therapy suggest that insulin should be considered as an early, rather than an end-stage, treatment.

CONCLUSIONS

Insulin is the most efficacious pharmacologic treatment for patients with diabetes. The long-awaited approval of metformin in the United States, and the introduction of new agents, such as the α-glucosidase inhibitors and the thiazolidinediones, are unlikely to decrease the need for insulin in many of the T2DM population, which is rapidly becoming the most common chronic disease in the world. Insulin is ultimately a more powerful drug than any of the other available treatments for T2DM, as well as the only naturally occurring substance used to treat it, and until the high failure rate with diet and oral agents can be abrogated, its frequent use is all but assured.

The anticipated benefits of achieving normoglycemia in T2DM, as in T1DM, should stimulate health care providers and patients alike to use the therapy that provides glycemic control as close to the nondiabetic range as safely possible. When dietary efforts fail, insulin may well be considered the most likely therapy to achieve and maintain those levels of glycemia that are likely to prevent and/or delay long-term complications. Although the best regimen for insulin use in T2DM has yet to be firmly established, a large number of permutations have been investigated. Insulin therapy, with adequate doses and in concert with careful attention to reducing all cardiovascular risk factors, should remain a mainstay of T2DM therapy.

ADDITIONAL READINGS

Cusi K, Cunningham ER, Comstock JP: Safety and efficacy of normalizing fasting glucose with bedtime NPH insulin alone in NIDDM. *Diabetes Care* 1995;18:843.

Ilkova H, Glaser B, Tunckale A, et al: Induction of long-term glycemic control in newly diagnosed type 2 diabetic patients by transient intensive insulin treatment. *Diabetes Care* 1997;20:1353.

Nathan DM: Initial management of glycemia in type 2 diabetes mellitus. *N Engl J Med* 2002;347:1342.

UK Prospective Diabetes Study Group. Intensive blood-glucose control with sulphonylureas or insulin compared with conventional treatment and risk of complications in patients with type 2 diabetes. *Lancet* 1998;352:837.

Yki-Jarvinen H, Ryysy L, Nikkila K, et al: Comparison of bedtime insulin regimens in patients with type 2 diabetes mellitus: A randomized, controlled trial. *Ann Int Med* 1999;139:389.

For a more detailed discussion of this topic and a bibliography, please see Porte *et al: Ellenberg & Rifkin's Diabetes Mellitus,* 6th ed., Chapter 30.

Hypoglycemia

Pierre J. Lefèvre   André J. Scheen

Strictly speaking, the definition of hypoglycemia is biochemical; i.e., hypoglycemia is present when the blood glucose level falls below the lowest limit of normal physiologic fluctuations (Table 11-1). In addition, one observes a constellation of symptoms and signs in clinical practice that point to the diagnosis.

In adults, the symptoms of hypoglycemia are caused by adrenergic reaction to a rapid fall in blood glucose or to cellular malnutrition at the neurologic level ("the supply of metabolizable carbohydrates to the neuron is inadequate for normal function"), with associated symptoms more prominent when hypoglycemia develops slowly. In a given patient, the symptoms associated with hypoglycemia tend to be repetitive and stereotyped.

It should be noted that recurrent episodes of severe hypoglycemia may result in cumulative and permanent cognitive impairment, although this has recently been challenged. Furthermore, repetitive episodes of hypoglycemia, particularly at night, induce *hypoglycemia unawareness,* a situation in which the patient with diabetes does not experience appropriate autonomic warning symptoms before development of neuroglycopenia. Glycemic thresholds for hypoglycemic cognitive dysfunction, like those for autonomic and symptomatic responses to hypoglycemia, shift to lower plasma glucose levels after recent antecedent hypoglycemia in patients with type 1 diabetes mellitus (T1DM).

ETIOLOGY OF HYPOGLYCEMIA

There are two principal forms of hypoglycemia: exogenous hypoglycemia attributable to injection or ingestion of a hypoglycemic compound, and endogenous hypoglycemia (Table 11-2).

Exogenous Hypoglycemia

Insulin

Insulin is the most frequent cause of hypoglycemia, occurring in both diabetic and nondiabetic patients. The EURODIAB IDDM Complications Study indicated that the proportion of T1DM patients with one or more severe hypoglycemic attacks in 1 year averaged 32%, with a minimum of 12% in one center and as many as 48% in another. Predictors of severe hypoglycemia in patients with T1DM include previous severe hypoglycemia, patient's determination to achieve normoglycemia, (lower) social class, and C-peptide negativity.

In diabetic patients, hypoglycemia may result from administration of an insulin overdose or from the concomitant administration of drugs that, when given alone, favor hypoglycemia. The overdose may be absolute or relative: mistake in the evaluation of the dose, injection repeated by mistake (by the patient or by the nursing staff), poor comprehension of medical instructions, lack of sufficient food intake (gastrointestinal problems, ritual or presurgical fast, etc.), physical exercise, or decreases in insulin requirements (immediately postpartum, after weight loss, after steroid tapers, etc.).

TABLE 11-1 Signs and Symptoms of Hypoglycemia

Blood glucose:	
Adults	50 mg/dL (2.8 mmol/L)
During first 48 hours of life	30 mg/dL (1.7 mmol/L)
Small-for-date newborns	20 mg/dL (1.1 mmol/L)
Symptoms:	
Adults	*Adrenergic:* Pallor, sweating, tachycardia, palpitations, sensation of hunger, restlessness, anxiety *Neuroglycopenic:* Fatigue, irritability, headache, loss of concentration, somnolence, psychiatric or visual disorders, transient sensory or motor defects, confusion, convulsions, coma
Older children	Frequent yawning, episodic staring, bizarre behavior, twitching, pallor, remoteness, paresthesias, visual disturbances, loss of concentration
Newborns	High-pitched cry, skin pallor or cyanosis, respiratory distress, apnea, sluggishness, irritability, hypotonia or intermittent twitching, occasionally grand mal seizures

Glucagon secretory responses to plasma glucose decrements become deficient early in the course of T1DM in the vast majority of patients, often within a few years following diagnosis. However, because epinephrine compensates for deficient glucagon secretion, counterregulation is adequate in many of these patients. Nevertheless, the epinephrine secretory response to plasma glucose decrements typically becomes deficient later in the course of the disease. Patients with combined glucagon and epinephrine deficiencies are at substantially increased risk of severe hypoglycemia, at least during intensive therapy. Patients who have defective counterregulatory responses to insulin-induced hypoglycemia have a 20- to 25-fold greater chance of developing severe hypoglycemia than those who counterregulate correctly.

In the Diabetes Control and Complications Trial (DCCT), the incidence of severe hypoglycemia was approximately three times higher in the intensive-therapy group than in the conventional-therapy group. In fact, in the intensive-therapy group, there were 62 hypoglycemic episodes per 100 patient-years in which assistance was required in the provision of treatment, as compared to 19 such episodes per 100 patient-years in the conventional-therapy group. This included 16 and 5 episodes of coma or seizure per 100 patient-years in the respective groups. Particularly severe hypoglycemia has been reported in some patients treated with continuous subcutaneous insulin infusion (CSII, insulin pumps). During CSII, the incidence of severe hypoglycemic episodes ranges between 0.1 and 1.2 per patient per year.

A recent meta-analysis of the effect of the rapid-acting insulin analog, lispro, on severe hypoglycemia in patients with T1DM has shown a slight but significant reduction in the incidence of severe hypoglycemia as compared with regular insulin therapy; of 2327 patients receiving lispro, 72 (3.1%) had a total of 102 severe episodes, compared to a group of 2339 receiving regular human insulin, in which 102 (4.4%) had a total of 131 episodes ($p = 0.024$).

TABLE 11-2 Etiology of Hypoglycemia

Exogenous hypoglycemia
  Insulin
  Oral antidiabetic agents
  Alcohol
  Other exogenous agents
    Salicylates
    Hypoglycins
    Pentamidine
    Perhexilin
    β-Receptor-blocking drugs
    Other drugs

Endogenous hypoglycemia
  Organic hypoglycemias
    Insulinomas and related disorders
      Insulinoma
      Nesidioblastosis and β-cell hyperplasia
    Extrapancreatic neoplasms
    Inborn errors of metabolism
      Hereditary fructose intolerance
      Fructose-1,6-diphosphatase deficiency
      Galactosemia
      Phosphoenolpyruvate carboxykinase deficiency
      Inborn errors in glycogen metabolism

Functional hypoglycemias
  Alimentary hypoglycemia
  Spontaneous reactive hypoglycemia
  Alcohol-promoted reactive hypoglycemia
  Posthyperalimentation hypoglycemia
  Endocrine deficiency states
    Hypoglycemia due to glucocorticoid deficiency
    Hypoglycemia in GH deficiency
    Hypoglycemia and catecholamine deficiency
    Hypoglycemia and glucagon deficiency
  Severe liver deficiency
  Profound malnutrition
  Prolonged muscular exercise
  Autoimmune insulin syndrome
  Antibodies against the insulin receptor
  Functional or transient hypoglycemia in infancy
    Transient neonatal hypoglycemia
    Infants of diabetic mothers
    Erythroblastosis fetalis
    Leucine-induced hypoglycemia
    Ketotic hypoglycemia
    Maple syrup urine disease
    Adrenal hyporesponsiveness

The hypoglycemic effect of insulin can be exacerbated by the simultaneous ingestion of ethanol (discussed later) or of numerous drugs. These include sulfonylureas, biguanides, thiazolidinediones, nonselective β-receptor-blocking agents such as propranolol, monoamine oxidase inhibitors (MAOIs), angiotensin-converting enzyme (ACE) inhibitors, salicylates, and tetracyclines. When β-receptor blockade is needed in diabetics for cardiovascular reasons, selective β_1-receptor-blocking agents (e.g., atenolol, metoprolol, bisoprolol, acebutolol) should be used. Potentiation of the hypoglycemic effect of insulin in diabetic patients can be observed in coexisting adrenocortical or pituitary insufficiency. Of historical interest, pituitary ablation, irradiation, and cryoablation have been used in the past for the treatment of advanced diabetic retinopathy. These procedures frequently resulted in increased insulin sensitivity and, as a result, the risk of hypoglycemia.

In nondiabetics as well as in diabetic patients, insulin has been used for homicidal or suicidal purposes. Severe unexplained hypoglycemia in a nondiabetic individual should always raise the possibility of the purposeful overadministration of exogenous insulin. Thus, factitious hypoglycemia due to clandestine self-use or the criminal administration of insulin must always be considered in the differential diagnosis of hypoglycemia.

Oral Antidiabetic Agents

Diabetic patients can become hypoglycemic while taking oral antidiabetic agents. Overdose or insufficient food intake often explains the occurrence of hypoglycemia. Patients with renal or hepatic insufficiency, which may interfere with excretion or metabolism (or both) of these drugs, are especially susceptible to hypoglycemia, as are those taking long-acting sulfonylureas (e.g., chlorpropamide, glibenclamide) or highly potent sulfonylureas (e.g., glibenclamide, glyburide, or glipizide).

Potentiation of the hypoglycemic properties of sulfonylureas may occur when other drugs are used simultaneously. Table 11-3 summarizes the various mechanisms involved, and Table 11-4 lists the specific pharmacological agents to consider.

Because of their rapid metabolism, the newer nonsulfonylurea insulin secretagogues (repaglinide, nateglinide) appear to result in a decreased risk of hypoglycemia compared to conventional sulfonylureas. In contrast to sulfonylureas, biguanides, when taken alone, infrequently cause hypoglycemia, except in the case of simultaneous prolonged fasting or severe caloric and carbohydrate restriction. Similarly, α-glucosidase inhibitors or thiazolidinediones used in monotherapy do not cause hypoglycemia. However, when combined with insulin secretagogues, they certainly may.

TABLE 11-3 Mechanisms by Which Various Drugs Increase the Hypoglycemic Effect of Sulfonylureas

1. Increase in half-life due to inhibition of metabolism or excretion rate: ethanol, phenylbutazone, coumarin anticoagulants, chloramphenicol, doxycycline, antibacterial sulfonamides, phenyramidol, allopurinol
2. Competition for albumin-binding sites: phenylbutazone, salicylates, antibacterial sulfonamides
3. Inhibition of gluconeogenesis, increase in glucose oxidation, or stimulation of insulin secretion: ethanol, β-adrenergic drugs, monoamine oxidase inhibitors, tranylcypromine, tromethamine

TABLE 11-4 Drugs Capable of Inducing Hypoglycemic Episodes
in Diabetic Patients Treated with Sulfonylureas

Antibacterial sulfonamides: sulfaphenazole, sulfamethoxime, sulfadimidine, sulfathiazole, sulfadiazone, sulfisoxazole, etc.
Analgesics and anti-inflammatory drugs: salicylates, phenylbutazone, oxyphenbutazone
Drugs affecting plasma lipoprotein concentration: clofibrate, fenofibrate
Antibiotics: chloramphenicol, novobiocin, tetracyclines, doxycycline
Miscellaneous: allopurinol, probenecid, phenyramidol, monoamine oxidase inhibitors, tromethamine, isoniazid, sulfinpyrazone, angiotensin-converting enzyme (ACE) inhibitors

Alcohol

Alcohol can not only induce hypoglycemia, it can also promote reactive hypoglycemia (discussed in the section on functional hypoglycemias). Alcohol-induced fasting hypoglycemia characteristically develops in chronically malnourished or more acutely food-deprived individuals within 6–36 hours of ingesting a moderate to large amount of alcohol. Alcohol-induced fasting hypoglycemia results primarily from decreased hepatic glucose output due to impaired gluconeogenesis. As noted previously, alcohol also potentiates the hypoglycemic effects of insulin and oral hypoglycemic agents.

Other Exogenous Agents

Numerous other exogenous agents or drugs may cause hypoglycemia.

Salicylates: Salicylic acid, salicylate, and their derivatives have hypoglycemic properties associated with increased utilization of glucose by peripheral tissues and reduction of gluconeogenesis. In salicylate poisoning, particularly in children below the age of 2 years, hypoglycemia may be observed together with the more common alteration of the acid–base equilibrium: initial respiratory alkalosis due to stimulation of the respiratory center and subsequent metabolic acidosis caused by the drug itself. Children with fever and dehydration are particularly prone to intoxication from relatively small doses of salicylate. Hypoglycemia can be observed in adults taking aspirin, mainly under exceptional circumstances such as when large doses are given to patients with renal failure. Salicylates potentiate the hypoglycemic effects of sulfonylureas.

Hypoglycins: Hypoglycins are compounds found in the unripe tropical fruit *Blighia sapida.* They are responsible for the Jamaican vomiting sickness, a syndrome characterized by vomiting, shock, and hypoglycemic coma; death is common. Hypoglycemia results from inhibition of hepatic gluconeogenesis and increased peripheral glucose utilization; these alterations apparently result from inhibition of long-chain fatty acid oxidation caused by the toxic agent.

Quinine: Administration of quinine stimulates insulin secretion. As a consequence, severe hypoglycemia and hyperinsulinemia can occur in patients with malaria who are treated with intravenous quinine.

β-Receptor-blocking agents: β-Blockers may promote hypoglycemia by their inhibitory effect on adipose tissue lipolysis, which provides alternative fuels when the glucose concentration is low. Hypoglycemia has been observed in young children taking β-blockers, usually after a 6- to 10-hour fast. Maternal therapy with β-blockers may affect the fetus and exaggerate neonatal hypoglycemia. Nonselective β-receptor-blocking agents potentiate the hypoglycemic action of both insulin and sulfonylurea-type drugs.

Pentamidine: Pentamidine, now uncommonly used in the treatment of *Pneumocystis carinii* infection, an opportunistic infection frequently seen in patients with acquired immunodeficiency syndrome (AIDS), causes cytolysis of the β-cells, leading to temporary hyperinsulinemia and hypoglycemia often followed by insulinopenic diabetes.

Miscellaneous drugs that may cause hypoglycemia: Ouabain, mebendazole, isoproterenol, tris(hydroxymethyl) aminomethane (THAM), mesoxalate, disopyramide, tranylcypromine, and possibly MAOIs may cause hypoglycemia by stimulating insulin release. Potassium *para*-aminobenzoate, haloperidol, propoxyphene, anabolic steroids, perhexilin, and guanethidine have been incriminated as possible causes of hypoglycemia through unknown mechanisms. Clofibrate and ACE inhibitors potentiate the hypoglycemic properties of oral antidiabetic agents.

Endogenous Hypoglycemia

Endogenous hypoglycemia may be organic (insulinoma, extrapancreatic neoplasms, due to inborn errors of metabolism) or functional.

Organic Hypoglycemias
Insulinomas and related disorders
Insulinoma: Insulinomas are uncommon neuroendocrine neoplasms derived from pancreatic β-cells. The majority (up to 85%) of these tumors are single, benign adenomas; multiple adenomas or scattered microadenomas are observed in 10–19% of the cases; and islet cell carcinomas are less frequent (2–11% of cases). Insulinoma may sometimes be seen as part of multiple endocrine neoplasia (MEN) syndrome, type 1.

Nesidioblastosis and β-cell hyperplasia: Nesidioblastosis is a rare disease leading to persistent hyperinsulinemic hypoglycemia of infancy. It is characterized histologically by the budding off from duct epithelium of endocrine cells and by the presence in the pancreas of microadenomata. Congenital hyperinsulinism with focal or diffuse nesidioblastosis can be associated with several genetic mutations affecting the β-cell. Symptoms may occur during the first days of life, but most commonly appear within the first 6 months. In a small series, partial pancretectomy cured the majority of neonates who underwent the procedure.

Extrapancreatic neoplasms: Non–islet cell tumors are rare causes of hypoglycemia. Almost half of these tumors have a mesenchymal origin (Doege-Potter syndrome), 23% are hepatomas (Nadler-Wolfer-Elliott syndrome), 10% are adrenocortical carcinomas (Anderson's syndrome), 8% are gastrointestinal tumors, 6% are lymphomas and leukemias, and 8% are miscellaneous. Tumor hypoglycemia may occur in any age group, but is most common in adults between 40 and 70 years of age. A form of insulin-like growth factor-II (IGF-II) is likely responsible for the hypoglycemia (by direct insulin-like action on nonhepatic tissues and suppression of growth hormone secretion). Severe hypoglycemia caused by elevated IGF-II levels has also been reported in patients with acinar cell carcinoma of the pancreas, solitary fibrous tumor of the pleura, metastasis from a meningeal hemangiopericytoma, and disseminated breast cancer.

Inborn errors of metabolism: Although some of the inborn errors of metabolism may be considered functional, we have classified them as a cause of organic hypoglycemia because they are characterized by a well-defined enzymatic defect and thus are organic at the molecular level. Hereditary defects in metabolism include hereditary fructose intolerance, fructose-1,6-disphosphatase deficiency, galactosemia, phosphoenolpyruvate carboxykinase deficiency, and glycogen storage diseases. Among the 11 varieties of glycogen storage diseases now recognized, only a few (types I [von Gierke's disease], III [Forbe's disease], VI [Her's disease], and IXb) lead to hypoglycemia.

Functional Hypoglycemias

Alimentary hypoglycemia: Rapid gastric emptying, as may be seen following gastrectomy and in hyperthyroidism, results in early hyperglycemia followed by reactive hyperinsulinemia and alimentary hypoglycemia. In addition, several gut factors (i.e., secretin, glucagon-like peptide-1 [GLP-1], cholecystokinin, gastric inhibitory polypeptide [GIP]) released after glucose ingestion act in concert with glucose, or even before glucose, to stimulate insulin secretion.

Reactive hypoglycemia: The term *spontaneous reactive hypoglycemia* is usually applied to a syndrome with the following features: (1) symptoms similar to those seen in insulin-induced hypoglycemia (diaphoresis, tachycardia, tremulousness, and headache, among others) and often accompanied by other symptoms less typical of hypoglycemia (e.g., fatigue, drowsiness, feelings of incipient syncope, depersonalization, irritability, and lack of motivation); (2) symptoms that may be episodic, and are sometimes aggravated by carbohydrate-rich meals; and (3) plasma glucose concentration that drops to 45 mg/dL (2.5 mmol/L) or less in at least one half-hourly sample taken during a 5- to 6-hour oral glucose tolerance test (OGTT). Since the latter occurs in up to 30% of apparently healthy individuals without hypoglycemia symptoms, the diagnosis should be restricted to individuals with low glucose levels at the time of symptoms and following meals that produce symptoms (not following OGGT).

The cause of reactive hypoglycemia has been evaluated. Some patients have an altered glycemic threshold (a higher glucose level) for eliciting an adrenergic response, which results in confusion. Increased insulin sensitivity has also been documented, whereas abnormalities in counterregulatory hormones have not.

Alcohol-promoted reactive hypoglycemia: Moderate amounts of alcohol (50 g) increase the insulin response elicited by the ingestion of insulinotropic carbohydrates, such as saccharose, but not of noninsulinotropic ones, such as fructose. Thus, drinks that contain both alcohol and glucose or saccharose (beer, gin and tonic, rum and cola, whisky and ginger ale, among others) are more likely to provoke hypoglycemia on an empty stomach than those containing only alcohol and saccharin or alcohol and fructose. Acute ingestion of alcohol impairs the epinephrine response and markedly suppresses the release of growth hormone in response to a fall in blood glucose levels.

Posthyperalimentation hypoglycemia: Hypoglycemia has been reported following discontinuation of total parenteral alimentation (TPA). It is considered to be secondary to residual effects of insulin from chronically stimulated islet cells.

Endocrine deficiency states: Hypoglycemia due to glucocorticoid deficiency: Glucocorticoid deficiency may cause fasting hypoglycemia as a result of defective gluconeogenesis. This condition may be encountered in acute or chronic adrenal insufficiency (Addison's disease), in congenital adrenal hyperplasia, as a consequence of removal or destruction of the adrenals, in panhypopituitarism, in isolated ACTH deficiency, and other conditions. Spontaneous hypoglycemia in patients with glucocorticoid deficiency occurs mainly if other precipitating factors such as alcohol ingestion, pregnancy, or prolonged fasting are present. Insulin or sulfonylurea administration may be dangerous to any patient with adrenal insufficiency.

Hypoglycemia in growth hormone deficiency: Growth hormone deficiency, either isolated or as part of panhypopituitarism, leads to increased insulin sensitivity and hypoglycemia during prolonged fasts. The prevalence of fasting hypoglycemia is approximately 20% in children with hypopituitarism. It is not seen in adults with isolated growth hormone deficiency, however. As noted previously, hypophysectomy, which leads to inadequate glucocorticoid as well as growth hormone secretion, results in increased insulin sensitivity, and therefore reduced insulin requirements.

Hypoglycemia and catecholamine deficiency: For many years epinephrine deficiency has been considered a possible cause of hypoglycemia in children. The so-called Zetterström syndrome is observed predominantly in male infants of low birthweight who do not increase their urinary catecholamine excretion in response to insulin-induced hypoglycemia.

Severe liver disease: Fasting hypoglycemia may result from insufficient liver glucose output following severe liver damage. Risk of hypoglycemia should be considered in patients with hepatitis (hepatitis fulminans), ingestion of various poisons (carbon tetrachloride, chloroform, benzene derivatives, *Amanita phalloides* toxin, hypoglycins, and others), primary carcinoma of the liver, or thrombosis of the subhepatic veins (Budd-Chiari syndrome).

Profound malnutrition: Extreme malnutrition leads to hypoglycemia. It is also found with relative frequency in kwashiorkor. In infants, hypoglycemia may result from acute or chronic diarrhea.

Prolonged exercise: During prolonged exercise, glucose turnover is markedly increased. If nutrient intake and carbohydrate stores are insufficient, hypoglycemia can develop.

Autoimmune insulin syndrome: Since the description of the first case of autoimmune insulin syndrome in 1970, more than 200 patients with this syndrome have been reported, mainly in Japan. At least one-third of the patients with the syndrome have been treated with a drug containing a sulfhydryl group, such as methimazole or penicillamine. Patients with the syndrome spontaneously develop antibodies against insulin, and hypoglycemia results from inappropriate release of insulin from insulin–antibody complexes. The affinity constant of the antibodies of patients with the autoimmune insulin syndrome is usually much smaller than that of insulin-treated diabetes.

Antibodies against the insulin receptor: Autoantibodies against the insulin receptor are usually observed in patients with acanthosis nigricans and associated insulin resistance. Hypoglycemia is attributed to an insulinomimetic action of the antibody.

Functional or transient hypoglycemia in infancy: Hypoglycemia at birth and in infancy has been comprehensively reviewed by Lteif and Schwenk. Many of the causes of neonatal or infant hypoglycemia have already been mentioned. Other causes of neonatal or infant hypoglycemia will be discussed briefly below.

Transient neonatal hypoglycemia: Transient neonatal hypoglycemia (during the first 3 days of life) can be observed in about 10% of live births, with 30% being symptomatic.

Infants of diabetic mothers: Infants of diabetic mothers frequently develop severe hypoglycemia during their first hours of life. It results from hyperinsulinemia caused by β-cell hyperplasia, which is induced by fetal hyperglycemia of maternal origin. Relative hypoglucagonemia may be a contributing factor.

Erythroblastosis fetalis: Hypoglycemia is frequently associated with erythroblastosis fetalis, a consequence of rhesus immunization. Islet cell hyperplasia leads to hyperinsulinemia and associated hypoglycemia.

Leucine-induced hypoglycemia: Certain infants develop hypoglycemia when given leucine or a leucine-containing food. Of note, cow's milk is richer in leucine than mother's milk. Excessive insulin response to leucine is characteristic of the syndrome, and relative basal hyperinsulinism is also observed when fasting hypoglycemia is present. Islet cell hypertrophy and hyperplasia are common. In most cases, symptoms are appreciated during the first 6 months of life. Severe mental retardation occurs if diagnosis is delayed.

Ketotic or ketogenic hypoglycemia: This form of childhood hypoglycemia is characterized by sporadic attacks of hypoglycemia and ketosis, occurring preferentially after food deprivation between the ages of 1 and 8 years, usually with spontaneous recovery before 10 years of age. Ketotic hypoglycemia is not a specific entity, but may represent a metabolic derangement in the presence of various biochemical abnormalities (e.g., disturbance of the gluconeogenic mechanism, due either to an enzymatic block or to diminished availability of substrate). In addition to the idiopathic form, ketotic or ketogenic hypoglycemia has been reported in fructose-1,6-diphosphatase deficiency, hypoalaninemia, growth hormone deficiency, adrenal medullary hyporesponsiveness, adrenal cortical insufficiency, branched-chain aminoacidemia, glucose-6-phosphatase deficiency, and amylo-1,6-glucosidase deficiency.

Maple syrup urine disease: Hypoglycemia is frequently encountered in patients with maple syrup urine disease. Its mechanism is still obscure, but usually clears with appropriate dietary treatment.

Adrenal hyporesponsiveness: Hypoglycemia with adrenal hyporesponsiveness is observed most frequently in small-for-date children born after a complicated pregnancy. The hypoglycemic attacks occur sporadically between 0.5 and 5 years of age, without pallor or perspiration. Insufficient rise in urinary epinephrine during hypoglycemia, often associated with insufficient cortisol rise, suggests dysfunction of the hypothalamic hypoglycemia center.

INVESTIGATION OF A PATIENT WITH POSSIBLE HYPOGLYCEMIA

Hypoglycemia should be suspected in all patients exhibiting the following signs and symptoms:

1. Presenting with the symptoms already noted (Table 11-1)
2. Seizures or episodic psychiatric syndromes
3. Coma of unknown origin

4. Stereotyped symptom patterns relative to similar or identical circumstances, such as in the fasting state, after muscular exercise, or a few hours after a meal
5. And, in any patient at risk of developing hypoglycemia (diabetic patients treated with insulin or sulfonylureas, alcoholics, etc.)

However, before a detailed investigation is conducted, hypoglycemia must always be confirmed by an accurate measurement of blood glucose concentration.

History

A complete history is essential in patients with a possible hypoglycemic disorder (Table 11-5). For example, if the symptoms occur after a meal, hypoglycemia is probably alimentary or reactive, whereas those occurring during fasting or after exercise suggest organic hypoglycemia.

In a patient suspected of an insulinoma, the history frequently reveals that hypoglycemic symptoms are precipitated by fasting or exercise and relieved by food or sugar ingestion. This situation is also encountered in patients with extrapancreatic tumor hypoglycemia. In these patients, however, the discovery of the tumor often precedes the symptoms of hypoglycemia. Symptoms occurring early after food ingestion suggest alimentary hypoglycemia, whereas symptoms occurring 90 minutes to 5 hours after a meal suggest reactive hypoglycemia. The content of drink mixtures and cocktails consumed will permit diagnosis of alcohol-promoted reactive hypoglycemia.

The interrogation of parents of infants presenting with hypoglycemia may lead to a diagnosis. For instance, symptoms occurring after ingestion of milk suggest leucine-induced hypoglycemia or galactose intolerance, whereas the abrupt occurrence of vomiting and hypoglycemia when a breastfed child is given his first drink of orange juice strongly suggests fructose intolerance. By definition, history is often misleading in factitious hypoglycemia.

In a patient suspected of an autoimmune insulin syndrome, previous intake of drugs containing sulfhydryl groups (e.g., methimazole, penicillamine) should be carefully probed.

Physical Examination

Certain observations made during a physical examination may suggest hypoglycemia. One should pay special attention to the following signs:

TABLE 11-5 Investigation of Hypoglycemia: Patient History

Nature, quantity, and timing of food ingestion
Nature and timing of symptoms
Type, intensity, and timing of physical activity
Timing of symptoms/symptom relief relative to other events (meals, fasting, exercise)
Ingestion of alcohol (quantity and timing)
Ingestion of drugs (specific questions about drugs that may increase the hypoglycemic activity of antidiabetic agents)
Use of insulin (dose, frequency, site of administration)
Use of oral antidiabetic agents (dose and timing of administration)

- Weight gain may occur in certain patients if hypoglycemic episodes are frequent; this has been reported in both organic (e.g., insulinoma) and functional (e.g., alimentary or reactive) hypoglycemia.
- Weight loss can be seen in hypoglycemia associated with nonpancreatic tumor as well as pituitary or adrenal insufficiency.
- Possible sites of subcutaneous or intramuscular injection should be sought in factitious, suicidal, or criminal hypoglycemia.
- Acanthosis nigricans may be present in patients presenting with hypoglycemia due to insulin receptor antibodies with insulinomimetic properties.
- Hepatomegaly is usually present in the Nadler-Wolfer-Elliott syndrome and in various hypoglycemias of childhood (e.g., galactosemia and types I, VI, IX, and X glycogenosis).
- Evidence of abdominal and thoracic masses should be sought in tumor-associated hypoglycemia.
- Psychoneurotic symptoms are frequently associated with reactive hypoglycemia.

Laboratory and Technical Investigations in Endogenous Hypoglycemia

Suspected Insulinoma

An insulinoma should be suspected in any patient presenting with the triad described by Whipple: symptomatic hypoglycemia, symptoms precipitated by fasting or exercise, and relief of symptoms by glucose. However, the cornerstone of the diagnosis is hyperinsulinism, in which endogenous plasma insulin levels are inappropriately high based on the prevailing blood glucose levels.

Basal plasma levels of glucose and insulin: Relative basal hyperinsulinism can often be demonstrated by the repeated (5–12 times) simultaneous determination of blood glucose and plasma insulin after an overnight fast. In normal individuals, fasting plasma glucose concentration is usually between 70 and 110 mg/dL (3.9–6.1 mmol/L), with plasma insulin concentrations usually ranging between 5 and 15 µU/mL. In obese individuals, basal plasma insulin is usually increased as a result of insulin resistance, and values up to 40–50 µU/mL have been reported.

Circulating levels of glucose, insulin, and C-peptide during a prolonged fast: A 24- to 48-hour fast in normal individuals is accompanied by a modest decline in blood glucose and a significant decline in plasma insulin and C-peptide. In patients with insulinoma, blood glucose declines markedly during fasting, while insulin and C-peptide plasma levels remain stable or decline only very moderately, resulting in relative hyperinsulinism. An insulin level >5 µU/mL and/or a C-peptide plasma level above 0.2 nmol/L at the end of a prolonged fast is highly suggestive of the presence of an insulinoma. In most patients with an insulinoma, symptomatic hypoglycemia will occur within 8–24 hours of food deprivation. In some, however, a formal extension of the fast for 72 hours may be necessary.

Insulin suppression tests: Suppression of endogenous insulin secretion by insulin-induced hypoglycemia is an elegant means to differentiate between insulin secretion under physiologic control and uncontrolled insulin release by tumor. In normal subjects, insulin-induced hypoglycemia results in >50% reduction of circulating C-peptide levels, indicating inhibition of endogenous insulin secretion. Such inhibition is not observed in 90% of insulinoma cases. Diazoxide infusion (600 mg over 1 hour in 500 mL saline) or oral (600 mg) administration tests can provide confirmation (i.e., showing suppression of insulin and a correction of fasting hypoglycemia). These tests may be useful in forecasting the effectiveness of chronic diazoxide therapy when surgical removal of the tumor cannot be realized. The intravenous somatostatin test has little value in the diagnosis of insulinoma.

Other determinations: In normal subjects, plasma proinsulin represents only 10–15% of total immunoreactive insulin. In 85% of patients with insulinoma, the proinsulin component is elevated (>25% of total fasting insulin immunoreactivity). Values up to 80% have been reported in malignant insulinomas. Plasma levels of glucagon and pancreatic polypeptide may be elevated, and low HbA$_{1c}$ levels have been reported in 25% of patients with insulinoma.

Localization of the tumor: The usually small size of insulinomas makes diagnosis by radiologic examination difficult. Selective arteriography via the celiac axis and the superior mesenteric artery localizes the tumor(s) in approximately 50% of cases. Tomodensitometry and ultrasonography help in the diagnosis of relatively large tumors (diameter >2–3 cm). Magnetic resonance imaging (MRI) using a high-gradient-power 0.5-T magnet has recently been shown to be very useful in the preoperative localization of insulinomas. Endoscopic ultrasound may also be helpful. Percutaneous transhepatic catheterization of the splenic and portal veins can be used for selective retrograde venous angiography and for selective blood sampling and subsequent insulin plasma measurements: higher plasma insulin levels are found in the vein or veins draining the tumor. Of note, there is more than one insulin-secreting tumor in about 10% of cases. In view of the performance of the combination of surgical operation and intraoperative ultrasonography, some now consider that preoperative localization of insulinomas is not necessary.

Suspected Non–islet Cell Tumor Hypoglycemia

Basal and fasting levels of glucose and insulin: As in patients with insulinoma, patients with non–islet cell large tumor hypoglycemic syndrome usually have low fasting blood glucose, and blood glucose falls continuously in a starvation test. In contrast to patients with insulinoma, insulin plasma levels are low and decrease to almost zero during fasting.

Dynamic tests: Insulin suppression and stimulation tests have little value. Insulin is usually markedly suppressed by the prevailing hypoglycemia. In provocative tests (with tolbutamide, glucagon, or leucine), the insulin response is usually low. In the OGTT, abnormal glucose tolerance with low insulin response is frequently observed. The glycemic response to glucagon is usually normal, indicating the persistence of significant amounts of glycogen stores.

Other determinations: IGF-II levels can be measured in rare malignancies when hypersecretion of this hormone is suspected to be responsible for the hypoglycemia.

Localization of the tumor: Most of these tumors are large or very large and are easy to localize on the basis of careful clinical examination, routine X-ray investigation (chest or abdominal roentgenogram), MRI, or ultrasonography.

Suspected Alimentary or Reactive Hypoglycemia

As stated earlier, it would be ideal to restrict the diagnosis of alimentary or reactive hypoglycemia to individuals in whom hypoglycemia can be demonstrated in blood samples taken in everyday life or after the typical meals that are said to induce the symptoms. For practical reasons, however, this is rarely the case, and the OGTT is still used routinely for the diagnosis of postprandial hypoglycemia.

The oral glucose tolerance test: In the OGTT, one or more blood glucose values below 45 mg/dL are found in these patients. The glucose nadir may occur early, at 90 or 120 minutes, and when this occurs it is usually preceded by an excessive early rise in alimentary hyperglycemia. In reactive hypoglycemia, the glucose nadir is usually found 3–5 hours after the ingestion of glucose. In the late phase of the OGTT, an unequivocal rise in cortisol, glucagon, and growth hormone occurs following the glucose nadir.

Investigation of gastric emptying: Rapid gastric emptying, the causative factor in alimentary hypoglycemia, can be demonstrated by X-ray or isotopic studies of the upper gastrointestinal tract.

Suspected Factitious Hypoglycemia

Surreptitious self-administration of insulin or sulfonylureas is difficult to detect and can lead to a false diagnosis of islet cell disease.

C-peptide measurements: The association of low blood glucose with high plasma insulin and low C-peptide levels strongly suggests exogenous administration of insulin, in contrast to endogenous insulin overproduction, in which low blood glucose and high plasma insulin levels are accompanied by normal or high C-peptide levels.

Detection of factitious hypoglycemia due to sulfonylurea ingestion: Clandestine ingestion of sulfonylurea compounds may mimic an insulinoma both clinically and biologically. Screening of plasma and urine for sulfonylurea compounds may establish the diagnosis.

Recognizing Hormone Deficiency as a Cause of Hypoglycemia

Routine endocrinologic investigations will easily confirm a suspected diagnosis of glucocorticoid or growth hormone deficiency, panhypopituitarism, and catecholamine deficiency. Apparently extremely rare, the syndrome of glucagon deficiency could be diagnosed on the basis of a lack of glucagon rise during an insulin tolerance test, as well as in response to an alanine or arginine intravenous infusion.

The insulin tolerance test is the most commonly used procedure for revealing a state of increased insulin sensitivity, as well as for measuring the responses of the various counterregulatory hormones. The test is performed after an overnight fast. Insulin is administered (0.1 U/kg body weight in adults and 4 U/m^2 in children), and multiple plasma samples are taken between 20 and 120 minutes after injection for measurements of ACTH, cortisol, and 18-OH desoxycorticosterone, adrenaline and noradrenaline, and growth hormone and glucagon. Urinary catecholamine excretion during the 3 hours following insulin administration gives an overall picture of the sympathicoadrenomedullary responsiveness, mainly in young children. In adults suspected of presenting with growth hormone or glucocorticoid deficiency, an initial test can be performed using 0.05 U/kg body weight of insulin to avoid severe hypoglycemia.

TREATMENT OF HYPOGLYCEMIA

Prevention of Hypoglycemia

In many circumstances, hypoglycemia is preventable. Among insulin-treated patients with diabetes, appropriate education is of paramount importance; they should know how to adjust their insulin regimen according to their daily needs, their food intake, and their physical activity. The use of continuous subcutaneous insulin infusion has been advocated in adolescents to lower the risk of severe hypoglycemia, improve metabolic control, and enhance coping. An appreciation of the pharmacologic interactions between many drugs and both insulin and oral antidiabetic agents will permit the necessary dosage adjustments when interfering compounds are prescribed simultaneously.

Alcohol-induced fasting hypoglycemia can be prevented by advising the patient to consume an adequate amount of carbohydrate within 6–36 hours of ingesting moderate or large amounts of alcohol. In patients suffering from alcohol-provoked reactive hypoglycemia, the incidence and severity of symptoms are reduced by decreasing the amount of sucrose (or glucose) ingested and by replacing it with either saccharin or fructose.

The administration of acetylsalicylic acid in children below the age of 2 years should be avoided; if used, the daily dose should not exceed 10–20 mg/kg body weight every 6 hours. One must be particularly cautious in dehydrated children. In children who are prone to ketotic hypoglycemia, attacks can be avoided by insisting on a nighttime carbohydrate-rich snack and consumption of frequent, small-to-moderate amounts of carbohydrate-rich foods, particularly during periods of mild illness.

Prevention of neonatal hypoglycemia requires the prenatal identification of infants at risk (e.g., infants of diabetic mothers; those suffering from erythroblastosis, who are small for dates, or preterm; smaller of twins). Measures to prevent hypoglycemia in at-risk infants include: reduce nonessential caloric expenditure, effect heat conservation by having the infant nursed in an appropriate thermal environment, and ensure adequate caloric intake through a regimen of early feeding. Specific dietary changes can prevent hypoglycemic attacks in patients with fructose intolerance (removal of sucrose, fruit, and fruit juices), galactosemia (galactose-free diet), and leucine-induced hypoglycemia.

Frequent feeding (every 2–3 hours) prevents severe hypoglycemia in type I glycogen storage disease; portacaval transposition gave promising results in a few cases. Hypoglycemia following TPN is prevented by starting an IV infusion of 10% glucose at the time of discontinuation and gradually decreasing the IV glucose load over 12 hours.

Management of Acute Hypoglycemia

When the patient remains conscious, ingestion of some form of sugar (soft drinks containing saccharose, sugar cubes, glucose tablets, or solution equivalent to 5–20 g of carbohydrate) is usually followed by rapid relief of symptoms. In the unconscious patient, intravenous injection of glucose should be given, approximately 0.5 g/kg body weight in children. In diabetics with severe hypoglycemia, glucose doses in the range of 25–50 mL of 30–50% solution should be given. Intravenous glucose should be maintained as long as necessary (possibly days in hypoglycemia due to long-acting sulfonylureas) until persistent euglycemia or slight hyperglycemia is present.

The symptoms of hypoglycemia will resolve almost immediately following intravenous glucose unless hypoglycemia has been sufficiently prolonged to induce organic changes in the brain. If a patient in a prolonged hypoglycemic coma remains unconscious despite blood glucose levels of about 200 mg/dL, blood glucose should be maintained at that level by a glucose drip to which 100 mg hydrocortisone should be added every 4 hours for the first 12 hours to minimize cerebral edema. In patients with type 1 diabetes, sufficient insulin should be given to prevent ketosis. Finally, rapid recovery of consciousness has been described in cases that are refractory to glucose and hydrocortisone following slow intravenous infusion of 200 mL of a 20% mannitol solution. The possible side effects of this treatment must be considered.

Intravenous, subcutaneous, or intramuscular glucagon (0.5–1.0 mg) can also be used to treat severe hypoglycemic reactions in insulin-treated diabetic patients. The patient will often become conscious within 5–20 minutes of glucagon administration; if not, a second dose may be given. Since glucagon is effective for only 1–1.5 hours, the patient should eat a snack or a meal (≥ 20 g of carbohydrates) immediately after regaining consciousness, to prevent hypoglycemia from recurring. Glucagon is less suitable for treating hypoglycemic attacks in sulfonylurea-treated patients, because hypoglycemia in this circumstance is prolonged.

Etiologic Management and Particular Cases

Insulinoma

Single benign adenomas are most common, and their removal by pancreatic surgery is the first and obvious choice of treatment. Preoperative localization of the tumor is recommended. The risk of the operation is related to the location of the tumor, being minimal with enucleation of the adenoma or distal pancreatic resection, and increasing if subtotal pancreatectomy, or particularly, pancreatoduodenectomy is performed. Laparoscopic excision has been reported. Medical management of a benign tumor is reserved for patients who refuse surgery or in whom major contraindications for the operation exist. In those cases, management will often include diet with frequent meals, diazoxide, which directly inhibits the release of insulin by β-cells and also has extrapancreatic hyperglycemic effects, and a thiazide diuretic. Diazoxide daily doses range from 150 to 600 mg; higher doses induce sodium retention and edema, which are counteracted by thiazides. In some cases of insulinoma, the anticonvulsant diphenylhydantoin (300–600 mg/day) has been used successfully to control refractory hypoglycemia.

Neonatal Hyperinsulinism Due to Nesidioblastosis

Initial treatment consists of glucose (up to 15–25 mg/kg/min), hydrocortisone (10 mg/kg/day), and diazoxide (20 mg/kg/day), as well as intermittent glucagon injections (0.1 mg/kg IM). If the situation is unstable with this therapy, removal of 75%, and sometimes, in a second operation, of 95–100%, of the pancreas may be necessary to prevent severe hypoglycemia and secondary mental retardation.

Autoimmune Insulin Syndrome

Drugs that accelerate the production of insulin antibodies include methimazole, thiopronin, glutathione, and penicillamine. Use of these drugs should be avoided in patients with autoimmune insulin syndrome because immediate recurrence of the syndrome has been reported after readministration of the incriminated drug.

Anti–Insulin Receptor Antibodies

Prognosis is poor in patients who present with fasting hypoglycemia due to insulin receptor antibodies having insulinomimetic properties. Remissions can be obtained by plasmapheresis, immunosuppression with alkylating agents, or glucocorticoid therapy.

Malignant Tumors

Streptozocin, in combination with fluorouracil or doxorubicin, is the most effective antitumor agent for treating metastatic malignant insulinoma, possibly after surgical reduction of the tumor mass and/or removal of liver metastases. Streptozocin causes selective destruction of the pancreatic β-cell, leading to control of hypoglycemia for many and a measurable decrease in tumor size in up to half of cases. Medical treatment often involves diazoxide and a thiazide diuretic, the doses required often being higher than for benign tumors. Other compounds capable of alleviating hypoglycemia include glucocorticoids, which increase gluconeogenesis and insulin resistance, and high doses of propranolol or chlorpromazine, which have reduced plasma insulin levels in a small number of patients. Some patients with malignant insulinoma can be improved with the somatostatin analog octreotide or by radiotherapy.

Alimentary and Reactive Hypoglycemia

Dietary changes are the first treatment of alimentary and reactive hypoglycemia. Simple sugars should be omitted and replaced by complex carbohydrates. Alcohol consumption should also be limited. If symptoms persist, small but frequent meals (usually six) with high-protein, low-carbohydrate content should be consumed. When dietary management is insufficient, dietary fiber or anticholinergic drugs (such as atropine or propantheline) or both can be used to decrease gastric emptying and the carbohydrate absorption rate. This is often necessary in patients who have undergone gastric surgery. Biguanides (such as metformin) may help some patients. In our experience the treatment of choice is acarbose, an α-glucosidase inhibitor that delays carbohydrate digestion and intestinal glucose absorption. With a dose of 50–100 mg at the beginning of the meal, acarbose significantly reduces postprandial hypoglycemia.

Leucine-Sensitive Hypoglycemia

The treatment of leucine-sensitive hypoglycemia consists of frequent feeding and a low-leucine diet. In some cases, it is necessary to prescribe diazoxide, at doses ranging between 5 and 10 mg/kg/day. Hirsutism may complicate long-term treatment with diazoxide.

ADDITIONAL READINGS

Bolli CB, Pampanelli S, Porcellati F, et al: Recovery and prevention of hypoglycaemia unawareness in type 1 diabetes mellitus. *Diabetes Nutr Metab* 2002;15(6):402.

Cryer PE: Hypoglycaemia: the limiting factor in the glycaemic management of type I and type II diabetes. *Diabetologia* 2002;45:937.

Cryer PE, Davis SN, Shamoon H: Hypoglycemia in diabetes. *Diabetes Care* 2003;26:1902.

Smith D, Amiel SA: Hypoglycaemia unawareness and the brain. *Diabetologia* 2002;45:949.

Yki-Jarvinen H: Strategies to prevent hypoglycaemia during insulin therapy in type 2 diabetes. *Diabetes Nutr Metab* 2002;15:411.

For a more detailed discussion of this topic and a bibliography, please see Porte *et al: Ellenberg & Rifkin's Diabetes Mellitus,* 6th ed., Chapter 58.

12 | The Oral Antidiabetic Agents

Sunder Mudaliar   Robert R. Henry

Three major pathophysiologic abnormalities are associated with type 2 diabetes mellitus (T2DM): impaired insulin secretion, excessive hepatic glucose output, and insulin resistance in skeletal muscle, liver, and adipose tissue. The treatment goals are the alleviation of symptoms through normalization of blood glucose levels and the prevention of acute and long-term complications. These goals can be achieved through pharmacologic and nonpharmacologic means. Nonpharmacologic measures include diabetes education and life-long diet management, exercise, and weight loss. Although diet and exercise remain the cornerstones of treatment, in the vast majority of patients with T2DM, pharmacologic agents are invariably needed to achieve optimal glycemic control and reduce the incidence of microvascular and possibly macrovascular complications, as shown in the United Kingdom Prospective Diabetes Study (UKPDS).

Four major classes of oral pharmacologic agents are available for treatment. They act as follows at the major sites of defects in T2DM: (1) by increasing insulin availability (the secretagogues, i.e., sulfonylureas and meglitinides); (2) by suppressing excessive hepatic glucose output (the biguanides, i.e., metformin); (3) by improving insulin sensitivity (thiazolidinediones or glitazones, i.e., rosiglitazone and pioglitazone); and finally (4) by delaying gastrointestinal glucose absorption (the α-glucosidase inhibitors acarbose and miglitol) (Fig. 12-1).The therapeutic objectives recommended by the American Diabetes Association (ADA) include fasting plasma glucose (FPG) of 90–130 mg/dL, peak postprandial plasma glucose < 180 mg/dL, and glycosylated hemoglobin (HbA$_{1c}$) < 7%[4] (Table 12-1). All of the above agents are effective as monotherapy in suitable patients and help to maintain optimal glycemic control in the initial stages. However, since T2DM is a progressive disease, over a period of time glycemic control inevitably deteriorates, and eventually combination oral therapy or (in many patients) insulin therapy will be needed to achieve optimal glycemic levels. This was clearly demonstrated in the UKPDS. Here we review the pharmacology, mode of action, and clinical applications of the various antidiabetic agents alone and in combination.

INSULIN SECRETAGOGUES

The insulin secretagogues have potent hypoglycemic effects through stimulation of insulin secretion from the pancreatic β-cell. This class of agents includes the sulfonylureas and the meglitinides.

Sulfonylureas

Sulfonylureas have been available for the treatment of T2DM since the 1950s. They continue to be used as initial pharmacologic therapy, particularly when hyperglycemia is pronounced and evidence of impaired insulin secretion is present. Furthermore, sulfonylureas are often the foundation of combination therapy because of their ability to increase or maintain insulin

167

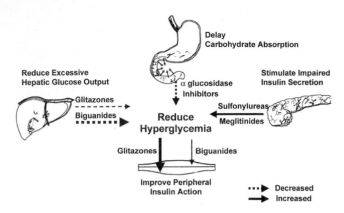

FIG. 12-1 The major sites of action of the various classes of oral antidiabetic agents.

secretion. They have a long history of use and few serious side effects (including hypoglycemia) and are relatively inexpensive. The major disadvantage is secondary failure, which may occur with all oral agents as a result of the progressive nature of T2DM. A list of the sulfonylureas is given in Table 12-2.

Mechanism of Action

The hypoglycemic action of the sulfonylureas is due to stimulation of ATP-dependent K^+ channels (K_{ATP} channels) in the pancreatic islet cells. When sulfonylureas bind to the receptors, they close these K_{ATP} channels. This results in a decrease in K^+ permeability of the β-cell membrane, depolarizes the membrane, and opens voltage-dependent Ca^{2+} channels, leading to an increase in intracellular calcium. The calcium ions bind to calmodulin, resulting in the exocytosis of insulin-containing secretory granules. Recently, it has been demonstrated that the K_{ATP} channel is a complex of a 140-kd sulfonylurea receptor (SUR) and an inward rectifier-channel protein (KIR 6.2). The K_{ATP} channels are also inhibited by glucose and other islet ATP-generating fuels. Incidentally, ATP-dependent K^+ channels binding sulfonylureas are also present in the myocardium, vascular smooth muscle, adipose tissue, and brain, in addition to the β-cell. The role of these receptors in vascular and cardiac tissue is discussed below; the significance of sulfonylurea binding in the brain remains to be defined.

TABLE 12-1 Goals for Glycemic Control

Biochemical index	Goal
Fasting/preprandial plasma glucose (mg/dL)	90–130
Peak postprandial plasma glucose (mg/dL)	<180
Glycosylated hemoglobin (%) (normal range 4–6)	<7

Source: American Diabetes Association: Clinical practice recommendations. *Diabetes Care* 2002;25(suppl1):S33.

TABLE 12-2 First- and Second-Generation Sulfonylurea Compounds

Name	Initial dose (mg/day)	Daily dose range (mg/day)	Recommended maximum daily dose (mg/day)	Doses/day
First generation				
Tolbutamide	500–1500	500–3000	3000	2–3
Chlorpropamide	100–250	100–500	500	1
Tolazamide	100–250	100–1000	1000	1–2
Acetohexamide	250–500	250–1500	1500	1–2
Second generation				
Glyburide	1.25–2.50	1.25–20	20	1–2
Micronized formulation	0.75–1.50	0.75–12	12	1
Glibenclamide	1.25–2.50	1.25–2.50	20	1–2
Glipizide	2.5–5	2.5–40	40	1–2
Glipizide XL	5	5–20	20	1
Gliclazide	40	40–320	320	1–2
Glimepiride	1–2	4–8	8	1

Pharmacokinetics

All the sulfonylureas are rapidly absorbed from the GI tract after oral administration. The pharmacokinetics and metabolism of the sulfonylureas are shown in Table 12-3. It is noteworthy that the half-life of chlorpropamide is very long, ranging from 25 to 60 hours, with a duration of action of 24–72 hours.

Clinical Use and Efficacy

Sulfonylureas have been used as oral hypoglycemic agents for approximately 50 years, and despite the availability of multiple classes of oral agents, these drugs continue to be used frequently as initial pharmacologic therapy. Furthermore, because of their ability to increase or maintain insulin secretion, these agents are often the foundation of combination therapy. The plasma glucose-lowering effect is slightly better in patients who have been recently diagnosed. Placebo-controlled studies have shown that sulfonylureas reduce FPG levels by about 54–72 mg/dL and HbA_{1c} levels by 1.5–2% in patients with long-standing T2DM.

Although similar in efficacy to first-generation agents (tolbutamide, chlorpropamide, tolazamide, and acetohexamide), second-generation sulfonylureas (glyburide, glipizide, and glimepiride) are more potent and lack some of the side effects seen with older agents. As a result, they have largely replaced first-generation agents in the clinical setting. Glimepiride is the most potent sulfonylurea on a per-milligram basis and appears to be as effective as other sulfonylureas in reducing glucose levels when administered at 1–8 mg daily.

Since they have potent insulin secretory effects, primary failure of sulfonylurea therapy is uncommon if patients are carefully selected. It is possible that some patients who fail sulfonylurea therapy have unrecognized type 1 diabetes mellitus (T1DM). When they are recognized, these patients should always be treated with insulin. Secondary failure of sulfonylurea therapy is also a major long-term therapeutic problem and seems to relate mainly to the natural history of T2DM and decreasing β-cell function. The incidence of secondary failure is also difficult to ascertain since its definition varies from study to study, but it is generally reported to range from 5% to 10% per year. There have been suggestions that the secondary failure of sulfonylureas may be due to exhaustion of the pancreatic β-cells. This hypothesis, however, has

TABLE 12-3 Metabolism of Sulfonylureas

Compound and date of introduction	Biologic plasma half-life (hours)	Duration of hypoglycemic action (hours)	Mode of metabolism	Activity of metabolites	Excreted in urine (%)
Tobutamide	4–6.5	6–10	Hepatic carboxylation	Inactive	100
Chlorpropamide	36	60	Hepatic hydroxylation or side chain cleavage	Active	80–90
Tolazamide	7	2–14	Hepatic metabolism	Three inactive Three weak	85
Acetohexamide	4–6	12–18	Hepatic reduction to 1-hydroxyhexamide	2.5 × original	60
Glyburide (glibenclamide)	4–11*	24	Hepatic metabolites	Mostly inactive	50
Glipizide	2.5–4.7	Up to 24	Hepatic metabolites	Inactive	50
Gliclazide	8–11	Up to 24	Hepatic metabolites	Probably Inactive	60–70
Glimepiride	5–9	24	Hepatic metabolites	Mildly active	60

*Micronized in 4 hours.

Source: Data from Gerich JE: Oral hypoglycemic agents. *N Engl J Med* 1989;321:1231; Zimmerman BR: Sulfonylureas. *Endocrinal Metab Clin No Am* 1997;26:511.

no evidence to support it. In the UKPDS, β-cell deterioration occurred at the same rate in diet-treated, metformin-treated, and sulfonylurea-treated patients. It appears difficult to identify clinical features predicting secondary failure to sulfonylureas. The primary predictive factor appears to be the duration of diabetes. Studies conducted to see whether a temporary reduction in hyperglycemia with insulin therapy restores the effectiveness of sulfonylurea therapy have not been successful. Patients who fail to achieve ADA target goals should be started on combination therapy with one of the other oral agents or begin insulin.

Extrapancreatic Effects

In addition to their effects on the pancreatic β-cells, the sulfonylureas possess extrapancreatic actions that are independent of their ability to improve glycemia. These effects have been studied both *in vitro* and *in vivo,* in animal and human studies, and include effects on insulin sensitivity, cardiac effects, and effects on lipids. In human studies, Beck-Nielsen and colleagues demonstrated that sulfonylurea treatment of obese patients with T2DM enhances insulin-stimulated peripheral glucose utilization in both adipose tissue and skeletal muscle, in part through a potentiation of insulin action on adipose tissue glucose transport and lipogenesis and skeletal muscle glycogen synthase. On the other hand, Prigeon and colleagues, in their study in 15 patients with T2DM, found that glyburide treatment did not have any effect on peripheral glucose uptake, as measured by the insulin sensitivity index. Recently, Shi and coworkers have demonstrated that human adipocytes express a sulfonylurea receptor (SUR1) that regulates intracellular calcium and controls lipogenesis and lipolysis.

Ever since the results of the University Group Diabetes Program (UGDP) study were published, there has been controversy regarding the potentially harmful cardiac effects of sulfonylureas. This is because the myocardium K_{ATP} channels mediate ischemic preconditioning, which is critical to myocardial protection and limitation of infarct size. Sulfonylurea binding to these channels has been shown to inhibit the response to ischemia, potentially delay the recovery of contractile function, and increase infarct size during a myocardial infarction. In a recent study, sulfonylurea therapy was associated with an increase of in-hospital mortality among patients undergoing direct angioplasty for myocardial infarction.

On the other hand, several studies have reported no link between long-term sulfonylurea use and increased mortality. The UKPDS clearly documented that long-term sulfonylurea therapy is not associated with increased cardiovascular morbidity or mortality. A recent study from the Mayo Clinic did not find increased long-term mortality over 8.4 years in a group of 102 T2DM patients treated with either insulin or sulfonylureas at the time of admission to hospital with an acute myocardial infarction.

To add further to the controversy, it is known that the prevention of K_{ATP} channel opening during ischemia reduces potassium efflux from myocardial cells and also reduces the occurrence of ventricular fibrillation during ischemia. Indeed, in a recent study in Europe, sulfonylurea therapy was actually associated with reduced postinfarct morbidity and mortality in patients with diabetes. It is also possible that the increased cardiovascular risk may not be a class effect of sulfonylureas. There is also a variable efficacy with which the various sulfonylurea drugs inhibit cardioprotective K_{ATP} channels. Thus, the interaction between sulfonylurea drugs and K_{ATP} channels during metabolic stress is complex, with various factors governing sulfonylurea-inhibitory gating of the channel. The net clinical effects of the seemingly opposing myocardial actions of sulfonylureas may not be deleterious. Whether some sulfonylureas (glipizide or glimepiride) are more beneficial for the cardiovascular consequences of T2DM remains to be determined.

Effects on Lipids

Unlike the insulin sensitizers, sulfonylurea treatment probably does not possess lipid-lowering effects other than that due to improved glycemic control.

Dosing

The initial starting dose of the sulfonylurea agent depends on the prevailing level of hyperglycemia. If the initial FPG is <200 mg/dL, sulfonylureas should be started at the lowest dose and titrated upward at weekly intervals so as to achieve an FPG of 90–130 mg/dL. If the initial FPG is >200 mg/dL, higher initial doses of sulfonylureas may be used. If a patient presents with marked symptoms and hyperglycemia, the sulfonylurea agent may be started at the highest dose and the patient followed up closely. Studies have shown that the sulfonylureas are better absorbed and are more effective if given about 30 minutes before a meal. This may, however, create a compliance problem for patients. For once-daily agents, the dose should be given with breakfast or the main meal of the day. In elderly adults, over 65 years, patients with hepatic disease, or other patients who may be more sensitive to hypoglycemic drugs, the lowest initial dose should be used and dose adjustments should be made more conservatively.

Some patients with T2DM being treated with insulin can be switched successfully to oral sulfonylurea therapy. For patients being treated with <20 U of insulin per day, a lower starting dose of the sulfonylurea once daily may be tried. For patients being treated with 20–40 U of insulin per day, a higher starting dose (half-maximal) may be tried. For patients being treated with >40 U of insulin per day, it is recommended that the daily insulin dose be decreased 50% and the sulfonylurea be initiated at half-maximal dose, although it would be unlikely that such a patient could be removed completely from insulin therapy.

Side Effects

Sulfonylurea antidiabetic agents are generally well tolerated and have a low incidence of side effects. Hypoglycemia is the most common side effect during sulfonylurea therapy and manifests as hunger, pallor, nausea/vomiting, fatigue, diaphoresis, headache, palpitations, numbness of the mouth, tingling in the fingers, tremors, muscle weakness, blurred vision, hypothermia, uncontrolled yawning, irritability, mental confusion, sinus tachycardia, shallow breathing, or loss of consciousness. Hypoglycemia can be a result of excessive dosage, but it also could be due to other factors such as improper diet or excessive physical activity. Sulfonylurea-induced hypoglycemia can be severe and requires immediate reevaluation and adjustment of both dosage and the patient's diet. The risk of hypoglycemia is also increased in the elderly and when there is poor nutrition, alcohol intake, gastrointestinal disease, or impaired renal function.

Other adverse sulfonylurea effects occur infrequently, typically during the first 6 weeks of therapy. Mild GI effects are common, whereas skin reactions and hematologic complications are rare. Patients often experience some weight gain with use of sulfonylureas.

Contraindications

Sulfonylurea use is contraindicated in pregnancy because there are no adequate human studies of effects on the fetus, although animal reproduction studies have shown some adverse fetal effects. If they are used at all, the decision to administer sulfonylurea drugs must weigh the potential risks to the fetus against the potential benefits to the mother. Because abnormal glucose concentrations are themselves a risk factor for congenital abnormalities, insulin is recommended to maintain blood glucose as close to normal as possible. However, in a recent study, Langer and coworkers demonstrated that adequate control could be obtained with significantly less hypoglycemia with glyburide as compared to insulin in women with gestational diabetes diagnosed after 11 weeks of pregnancy. More important, there was no evidence of any of the complications feared to result from fetal or neonatal hyperinsulinemia due to transplacental passage of the sulfonylurea drug, and glyburide was not detected in the cord serum of any infant, despite measurable serum concentrations in some of their mothers. However, this study does not permit us to draw firm conclusions about the teratogenicity of oral hypoglycemic drugs in early pregnancy (when organogenesis occurs). Also, since it is not known whether sulfonylureas are excreted in breast milk, it is recommended that sulfonylureas not be used in women who are breastfeeding, to avoid hypoglycemia in nursing infants.

Renal impairment or hepatic disease can cause elevations in sulfonylurea blood concentrations, and hepatic disease can also reduce gluconeogenic capacity; both problems increase the risk of hypoglycemia, and sulfonylureas should be administered carefully in these patients. Some sulfonylureas, such as chlorpropamide and acetohexamide, can exacerbate hepatic porphyria and should be used cautiously in patients with a history of this condition.

Elderly patients may be more susceptible to the hypoglycemic effects of sulfonylureas. Chlorpropamide can cause prolonged and serious hypoglycemia in the elderly, as well as Syndrome of Inappropriate Anti-diuretic Hormone (SIADH). Therefore, this medication is not recommended for use in the geriatric population. The use of sulfonylureas has not been studied systematically in children with T2DM.

Drug Interactions

Although drug interactions for the second-generation sulfonylureas (glyburide and glipizide) are theoretically less of a concern than for the first-generation agents, caution should be used if any of the following drugs are prescribed to patients receiving oral sulfonylureas because of the potential for protein-binding interactions and hypoglycemia: clofibrate, salicylates, NSAIDs, and sulfonamides. Also, the interaction between oral anticoagulants and oral sulfonylureas is complex, and it is wise for clinicians to monitor coagulation parameters closely when sulfonylureas and warfarin are used together.

Repaglinide

Repaglinide is a carbamoylmethyl benzoic acid (CMBA) derivative that belongs to a new class of antidiabetic agents, structurally related to meglitinides. Like the sulfonylureas, repaglinide is an insulin secretagogue, and its mechanism of action involves ATP-sensitive K^+ channels. Repaglinide is unique in that it has a rapid onset and short duration of action; when taken just before meals, it replicates physiologic insulin profiles. It has been shown to lower HbA_{1c} levels by 1.6–1.9%.

Mechanism of Action

Repaglinide binds a characterizable site on the β-cells in the pancreas and closes ATP-dependent potassium channels. The intracellular uptake of repaglinide is very limited; however, intracellular uptake is not required to stimulate insulin secretion. Repaglinide's activity is both dose-dependent and glucose-dependent. From *in vitro* studies utilizing mouse islet cells, it has been observed that repaglinide was more potent at stimulating insulin secretion than the oral sulfonylurea glyburide in the presence of moderate concentrations of glucose; however, in the absence of glucose, glyburide, but not repaglinide, stimulated insulin secretion. Although repaglinide and glyburide are equally potent as potassium channel blockers, the activity of repaglinide on the potassium channel diminishes as glucose concentrations rise from moderate to high. In addition, repaglinide does not mimic a second action of glyburide on calcium-dependent insulin exocytosis. This secondary action of glyburide may explain why glyburide is more potent than repaglinide at high glucose concentrations.

Pharmacokinetics

Repaglinide is administered orally and is rapidly and completely absorbed from the GI tract. The mean absolute bioavailability is 56%, and peak plasma levels are achieved within 1 hour of administration. Caution should be used in patients with impaired hepatic function, and longer dosing intervals should be used to assess the extent of glucose control accurately.

Clinical Use and Efficacy

In clinical studies in the United States, repaglinide at doses of up to 4 mg QID has been shown to reduce FPG levels by ~50 mg/dl and HbA1C by 1.9% as compared to placebo. In other studies, repaglinide was shown to provide glycemic control that was at least as effective and potentially safer than that provided by glyburide. In this 1-year study, repaglinide efficacy was sustained over 1 year, and although overall safety and changes in lipid profile and body weight were similar with both agents, weight-gain data for the subset of pharmacotherapy-naive patients suggested that patients on repaglinide gained less weight than those given glyburide. Thus, patients in this study using repaglinide received the same therapeutic benefits as those using glyburide and may have received additional benefits.

In addition to its efficacy when used as monotherapy, repaglinide is also useful as combination therapy. Several studies have documented that combination treatment with repaglinide and metformin or the thiazolidinediones provides superior glycemic control compared with monotherapy with either agent alone.

Since repaglinide is quickly absorbed and has a short half-life, it may be advantageous in subjects who are prone to delayed or missed meals. Indeed, results from one study suggest that treatment with repaglinide in well-controlled T2DM patients who miss or delay a meal is superior to treatment with longer-acting sulfonylurea drugs (such as glyburide) with respect to the risk of hypoglycemic episodes.

Dosage

Since repaglinide has a rapid and short-acting pharmacodynamic profile, it is most effective when given before meals. For treatment-naive patients or patients whose HbA_{1c} is <8%, therapy may be initiated with a dose of 0.5 mg (immediately before a meal or 15 or 30 minutes before eating) and, depending on the response (aiming at peak postprandial plasma glucose <180 mg/dL), increased to 2 mg before meals up to four times a day. For patients who have taken oral hypoglycemic agents and whose HbA_{1c} is >8%, a higher initial dose of 1 or 2 mg may be used before each meal. After each dose adjustment, at least 1 week should elapse to assess effectiveness. The maximum dose of repaglinide is 4 mg taken with every meal up to four times a day (total 16 mg in a 24-hour period). If a sulfonylurea agent is to be replaced by repaglinide, repaglinide should be started the day after the final dose of the other agent is given. Since overlapping effects are possible, close monitoring for hypoglycemia should be maintained for up to 1 week. If monotherapy alone fails to achieve glycemic goals, combination therapy with metformin or with glitazones may be initiated.

Patients with Hepatic Impairment

Repaglinide is metabolized mainly in the liver, and its clearance is significantly reduced in patients with hepatic impairment. Also, hepatic disease can reduce gluconeogenic capacity, and hence repaglinide should be administered carefully in these patients to avoid the risk of hypoglycemia.

Patients with Renal Impairment

Repaglinide is safe and well tolerated in subjects with varying degrees of renal impairment. Although adjustment of starting doses of repaglinide is not necessary for renal impairment or renal failure, severe impairment may require more care when upward adjustments of dosage are made. Hemodialysis does not significantly affect repaglinide clearance.

Contraindications/Cautions

Repaglinide is contraindicated only in patients with known hypersensitivity to the drug and in patients with type 1 diabetes, as it is not effective in the absence of functioning pancreatic β-cells. There are no adequate human studies regarding the effects of this drug on the fetus, and repaglinide is contraindicated in pregnancy, as are all other oral antidiabetic agents. It should also not be used in conjunction with another insulin secretagogue.

Side Effects

Since repaglinide is an insulin secretagogue like the sulfonylureas, hypoglycemia is the most common side effect. During clinical trials, hypoglycemic occurrences due to repaglinide tended to be lower (16%) than those caused by sulfonylureas (20%). Due to its short metabolic half-life, hypoglycemia is rarely prolonged.

Drug Interactions

Repaglinide is metabolized in the liver by the cytochrome P-450 enzyme CYP3A4. Drugs that are involved in the induction or suppression of this enzyme system may alter the expected hypoglycemic action of this agent. Highly protein-bound agents may also potentiate the hypoglycemic effects of repaglinide. These include β-blockers, chloramphenicol, monoamine oxidase inhibitors (MAOIs), NSAIDs, probenecid, salicylates, sulfonamides, and warfarin, which may lower serum glucose levels when used concomitantly with repaglinide. In a recent study, plasma repaglinide concentration at 7 hours was increased 28-fold by gemfibrozil and 70-fold by the combination of gemfibrozil and itraconazole ($p < 0.001$). Thus, gemfibrozil alone and in combination with itraconazole considerably enhances and prolongs the blood glucose-lowering effect of repaglinide. Concomitant use of gemfibrozil and repaglinide is best avoided. If the combination is considered necessary, repaglinide dosage should be greatly reduced and blood glucose concentrations monitored carefully.

Nateglinide

Nateglinide (a D-phenylalanine derivative), like repaglinide, exerts its glucose-lowering effect by stimulating insulin secretion. Also like repaglinide, nateglinide's pharmacokinetic features include rapid absorption and elimination. However, its unique faster kinetics may be explained by the relatively low binding affinity of the drug for the SUR receptor.

Pharmacokinetics

Nateglinide is administered orally in doses of 60–120 mg given 10 minutes before a meal. Absorption is rapid, with a mean absolute bioavailability of ~75%, and peak plasma levels are achieved within 1 hour. When nateglinide is administered immediately after a meal, a reduced rate of absorption (35% decrease in peak plasma levels, 22% increase in time to peak levels) is observed. Nateglinide undergoes limited first-pass hepatic metabolism.

Effects on Glycemia

In clinical studies, as compared to placebo, nateglinide 120 mg before meals reduces HbA_{1c} by 0.6–1%. It must be emphasized that the predominant effect of nateglinide is to decrease postprandial hyperglycemia. When used in combination with metformin, while nateglinide decreases mealtime glucose levels, metformin primarily affects fasting plasma glucose. In one study, while nateglinide and metformin monotherapy reduced HbA_{1c} by 1% and 1.3%, respectively (compared to placebo), the combination of metformin and nateglinide resulted in additive effects, with further decreases in HbA_{1c} of 1.4% and FPG of 43 mg/dL. Thus nateglinide and metformin monotherapy each improved overall glycemic control, but by different mechanisms.

Patients with Renal Impairment

Dosage adjustment is unnecessary in patients with mild to severe renal insufficiency.

Patients with Hepatic Impairment

Nateglinide is metabolized mainly in the liver, and its clearance is reduced in patients with hepatic impairment. Also, hepatic disease can reduce gluconeogenic capacity, and hence nateglinide should be administered carefully in these patients, to avoid the risk of hypoglycemia.

Contraindications/Cautions

Nateglinide is contraindicated in patients with a known hypersensitivity to the drug and also in patients with T1DM. Further, nateglinide should not be used in combination with another insulin secretagogue. Like all other oral antidiabetic agents, nateglinide is contraindicated in pregnancy.

Drug Interactions

There are no significant drug interactions with nateglinide.

BIGUANIDES

Phenformin and metformin are oral biguanide agents that were introduced for the treatment of T2DM in the late 1950s. Phenformin was withdrawn from clinical use in the late 1970s because of a substantial association with lactic acidosis. The risk for lactic acidosis is considerably lower with metformin. Metformin was used in many other countries and was finally approved for use in the United States in 1995 for the treatment of T2DM, either as monotherapy or in combination with sulfonylureas, α-glucosidase inhibitors, or insulin. Subsequently, it has also been approved for use in combination with rosiglitazone, pioglitazone, and repaglinide.

Mechanism of Action

Although its mechanism of action has not been clearly determined, decreased hepatic gluconeogenesis is thought to be the primary therapeutic effect of metformin in T2DM. In addition, metformin appears to improve utilization of glucose in skeletal muscle and adipose tissue by increasing cell-membrane glucose transport. Other mechanisms may include decreased intestinal glucose absorption; however, this has only been observed in animals. Metformin has no direct effects on insulin secretion and hence, in contrast to sulfonylureas, which have a hypoglycemic effect, metformin does not generally cause hypoglycemia when given alone. In clinical practice, metformin demonstrates more of an antihyperglycemic action than a hypoglycemic action. Unlike phenformin, metformin does not inhibit the mitochondrial oxidation of lactate unless plasma concentrations of metformin become excessive (i.e., in patients with renal failure) and/or hypoxia is present. Recently, it has been reported that metformin's beneficial effects in decreasing hepatic glucose production and increasing peripheral glucose utilization involve AMP-activated protein kinase (AMPK), which is a major cellular regulator of lipid and glucose metabolism. In this study, activation of AMPK in hepatocytes by metformin resulted in reduced acetyl-CoA carboxylase (ACC) activity with induction of fatty acid oxidation and suppressed expression of lipogenic enzymes.

Pharmacokinetics

The bioavailability of metformin is 50–60%. Food decreases the extent and slightly delays the absorption of metformin; however, it should be taken with meals. Metformin is not metabolized by the liver, which may explain why the risk of lactic acidosis is much less for metformin than for phenformin. Metformin is excreted by the kidneys, largely unchanged, through an active tubular process. The plasma half life is increased in patients with renal impairment.

Clinical Use and Efficacy

Metformin is approved for use as monotherapy and also in combination with sulfonylureas, repaglinide, nateglinide, α-glucosidase inhibitors, and thiazolidinediones. Several controlled clinical studies of metformin monotherapy have demonstrated significant reductions in both fasting blood glucose levels (60–70 mg/dL) and HbA_{1c} levels (1–2%) compared with placebo in patients who were poorly controlled by diet alone. The efficacy of metformin in reducing plasma glucose levels in a predominantly overweight population is comparable to that seen with sulfonylureas. Because of its potential to ameliorate insulin resistance, prevent weight gain, and improve lipid levels, metformin may be best suited for initial monotherapy in obese patients with more severe insulin resistance and dyslipidemia. When monotherapy alone does not result in acceptable glycemic control, metformin should be combined with a sulfonylurea and/or other oral antidiabetic oral agents. The antihyperglycemic action of metformin is additive to that of the sulfonylureas. In sulfonylurea-treated patients with T2DM who do not achieve optimal control or who experience secondary failure, it is important not to discontinue sulfonylurea therapy, but to add metformin. Discontinuation of sulfonylurea therapy and substitution of metformin will not decrease the FPG below that observed with sulfonylurea monotherapy alone. The sulfonylurea is continued with metformin to maintain its effect on pancreatic insulin secretion.

Effects on Insulin Sensitivity

Most studies have documented an increase of ~20–30% in insulin-mediated glucose uptake with metformin therapy. This increase in glucose uptake is due mainly to stimulation of nonoxidative glucose disposal (primarily glycogen synthesis). In metformin-treated patients with diabetes, both fasting and postprandial insulin levels decreased secondary to the normal compensatory response of the pancreas to lower prevailing glucose levels and enhance insulin sensitivity.

Effects on Weight

Unlike the insulin secretagogues and the thiazolidinediones, metformin therapy does not result in weight gain in patients with T2DM who receive metformin alone and minimizes weight gain when used in combination with other oral agents or insulin. Most studies show modest weight loss (2–3 kg) during the first 6 months of treatment. Metformin therapy is also associated with weight loss in nondiabetic subjects. The exact mechanisms by which metformin prevents weight gain or induces weight loss have not been determined, but several mechanisms have been postulated. These include a decrease in food consumption, an increase in energy expenditure, and a reduction of hyperinsulinemia. Some animal studies suggest an anorectic effect, but in human studies it has not been possible to differentiate between a central effect of metformin in decreasing calorie intake versus an increase in energy expenditure.

Effects on Lipids

In addition to its glycemic effects, metformin is known to have favorable effects on plasma lipids, in both diabetic and nondiabetic subjects. As monotherapy, metformin decreases plasma triglyceride and low-density lipoprotein (LDL)-cholesterol levels by 10–15% and also reduces postprandial hyperlipemia, plasma free fatty acid (FFA) levels, and FFA oxidation. The decrease in plasma triglyceride concentration is independent of changes in the plasma glucose level, because metformin reduces triglyceride levels in nondiabetic patients with hypertriglyceridemia. Metformin therapy does not appear to affect high-density lipoprotein (HDL)-cholesterol levels consistently, which either do not change or increase slightly after metformin therapy.

Effects on Other Cardiovascular Risk Factors

Insulin resistance is known to be associated with a hypercoagulable state and an increase in many cardiovascular risk factors, including plasminogen activator inhibitor 1 (PAI-1). Metformin has many beneficial effects on cardiovascular risk factors. Elevated PAI-1 levels are decreased with metformin therapy in patients with and without diabetes. In the French Biguanides and the Prevention of the Risk of Obesity (BIGPRO) 1 trial, metformin therapy also reduced tissue-type plasminogen activator (tPA) antigen and von Willebrand factor (vWF) levels. These two factors are secreted mainly by endothelial cells, and metformin therapy appeared to have suppressive effects on the production or metabolism of these two hemostatic proteins. In another 18-month study, metformin treatment in elderly T2DM patients was associated with significant reductions in markers of platelet function, thrombin generation, and fibrinolysis inhibition (PAI-1 activity, PAI-1 antigen). However, in this study, increases in some fibrinolytic activation markers (tPA and antithrombin (AT)-III; $p < 0.01$) were also observed.

Effects on Cardiovascular Disease

The long-term effects of metformin on serum lipids and other metabolic risk factors appear to have cardiovascular benefits. In the UKPDS, metformin therapy in obese, newly diagnosed patients with T2DM was associated with a significant decrease in cardiovascular and all-cause mortality. Whether this benefit with metformin treatment was due to the absence of weight gain or other beneficial effects on the metabolic syndrome of diabetes remains to be determined.

Effects on Polycystic Ovary Syndrome (PCOS)

Women with PCOS are characterized by chronic anovulation and infertility due to excessive androgen production. There is evidence to suggest that this hyperandrogenism may be secondary to insulin resistance and chronic hyperinsulinemia. Several, but not all, studies have shown that in patients with PCOS, metformin improves glucose tolerance and insulin sensitivity and also normalizes plasma sex hormone binding and free testosterone levels. In a recent study in 43 amenorrheic women with PCOS, metformin treatment for 6 months was found to reduce the endocrinopathy of PCOS and allow resumption of normal menses in most (91%) previously amenorrheic women with PCOS.

Dosing

Metformin should be taken with meals, and the starting dose (500 or 850 mg with breakfast or 500 mg with breakfast and dinner) and be increased slowly at weekly or biweekly intervals to minimize GI side effects.[6] Metformin lowers fasting plasma glucose and HbA$_{1c}$ in a dose-related manner, and although benefits are observed at lower doses, significant glycemic responses to metformin are usually seen at doses of approximately 1500 mg/day or greater. Data from one study suggest that most patients will achieve maximal efficacy at a daily dosage of 2000 mg (1000 mg bid), although some patients may achieve additional benefit if the dosage is increased to 2500 mg. The maximum daily dose of metformin is 2550 mg. Doses above 2000 mg daily may be better tolerated when given three times a day with meals. The glycemic goal should be an FPG between 80 and 120 mg/dL and $HbA_{1c} < 7\%$. If adequate glycemic control is not achieved with maximum doses of metformin ($HbA_{1c} > 8\%$), combination therapy should be considered.

Side Effects

Adverse GI effects are seen in at least 30% of patients taking metformin. These include anorexia, nausea/vomiting, abdominal discomfort, dyspepsia, flatulence, diarrhea, and metallic taste. These side effects tend to decline with continued use and can be minimized by initiating therapy with low doses of metformin. The risk of hypoglycemia is much less common with metformin than with the sulfonylureas. Hypoglycemia is more common when metformin is co-administered with other oral hypoglycemic agents, especially insulin secretagogues, or when there is deficient caloric intake or strenuous exercise not compensated by caloric supplementation. Asymptomatic vitamin B_{12} deficiency was reported with metformin monotherapy in 9% of patients during clinical trials. Serum folic acid concentrations did not decrease significantly. Weight loss may occur during therapy with metformin, perhaps as a result of its ability to cause anorexia. In contrast, sulfonylureas and insulin tend to cause weight gain. Up to 5% of patients cannot tolerate metformin and require discontinuation of this medication.

Contraindications/Cautions

Since metformin is largely eliminated unchanged in the urine via glomerular filtration and tubular secretion, it is contraindicated in patients with renal disease or renal impairment (serum creatinine >1.5 mg/dL in men and >1.4 mg/dL in women). In patients with reduced muscle mass, such as elderly patients (especially those older than 80 years of age), the serum creatinine concentration may underestimate the glomerular filtration rate, and creatinine clearance should be determined. If the creatinine clearance is <70 mL/min, metformin should not be given. Renal dysfunction also increases the risk of adverse reactions such as lactic acidosis from metformin. Lactic acidosis can also occur in patients predisposed to lactic acidosis, such as those with hepatic disease, cardiac disease (e.g., heart failure or acute myocardial infarction), severe infection, severe trauma, dehydration, severe burns, hyperosmolar nonketotic coma, major surgery, or alcoholism. Metformin is contraindicated in these patients.

Metformin should also not be used in diabetic patients with congestive heart failure requiring pharmacologic therapy because in this situation, decreased renal perfusion and glomerular filtration rate can impair metformin excretion. Metformin should also be withheld at the time of or prior to the performance of X-ray procedures involving intravenous radiographic contrast agents because of an increased risk of renal impairment and possible lactic acidosis. Metformin should be reinstituted only after renal function has been reevaluated after 48 hours and found to be normal.

The safety of metformin in pregnant and lactating women has not been established. Recently, metformin has received approval from the U.S. Food and Drug Administration (FDA) for use in adolescents with T2DM.

Drug Interactions

Metformin can also inhibit the absorption of cyanocobalamin (vitamin B_{12}) by competitively blocking the calcium-dependent binding of the intrinsic factor–vitamin B_{12} complex to its receptor. Patients should be monitored for possible development of anemia.

α-GLUCOSIDASE INHIBITORS

Two α-glucosidase inhibitors, acarbose and miglitol, are currently marketed in the United States. At recommended doses, both agents have only modest effects on HbA_{1c} levels (mean 0.5–1.0% reductions). α-Glucosidase inhibitors are suitable alternatives in patients with mild to moderate hyperglycemia (especially postprandial hyperglycemia) and, because of their relative safety, are often useful as monotherapy in elderly patients with mild T2DM. In addition, although it is not FDA-approved for T1DM, acarbose has been utilized as an adjunct to insulin therapy to reduce postprandial plasma glucose levels in these patients.

Mechanism of Action

Acarbose and miglitol are potent inhibitors of the α-glucosidase enzymes present in the brush border of the enterocytes located in the proximal portion of the small intestine. Clinically, this leads to delayed intraluminal production of monosaccharides (i.e., glucose), delayed and prolonged postprandial rises in plasma glucose, and a blunted plasma insulin response. When used as monotherapy, both agents do not enhance insulin secretion and in overdose will not result in hypoglycemia.

Pharmacokinetics

The two agents differ significantly in their rate of systemic absorption. Systemic absorption of active acarbose is only about 2%, whereas after oral administration of a 25-mg dose of miglitol, there is rapid and nearly complete systemic absorption of the drug. Low systemic absorption of acarbose is therapeutically desirable, since the drug acts locally in the GI tract. Acarbose is metabolized within the GI tract, and metabolism occurs principally by intestinal microbial flora, intestinal hydrolysis, and the activity of digestive enzymes. Plasma elimination half-life of acarbose is about 2 hours in healthy adults, and most of an oral dose (~51%) is excreted through the feces.

Unlike acarbose, miglitol is absorbed systemically via a jejunal transport mechanism similar to that of glucose absorption. Oral absorption of miglitol is saturable at high doses; only 50–70% of a 100-mg dose is absorbed systemically. There is no evidence at this time that systemic absorption is required for miglitol activity, but it appears that miglitol concentrates in intestinal enterocytes to exhibit its action locally in the GI tract. Unlike acarbose, miglitol is not metabolized in any way and is excreted unchanged by the kidneys. In patients with severe renal impairment (i.e., CrCl < 25mL/min), both acarbose and miglitol attain higher systemic peak and area-under-the-curve (AUC) concentrations than in patients with normal renal function. Thus, patients with renal failure are expected to accumulate both drugs to some degree. The pharmacokinetics of acarbose have not been studied in patients with cirrhosis. Because miglitol is not metabolized by the liver, the pharmacokinetics in patients with cirrhosis are not altered. For both drugs, no significant differences in pharmacokinetics have been observed based on age, race, or gender.

Clinical Use and Efficacy

Acarbose is approved for use as monotherapy or in combination with insulin, metformin, or sulfonylureas. Miglitol is approved only for use as monotherapy and in combination with sulfonylureas. To be maximally effective, both drugs must be administered at the start of a main meal. This is because they are competitive inhibitors and must be present at the site of enzymatic action at the same time the carbohydrates are present in the small intestine. Taking the medication before or more than 15 minutes after the start of the meal reduces the impact of the medication on postprandial blood glucose. Also, to be clinically effective, the patient must be consuming a diet that is high in complex carbohydrates (roughly ≥ 50% of calories), since the glycemic response to acarbose and miglitol is dependent on the carbohydrate content of the diet. Several randomized, double-blind, placebo-controlled trials have demonstrated that the addition of acarbose or miglitol to diet therapy significantly reduces postprandial glucose and HbA_{1c} levels compared with placebo. Monotherapy with these agents lowers mean postprandial glucose levels by ~40–60 mg/dL and mean fasting glucose levels by 10–20 mg/dL; overall, mean HbA_{1c} levels are reduced 0.5–1.0%.

In combination therapy with sulfonylureas, metformin, and insulin, acarbose further reduces mean HbA_{1c} between 0.3% and 0.5% and mean postprandial glucose between 25 and 30 mg/dL from baseline. Miglitol in combination therapy with sulfonylureas reduces mean HbA_{1c} by 0.7% and mean 1-hour postprandial glucose by ~60–70 mg/dL. Compared with sulfonylureas or metformin, acarbose and miglitol possess less potent effects on fasting glucose and are typically reserved for use as monotherapy in patients with mild to moderate hyperglycemia, particularly postprandial hyperglycemia. In addition, the absence of hypoglycemia with these agents when used as monotherapy makes them particularly useful and relatively safe in elderly T2DM patients.

Effects in Reactive Hypoglycemia and the Dumping Syndrome

α-Glucosidase inhibitors appear to have beneficial effects in people with reactive hypoglycemia and those with the dumping syndrome. In one study of 21 nonobese patients (6 males, 15 females) with reactive hypoglycemia, acarbose treatment for 3 months blunted post-OGTT increases in insulin and C-peptide levels and reduced the frequency of hypoglycemic attacks from four times a week to one. Similar beneficial effects were reported in another study.

Effects on Weight

Due to polysaccharide metabolism by colonic microflora and the capacity of the large bowel to conserve calories, there is minimal calorie loss associated with acarbose and miglitol therapy. Weight loss, if it occurs, is typically mild (i.e., 0.8–1.4 kg over 1 year in clinical studies). In humans, acarbose and miglitol also appear to offset the insulinotropic effects and weight gain associated with sulfonylurea treatment when they are added to combination therapy. The exact metabolic or pharmacologic mechanism(s) responsible for α-glucosidase–induced weight loss remains unknown.

Effects on Lipids

In some studies, α-glucosidase inhibitors are associated with decreases in triglyceride levels. There is also evidence that acarbose may reduce triglyceride levels in nondiabetics, and the drug may be a useful adjunct to dietary therapy in nondiabetic patients affected by severe hypertriglyceridemia.

Dosage

Acarbose and miglitol are administered with the first bite of each main meal. If patients do not have oral dietary intake, they should not take these agents. To minimize GI side effects, both acarbose and miglitol should be started at 25 mg PO, three times per day, taken with the first bite of each main meal. To reduce GI side effects further, some patients may benefit from an initial dose of 25 mg PO once daily for 1 week, titrated up as tolerated to 25 mg PO three times per day. After 4–8 weeks of the 25-mg-PO, three-times-daily dose, the dosage may be increased if needed to 50 mg PO three times daily. One-hour postprandial glucose levels throughout treatment and an HbA_{1c} level at 3 months should be used to determine response to therapy. If at 3 months the HbA_{1c} level is not satisfactory, the dose may be titrated to the maximum recommended dose of 100 mg PO three times per day. The usual maintenance dose range is 50–100 mg PO three times per day. One-hour postprandial glucose levels should be used to determine response to therapy and to titrate dose. In adults weighing <60 kg, the maximum recommended dose of acarbose is 50 mg TID. Patients who do not respond to monotherapy should be changed to another form of therapy or considered for oral combination therapy in order to achieve optimal glycemic goals.

Patients with Renal Impairment

There is no experience with either acarbose or miglitol in patients with serum creatinine > 2 mg/dL, and treatment of these patients with acarbose or miglitol is not recommended.

Contraindications

Acarbose and miglitol are contraindicated in patients with inflammatory bowel disease, colonic ulceration, ileus, partial or predisposition to GI obstruction, or GI disease involving disorders of absorption or digestion. If a patient has poor oral intake, continual vomiting, or diarrhea, acarbose and miglitol therapy should be withheld until adequate oral dietary intake resumes. Since miglitol elimination is dependent on glomerular filtration, the drug may accumulate in patients with renal impairment. Hence the drug should not be used in patients with CrCl < 25 mL/min or serum creatinine > 2.0 mg/dL. Acarbose is contraindicated for use in patients with cirrhosis. If hepatic enzyme elevations occur during acarbose therapy, dose reduction or discontinuation of acarbose may be necessary, particularly if such elevations persist. However, there are two studies whose results document the good tolerability and efficacy of acarbose therapy in patients with chronic liver disease.

Acarbose and miglitol have not been studied in pregnancy and should not be used in pregnant or lactating women.

Side Effects

Hypoglycemia

When used as monotherapy, acarbose and miglitol do not cause hypoglycemia. However, when these agents are used in combination with insulin or other insulin secretagogues (sulfonylureas or repaglinide), hypoglycemia may occur. It is important to remember that this hypoglycemia associated with the use of acarbose or miglitol plus insulin or an insulin secretagogue should be treated with oral glucose (dextrose) and not sucrose or other complex carbohydrates, which may be ineffective. The hydrolysis of sucrose (cane sugar) to fructose and glucose is inhibited by acarbose, and thus products containing sucrose are unsuitable for the rapid correction of hypoglycemia. Patients should be aware of the need to have a readily available source of glucose (dextrose, d-glucose) to treat hypoglycemic episodes.

Gastrointestinal

The most common adverse reactions to acarbose and miglitol are gastrointestinal in nature, including abdominal discomfort, increased flatulence, and diarrhea. These symptoms occur with the highest incidence during initiation of therapy and abate or decrease in intensity with continued use. At least 50–60% of patients receiving acarbose and miglitol experience the above adverse GI reactions, which are caused primarily by an increase in gas formation secondary to fermentation of unabsorbed carbohydrate in the large intestine. In clinical trials, the use of antacids or fibrous substances to modify the adverse GI side effects of acarbose has not been successful. Proper dosage titration, however, may help improve patient tolerance of GI-related adverse events (see Dosage above).

Systemic adverse events with acarbose are relatively rare. In one U.S. study, asymptomatic elevations of hepatic enzymes occurred in 3.8% of patients receiving acarbose versus 0.9% of those receiving placebo. Serum transaminase elevations appear to be dose-related, with an increased frequency in those on >300 mg/day.

Drug Interactions

Digestive enzyme preparations containing carbohydrate-splitting enzymes (e.g., amylase, pancreatin, and pancrelipase) may reduce the pharmacologic effect of α-glucosidase inhibitors (e.g., acarbose or miglitol) and should not be administered concurrently. It is also possible that concomitant administration of acarbose or miglitol with bile acid sequestrants, such as cholestyramine or colestipol, may decrease the effects of these antidiabetic agents. Also, oral neomycin may eliminate gut bacteria responsible for metabolism of carbohydrates and therefore enhance the reduction in postprandial glucose as well as exacerbate GI adverse effects. Clinical documentation of such interactions, however, is lacking. Antacids are not known to affect acarbose action.

α-Glucosidase inhibitors may impair the oral absorption of digoxin and lead to subtherapeutic serum digoxin concentrations in some patients. It is recommended that these agents be administered 6 hours after an oral digoxin dose to ensure time for adequate digoxin absorption. In addition, patients should be closely observed for the loss of clinical effect of digoxin therapy if either acarbose or miglitol is added to the medication regimen. In some cases, digoxin serum concentration monitoring may be helpful. Caution should also be exercised in patients on concomitant warfarin therapy, and prothrombin times should be closely observed during the first month of acarbose and miglitol therapy.

The combination of acarbose with acetaminophen and ethanol should be avoided, since both alcohol and acarbose augment the activity of the hepatic isoenzyme CYP2E1, which is responsible for metabolism of acetaminophen to a toxic reactive metabolite.

THIAZOLIDINEDIONES

The thiazolidinediones or glitazones are oral antidiabetic agents that are also termed *insulin sensitizers;* they act primarily by reducing insulin resistance, which is thought to be central to the development of T2DM and its cardiovascular complications. These agents are chemically and functionally unrelated to the other oral antidiabetic agents. Two compounds in this class are presently approved for use in the United States: rosiglitazone and pioglitazone. The first agent in this class, troglitazone, was marketed in the United States from March 1997 until it was withdrawn in March 2000, when the FDA determined that the risk of idiosyncratic hepatotoxicity associated with troglitazone therapy outweighed its potential benefits. In clinical use so far, rosiglitazone and pioglitazone appear to be devoid of fulminant hepatotoxicity. Monotherapy with the glitazones results in significant improvements in FPG by 59–80 mg/dL and in HbA_{1c} by 1.4–2.6% compared with placebo. Rosiglitazone and pioglitazone are approved for use as monotherapy and also in combination with insulin, metformin, or secretagogues.

Mechanism of Action

The thiazolidinediones are highly selective and potent agonists for the peroxisome proliferator-activated receptor γ (PPARγ). PPARγ receptors are found in key target tissues for insulin action such as adipose tissue, skeletal muscle, and liver, and evidence to date indicates that these receptors may be important regulators of lipid homeostasis, adipocyte differentiation, and insulin action. A close relationship has been shown to exist between the ability of various thiazolidinediones to stimulate PPARγ and its antidiabetic action.

The thiazolidinediones have been shown to stimulate the expression of several proteins which improve insulin sensitivity and improve glycemia, such as GLUT-1, GLUT-4, p85 α-phosphatidylinositol 3-kinase (p85αPI-3K) and uncoupling protein-2 (UCP). In addition, the glitazones also interfere with expression and release of mediators of insulin resistance, such as tumor necrosis factor-α (TNF-α), leptin, etc. The hypotensive and antiatherosclerotic effects of the glitazones may also occur through PPARγ agonism. Pharmacologic activation of PPARγ with the glitazones inhibits vascular smooth muscle cell proliferation and migration, with the potential to limit restenosis and atherosclerosis. Recently, great attention has been focused on adiponectin, which is a fat-derived hormone with antidiabetic and antiatherogenic properties. Hypoadiponectinemia seen in obesity is associated with insulin-resistant diabetes and atherosclerosis and several workers have shown that the thiazolidinediones increase plasma adiponectin levels by the transcriptional induction in adipose tissues. Recent studies have also shown that adiponectin increases insulin sensitivity by increasing tissue fat oxidation, resulting in reduced circulating fatty acid levels and reduced intracellular triglyceride contents in liver and muscle. Adiponectin also suppresses the expression of adhesion molecules in vascular endothelial cells and cytokine production from macrophages, thus inhibiting the inflammatory processes that occur during the early phases of atherosclerosis. Thus, the thiazolidinediones act, at least in part, by binding with PPARγ in various tissues to influence the expression of a number of genes encoding proteins involved in glucose and lipid metabolism, endothelial function, and atherogenesis.

Pharmacokinetics

After oral administration, both rosiglitazone and pioglitazone are rapidly absorbed, and peak serum concentrations occur within 1 hour for rosiglitazone and within 2 hours for pioglitazone. Food does not alter the pharmacokinetics of rosiglitazone, but it slightly delays the time to peak serum concentration of pioglitazone to 3–4 hours, although total absorption is unchanged. Steady-state serum concentrations of both drugs are achieved within 7 days and are highly protein-bound (>99%), primarily to serum albumin. Rosiglitazone is extensively metabolized, with no unchanged drug detected in urine. Metabolites are active but have significantly less activity than the parent compound. On the other hand, pioglitazone is extensively metabolized by hydroxylation and oxidation. The plasma half-life ranges from 3 to 4 hours for rosiglitazone and from 3 to 7 hours for pioglitazone and 16 to 24 hours for pioglitazone metabolites.

Clinical Use and Efficacy

Both rosiglitazone and pioglitazone are at present approved for use as monotherapy and in combination with metformin, secretagogues, and insulin. In clinical studies, rosiglitazone at doses of 4 and 8 mg/day (as a single daily dose or two divided daily doses) improved FPG by up to 55 mg/dL and HbA$_{1c}$ by up to 1.5% as compared with placebo. In these studies, when administered at the same daily dose, rosiglitazone was generally more effective in reducing FPG and HbA$_{1c}$ when administered in divided doses twice daily compared with once-daily doses. However, for HbA$_{1c}$, the difference between the 4-mg once-daily and the 2-mg twice-daily doses was not statistically significant. In another U.S. study, when compared directly with maximum stable doses of glyburide, rosiglitazone reduced FPG by 25 mg/dL (4 mg/day) and 41 mg/dL (8 mg/day), compared with a reduction of 30 mg/dL for glyburide (15 mg/day). Although the initial fall in FPG was greater with glyburide in this study, the improvement in glycemic control with rosiglitazone was maintained through week 52 of the study. The addition of 2–8 mg/day of rosiglitazone to existing sulfonylurea, metformin, or insulin therapy also achieves further reductions in FPG and HbA$_{1c}$ by ~50 mg/dL and ~1–1.3%.

The other currently marketed thiazolidinedione, pioglitazone, also possesses glucose-lowering properties similar to rosiglitazone when used as monotherapy and combination therapy in doses up to 45 mg once daily. In the absence of head-to-head studies, it is not possible to evaluate which glitazone is more potent in clinical use.

Other Beneficial Effects

The glitazones have been shown to have multiple beneficial effects not only on peripheral insulin sensitivity, hepatic glucose metabolism, and lipid metabolism, but also on endothelial function, atherogenesis, fibrinolysis, and ovarian steroidogenesis.

Effects on Insulin Sensitivity

Insulin resistance is a hallmark of type 2 diabetes, and in keeping with their role as insulin sensitizers, the thiazolidinediones, in addition to lowering blood glucose, also improve insulin sensitivity. Using the hyperinsulinemic, euglycemic clamp technique, several workers have demonstrated significant improvements in hepatic and muscle insulin sensitivity with both rosiglitazone and pioglitazone despite increases in body weight and adiposity. Although both metformin and the glitazones are classified as insulin sensitizers, in head-to-head studies, glitazone use is associated with more pronounced improvements in indicators of insulin sensitivity.

Effects on Lipids

In T2DM, the major quantitative change in lipid levels is an elevation in triglyceride-rich lipoproteins, a decrease in HDL cholesterol concentrations, and qualitative changes in the composition of the LDL molecule (including an increase in the proportion of small, dense LDL, which is prone to glycation and oxidation and which has the potential to make it more atherogenic). This diabetic dyslipidemic profile is closely related to underlying insulin resistance and may be partly responsible for the increased cardiovascular morbidity and mortality in T2DM patients. By improving glucose tolerance and reducing insulin resistance, the glitazones have the potential to influence diabetic dyslipidemia favorably. In a recent randomized, placebo-controlled study, pioglitazone at 30 and 45 mg daily reduced triglycerides by 5% and16% and increased HDL levels by 16 and 20%, respectively. In the case of rosiglitazone, however, despite a significant decrease in FFA levels by up to 22%, initial studies demonstrated no significant lowering of triglycerides, although HDL levels do increase by up to 19%. The reasons for these differences are not clear at present. In the absence of head-to-head studies, it is not possible to say whether the differences seen in the clinical studies are due to differences in the intrinsic properties of the drugs themselves or due to differences in the study population. In addition, although in most of the studies with the glitazones so far there is an approximately 10–15% increase in LDL-cholesterol levels, this concern is offset by the fact that studies have established that, following glitazone treatment, the LDL particles become larger and more buoyant. Also of note is the fact that recent reports document a small but significant increase in lipoprotein (a) [Lp(a)] levels with glitazone treatment. Since Lp(a) may be associated with the development of coronary artery disease, further larger, long-term studies are needed to assess the impact of glitazone therapy on atherosclerosis and cardiovascular mortality. In the short term, however, glitazone treatment has been associated with improvement in surrogate markers of atherosclerosis such as carotid intimal media thickness and coronary restenosis as assessed by intravascular ultrasound (discussed below).

Effects on Adipose Tissue

Glitazone use is associated with an increase in adipogenesis and in some patients an increase in body weight. Thus, it appears paradoxical that, on the one hand, the thiazolidinediones, as PPARγ agonists, increase adipogenesis, which leads to an increase in body fat and body weight and potentially worse insulin sensitivity, while on the other hand, clinical use of these agents results in significant improvements in insulin sensitivity and glucose tolerance. There are several possible mechanisms by which this paradox might be explained. At the tissue level, the glitazones have been demonstrated to specifically promote the differentiation of preadipocytes into adipocytes only in subcutaneous, not in omental fat. In clinical studies also, glitazone treatment results in a shift of fat distribution from visceral to subcutaneous adipose depots. In studies with rosiglitazone, there was also a significant decrease in hepatic and skeletal muscle triglyceride content as measured by MRI analysis. Thus it is possible that the reduction in visceral adipocytes leads to lower levels of molecules which promote insulin resistance like TNF-α and leptin and the increase in the size of the more metabolically active SQ adipose tissue leads to lower plasma fatty acid concentrations and a redistribution of intracellular lipid from insulin-responsive organs (such as the liver and muscle) into peripheral adipocytes.

Hypertension and Cardiac Function

The prevalence of hypertension in diabetic patients is 1.5–2-fold higher than in nondiabetic individuals, and hypertension is one of the components of the insulin-resistance syndrome. In T2DM and other insulin-resistant states, there is impaired insulin-induced vasodilation, and it is possible that by enhancing insulin action, the thiazolidinediones may enhance the tonic vasodilator response to insulin and thereby reduce peripheral vascular resistance and blood pressure. Additionally, by reducing hyperinsulinemia and plasma insulin levels, these agents may reduce the potential blood pressure-raising actions of insulin, such as renal sodium retention and increased sympathetic activity. Data are now accumulating that the glitazones have modest beneficial effects on both systolic and diastolic blood pressure.

Effects on Atherogenesis

Patients with diabetes mellitus have an increased risk of developing extensive atherosclerosis and premature coronary artery disease. During plaque development, vascular cells, such as monocytes/macrophages, T-cells, endothelial cells, and vascular smooth muscle cells, release inflammatory mediators such as cytokines, including interleukin-6 (IL-6), tumor necrosis factor-α, soluble adhesion molecules, and downstream acute-phase reactants such as C-reactive protein (CRP), all of which orchestrate an ongoing inflammatory response in the vessel wall. In addition to these chemokines, matrix-degrading matrix metalloproteinases (MMPs), such as MMP-2, -8, and -9, have also been implicated in plaque rupture. Recent experimental data suggest that the thiazolidinediones exhibit potent anti-inflammatory properties in the vessel wall. In addition, in preliminary clinical studies, the glitazones have been shown to decrease carotid intimal medial thickness and also coronary intimal hyperplasia in patients with and without coronary stents. This effect of the glitazones, if shown to persist in the long term, could be highly beneficial, delaying or preventing development of the accelerated atherosclerosis of diabetes.

Effects on β-Cell Function

Along with insulin resistance, β-cell dysfunction is one of the cardinal features of type 2 diabetes. The thiazolidinediones, in addition to being insulin sensitizers, also have favorable effects on the β-cells. In one study, although 3 months of rosiglitazone treatment in patients with type 2 diabetes did not alter insulin secretory capacity (as assessed by a panel of different β-cell tests), rosiglitazone therapy did improve the ability of the β-cell to sense and respond to changes in glucose concentrations, suggesting a protective role of rosiglitazone treatment on the β-cell, either via improved metabolic control or through direct drug actions. In another study, treatment with troglitazone delayed or prevented the onset of type 2 diabetes in high-risk Hispanic women with a history of gestational diabetes. This protective effect was associated with the preservation of pancreatic β-cell function and appeared to be mediated by a reduction in the secretory demands placed on β-cells by chronic insulin resistance.

Dosage

The usual starting dose of rosiglitazone is 4 mg PO given as either a single dose once daily or in divided doses twice daily. For patients who respond inadequately after 12 weeks of initial treatment with rosiglitazone, the dose may be increased to 8 mg PO given as a single dose once daily or in divided doses twice daily. For pioglitazone, therapy may be initiated at 15 or 30 mg PO once daily. For patients who respond inadequately to the initial dose, the dose can be increased in increments up to 45 mg PO once daily. Patients who do not respond adequately to monotherapy with either rosiglitazone and pioglitazone should be considered for combination therapy with other antidiabetic agents. The safety and efficacy of both drugs in adolescents and children have not yet been established.

Patients with Hepatic Impairment

If a patient exhibits clinical or laboratory evidence of active liver disease or increased serum transaminase levels (ALT > 2.5 times the upper limit of normal) at start of therapy, rosiglitazone or pioglitazone therapy should not be initiated (see Contraindications below).

Patients with Renal Impairment

There are no clinically relevant differences in the pharmacokinetics of rosiglitazone or pioglitazone in patients with mild to severe renal impairment or in hemodialysis-dependent patients compared with patients who have normal renal function. Hence dosage adjustments are not required in patients receiving these agents alone. However, since metformin is contraindicated in patients with renal impairment, concomitant administration of rosiglitazone or pioglitazone with metformin is also contraindicated in patients with renal impairment.

Side Effects

The glitazones increase plasma volume by 6–7%, and edema is often associated with their use. From the available evidence, it appears that edema is a class effect of the thiazolidinediones and is multifactorial in origin. The incidence of edema in U.S. clinical trials varied from about 3% to 7.5% with the thiazolidinediones compared to 1–2.2% with placebo or other antidiabetic agents. Of note, the highest incidence of edema has been reported when the thiazolidinediones are used in combination with insulin. In clinical studies, these patients have an incidence of edema of 15.3% when treated with insulin plus pioglitazone and 14.7% when treated with insulin plus rosiglitazone, compared to 7.0% and 5.4% in the insulin-plus-placebo–treated patients, respectively. In addition to peripheral edema, there have also been anecdotal reports of pulmonary edema associated with the thiazolidinedione agents. Hence, therapy with the glitazones should be initiated at low doses and patients should be evaluated early for edema and also for congestive heart failure in the first few weeks. Caution should be exercised when using thiazolidinediones in those at risk for or with a history of heart failure and in those with New York Heart Association (NYHA) Class I and Class II heart failure. At present, these agents should not be used in patients with NYHA Class III and Class IV heart failure. Management of pedal or generalized edema may vary depending on individual patient characteristics and is best determined by the treating clinician. Options include dose reduction, drug discontinuation, and symptomatic therapy with diuretics. Further studies are clearly needed to elucidate the mechanism(s) responsible for the causation of edema in patients with type 2 diabetes treated with thiazolidinediones, and to determine if it is possible to predict those patients susceptible to development of edema, and especially congestive heart failure.

Weight gain in a dose-related manner has also been reported more frequently with glitazone therapy. Both rosiglitazone and pioglitazone treatment are associated with weight gain, whether these agents are used as monotherapy or in combination therapy. Of note, the weight gain is blunted when metformin is used in combination with glitazones, and there is increased weight gain when glitazones are used in combination with insulin. In U.S. clinical trials, rosiglitazone treatment was associated with a median weight gain between 0.8 and 5.4 kg, while pioglitazone treatment was associated with a median weight gain between 0.9 and 3.6 kg.

As a result of increases in plasma volume and a dilutional effect, decreases in hemoglobin and hematocrit also occur in a dose-related fashion in patients treated with rosiglitazone and pioglitazone alone or in combination. These changes occur primarily during the first 4–12 weeks of therapy and remain relatively constant thereafter. These changes have not been associated with any significant hematologic clinical effects.

In preapproval clinical trials, there were no cases of idiosyncratic drug reactions leading to hepatic failure reported for either rosiglitazone or pioglitazone.

The thiazolidinediones do not stimulate insulin secretion and hence when used as monotherapy are not expected to cause hypoglycemia. However, mild to moderate hypoglycemia can occur and has been reported during combination therapy with sulfonylureas or insulin.

Drug Interactions

The oxidative metabolism for rosiglitazone and pioglitazone occurs by distinct cytochrome pathways: pioglitazone involves CYP 3A4 and CYP 2C8, whereas rosiglitazone is metabolized principally by CYP 2C8. Pioglitazone may reduce the bioavailability of oral contraceptives containing ethinyl estradiol and norethindrone by induction of CYP3A4, and co-administration of pioglitazone with oral contraceptives may reduce the effectiveness of these agents. Oral contraceptive concentrations were reduced by up to 30% with the co-administration of troglitazone. Higher-dosage oral contraceptive formulations may be needed to increase contraceptive efficacy during pioglitazone use. Alternatively, the use of an alternative or additional method of contraception is recommended. On the other hand, studies with rosiglitazone have not shown any clinically relevant effect on the pharmacokinetics of oral contraceptives (ethinyl estradiol and norethindrone).

Repeat dosing with rosiglitazone had no clinically relevant effect on the steady-state pharmacokinetics of other, commonly used drugs.

Contraindications/Precautions

In clinical trials with rosiglitazone and pioglitazone, the incidence of hepatotoxicity and liver enzyme elevations has been similar to that of placebo. In clinical use to date, there have been a few reports of hepatotoxicity associated with both rosiglitazone and pioglitazone use. Thus, although the risk of hepatotoxicity is much lower, it is prudent that rosiglitazone and pioglitazone be used cautiously in patients with hepatic disease, since both rosiglitazone and pioglitazone are structurally very similar to troglitazone.

Liver enzymes should be checked before the initiation of therapy with rosiglitazone or pioglitazone in all patients. Therapy with glitazones should not be initiated in patients with increased baseline liver enzyme levels (ALT > 2.5 times the upper limit of normal). In patients with normal baseline liver enzymes, following initiation of therapy with rosiglitazone or pioglitazone, it is recommended that liver enzymes be monitored every 2 months for the first 12 months and periodically thereafter. Recently, the requirements for LFT monitoring during pioglitazone therapy has been modified, and after baseline evaluation of serum ALT, thereafter ALT levels only need to be measured periodically per the clinical judgment of the health care professional. Patients with mildly elevated liver enzymes (ALT levels 1–2.5 times the upper limit of normal) at baseline or during therapy with rosiglitazone or pioglitazone should be evaluated to determine the cause of the liver enzyme elevation. Initiation of, or continuation of, therapy with a glitazone in patients with mild liver enzyme elevations should proceed with caution and should include appropriate close clinical follow-up, including more frequent liver enzyme monitoring, to determine whether the liver enzyme elevations resolve or worsen.

If at any time ALT levels increase to more than three times the upper limit of normal in patients on therapy with rosiglitazone or pioglitazone, liver enzyme levels should be rechecked as soon as possible. If ALT levels remain more than three times the upper limit of normal, glitazone therapy should be discontinued. If any patient develops symptoms suggesting hepatic dysfunction, which may include unexplained nausea, vomiting, abdominal pain, fatigue, anorexia, and/or dark urine, liver enzymes should be checked. The decision of whether to continue the patient on therapy with rosiglitazone or pioglitazone should be guided by clinical judgment pending laboratory evaluations. If jaundice is observed, drug therapy should be discontinued.

Caution should also be exercised when using pioglitazone or rosiglitazone in premenopausal anovulatory females with insulin resistance who may resume ovulation as a result of glitazone therapy. These patients may be at risk of becoming pregnant if adequate contraception is not used. In the case of pioglitazone, those who use oral contraceptive therapy may also be at risk due to CYP3A4 enzyme induction (see above).

Because of increases in plasma volume, both glitazones should be used cautiously in patients with peripheral edema or early congestive heart failure (especially when used in combination with insulin). Patients with severe congestive heart failure, defined as NYHA functional Class III and IV heart failure, should not receive glitazones unless the expected benefit is judged to outweigh the potential risk.

Rosiglitazone and pioglitazone are contraindicated in pregnancy. Although animal data suggest no teratogenic effects, there are no adequate and well-controlled studies in pregnant women. Also, it is unknown whether these drugs are secreted in human milk, and hence they should not be administered to breastfeeding women.

Thiazolidinediones are active only in the presence of insulin. They are not indicated for patients with T1DM.

TREATMENT STRATEGIES IN TYPE 2 DIABETES

Insulin resistance is a major abnormality in patients with T2DM, and in addition to hyperglycemia, diabetic patients often manifest hyperlipidemia, hypertension, and a hypercoagulable state. These abnormalities have collectively been referred to as the "deadly quartet" and comprise the *insulin resistance syndrome* or the *metabolic syndrome*. Hence, in addition to treating hyperglycemia in these patients, we must also strive to ameliorate the other abnormalities of the metabolic syndrome. The goal for glycemic control is an HbA_{1c} of <7%; the goal for lipid control is LDL < 100 mg/dL, HDL > 40 mg/dL in men and > 50 mg/dL in women, triglycerides < 200 mg/dL (statins are possible first-line agents); the goal for blood pressure control is <130/80 mmHg or 120/70 mmHg (if there is proteinuria; ACE inhibitors are probable first-line agents); and for the hypercoagulable state, all T2DM patients >40 years old should be on aspirin (if not contraindicated).

The first line of therapy for T2DM includes the use of diet management to provide both optimal composition and caloric content so as to assist in achieving desirable body weight. Diet therapy with weight loss is the most effective form of therapy in the obese T2DM patient, but long-term compliance remains poor. Exercise therapy has additional and independent benefits on the metabolic syndrome of diabetes and facilitates the success of diet. When diet, exercise, and weight loss are unable to achieve the glycemic goals outlined above, the usual next step is to proceed to oral antidiabetic medications, alone or in combination. When adequate glycemic control cannot be achieved with oral agents, insulin is then added or substituted as sole therapy.

Monotherapy

The choice of initial oral agents in patients with diabetes is dictated by many factors, including patient profile, initial level of hyperglycemia, and economic and formulary considerations (Fig. 12-2 and Table 12-4). A summary of the reported glucose-lowering effects of monotherapy is given in Table 12-5. Since these were not simultaneous trials, the comparative data are only a rough approximation of the relative effectiveness of these agents.

In general, patients with marked hyperglycemia (>300 mg/dL), ketonuria, or ketonemia, pregnant patients, and patients with acute myocardial infarction

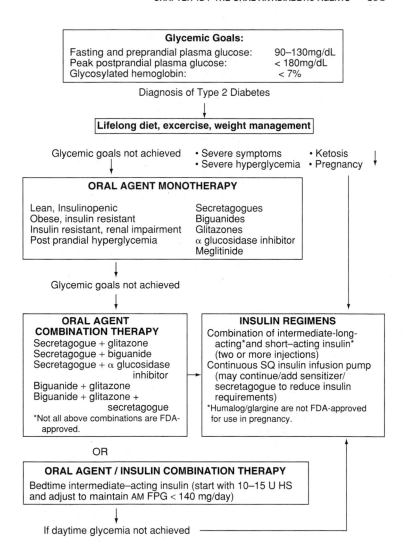

FIG. 12-2   Suggested algorithm for the treatment of type 2 diabetes.

and all acute situations should all be treated with insulin. In most other patients, a sulfonylurea (in lean patients) or metformin (in obese patients) may be initiated and titrated upward every 1–2 weeks depending on the response. It is extremely important that patients regularly monitor their fingerstick blood glucose. The goal for fasting capillary blood glucose is between 80 and 120 mg/dL and that of peak postprandial capillary blood glucose < 160 mg/dL. In elderly patients and those with irregular meal profiles, a short-acting secretagogue such as repaglinide may be preferable to a sul-

TABLE 12-4 Oral Antidiabetic Agents as Initial Monotherapy

Agent	Major mechanism(s) of action	Most suitable patient profile	Glycemic benefit
Insulin secretagogues			
Sulfonylureas	↑↑ Day-long pancreatic insulin secretion	Lean/insulinopenic	Fasting and postprandial glycemia
Meglitinides	↑↑ Postprandial pancreatic insulin secretion	Lean/insulinopenic	Postprandial glycemia
Biguanide (metformin)	↓↓ Hepatic glucose production ↑ Peripheral glucose utilization	Obese/insulin-resistant	Fasting and postprandial glycemia
α-Glucosidase inhibitors (acarbose/miglitol)	↓ Postprandial carbohydrate absorption	Lean/insulinopenic or obese/insulin-resistant	Postprandial glycemia
Thiazolidinediones/glitazones (rosiglitazone/pioglitazone)	↑↑ Peripheral glucose utilization ↓ Hepatic glucose production	Obese/insulin-resistant	Fasting and postprandial glycemia

TABLE 12-5 Relative Efficacy of Oral Antidiabetic Agents as Monotherapy (Change from Placebo)*

Agent	Reduction in fasting plasma glucose (mg/dL)	Reduction in HbA$_{1c}$ (%)	Reduction in postprandial plasma glucose (mg/dL)
Insulin secretagogues			
Sulfonylureas (various agents/doses)	54–70	1.5–2.0	92
Repaglinide	61	1.7	104
Nateglinide	—	0.6–1.0	—
Metformin (2550 mg/day)	59–78	1.5–2.0	83
Rosiglitazone (8 mg/day)	62–76	1.5	—
Pioglitazone (45 mg/day)	59–80	1.4–2.6	—
Acarbose (300 mg/day)	20–30	0.5–1.0	40–50
Miglitol (300 mg/day)	—	0.5—0.8	40–60

* These data were not obtained from simultaneous trials, so the comparisons are only a rough approximation of the relative effectiveness as stage; severity of hyperglycemia and type of patients studied varied in the studies from which these data were derived.

fonylurea, which may cause hypoglycemia if meals are missed. In patients with predominant postprandial hyperglycemia, acarbose or miglitol may be good choices, especially in those with high carbohydrate intake. Obese patients with renal insufficiency may be started with a glitazone instead of metformin, which is contraindicated in these patients. Summaries of the metabolic effects and safety of the oral antidiabetic agents used as monotherapy are shown in Tables 12-6 and 12-7.

Unfortunately, because of the progressive nature of T2DM and the continued decline in β-cell function, most monotherapy studies demonstrate eventual failure to provide adequate glucose control in most patients with T2DM, and combination therapy is frequently a necessity, especially if one is to achieve optimal glycemic control (HbA$_{1c}$ < 7%). This strategy of treating patients with increasing doses of an oral agent and slowly adding agents when glycemic control deteriorates has been termed the "treat to failure" strategy. In the UKPDS, the progressive deterioration of glucose control was such that after 3 years, only about 50% of subjects attained a goal of HbA$_{1c}$ < 7% with monotherapy, and after 9 years this declined to < 25%. It is important to rule out first the possibility that secondary treatment failure is due to noncompliance; doing so will avoid the need for additional agents.

TABLE 12-6 Metabolic Effects of Oral Antidiabetic Agents as Monotherapy

	Sulfonylureas/ Meglitinides	Acarbose	Metformin	Rosiglitazone/ Pioglitazone
Weight	↑	↔	↓ or ↔	↑
LDL cholesterol	↔	↔	↓	↔ or ↑
HDL cholesterol	↔	↔	↑ or ↔	↑↑
Triglycerides	↔	↔	↓	↔ or ↓

TABLE 12-7 Relative Efficacy of Oral Agents in Combination

Agents	Reduction in fasting plasma glucose (mg/dL)	Reduction in HbA$_{1c}$ (%)	Reduction in postprandial plasma glucose (mg/dL)
Sulfonylurea + metformin	64	1.7	87
Sulfonylurea + acarbose	—	0.5 to 1.0	85
Sulfonylurea + rosiglitazone (8 mg)	38	0.9	—
Sulfonylurea + pioglitazone (30 mg)	52	1.2	—
Metformin + acarbose	—	0.8	38
Metformin + repaglinide	39	1.4	—
Metformin + nateglinide	—	0.9	—
Metformin + rosiglitazone (8 mg)	54	1.3	—
Metformin + pioglitazone (30 mg)	38	0.8	—

There is also an emerging concept that it may be advantageous to begin combination therapy earlier in the course of the disease rather than escalate the dose of a single current agent in order to achieve greater glucose-lowering effect. Such a practice is based on the belief that therapy directed at more than one mechanism of action may provide more rapid, sustained, and cost-effective glycemic control. Further studies will be necessary to confirm the clinical utility of this practice.

Combination Therapy

The goal of combination therapy is to take advantage of the differing mechanisms of action of the various pharmacologic agents and create an individualized treatment plan for achieving effective glycemic control. The combination of two agents may often result in a synergistic rather than a mere additive glucose-lowering effect. In some cases, lower doses of both agents can be used, which can further minimize side effects. Oral combination therapy is advantageous because it can often delay the need for insulin. Ideally, combination therapy should be instituted before manifestation of hyperglycemic symptoms. A comparison of some of the trials is shown in Table 12-7. It must be emphasized that heterogeneity of patients and severity and stage of disease make comparisons only approximate.

Combination of an Insulin Secretagogue and an Insulin Sensitizer

The combination of a secretagogue and an insulin sensitizer can be synergistic and addresses two of the major pathophysiologic abnormalities in T2DM. If monotherapy with a sulfonylurea or metformin fails to achieve the desired level of glycemic control, the other, second oral agent (if not contraindicated) should be added, with dose escalation over 4–8 weeks to the maximum. Indeed, the use of a sulfonylurea plus metformin is the most widely and extensively studied combination of oral agents and lowers HbA$_{1c}$ by an additional 1.7%. The combination of a sulfonylurea and a glitazone is also useful. The addition of rosiglitazone 4 mg BID to a sulfonylurea resulted in a reduction of FPG by 38 mg/dL and the HbA_{1c} by 0.9% over 6 months. Similarly, 30 mg of pioglitazone daily, when added to a sulfonylurea, decreased FPG by 52 mg/dL and HbA_{1c} by 1.2% after 26 weeks.

When a glitazone is used in combination with a sulfonylurea, the current dose of the sulfonylurea should be continued, and the glitazone should be initiated at the lowest dose. If the response is not adequate, the dose can be increased after approximately 2–4 weeks to the maximum. If patients experience hypoglycemia in combination with a sulfonylurea, the sulfonylurea dose may be lowered as necessary to optimize therapy. The addition of the non-sulfonylurea secretagogues repaglinide and nateglinide to metformin or a glitazone has also been shown to confer significantly better glycemic control than monotherapy with either agent.

Combination of Two Insulin Sensitizers

Since metformin and the glitazones act through different mechanisms, their combination may be expected to be more efficacious. Moreover, since metformin predominantly restrains hepatic glucose production and the glitazones act primarily on insulin resistance in muscle and adipose tissue, their combination also ameliorates two major pathophysiologic abnormalities in T2DM. The combination of metformin and rosiglitazone, 8 mg daily for 26 weeks, reduced FPG by 54 mg/dL and HbA_{1c} by 1.3% compared with placebo. The combination of metformin and pioglitazone, 30 mg daily, decreased FPG by 38 mg/dL and HbA_{1c} by 0.8%, compared with placebo, after 26 weeks.

Other Oral Combinations

The addition of acarbose to sulfonylurea or metformin therapy represents another option for improving glycemic control in patients with T2DM, particularly those with significant postprandial hyperglycemia; it also lowers HbA_{1c} a further 0.5–1%. It should be reiterated that although acarbose monotherapy does not cause hypoglycemia, combination with sulfonylureas may increase the hypoglycemic potential of the sulfonylurea. This hypoglycemia should be treated with dextrose, and not sucrose, which, as mentioned earlier, may not be effective.

Some physicians may choose to add bedtime insulin to oral agent monotherapy rather than add a second oral agent. However, it has been shown that the addition of metformin to ongoing sulfonylurea therapy in patients experiencing secondary failure achieves reductions in FPG and HbA_{1c} that are not statistically different from those achieved with the addition of insulin to the current therapy or complete switchover to insulin. Thus, use of this combination may delay the need to use insulin.

If combination therapy with two oral agents does not achieve the desired goal, available options include (1) adding a third oral agent; (2) adding bedtime insulin while maintaining therapy with one or both oral agents; or (3) switching the patient to a mixed-split (short-acting plus long-acting insulin given in two to four daily injections) insulin regimen. Although the use of combination therapy may require greater patient adaptability and compliance, most patients prefer combination therapy to the alternative of exclusive insulin use. Thus, it is important to individualize therapy on the basis of patient preferences.

Triple Oral Combination Therapy

The combination of a sulfonylurea, metformin, and a glitazone, or a sulfonylurea, metformin, and acarbose, is often used in clinical practice. The unique mechanisms of action of these agents can potentially complement each other to improve glycemic control in patients with T2DM. This combination may obviate the need for insulin therapy, but issues of effectiveness, cost, benefit, and compliance have yet to be determined. Future studies will be required to test the efficacy of these various combinations.

Adding Insulin to Oral Therapy

In the not-so-distant past, patients who were not adequately controlled with sulfonylureas were switched over to insulin exclusively. Numerous studies in the late 1980s and in the early part of this decade demonstrated a modest yet significant improvement in glycemic control with combined sulfonylurea-insulin therapy over that seen with insulin alone. Continuation of the sulfonylurea in this instance resulted in better glycemic control, primarily due to the effect of evening insulin in restraining hepatic glucose output during the night and early morning periods (a characteristic feature of T2DM). Once fasting hyperglycemia is controlled, it appears that the daytime sulfonylureas are better able to maintain daytime postprandial glycemia. The use of these two agents simultaneously allows one to start with a low dose of insulin and results in better glycemic control during the transition. Combination sulfonylurea–insulin therapy also reduces day-to-day variability in fasting glucose levels compared with a single daily insulin injection.

The addition of intermediate insulin at bedtime to ongoing sulfonylurea therapy has been shown to offer glycemic control comparable to that of various insulin regimens and insulin–sulfonylurea combinations. Moreover, administration of insulin at bedtime resulted in less weight gain and reduced hyperinsulinemia. This regimen, known as bedtime-insulin/daytime-sulfonylurea (BIDS) therapy, may be better than daytime insulin therapy because hepatic glucose overproduction is typically most abnormal during the night.

Patient selection is an important determinant in the success of a BIDS regimen and is more likely to be successful in obese patients who have been diagnosed with diabetes after the age of 35, have had diabetes for less than 10–15 years, and have glucose values consistently <250–300 mg/dL. To implement BIDS therapy, the patient's current sulfonylurea therapy is continued, and intermediate-acting insulin (0.1–0.2 U/kg) is administered at bedtime (usually 9–11 P.M.). The insulin dose is adjusted until the morning FPG level is <120 mg/dL. The sulfonylurea dose should be reduced if daytime hypoglycemia is a problem. Patients who continue to experience hyperglycemia before supper despite acceptable fasting glucose levels may require a switch to multiple insulin injections and discontinuation of the sulfonylurea. There are few, if any, apparent benefits to maintaining sulfonylureas when patients are on multiple doses of insulin. The above regimen is also suitable for use in those patients who have failed a combination of a sulfonylurea and metformin. Metformin is retained in this regimen because its insulin-sparing effect, along with its favorable effect on the lipid profile, may be beneficial in ameliorating cardiovascular risk.

Adding Oral Agents to Insulin Therapy

If the oral agent–insulin combination therapies described above fail, the patient is typically switched over to insulin exclusively; intermediate-acting insulin (NPH or Lente™) may be administered twice daily (morning and bedtime). However, a combination of intermediate-acting and regular insulin (morning and supper) is more commonly used for optimal control. In some cases, multiple (three or more) injections may be necessary to achieve acceptable glycemic control. Several specific insulin regimens to treat T2DM are available.

Until recently, the only option for patients who were not adequately controlled with insulin was to increase their insulin dose. However, this practice further increases the likelihood of hyperinsulinemia and weight gain. There has been ongoing research in this area, and it appears that adding oral agents such as acarbose, metformin, or a glitazone to insulin therapy—alone or in combination—is a feasible way of improving or normalizing glycemic control in a significant number of patients. It may even be possible to discontinue insulin therapy in selected patients and reinitiate combination oral hypoglycemic treatment.

Insulin and metformin: Metformin may be a useful adjunct in patients who are poorly controlled with insulin after sulfonylurea agents have achieved maximal effect. In these patients, metformin offers an advantage in that it does not stimulate insulin secretion and thereby exacerbate hyperinsulinemia. Metformin also does not contribute to weight gain, which can exacerbate insulin resistance. Combination therapy with bedtime insulin plus metformin not only prevents weight gain but also seems superior to other bedtime insulin regimens with sulfonylureas with respect to improvement in glycemic control and frequency of hypoglycemia.

In a patient on a full insulin regimen achieving suboptimal glycemic control, one can attempt to initiate and titrate metformin up to 500 mg three times a day. If the FPG remains >120 mg/dL consistently, the dose of metformin can be further increased gradually to a maximum of 850 mg three times a day (or 1000 mg twice a day). If glycemic control is adequate (FPG remains <120 mg/dL on two consecutive days), one can attempt to reduce the dose of insulin by 25% and closely monitor blood glucose values for decompensation. If this occurs or if glycemic control is not adequate on the maximum dose of metformin and lower doses of insulin, there is the option of adding a once-daily sulfonylurea (extended-release glipizide or glimepiride) and titrating the dose as required. The addition of a glitazone and acarbose to the above regimen also remains an option to the alternative of exclusive insulin treatment. The issues of cost effectiveness and compliance remain to be determined.

Insulin and acarbose: Addition of acarbose to insulin therapy may be an option when postprandial hyperglycemia continues to be a problem Acarbose may decrease HbA_{1c} by approximately 0.4% in patients who are poorly controlled on insulin therapy. Acarbose may be initiated in patients on insulin treatment by starting with a low dose of 25 mg with breakfast and titrating up by 25 mg weekly to 50–100 mg three times daily with meals (100-mg TID dose for patients more than 60 kg in weight), depending on GI tolerance and efficacy.

Insulin and a glitazone: Glitazones primarily improve insulin sensitivity and thus can be beneficial for combination with insulin. When initiating glitazone treatment in T2DM subjects on insulin who have suboptimal glucose control, the current insulin dose should be continued and the lowest dose of a glitazone (4 mg of rosiglitazone or 30 mg of pioglitazone) should be added once daily. If FPG levels remain consistently above 120 mg/dL, the dose of the glitazone should be increased every 2–4 weeks, up to a maximum of 8 mg daily for rosiglitazone and 45 mg daily for pioglitazone, until FPG levels are consistently within the target range. At that time, one may attempt to lower the total daily dose of insulin by 10–25%. Increased weight gain has been observed with this combination.

Reinitiation of Oral Therapy in Insulin-Treated Patients

The recent availability of newer oral antidiabetic agents has allowed the possibility of discontinuing insulin treatment and reinitiating oral agents in selected patients with T2DM. This therapeutic strategy, however, is still under investigation. In a recent pilot study, of 55 patients with T2DM who were on twice-daily insulin treatment for more than 10 years and had a random C-peptide level >0.8 ng/mL, 42 patients were successfully able to switch over to a combination of glyburide and metformin and discontinue insulin treatment. This change to a combination of oral agents was accomplished with significantly better glycemic control (a decrease in HbA_{1c} of 1.3%) and decrease in body weight (5 lb) over 6 weeks. In this study, significant factors predicting a successful switch to oral agents in the responders included a lower body mass index ratio (30 versus 34.8), lesser duration of insulin treatment (5.0 versus 8.6 years), and lesser total daily dose of insulin (0.8 versus 1.2 U/kg body weight).

CONCLUSIONS

Until 1994, the pharmacologic management of T2DM (non-insulin-dependent diabetes mellitus [NIDDM], as it was then called) was quite straightforward. Only two classes of agents were available. Upon initial diagnosis, a sulfonylurea was prescribed, and when patients became too symptomatic or were markedly hyperglycemic, insulin treatment was added or substituted. In the last 10 years, however, two major developments have occurred. First, we now have unequivocal evidence from major long-term studies such as the UKPDS that tight control of hyperglycemia in T2DM has significant benefits on the prevention and progression of microvascular and possibly macrovascular disease. Second, to achieve this optimal control, several new classes of oral antidiabetic agents have become available for use as monotherapy: insulin secretagogues (sulfonylureas, repaglinide, nateglinide), biguanides (metformin), α-glucosidase inhibitors (acarbose and miglitol), and thiazolidinediones (rosiglitazone and pioglitazone). However, T2DM is a progressive disease, and over the years tight control of blood glucose often involves combination therapy as a means of optimizing glycemic control. Combinations of oral agents can often delay the need for insulin. Oral agents can also be used in combination with insulin to aid in achieving glycemic goals and reducing hyperinsulinemia.

Which combination of oral agents or insulin is more beneficial is at present not clear, and studies to answer this question are in progress. Several new insulin sensitizer agents are also in development, and the feasibility of inhaled or even buccal insulin may soon become a reality. The ultimate objective, of course, is the prevention of diabetes. Several recent studies have demonstrated that both lifestyle and pharmacologic measures are successful in preventing the progression to type 2 diabetes in subjects with impaired glucose tolerance. Whether the strategies used in these two studies can be translated into a "real-world" scenario in both developed and developing nations, and in all ethnic groups, is not clear at present. Nevertheless, the fact that type 2 diabetes can be prevented (or at least delayed) with intensive lifestyle or pharmacologic measures is an exciting development for those who take care of patients at high risk for the development of T2DM.

ACKNOWLEDGMENTS

This work was supported by the Department of Veterans Affairs and the VA San Diego Healthcare System, California.

ADDITIONAL READINGS

American Diabetes Association: Clinical Practice Recommendations. *Diabetes Care* 2004;27:S15.

Inzucchi SE: Oral antihyperglycemic therapy for type 2 diabetes: Scientific review. *JAMA* 2002;287:360.

Moller DE: New drug targets for type 2 diabetes and the metabolic syndrome. *Nature* 2001;414:821.

UK Prospective Diabetes Study (UKPDS) Group. Intensive blood-glucose control with sulphonylureas or insulin compared with conventional treatment and risk of complications in patients with type 2 diabetes (UKPDS 33). *Lancet* 1998;352:837.

UK Prospective Diabetes Study (UKPDS) Group. Effect of intensive blood-glucose control with metformin on complications in overweight patients with type 2 diabetes (UKPDS 34). *Lancet* 1998;352:854.

For a more detailed discussion of this topic and a bibliography, please see Porte *et al: Ellenberg & Rifkin's Diabetes Mellitus,* 6th ed., Chapter 32.

---

13 | The Mother in Pregnancies Complicated by Diabetes Mellitus

Boyd E. Metzger   *Richard L. Phelps*
Sharon L. Dooley

Pregnancy affects a wide range of physiologic functions increasingly from conception until delivery. Intermediary metabolism is no exception. The alterations are pronounced, resulting in differences in the expression of diabetes mellitus and requiring modifications in its treatment.

METABOLIC ADAPTATIONS IN NORMAL PREGNANCY

Clinical Features of Carbohydrate Metabolism in Pregnancy

Alterations in carbohydrate metabolism are especially prominent in the second half of pregnancy. Disposition of administered glucose is only minimally altered, whereas the hypoglycemic response to insulin is markedly reduced. This indicates that an increased amount of insulin is required to maintain normal glucose tolerance. Pregnancy is, therefore, a physiologic challenge to insulinogenic reserve. Maternal islet cell hyperplasia during normal gestation and clinical experience in subjects with diminished or absent pancreatic β-cell reserve are consistent with this premise. Thus, pregnancy may be attended by onset or first recognition of carbohydrate intolerance (i.e., gestational diabetes mellitus [GDM]), and substantial increases in the requirements for insulin usually occur in women with insulin-requiring pregestational diabetes mellitus (PGDM). The changes parallel the growth of the fetus and placenta: they increase rapidly as the conceptus increases in size from weeks 20–24 of pregnancy onward, and they are promptly reversed following delivery. In the immediate postpartum period, normal glucose tolerance returns in most women with GDM, and insulin requirements decline precipitously in patients with insulin-requiring PGDM. These temporal correlations have implicated the conceptus in the diabetogenic effects of pregnancy.

Effects of the Conceptus on Maternal Metabolism

Several functional properties of the conceptus exert metabolic effects during its development. These properties and resultant impact on maternal metabolism are summarized briefly below.

Insulin Kinetics and Turnover

Intraplacental degradation is responsible for a modest increase in the clearance of maternal insulin.

Insulin Action

Dramatic changes occur in insulin sensitivity and insulin secretion.

Insulin sensitivity: Insulin sensitivity begins to decrease by the end of the first trimester of pregnancy and is greatly reduced in late gestation. Insulin resistance is present in liver, adipose tissue, and skeletal muscle. The binding of insulin to its receptors is not diminished in human pregnancy; instead, insulin resistance is due to intracellular factors.

Insulin secretion: In early pregnancy, basal insulin concentrations are unchanged, and insulin response to oral or intravenous glucose is minimally increased. Basal and stimulated insulin secretion increase greatly in late pregnancy (two- to threefold) to offset the marked reduction in insulin action.

Placental Hormones

The placenta secretes estrogen, progesterone, and human placental lactogen (HPL; human chorionic somatomammotropin [HCS]) in amounts that parallel its increasing size through the course of pregnancy. Each hormone can promote insulin secretion and decrease the sensitivity to insulin in the periphery. Prolactin of pituitary and decidual origin and the human growth hormone variant (hGH-V) of placental origin may also contribute to the insulin resistance of pregnancy. Potential roles of tissue necrosis factor-α and leptin are being investigated intensively. However, the precise role and magnitude of these effects remain to be defined.

Other Changes in Endocrine Function

Some endocrine changes, not directly of intrauterine origin, may also be important. Serum glucocorticoid concentrations increase twofold in late pregnancy, and circulating maternal free cortisol is also increased. It is unlikely that the glucocorticoids are of fetal origin or controlled by placental corticotrophin-releasing factor, since normal diurnal rhythms of cortisol secretion are preserved. Instead, maternal hypothalamic-pituitary feedback may operate at a higher setting, perhaps as a result of the increased availability of sex steroids.

Maternal Nutrient Metabolism

Transfer of maternal fuels to the growing conceptus occurs continuously. Many nutrients are transferred from mother to fetus in a concentration-dependent manner and are used for structural growth and development as well as oxidative needs. The fluxes are considerable and challenge maternal mechanisms for conserving key intermediary metabolic substrates as fuel needs of the placenta and fetus escalate.

Accelerated starvation: Fasting in the last half of pregnancy results in rapid mobilization and oxidation of fatty acids and marked increases in plasma and urinary ketones. A larger and more rapid decline in maternal blood sugar and amino acids is also seen. The fall in blood glucose may progress to frank hypoglycemia. This has been viewed as a failure of amino acid mobilization to provide enough gluconeogenic substrates to match rates of glucose removal. These changes in fasting metabolism in late pregnancy are designated "accelerated starvation." The practical implications of "accelerated starvation" in ordinary clinical practice have been questioned. However, significant increases in plasma free fatty acids (FFAs), glycerol, and ketones, and reductions in plasma glucose and amino acids, were found by noon in pregnant women skipping breakfast. Thus, this clinical practice that is commonly used in scheduling laboratory tests or other procedures may have meaningful metabolic consequences in late pregnancy.

Facilitated anabolism: Metabolic alterations are also seen after eating (the fed state). In pregnancy, the increase in plasma glucose is higher and lasts longer; a larger increase in plasma very-low-density lipoprotein is seen, and the concurrent fall in plasma glucagon is greater than in nongravid subjects. Insulin resistance is instrumental in these changes that are enhanced by higher free fatty acids levels (due to incomplete suppression of lipolysis by insulin). Since transplacental transfer of glucose is concentration-dependent, more prolonged hyperglycemia after oral intake in late pregnancy results in greater availability of glucose for delivery to the fetus. Increased plasma triglycerides can serve as an alternative oxidative fuel in the mother, "sparing" glucose for transplacental flux. Finally, the greater suppression of glucagon may also play a role by blunting gluconeogenesis and ketogenesis and so spare ingested amino acids for maternal or fetal needs. The metabolic pattern summarized above is designated "facilitated anabolism."

PATHOPHYSIOLOGY OF DIABETES AND PREGNANCY

A pregnant woman with diabetes and her offspring are both at risk for morbidity and mortality. In the pre-insulin era, pregnancy was uncommon, few fetuses survived, and maternal mortality approached 25%. Now, under optimal circumstances maternal deaths are rare, intrauterine fetal deaths are uncommon, and the incidence of neonatal deaths (except those due to major congenital malformations) approaches that of the general obstetric population. However, other less extreme morbid outcomes are still commonly seen.

Effects of Diabetes on Pregnancy

It appears that morbidities in the offspring are due to abnormalities in the maternal metabolic environment rather than genetic influences, because offspring of diabetic fathers develop normally. The specific morbidities that result are dependent on the time in pregnancy when the metabolic disturbances are present. This concept, designated "fuel-mediated teratogenesis" (Fig. 13-1), was formulated by the late Norbert Freinkel in his 1980 Banting Lecture. See Chapter 14 for more details.

Effects of Pregnancy on Diabetes

Glycemic Control

In normal pregnancy, insulin resistance is overcome by major increases in maternal insulin production that result in blood glucose concentrations close to those found in nongravid women. With insulin deficiency, substantial increases in blood glucose and other insulin-sensitive fuels occur unless counterbalanced by increased doses of insulin.

Effects of altered insulin sensitivity: As noted previously, normal control subjects have a small but significant reduction in insulin sensitivity by late in the first trimester (Fig. 13-2). Women with previous GDM and normal glucose tolerance are insulin-resistant before pregnancy but show a small though

POTENTIAL TERATOLOGY:

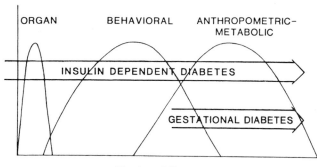

FIG. 13-1   The hypothesis of "fuel-mediated teratogenesis." It has been postulated that phenotypic gene expression in the newly forming cells of the conceptus may be modified by ambient fuels and fuel-related products during intrauterine development. Potential long-range effects will depend on the period in gestation during which maternal fuels and fuel-related products are aberrant and the cells that are undergoing development at that time. *(Adapted from Freinkel N: Diabetes 1980; 29:1023.)*

significant increase in insulin sensitivity late in the first trimester. Some women with type 1 diabetes experience more frequent, severe hypoglycemia near the end of the first trimester, necessitating temporary reduction in insulin doses. Aggressive efforts to achieve satisfactory glycemic control as quickly as possible may contribute to this tendency. In others, morning sickness may result in erratic, unpredictable caloric intake, marked swings in glycemic control, and episodes of severe hypo- and/or hyperglycemia. Whatever the factors responsible, clinicians should be aware of the tendency for less stable metabolic control in early pregnancy.

During the second trimester, insulin needs usually increase steadily, often to doses that are two- to threefold greater than in early pregnancy. In the last several weeks of pregnancy, glycemic control is often quite stable, requiring only minor modifications of insulin doses. In the 1–2 weeks before delivery, some patients again experience hypoglycemia and insulin doses may need to be reduced. Immediately postpartum, normal or supranormal insulin sensitivity is restored. Dramatic reduction of insulin doses (75–90%) may be necessary for several days. After that, insulin requirement usually becomes similar to what was needed before pregnancy.

Microvascular Disease

Retinopathy: Severe deterioration in diabetic retinopathy during pregnancy has been reported. Vision-threatening change is found primarily in patients with severe background or untreated proliferative retinopathy already present before pregnancy. Major progression rarely occurs during gestation in women with proliferative retinopathy previously treated with photocoagulation and deemed "inactive" prior to conception. Associations have been found between worsening retinopathy during pregnancy and duration of diabetes, severity of hyperglycemia at enrollment, magnitude of improvement in diabetic control

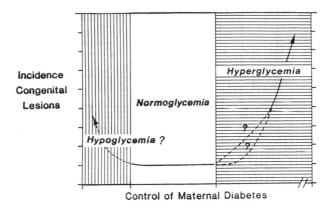

FIG. 13-2   Therapeutic dilemma in treatment with insulin during early human pregnancy. Hypoglycemia during the period of glycolytic dependence in the rodent embryo has been shown to be teratogenic. Whether the human embryo is similarly vulnerable during the corresponding developmental interval (i.e., about day 16–18 to day 24–25 postconception) has not been established. Moreover, the thresholds for the various factors in maternal serum that account for teratogenesis of diabetes (broadly designated above as "hyperglycemia") have not been ascertained. Thus, the optimal target for metabolic regulation prior to and during the first 4–6 weeks following conception is not yet precisely established. *(Adapted from Freinkel N: Horm Met Res 1988; 20:463–475.)*

achieved in the first half of gestation, and the presence of maternal hypertension. Data from the Diabetes Control and Complications Trial (DCCT) indicate that pregnancy also contributes to the risk of transient progression of retinopathy and that retinopathy can continue to progress after pregnancy or first appear as late as 6–12 months postpartum. However, the tendency for progression during gestation appears to be transient, since no permanent adverse affect of pregnancy on retinal status was found. Although photocoagulation therapy can be used effectively during gestation, it is best to delay conception in women with active retinopathy until it has been stabilized by treatment.

Nephropathy: Normal physiologic adaptations of pregnancy lead to glomerular hyperfiltration. This may be maladaptive in the presence of preexisting renal disease and/or hypertension. Pregnancy is also associated with more urinary tract infections and pyelonephritis. Mild preexisting diabetic nephropathy or mild renal insufficiency (creatinine < 1.4 mg/dL [124 mmol/L]) apparently does not accelerate nephropathy permanently, though transient worsening of proteinuria and/or creatinine clearance may occur during pregnancy. However, in diabetic patients with more severe renal insufficiency (creatinine > 1.4 mg/dL [124 mmol/L]), there is evidence that pregnancy may accelerate deterioration of renal function, as has been seen with moderate renal insufficiency of nondiabetic etiology. Nephropathy is associated with higher risks of hypertension/preeclampsia, acceleration of retinopathy, and fetal/neonatal morbidities, e.g., prematurity and intrauterine growth retardation (IUGR). Efforts to preserve renal function should include optimal glycemic and blood pressure control and close scrutiny for, and prompt treatment of, urinary tract infections.

Neuropathy: Little has been reported about effects of pregnancy on diabetic neuropathy. However, the presence of autonomic neuropathy, in particular gastroparesis, may have potentially adverse effects on maternal morbidity and pregnancy outcome. Irregular gastric emptying may result in inadequate nutrition, marked fluctuation in blood glucose, or maternal aspiration. Patients with bladder dysfunction are at risk for recurrent urinary tract infections.

Macrovascular Disease

Patients with macrovascular disease have significant risks of maternal and fetal morbidity. Pregnancy may exacerbate preexisting vascular disease. In the small number of cases reported as early as three decades ago, myocardial infarction in pregnancy was associated with a 50% mortality rate. Hopefully, outcome would be better with currently available options for management of coronary artery disease.

CLASSIFICATION OF DIABETES IN PREGNANCY

Pre-existing insulin-treated diabetes complicates approximately 0.2–0.5% of all pregnancies in the United States. In some populations, half or more of such pregnancies are in women with type 2 diabetes mellitus (T2DM). GDM affects an additional 3–8%. These figures are likely to rise in the future, because the incidences of obesity and T2DM are increasing in adolescents and young adults, especially among minority populations. Since there are more than 3,000,000 live births in the United States each year, diabetes during pregnancy constitutes an appreciable and increasing public health problem.

Gestational diabetes, defined as "carbohydrate intolerance with onset or first recognition during the present pregnancy," is subdivided by the severity of the metabolic disturbance using the level of fasting plasma glucose (FPG) to do so (Table 13-1). GDM is designated Class A_1 when FPG remains in the normal range for pregnancy (<95 mg/dL [5.3 mmol/L]) and Class A_2 when values equal or exceed this limit.

For epidemiologic purposes, pregnant women with abnormal glucose tolerance who had GDM in a prior pregnancy are not classified as GDM in the current pregnancy. Rather, they are designated "previous GDM" and subdivided on the basis of FPG concentration into Class A_1 or Class A_2 (Table 13-1).

We attempt to distinguish those patients with pregestational diabetes who have type 1 diabetes mellitus (T1DM) from those with T2DM. Standard clinical yardsticks are usually adequate for this purpose. The most important determinants of maternal and fetal outcome are the presence or absence of maternal vascular complications from diabetes and the degree of metabolic control achieved throughout pregnancy. Pregnancies are therefore classified as T1DM or T2DM, with or without complications (see Table 13-1). Maternal age at diagnosis and duration of diabetes no longer appear to be major independent risk factors for pregnancy complications. Accordingly, the traditional White Classification, devised over 50 years ago, currently has limited utility.

MANAGEMENT

Pregestational Diabetes

Preconception Counseling

Optimally, the management of pregnancy complicated by diabetes begins before pregnancy is contemplated. Beginning at puberty, potential complica-

TABLE 13-1 Classification of Carbohydrate Intolerance during Pregnancy

Class	Classification criteria
Gestational diabetes mellitus (GDM)	See text for diagnosis
Class A$_1$ (GDM)	Normal FPG* (<95 mg/dL)
Class A$_2$ (GDM)	Elevated FPG (≥95 mg/dL)
Previous gestational diabetes (Prev GDM)	Patients with diabetes only during a previous pregnancy
Class A$_1$ (Prev GDM)	Normal FPG (<95 mg/dL)
Class A$_2$ (Prev GDM)	Elevated FPG (>95 mg/dL)
Pregestational diabetes mellitus (PGDM)	Diagnosis of diabetes mellitus made prior to the present pregnancy
Type 1 diabetes mellitus:	
Uncomplicated	Absence of retinopathy, nephropathy, neuropathy, hypertension, coronary artery, and peripheral artery disease
Complicated	Presence of one or more of above
Type 2 diabetes mellitus:	
Uncomplicated	Same as for T1DM
Complicated	Same as for T1DM

*FPG = fasting plasma glucose.

tions of pregnancy for mother and offspring should be made known to all women with diabetes mellitus. It must be emphasized that pregnancy requires that special precautions be taken *in advance*. Thus, a discussion of family planning is carried out at each office visit. It is stressed that planned conception after medical assessment and improvement of metabolic control greatly reduces the risk of spontaneous abortion and fetal malformations.

Medical assessment: Evaluation of maternal health status, emphasizing possible diabetic vascular complications, is carried out whenever women seek advice before conception. A complete physical examination, including pelvic examination and, in most cases, examination by an ophthalmologist, is recommended. Measurements of glycohemoglobin, thyroid-stimulating hormone, 24-hour creatinine clearance and quantitative urinary protein excretion, CBC, and an automated chemistry screen are performed. Immunity to rubella is assessed, with immunization as necessary. Lifestyle issues are reviewed, including assessment of stress, tobacco, drug, or alcohol use. Some prescription drugs may need to be discontinued, in particular, angiotensin-converting enzyme (ACE) inhibitors, agents known to affect the fetus adversely.

Specific diabetes-related issues: Information about potential effects of diabetes on fetal growth and development (see Chapter 14) is reviewed with the prospective parents. It is stressed that the risks of spontaneous abortion and congenital malformations are linked to altered maternal metabolism around the time of conception and the following 7–8 weeks (Fig. 13-1). Although the metabolic factor or factors responsible are not precisely known, (Fig. 13-3), clinical studies have documented a marked reduction in the incidence of these events when efforts to effectively control diabetes are initiated before conception. Also discussed is the possibility that obesity, T2DM, and neurobehavioral deficits may be more prevalent in later life in offspring of diabetic mothers, particularly if metabolic control is not optimal throughout pregnancy. The possibility of deleterious effects of pregnancy on maternal vascular complications is also discussed as the mother's clinical condition warrants. Finally, the patient and significant other(s) are reminded that prenatal care is intensive and involves a significant time commitment and possibly a reordering of priorities before and through the pregnancy.

General strategies: To minimize the likelihood of birth defects and spontaneous abortions, we aim for good, stable metabolic control *before* conception (Fig. 13-3). This requires renewed effort for patients already familiar with intensive management and introduction to the concept of *tight control* for others. Periconceptional supplementation with folic acid may reduce the risk of neural tube birth defects, which occur more often when pregnancy is complicated by diabetes. A multivitamin containing 0.8 mg folic acid is prescribed prior to conception and continued through the first 6 weeks of gestation.

Toward optimal metabolic control: Glycemia is self-monitored by capillary blood sugar measurements, and estimates of hemoglobin A1c (HbA_{1c}) are performed serially. Diet prescriptions are based on an "exchange system." Multiple-dose insulin injection algorithms are developed. Results of capillary blood glucose tests are reviewed weekly. To varying degrees, women are familiar with "carbohydrate counting" wherein the premeal dose (bolus) of short-acting insulin is determined mainly by the grams of carbohydrate to be ingested. Many use this effectively while maintaining a balanced intake of protein, fat, and micronutrients. We encourage patients to maintain more day-

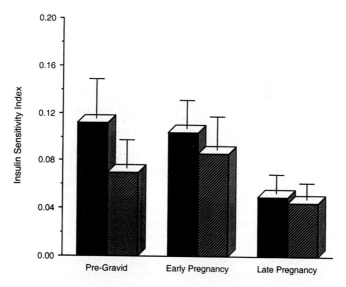

FIG. 13-3 Longitudinal changes in insulin sensitivity in women with normal pregnancy or gestational diabetes mellitus. Data from before pregnancy (pregravid), early, and late pregnancy are expressed as "insulin sensitivity index" (mean ± SD). Results from "Controls" are illustrated in the solid bars; those from women who developed GDM are shown by the hatched bars. *(Reproduced with modifications from Catalano PM, Tyzbir ED, Wolfe RR, et al: Am J Physiol 1993; 264:E60.)*

to-day consistency in mealtime and size than they may have done previously. Others need more guidance to ensure intake of adequate calories and optimal nutrient balance. We aim to have the HbA_{1c} concentration within or near the normal range before contraception is discontinued. In many cases this requires 3–6 months.

Management after Conception

Type 1 diabetes complicates pregnancy infrequently, and expertise in management can only be achieved if sufficient numbers of patients are seen on an ongoing basis. For this reason, care is usually best provided in a specialized referral clinic, employing a well-integrated team that, depending on the population served, consists of physicians, nurse educators, nutritionists, and social workers.

Diet

Basic approach: Diabetes does not alter the basic dietary recommendations for pregnancy, except that complex carbohydrates should be substituted for "simple" sugars. Because of the heightened propensity for accelerated starvation, evening snacks are usually recommended. Carbohydrate intake is seldom restricted below 180 g/day, and food intake is distributed to avoid periods of fasting in excess of 4–5 hours, except overnight. The proportion of the diet given at specific times is individualized according to patient preference and may also be manipulated to effect stability of metabolic control. However, whatever meal schedule is selected, day-to-day consistency is essential.

Meals and snacks: In the interest of simplicity, which enhances compliance, diets consist of three major meals and a bedtime snack. Some caregivers recommend multiple small feedings (six to seven) to dampen postmeal hyperglycemia. Whether the mean 24-hour blood glucose is lower with such regimens is unknown. Some reports based on retrospective analysis have shown stronger correlation between postprandial glycemia and birthweight than between fasting and premeal glycemia and birthweight. It is also not certain what influence the magnitude of blood glucose fluctuations, in contrast to the average level of glycemia, may have on perinatal outcome.

Goals for weight gain: Dietary prescriptions are individualized and often modified over the course of gestation. We recommend that weight gain be inversely proportional to the degree of adiposity in the mother before conception, which is judged by body mass index (BMI), defined as weight/height^2. A prepregnancy BMI of 20–26.0 kg/m^2 is considered normal, in which case a 25–35-pound (11–16-kg) weight gain is judged desirable. For those who are slender with BMI < 20 kg/m^2, the recommended weight gain is 28–40 pounds, and for those who are obese (BMI > 26 kg/m^2) it is 15–25 pounds. Some experts have estimated that the caloric cost of pregnancy may be only 100–150 kcal/day above requirements outside of pregnancy, substantially less than 250–300-kcal/day that was widely accepted in the past. Thus, it is important to monitor weight gain closely during pregnancy and to modify caloric intake to reach the goals summarized above.

Initial strategy: Before conception and during the first trimester, diet prescriptions are based on an estimate of the woman's weight-maintaining caloric intake, if reliable, or 32-kcal/kg ideal body weight (IBW). This is increased to 35–38 kcal/kg IBW after the first trimester, depending on appetite, physical activity, and weight gain. Dietary protein accounts for 1.5–2.0 g/kg IBW, carbohydrates comprise 50–55% of total calories, and fat comprises 30–35%.

Women who focus on carbohydrate counting must take care to achieve an adequate intake of the full spectrum of nutrients needed for pregnancy.

Modifications to meet goals: Variations in total calories as great as 25–30% may be necessary to attain optimal weight gain as described above. For many women with T2DM who are overweight, moderate calorie restriction (20–25% below the figure cited above) may reduce hyperglycemia without increasing ketonemia or ketonuria. However, when caloric intake is restricted further (e.g., 33% reduction), significant elevations of FFAs and plasma ketones may develop, and this degree of caloric restriction should be avoided. High-fiber diets have not been found to consistently reduce postprandial hyperglycemia during pregnancy. "Isocaloric diets" containing only 30–40% of calories as carbohydrate (rather than the 50–55% cited above) do lessen hyperglycemia, but the effects of the concomitant increase in dietary protein and fat on maternal amino acids, lipids, and ketones have not been investigated.

Insulin: Optimal therapy requires an individualized approach.

Choice of insulin preparations: In most cases, longer-acting insulin (e.g., NPH) is given at breakfast, supper, or bedtime to maintain *basal* insulinization, and more short-acting preparations (regular insulin, or the rapid insulin analogs, lispro, or aspart) are given prior to meals. Postinjection profiles of the above insulin analogs mimic the profiles of secreted insulin in normal subjects more closely than the pattern seen after injection of regular human insulin. In nonpregnant subjects, the superiority of the rapid insulin anaologs has been demonstrated for controlling postprandial hyperglycemia while achieving a parallel reduction in the frequency of hypoglycemia in some cases. In some patients, bolus injections of lispro or aspart insulin must be supplemented with low doses of intermediate-acting insulin or regular insulin to prevent hyperglycemia before the next meal, due to the complete disappearance of the insulin analog by that time. A long-acting insulin analog, glargine insulin (Lantus™), has been introduced as an alternative for delivery of *basal* insulin. No clinical trials in pregnant subjects are available, and its use during gestation should be considered only after full discussion of the potential benefits and the largely unknown potential risks. Some concerns have been raised about potential stimulation of IGF receptors from limited studies in experimental animals.

Specific treatment strategies: Doses of insulin are adjusted to achieve fasting and premeal blood glucose concentrations of 65–85 mg/dL (3.6–4.7 mmol/L) and 1- or 2-hour postprandial values of <140–150 and 120–130 mg/dL (7.7–8.3 and 6.7–7.2/L), respectively. Individually tailored algorithms are developed that provide guidelines for the dose of insulin at each injection time. These are altered as necessary by telephone contact or at clinic visits. Use of an insulin pump (continuous subcutaneous insulin infusion [CSII]) has not been shown to confer greater benefits in pregnancy than intensified conventional therapy. We encourage CSII therapy in patients who have been using it prior to conception; however, we seldom initiate its use during pregnancy.

Modifications for T2DM: Most patients with T2DM retain some endogenous insulin secretion, making it easier for them to achieve treatment goals than patients with T1DM. Treatment goals can often be achieved with a twice-daily "mixed" insulin regimen (combinations of short- and intermediate-acting insulin given before breakfast and supper). If the diet is carefully adhered to with respect to both time and content, blood glucose levels are quite stable and modifications of insulin dosage can be made every 1–2 weeks as needed.

Expectations: Patients with near-normal blood sugar values in the first trimester may experience a modest reduction in insulin needs at approximately 10–14 weeks. This is a time of vulnerability to severe hypoglycemia. Subsequently (in particular, during the interval between 20 and 30 weeks of gestation), insulin requirements increase substantially in most patients before stabilizing in mid to late third trimester at a level two- to threefold greater than before pregnancy. A reduction in insulin need is sometimes noted in the week or two before term. The challenge of therapy is to modify the insulin dose in parallel with these alterations in insulin sensitivity.

Monitoring diabetes control

Blood glucose testing: At each outpatient visit, measurements of plasma glucose and capillary blood sugar (by the patient with her meter and strips) are obtained simultaneously to check the accuracy of the metered measurements. Blood sugars are monitored at home before each meal and at bedtime; at least twice weekly, the patient also measures values 1 or 2 hours after each meal. We have found measurements of both premeal and postprandial blood sugar are often needed to determine optimal doses of rapid-acting insulin. The limiting factor in the dose of rapid-acting insulin that can be given before a meal is the nadir blood sugar level that occurs prior to the subsequent meal, regardless of the magnitude of the between-meal peak. Measurement of premeal blood sugar is particularly important in patients who have "hypoglycemia unawareness." When postprandial hyperglycemia is present despite acceptable premeal levels, adjustments in meal size and/or frequency of feedings are recommended. As mentioned above, when using lispro or aspart insulin, premeal glucose concentrations higher than optimal can reflect either a need for a larger bolus of short-acting insulin with the preceding meal or a need for more longer-acting insulin.

Hemoglobin A1c: Measurements of glycosylated hemoglobin are secured at the first visit during pregnancy and at 4–6-week intervals thereafter. The initial value for glycosylated hemoglobin provides an index of the degree of maternal metabolic control at the time of conception and an indication of the risk of major congenital malformations. Measurements of fructosamine or glycosylated albumin may be desirable when the value for HbA_{1c} is not a reliable indicator of glycemia (e.g., in the presence of hemoglobinopathy or hemolysis).

Ketones: Patients are asked to test urine for ketones in the first morning urine specimen each day and at any time that premeal estimates of blood glucose exceed 200–250 mg/dL. Some patients now do blood tests for β-hydroxybutyrate at these times. Testing ketone levels is useful in detecting inadequate dietary intake, particularly of carbohydrate, and metabolic decompensation before diabetic ketoacidosis (DKA) occurs. Monitoring urine glucose is of little value.

Obstetric surveillance: In addition to routine obstetrical surveillance, women with diabetes mellitus are offered a comprehensive fetal anatomic survey by ultrasound because of the increased risk of diverse fetal anomalies, best performed after 18 weeks. The detection rate varies by anomaly.

Surveillance by ultrasound for gestational age and biometry is performed for the following reasons:

• Confirmation of gestational age is most accurate between 6 and 12 weeks of gestation.

- The presence of evolving fetal macrosomia can be detected by serial measurements of fetal head and abdominal circumferences in conjunction with estimated fetal weight in the late second and third trimesters of pregnancy.

Biophysical surveillance of fetal well-being may reduce the already low risk of fetal death that is seen with excellent metabolic control. Weekly testing is usually initiated by 32 weeks, but earlier and more frequent testing is indicated if there is significant hypertension, vascular disease, or other pregnancy complications.

- The mainstay of assessment is the nonstress test; the observation of two or more accelerations in response to fetal movement during 20 minutes of continuous fetal heart rate monitoring, designated a reactive test, is highly predictive of the absence of fetal death for the subsequent week.
- An alternative modality is the biophysical profile by ultrasound, which is also used as a backup test in the event of a nonreactive nonstress test; a scoring system is used in the assessment of fetal activity, fetal tone, fetal breathing, and amniotic fluid volume.

Meticulous surveillance for pregnancy complications is practiced at frequent prenatal visits, usually on a weekly basis after 30–32 weeks, especially for pre-eclampsia, which is more prevalent in pregnancy complicated by diabetes mellitus, particularly in those with preexistent vasculopathy.

The traditional clinical criteria utilized for the diagnosis of pre-eclampsia are an abrupt rise in blood pressure and appearance of proteinuria of >300 mg in 24 hours; the diagnosis thus may be difficult to make in women with hypertension and nephropathy.

The diagnosis of pre-eclampsia in a preterm gestation warrants hospitalization for close observation of fetal and maternal status; the diagnosis at or near term warrants consideration of delivery.

Delivery and Postpartum Care

Diabetic aspects: Medical management during labor consists of monitoring blood sugar every 1–4 hours and continuous intravenous infusions of glucose (5–10 g/h). Insulin is administered as either an intravenous infusion via a separate line at the rate of 0.01–0.04 U/h/kg actual body weight (i.e., 0.7–2.8 U/h in a 70-kg woman) or by subcutaneous injection of short-acting (regular, lispro, aspart) insulin every 3–6 hours, or CSII in subjects using an insulin pump. The objective is to keep blood glucose in the physiologic range (70–120 mg/dL [3.9–6.7/L]). A relationship between higher cord blood glucose at delivery and subsequent neonatal hypoglycemia, noted in the past, has not been found when third-trimester control of diabetes in the mother is optimal.

Elective cesarean delivery: Neither glucose nor additional insulin is administered before elective cesarean delivery if blood sugar is in the range of 70–140 mg/dL (3.9–7.8/L). Blood sugar values outside this range necessitate infusion of glucose, insulin, or both. Insulin requirement declines dramatically immediately following delivery (by as much as 75–90%), and the administered dose may have to be reduced for a few days to 25% or less of the antepartum dose. Failure to observe this fall in insulin requirement may be a forewarning of events such as endometritis or retained placenta. After a variable period, insulin requirements return to prepregnancy levels.

Breastfeeding: Women who wish to breastfeed are maintained at or up to 300 cal above their caloric intake during pregnancy. Because oral agents may be secreted in breast milk and cause hypoglycemia in the infant, they should not be used postpartum in women with T2DM wishing to breastfeed without consulting with the patient's pediatrician. Women who do not plan to nurse are returned immediately to a diet appropriate for nongravid women (30–32 kcal/kg IBW [125–135 kJ/kg]). Patients are encouraged to use the diabetes management skills they acquired during gestation.

Obstetric aspects: The goal of obstetric management is vaginal birth of a term infant assuming an uncomplicated pregnancy.

• Cesarean delivery should be reserved for standard obstetric indications because of greater maternal morbidity.
• Induction is planned at >38 weeks when the cervix is considered favorable; cervical ripening should be considered by 40 weeks.
• The sequelae of prematurity are more prevalent in infants of diabetic mothers compared with age-matched infants of nondiabetic mothers; thus, amniocentesis should be utilized if the estimated due date is uncertain or if elective delivery is performed at <38 weeks of gestation (<39 weeks if elective cesarean delivery).

Infants are at approximately twofold risk of shoulder dystocia compared with normal infants if there is an asymmetric increase in abdominal and chest girth relative to head size. Shoulder dystocia incurs risk of brachial plexus injury, usually presenting as Erb's palsy; fortunately >90% of palsies resolve. Use of a protocol to avoid shoulder dystocia by elective cesarean delivery at a threshold of estimated fetal weight, e.g., >4500 g, is not a wholly effective strategy given that formula-based estimates of size by ultrasound lack precision with 95% confidence limits of ±15–20%; a combination of ultrasound estimate and clinical judgment should be utilized.

Gestational Diabetes Mellitus

Definition and Magnitude of the Problem

Gestational diabetes mellitus, defined as "carbohydrate intolerance of variable severity with onset or first recognition during pregnancy," may complicate as many as 3–8% of pregnancies in North American centers, making it approximately 10 times more common than pregestational diabetes. Even higher figures (up to 20%) have been reported in some racial/ethnic populations, especially when other diagnostic criteria are used.

Studies in the 1970s and early 1980s found the risk of perinatal loss and neonatal morbidity to be increased in women with GDM. However, recent studies have not found an increase in perinatal loss or in the frequency of some neonatal morbidities (hypoglycemia, hypocalcemia, polycythemia, and hyperbilirubinemia). This may reflect an overall improvement in obstetric practice, or current approaches to diagnosis and treatment of GDM. Despite such improvements in outcome, offspring of mothers with GDM remain at risk for fetal hyperinsulinism and attendant excess fetal size (macrosomia), increasing the likelihood of birth trauma and cesarean delivery, and possibly the of risk for long-range abnormalities (see above).

There appears to be little, if any increased risk of congenital anomalies in GDM. When increased risk has been found, it has been in populations where unrecognized pregestational T2DM is more common. The above considerations provide incentives for the detection and treatment of GDM using current methods, as well as justification for clinical trials of earlier and more aggressive treatment.

Screening and Diagnosis

GDM is almost always asymptomatic, and selective screening for glucose intolerance on the basis of clinical "risk factors" and/or past obstetric history fails to identify one-third to one-half of affected subjects. Random estimates of blood glucose and measurements of glycosylated hemoglobin or fructosamine do not provide acceptable diagnostic sensitivity. Although measurement of second-trimester amniotic fluid insulin content offers reasonable sensitivity for early diagnosis of GDM, this approach is costly, invasive, and carries risk.

Risk assessment: All pregnant women should undergo blood glucose testing for GDM, with the exception of those who are at very low risk. It is recommended that risk assessment be done at the first prenatal visit (see Table 13-2). Low-risk subjects not requiring blood glucose testing must have *all* of the characteristics indicated in the table. Those considered to be at high risk for GDM are tested immediately and again at 24–28 weeks if the initial test is not diagnostic of GDM. All others should be screened at 24–28 weeks of gestational age.

Glucose challenge test: In North America, a two-step screening-diagnostic strategy is most commonly applied. Step 1, a 50-g oral glucose challenge (GCT), is given without regard to time of the last meal or time of day. Venous plasma glucose is measured 1 hour later and a value $\geq$ 140 mg/dL

TABLE 13-2 Screening Strategy for Detecting GDM

GDM risk assessment should be ascertained at the first prenatal visit

Low risk	Blood glucose testing not routinely required if *all* of the following characteristics are present:
	• Member of an ethnic group with a low prevalence of GDM
	• No known diabetes in first-degree relatives
	• Age < 25 years
	• Weight normal before pregnancy
	• No history of abnormal glucose metabolism
	• No history of poor obstetric outcome
Average risk	Perform blood glucose testing at 24–28 weeks using either:
	• Two-step procedure: 50 g glucose challenge test (GCT) followed by a diagnostic oral glucose tolerance test in those meeting the threshold value in the GCT (see text for details)
	• One-step procedure: Diagnostic oral glucose tolerance test performed on all subjects
High risk	Perform blood glucose testing as soon as feasible, using the procedures described above.
	• If GDM is not diagnosed, blood glucose testing should be repeated at 24–28 weeks, or at any time a patient has symptoms or signs that are suggestive of hyperglycemia

(7.8 mmole/L) is considered positive. Lowering the screening threshold to 130 mg/dL (7.2 mmole/L) increases the yield of cases with GDM modestly but increases the proportion that require further testing from 15–18% to 23–25% of all women. Although convenient and rapid, measurement of finger-stick capillary blood sugar should not be used for the GCT because of the relatively low precision of the procedure resulting from intratest variability of 10–15%.

100 g Oral glucose tolerance test: A positive screening for GDM is followed by an oral glucose tolerance test (OGTT) for definitive diagnosis. In the United States, a 100-g dextrose load is usually used for OGTTs, and venous plasma glucose results are interpreted according to the criteria of O'Sullivan and Mahan. These criteria were originally developed to identify women who were at high risk for developing diabetes mellitus postpartum. There are no criteria based on the relationships between hyperglycemia and adverse perinatal outcome. The criteria originally used for the diagnosis of GDM were based on measuring the concentration of glucose in whole blood. Subsequently, values for plasma glucose have been extrapolated to conform to contemporary laboratory methodology. Carpenter and Coustan adjusted the values to approximate values that are obtained with enzymatic assays used in most laboratories today (Table 13-3). Data from several populations indicate that in cases diagnosed by Carpenter-Coustan criteria, risks for perinatal morbidities are similar to GDM diagnosed with the NDDG criteria. Thus, the Fourth International Workshop Conference on GDM concluded that the Carpenter-Coustan derivation of the O'Sullivan study may be recommended for the interpretation of a 100-g OGTT in pregnancy.

Etiology and Pathogenesis

Heterogeneity: Women with GDM are heterogeneous with respect to both genotype and phenotype. The *severity* of carbohydrate intolerance at diagnosis represents one form of phenotypic heterogeneity, and is the basis for using FPG to subclassify GDM (Table 13-1). It is also an important predictor of risk for progression to diabetes following pregnancy. Though women with GDM tend to be older and heavier than their nondiabetic peers, there is appreciable heterogeneity among cases with regard to age and weight. Finally, GDM is heterogeneous with respect to insulin resistance and β-cell function.

TABLE 13-3 Diagnosis of GDM: 100 g Oral Glucose Tolerance Test*

	O'Sullivan-Mahan whole-blood Somogyi-Nelson (mg/dL [mmol/L])	NDDG plasma AutoAnalyzer (mg/dL [mmol/L])	Carpenter-Coustan plasma glucose oxidase (mg/dL [mmol/L])
Fasting	90 [5.0]	105 [5.8]	95 [5.3]
1 hour	165 [9.2]	190 [10.6]	180 [10.0]
2 hour	145 [8.1]	165 [9.2]	155 [8.6]
3 hour	125 [6.9]	145 [8.1]	140 [7.8]

*The 100-g oral glucose tolerance test is performed in the morning after an overnight fast of at least 8 hours, but not more than 14 hours, and after at least 3 days of unrestricted diet (≥ 150 g carbohydrate/day) and physical activity. The subject should remain seated and should not smoke throughout the test. Two or more of the venous plasma concentrations must be met or exceeded for a positive diagnosis.

Insulin resistance: As indicated above, insulin resistance is characteristic of pregnancy. Women with previous GDM but normal glucose tolerance have been found to be insulin-resistant compared with age- and BMI-matched controls. In late gestation, both normal control subjects and those with GDM are very insulin-resistant, but on average, it is greater in women with GDM.

β-*Cell function:* Women with normal carbohydrate metabolism compensate for the insulin resistance in late gestation with augmentation of β-cell function (increased insulin secretion). By contrast, those with GDM fail to increase β-cell function adequately to maintain normal glucose tolerance.

Management

Diet: Nutritional therapy is the cornerstone of management and should be started promptly after the diagnosis of GDM is established. Dietary recommendations in the latter half of pregnancy are the same for GDM as in normal pregnancies and in pregnancies complicated by pregestational diabetes (see discussion above).

Insulin: The precise place for insulin in the therapy of GDM is not fully defined.

Glycemia-based indications for use of insulin: In patients with fasting hyperglycemia diagnostic of diabetes (i.e., fasting plasma glucose [FPG] > 126 mg/dL [7.0 mm/L]), there is little if any controversy, and treatment is started with insulin immediately because neonatal risks equal those for patients with pregestational diabetes. Most authors also prescribe insulin therapy for GDM when FPG falls between 105 and 126 mg/dL (5.8 and 7.0 mmol/L) on two successive measurements following a brief trial of dietary therapy. The use of insulin therapy is more controversial in women with GDM in whom FPG is consistently normal (<95 mg/dL [5.3 mmol/L]), or near normal (<105 mg/dL [5.8 mmol/L]. Most patients with GDM fall into this category, and their offspring are at some risk for diabetic fetopathy and its consequences. Accordingly, some have recommended therapy with insulin in *all* women with GDM who are over 25 years of age. Others have applied strict goals for glycemic control, with the result that 50–85% of subjects with GDM receive insulin therapy. Such aggressive treatment has been shown to reduce average birthweight, but may also increase the frequency of small-for-gestational-age (SGA) infants. The cost/benefits for insulin treatment of mild GDM in terms of neonatal morbidity, childhood obesity, and glucose tolerance have not been explored. In the absence of such information, we favor a more conservative approach and restrict insulin treatment for GDM, in patients with FPG within or near the normal range, to those with 1-hour postbreakfast plasma glucoses ≥ 140 mg/dL or 2-hour values ≥ 120 mg/dL that persists despite diet therapy.

Other parameters for choosing insulin therapy: Defining the optimal criteria for insulin treatment solely by blood glucose values is problematic, because other metabolic factors and maternal nutrients also have an impact on fetal growth. The use of other indicators in addition to maternal blood sugar levels to determine the need for insulin therapy is being investigated. These include ultrasound measurements of various fetal dimensions to detect evolving macrosomia. Safety concerns restrict measurement of amniotic-fluid insulin levels (which reflect fetal insulin secretion) as a routine clinical tool. It is to be hoped that future controlled clinical trials will lead to more definitive recommendations concerning the use of ultrasound to direct insulin treatment.

Therapeutic algorithms: When insulin is used, doses ranging from 0.5 to 1.4 U/kg of body weight/day are required to maintain fasting and premeal glucose values of 65–85 mg/dL (3.6–4.7 mmol/L) and 1-hour postprandial values < 140 mg/dL (7.8 mmol/L). A twice-daily "mixed" insulin regimen is usually employed, although multiple injections may be used.

Sulfonylurea drugs: As a class, the sulfonylurea drugs have been avoided during pregnancy because some of them have been shown to cross the placenta, stimulate fetal insulin secretion, and promote neonatal hypoglycemia. Recently, Langer and coworkers have reported that the sulfonylurea glyburide does not cross the placenta in significant amounts late in gestation, and that it is as safe and efficacious as intensive insulin therapy. If these finding are confirmed, glyburide may become an important alternative for the treatment of GDM.

Exercise: Cardiovascular fitness training can increase insulin sensitivity and the disposal of glucose by recruitment of glucose transporters. It is often used in the treatment of suitable patients with diabetes. In pregnancy, concerns about increasing uterine contractility, IUGR, prematurity, fetal bradycardia, and ketonuria have overridden the potential beneficial effects of strenuous exercise. Studies employing moderate exercise regimens to reduce glycemia in GDM have produced inconsistent results.

Monitoring carbohydrate metabolism:

General monitoring procedures: Patients with GDM should monitor urinary or blood ketones before breakfast and supper to detect possible deficiencies in dietary carbohydrate. We obtain a fasting and 1-hour or 2-hour postbreakfast plasma glucose measurement at each office visit in patients who are not being treated with insulin. Many women on diet therapy choose to monitor capillary blood glucose values as well. Patients who are treated with insulin should monitor capillary blood sugar before meals (four times a day) and review results with the physician or nurse practitioner every 1–2 weeks.

Is there an optimal time to monitor? As described above for PGDM, we also recommended that patients monitor postprandial blood glucose levels on at least 2 days a week. Monitoring postprandial blood sugar exclusively to guide insulin dosage has been claimed to be superior to premeal testing. However, if appropriate target values are set and pursued with equal vigor, the two approaches may well be equivalent. To assess the accuracy on an ongoing basis, patients have plasma glucose measurements obtained at each office visit to compare with a simultaneously obtained finger-stick value performed by the patient. Some self-monitoring blood glucose systems may consistently over- or underestimate plasma glucose by as much as 10–15%. This must be determined on an individual basis and taken into account when insulin doses are modified.

POSTPARTUM FOLLOW-UP

Carbohydrate Metabolism

Rationale for Postpartum Evaluation

The diagnosis of gestational diabetes carries significant implications for long-term maternal health. During pregnancy, one cannot distinguish with certainty between evolving type 1 or type 2 diabetes and transitory glucose intolerance that will subside postpartum. Postpartum and long-term follow-up are therefore essential. Within the first year postpartum, a significant proportion of patients with GDM display impaired glucose tolerance or diabetes mellitus, and the proportion increases progressively with time. When FPG is elevated during pregnancy to the level that is diagnostic of diabetes (>125 mg/dL), the incidence of diabetes in the first year postpartum is very high (75–90%). It is likely that in many of these patients, abnormalities in glucose tolerance antedated pregnancy.

Prognostic Factors

Certain characteristics that have been identified during pregnancy increase the risk for postpartum glucose intolerance. These are: (1) relative insulin deficiency (lower basal insulin levels and blunted acute-phase insulin response to oral glucose); (2) severity of hyperglycemia; and (3) obesity. Other associations, such as early gestational age at diagnosis, racial/ethnic origin (increased in Hispanics), and family history of maternal diabetes, are probably mediated primarily through one or more of the factors noted above.

When and How to Test

Because of the risks outlined above, all women with GDM should be tested for glucose intolerance 6–12 weeks after delivery with either a fasting plasma glucose measurement or a 75-g OGTT and results interpreted as per the American Diabetes Association Expert Committee on the Diagnosis and Classification of Diabetes Mellitus. Those with glucose intolerance (impaired fasting glucose, impaired glucose tolerance test, or T2DM) should receive appropriate counseling and/or therapy. Individuals with a normal postpartum FPG or OGTT need annual fasting or postload glucose testing.

Toward a Healthier Lifestyle

Patients are advised to maintain ideal body weight, to exercise regularly, and to avoid the use of progestin-only oral contraceptives, thiazides, niacin, and oral corticosteroids if possible. It is also stressed that carbohydrate intolerance will likely worsen or recur with future pregnancies. Kjos and coworkers have identified postpartum characteristics that predict risks of progression to diabetes. These are higher level of glycemia at initial postpartum evaluation, further weight gain, use of progestin-only oral contraceptive pills, and subsequent pregnancy. Clinical trials designed to "prevent" or delay the development of diabetes in individuals at high risk (including women with previous GDM) with the use of pharmacologic agents, intensive lifestyle intervention, or both have confirmed the importance of these recommendations.

Contraception and Other Considerations

The postpartum period is an ideal time to reeducate patients about the importance of preconception care. The benefits of good metabolic control life-long, especially prior to a planned pregnancy, should be reinforced.

After Pregestational Diabetes

For the woman with T1DM, there are few substantive reasons for selecting one contraceptive method over another, and the woman's desires should be paramount in the decision.

- Barrier methods (condom, diaphragm) are less ideal choices because of a failure rate of at least 5% per woman-year.
- Intrauterine devices are effective and safe in women with diabetes mellitus and are an excellent choice for long-term contraception.

- Contemporary formulations of low-dose combination oral contraceptives have attenuated metabolic side effects and provide excellent contraception; transdermal delivery systems may increase compliance. Progestin-only preparations are also available, including levonorgestrel implants and depo medroxyprogesterone.
- Cardiovascular risks of hormonal contraceptives in nondiabetic women, particularly myocardial infarction, have been associated with concurrent smoking and higher dose formulations. There are no adequately controlled studies in women with diabetes mellitus, thus, the important benefit of avoiding unplanned pregnancy must be weighed against theoretical risks for the woman with vasculopathy.

After Gestational Diabetes

Although contraceptive counseling is similar to that for women with T1DM, there is the concern that oral contraceptives may result in a recrudescence of carbohydrate intolerance. This concern has not been borne out with use of contemporary low-dose formulations, although progestin-only oral contraceptive agents have been associated with some increased risk of diabetes after GDM. It is prudent to document normal postpartum carbohydrate tolerance before initiating any hormonal contraceptive and to recommend regular surveillance at 6–12-month intervals.

ADDITIONAL READINGS

Buchanan TA, Catalano PM: The pathogenesis of GDM: Implications for diabetes after pregnancy. *Diabetes Revs* 1995;3:584.

Freinkel N: The Banting Lecture 1980: Of pregnancy and progeny. *Diabetes* 1980; 29:1023.

Herman WH, Janz NK, Becker MP, et al: Diabetes and Pregnancy: Preconception care, pregnancy outcomes, resource utilization and costs. *J Reprod Med* 1999;44:33.

Kjos SL, Buchanan TA: Current concepts: Gestational diabetes mellitus. *N Engl J Med* 1999;341:1749.

Metzger BE, Coustan DR: The Organizing Committee. Summary and Recommendations of the Fourth International Workshop-Conference on Gestational Diabetes Mellitus. *Diabetes Care* 1998;21(suppl 2)161.

For a more detailed discussion of this topic and a bibliography, please see Porte *et al: Ellenberg & Rifkin's Diabetes Mellitus,* 6th ed., Chapter 38.

14 The Offspring of the Mother with Diabetes

Bernard L. Silverman   Edward S. Ogata
Boyd E. Metzger

PREGNANCY AS A "TISSUE CULTURE EXPERIENCE"

The importance of the intrauterine environment as a determinant of metabolic function throughout the life span is being increasingly recognized. Jorgen Pedersen was the first to propose a mechanism whereby maternal fuels may exert a direct effect on the fetus. He advanced the hyperglycemia-hyperinsulinism hypothesis, wherein he postulated that more maternal glucose gains access to the fetus whenever maternal insulin is inadequate, and that this extra glucose stimulates insulin release in the fetus and thereby produces an increase of fetal mass.

Subsequent work demonstrated that *all* maternal fuels may be maladjusted in even the mildest forms of gestational diabetes. Accordingly, the Pedersen hypothesis can be modified to include *maternal fuels besides glucose* that are also regulated by maternal insulin (Fig. 14-1). It is then expected that the growth-enhancing actions of these fuels would affect fetal insulin-sensitive structures to a greater degree than structures which are relatively insulin-insensitive. Thus the hallmark of diabetic macrosomia should be *asymmetrical* growth in which weight (as an index of adipose stores) would be affected more than biparietal diameter (as an index of cerebral growth) or length (as an index of skeletal growth). Thus pregnancy can be likened to a "tissue culture experience," since most of these fuels cross the placenta in concentration-dependent fashion so their concentrations in the maternal circulation may determine the quantitative as well as qualitative characteristics of the "incubation medium" in which the conceptus develops.

CLINICAL FEATURES OF SPECIFIC MORBIDITIES

Morbidities in infants of diabetic mothers (IDMs) are understood most readily in the context of the above alterations in the delivery of multiple building blocks from mother to conceptus and the attendant premature morphologic and functional development of the β-cells of the fetal pancreas leading to hyperinsulinism. Conversely, both the frequency and the severity of neonatal morbidities are reduced substantially when diabetes mellitus is well controlled throughout gestation.

Unexplained Fetal Loss during Late Gestation

Improvements in metabolic control of diabetes throughout pregnancy and in obstetric assessment of fetal well-being have markedly reduced the frequency of unexplained fetal loss in late gestation. The pathophysiologic sequences responsible for the increased risk of intrauterine fetal death, and for the poor ability to tolerate labor when pregnancy complicated by diabetes mellitus has not been optimally controlled, have not been elucidated.

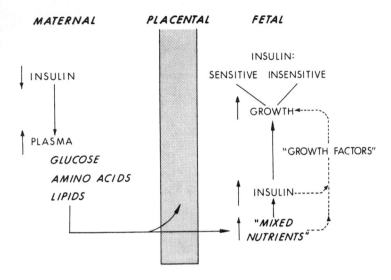

FIG. 14-1 Effect of maternal fuels on fetus development. The classical "hyperglycemia-hyperinsulinism" hypothesis of Pederson has been modified to include the contributions of other maternal fuels besides glucose that are also responsive to maternal insulin. All of these can influence the growth of the fetus and the maturation of fetal insulin secretion. Within this formation, growth will be disparately greater in insulin-sensitive than insulin-insensitive tissues in the fetus. *(From Freinkel N, Metzger BE: Pregnancy as a tissue culture experience: The critical implications of maternal metabolism for fetal development. In: Pregnancy Metabolism, Diabetes and the Fetus. CIBA Foundation Symposium No. 63. Excerpta Medica; 1979:3.)*

Birth Defects

Increased risks of congenital malformations and spontaneous abortions in pregnancies complicated by diabetes are linked to disturbances in maternal metabolism around the time of conception. However, when counseling and improved control of diabetes mellitus are initiated prior to conception, several groups have reported rates of major congenital malformations not higher than expected in the general obstetrical population. Unfortunately, in the United States, the majority of pregnant women with diabetes are not enrolled in regimens of tight metabolic control prior to conception. Consequently, major congenital malformations are still commonly encountered.

Neonatal Care of IDMs with Major Malformations

Infants of diabetic mothers with major malformations should be evaluated as if the cause of their malformations might not be maternal diabetes. For this reason, genetics consultation and studies of other organ systems (e.g., ultrasound imaging of the heart, kidneys, etc.) may be warranted. It is often appropriate to perform an imaging study of the brain to check for any gross abnormalities.

A multidisciplinary approach to support the family is critically important to address their emotional, social, and financial needs. If necessary, long-term-care plans must be devised and all aspects of discharge planning arranged well before the infant leaves the hospital.

Disturbances in Fetal Growth

As noted earlier, alterations in maternal metabolic fuels have a direct influence on the functional state of the fetal pancreatic ß-cells and the regulation of fetal growth. Normalization of the metabolic milieu throughout pregnancy is the key to prevention of fetal hyperinsulism and diabetic macrosomia. However, the incidence of large babies has tended to increase in recent years, especially in type 1 diabetes mellitus (T1DM). Better control of diabetes in early pregnancy (thus avoiding early growth retardation) and discontinuation of routine delivery before term may account for the rarity of intrauterine growth restriction and the increased prevalence of macrosomia. Rates of macrosomia as high as 30–40% have been reported in recent years, and the risk of birth trauma (shoulder dystocia) has increased.

Hypoglycemia

The normal human fetus at term is sufficiently metabolically mature to adapt to extrauterine life. It has adipose tissue, triglyceride stores, hepatic glycogen stores, and gluconeogenic capabilities. These depots interact in homeostatic fashion at birth as catecholamine and glucagon secretions surge while insulin secretion diminishes. The integrated relationships favor the production of endogenous glucose so the neonate can adapt to the sudden cessation of maternally derived glucose. Symptomatic hypoglycemia supervenes whenever this endogenous production of glucose is insufficient to sustain the fuel requirements of the brain.

From the screening of a large number of infants during the neonatal period, plasma glucose concentrations of 1.4–1.7 mmol/L (25–30 mg/dL) have often been used as benchmarks of neonatal hypoglycemia. However, it has been suggested that glucose provision to tissues may not always be adequate when plasma glucose concentrations are at these statistically derived lower limits, and that a value of 2.2 mmol/L (40 mg/dL) is more consistent with safe levels of glucose flux. Within that framework, approximately 20–25% of all IDMs experience neonatal hypoglycemia, usually during the first 4–6 hours. It must be emphasized that the level of plasma glucose concentration corresponding to inadequate provision of glucose to the brain is difficult to assess, and that the duration of hypoglycemia necessary to damage the central nervous system has not been determined. Within this framework, transient or persistent hypoglycemia (defined as two or more plasma glucose concentrations < 1.7 mmol/L [30 mg/dL] in the first 48 hours of life), when diagnosed and treated, does not adversely affect cognitive development in IDMs at 2–5 years of age. This emphasizes the importance of optimizing both maternal and neonatal care.

The potent role of hyperinsulinism in neonatal hypoglycemia is established. The clinical manifestations of neonatal hypoglycemia may vary substantially. Hypoglycemic infants may remain asymptomatic or become limp, obtunded, jittery, tremulous, sweaty, or cyanotic. Seizures may develop, and profound hypoglycemia may cause brain damage. If hypoglycemia is prolonged, myocardial contractility diminishes and congestive heart failure may develop. Accordingly, all IDMs should be screened for hypoglycemia hourly until the first full feeding and at frequent intervals during the first 24 hours of life. If reagent strips are used to screen for neonatal hypoglycemia, abnormal values must be confirmed with actual plasma or blood determinations in the laboratory. While awaiting laboratory documentation, asymptomatic infants who are capable of oral feeding may receive glucose solution to correct hypoglycemia. Symptomatic infants should be treated with 10–15 mL/kg of 10% glucose solution rather than with more concentrated solutions of glucose, which risk precipitating greater acute insulin release. Follow-up measurements of glucose must always be secured to assure adequacy of therapy and to screen for potential recurrence of hypoglycemia.

Respiratory Distress Syndrome (RDS)

Infants of diabetic mothers have been considered at increased risk for the development of RDS. However, much of this risk may be eliminated by tight control of maternal metabolism. The inordinate susceptibility of the offspring of the poorly regulated diabetic mother to RDS has been linked to a delay in the processes leading to fetal lung maturation. The advent of exogenous surfactant therapy has greatly improved the ability to treat RDS.

Hypocalcemia and Hypomagnesemia

Calcium concentrations should be measured after birth in both sick and healthy IDMs, since significant hypocalcemia may develop in the neonatal period. Hypomagnesemia, which limits parathyroid hormone secretion even in the presence of hypocalcemia, may be an important contributing factor. The hypomagnesemia develops in women with diabetes as a result of increased renal losses associated with glucosuria. This in turn causes fetal and neonatal hypomagnesemia.

Clinical signs of hypocalcemia include jitteriness, twitching, or seizures; arrhythmias may also occur. The neonate may not develop the characteristic prolongation of the QT interval associated with hypocalcemia in the adult.

Symptomatic hypocalcemia should be treated with an infusion of 10% calcium gluconate (2 mL/kg body weight over 5–10 minutes). During infusion, monitoring with an electrocardiogram is important. IDMs may require from 75 to 200 mg/kg elemental calcium/day, administered either enterally or parenterally. IDMs who are hypocalcemic on the basis of hypomagnesemia will not become normocalcemic until their hypomagnesemia is corrected. A 50% solution of magnesium at a dose of 0.25 mg/kg may be administered intramuscularly to correct hypomagnesemia.

Polycythemia/Hyperviscosity

IDMs are at increased risk for polycythemia and for the development of the neonatal polycythemia/hyperviscosity syndrome. Increased red cell mass is directly correlated with hyperviscosity. Hyperviscosity or red cell sludging can have severe consequences, including seizures and gastrointestinal injury. The primary therapy for the polycythemia/hyperviscosity syndrome is partial exchange transfusion to reduce red cell mass.

Hyperbilirubinemia

Neonatal hyperbilirubinemia occurs more frequently in IDMs because of increased red cell breakdown. In addition, the macrosomia of the IDM can increase the risk of bruising at delivery and thereby also augment bilirubin production.

Hypertrophic Cardiomyopathy

Many IDM neonates have a thickened interventricular septum and left or right ventricular wall. While most such infants are asymptomatic, some develop congestive heart failure as a result of left ventricular outflow obstruction. These abnormalities generally regress over 3–6 months.

"Lazy Left Colon"

A functional bowel anomaly unique to IDMs may present as neonatal gastrointestinal obstruction. Barium contrast studies are suggestive of aganglionic megacolon. However, normal bowel function eventually supervenes.

LONG-RANGE IMPLICATIONS OF THE INTRAUTERINE ENVIRONMENT: FUEL-MEDIATED TERATOGENESIS

Freinkel proposed that abnormal fuel delivery *in utero* could exert permanent long-range effects on the offspring ("fuel-mediated teratogenesis"). For example, maternal hyperglycemia, hyperaminoacidemia, or elevated free fatty acids during the second half of pregnancy, when fetal adipocytes, muscle cells, pancreatic cells, and neuroendocrine networks are undergoing proliferation and differentiation, might confer greater vulnerability for obesity or type 2 diabetes mellitus (T2DM) in later life; abnormal fuel mixtures during the first and second trimester when the brain is established and brain cells are being formed might result in subsequent neurologic, psychologic, or cognitive deficits; and disturbances in the early part of the first trimester during embryogenesis might compromise organogenesis and so produce birth defects (fuel-mediated organ teratogenesis).

Behavioral and Intellectual Functions

The possibility of long-term neurologic deficits in the offspring of diabetic mothers has been recognized for a number of years. Obvious factors, such as prolonged severe neonatal hypoglycemia, birth trauma, neonatal kernicterus, and others have been implicated in many such cases in the past. However, more subtle adverse effects have also been ascribed to fuel metabolism-related pathology.

The longitudinal observations of the Northwestern University Diabetes in Pregnancy Center have included detailed analysis of neuropsychologic development in offspring of diabetic mothers. On average, these offspring experienced minimally abnormal intrauterine fuel exposures. Significant mental deficiency was no different than national estimates in this group of offspring of mothers with well-controlled gestational and pregestational diabetes. Direct correlations were found between poorer maternal glucoregulation during the second and third trimesters and poorer performance at birth on the Brazelton Neonatal Behavioral Assessment Scales. Similarly, direct correlations between mild maternal ketonemia in the second and third trimesters and poorer performance on both the Mental Development Index of the Bayley Scales of Infant Development at age 2 and the Stanford-Binet Intelligence Scales at ages 3–5 years have been reported. Finally, average scores on the WISC-R Full Scale IQ at ages 7–11 years were inversely correlated with maternal HbA_{1c} in the second trimester and β-hydroxybuterate in the third trimester. Analysis of child educational achievement demonstrated lower scores on the arithmetic index that correlated with higher maternal third-trimester free fatty acids. The above correlations between intrauterine metabolism and development in childhood are not substantially different in gestational than in pregestational diabetes mellitus.

Data reported from Denmark are also consistent with the postulate of congenital fuel-mediated behavioral effects. In addition, Sells and colleagues compared neurodevelopment through 36 months of age in 109 infants of mothers with T1DM and 90 control infants. Mothers who were enrolled in a program of strict glycemic control before or within 21 days of conception had lower glycosylated hemoglobins than mothers enrolled later. Neurodevelopment of the offspring of earlier-enrolled mothers was similar to the control infants, whereas offspring of the later-enrolled mothers scored less well on tests of language development.

Such experiences have not been universal. Several retrospective surveys have failed to disclose an increased incidence of gross neurologic and/or IQ deficits in the offspring of diabetic mothers. However, negative reports need not necessarily exclude the possibility of small correlations between perturbations of maternal metabolism at key stages in pregnancy and long-range behavioral and/or intellectual performance.

Obesity

A number of analyses of the offspring of diabetic parents have disclosed disparities in weight relative to height during childhood and adolescence. It has been noted that the obesity is far more frequent in the offspring of diabetic mothers than diabetic fathers.

In the Northwestern University Diabetes in Pregnancy Center study, neonatal macrosomia in offspring of diabetic mothers disappeared by 1 year of age. After 2–3 years of age, offspring of diabetic mothers tend to gain weight faster than other children, and rapid weight gain is observed after 5 years of age. By 8 years of age almost half of the offspring of diabetic mothers in this cohort had a weight greater than the 90th percentile. This trend continues into adolescence, with rather dramatic increases in body mass index for the highest quartile (Fig. 14-2). Significant differences were not observed between offspring of mothers with gestational diabetes mellitus (GDM) when compared to offspring of mothers with pregestational diabetes mellitus (PGDM). Relative obesity in childhood, at ages 6–8 years, is significantly correlated with insulin secretion *in utero,* as is relative obesity in adolescence, ages 14–17 years.

In a study of 71 offspring of mothers with T1DM, Weiss and associates found correlations between amniotic fluid insulin measured at 31 ± 2 weeks gestation and body mass index at 5–15 years of age.

Further support for an effect of antepartum maternal glucoregulation on the subsequent anthropometric development of the offspring has come from studies of the Pima Indians, a relatively pure genetic group having the highest reported incidence and prevalence of type 2 diabetes mellitus.

Pettitt and coworkers have correlated the 2-hour response of Pima Indian mothers to oral glucose during pregnancy with the occurrence of obesity in their offspring. They have found that obesity is present at age 15–19 in two-thirds of the offspring whose mothers were diabetic during gestation. By con-

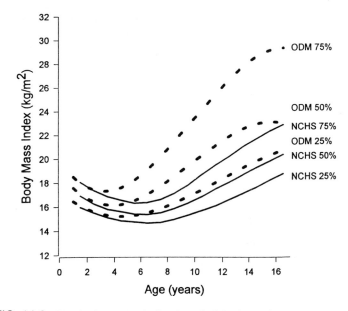

FIG. 14-2   Physical growth of offspring of diabetic mothers expressed as body mass index. Solid lines indicate percentiles for BMI of normal U.S. children as published by the National Center for Health Statistics; dashed lines depict 25th, 50th, and 75th percentiles for ODM. Data were smoothed by fitting to a third-order regression. *(From Silverman BL, Rizzo TA, Cho NH, et al: Long-term effects of the intrauterine environment: The Northwestern University Diabetes in Pregnancy Center. Diabetes Care 1998;21(Suppl 2):B142.)*

trast, they have encountered obesity in only 40% of the 15- to 19-year-olds whose mothers had the genetic propensity for obesity and diabetes, but did not become diabetic until after the pregnancy, and in 30% of the offspring whose mothers never became diabetic. Moreover, offspring of diabetic women were heavier than offspring of nondiabetic and prediabetic women, regardless of birthweight.

Abnormal Glucoregulation and Diabetes Mellitus

Diabetes has been classically viewed as a genetic disorder, and "diabetic genes" have been invoked to explain the increased incidence of diabetes in the offspring of diabetic parents. However, evidence from animal models and epidemiologic studies suggests that disturbance in islet function or development during intrauterine and early postnatal life also predispose to metabolic disturbances and impaired glucose tolerance in later life.

The offspring of gravidas enrolled in the Northwestern University Diabetes in Pregnancy Center long-term follow-up (ODM) are demonstrating an increased frequency of impaired glucose tolerance. At 14–17 years of age, mean fasting glucose and insulin concentrations in ODM are no different than in 80 control subjects, however, 2 hours after a glucose load, both glucose and insulin are elevated. The rate of impaired glucose tolerance is increased (Fig. 14-3). The relative risk of impaired glucose tolerance is 4.7 for offspring who had an elevated mean amniotic fluid insulin concentration. Plagemann and colleagues also report an increased incidence of impaired glucose tolerance in offspring of mothers with both gestational and type 1 diabetes (T1DM).

The Pima Indian studies provide additional evidence. Pettitt and associates reported that T2DM is present by age 20–24 in 45.5% of the offspring of "diabetic mothers," but in only 8.6% and 1.4% of the offspring of "prediabetic" or "nondiabetic mothers," respectively. In a study of Pima siblings born before or after the mother's development of diabetes, those exposed to maternal diabetes *in utero* had a 3.7-fold greater risk of developing diabetes.

Converse congenital relationships may also pertain in T1DM. Retrospective studies by Warram and coworkers have disclosed a two- to fivefold greater risk for the development of T1DM in the offspring of fathers than mothers with T1DM. These researchers have suggested that the seeming maternal protection against subsequent T1DM may be due to an induction of immunologic tolerance to the autoantigens of the β-cells during intrauterine development. Weiss and coworkers examined offspring of diabetic mothers at 5–15 years of age.

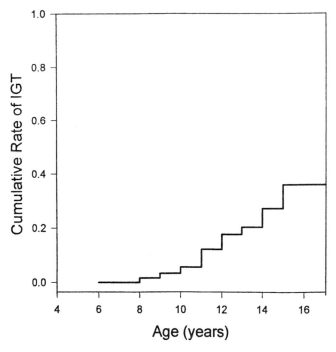

FIG. 14-3 Cumulative probability (Kaplan-Meir estimator) of impaired glucose tolerance (IGT) or diabetes in offspring of diabetic mothers. *(From Silverman BL, Rizzo TA, Cho NH, et al: Long-term effects of the intrauterine environment: The Northwestern University Diabetes in Pregnancy Center.* Diabetes Care *1998;21(Suppl 2):B142.)*

They find higher glucose, insulin, and C-peptide concentrations, especially in those offspring who had higher amniotic fluid insulin concentrations *in utero* at 31 ± 2 weeks. Thus, although the directional impacts may be different, current data indicate that nature (as embodied by genetic propensities) may be modified by nurture (as determined by congenital contributions via the intrauterine metabolic environment) in the pathogenesis of T1DM as well as T2DM.

Other Cardiovascular Risk Factors

In the Northwestern Diabetes in Pregnancy Center Study, body mass index, blood pressure, and lipid concentrations were examined in 99 offspring of diabetic mothers (ODM) and 80 controls. ODM were more obese, and had higher systolic and mean arterial blood pressure (BP), but similar diastolic BP compared to controls. ODM had lower fasting concentrations of low-density lipoprotein (LDL) and total cholesterol. In both groups, body mass index, triglycerides, and fasting and 2-hour glucose concentrations showed correlations with BP measurements. The increased prevalence of obesity, impaired glucose, and elevated blood pressure may predispose offspring of diabetic mothers to an increased risk of heart disease in adulthood.

General Relevance for Development in Later Life

The proposition that maternal fuel metabolism may exert long-range effects on development is being corroborated by many retrospective and prospective experiences. As such, there are now more reasons than ever to normalize maternal metabolism in all pregnancies complicated by diabetes and for viewing the success of pregnancy outcome in terms of the entire lifetime of the progeny as well as traditional perinatal criteria.

Moreover, these fuel-related phenomena need not be limited to pregnancies complicated by diabetes. The same relationships between ambient fuels, fetal insulin secretion, and gene expression *in utero* may well apply to all pregnancies, so the potential for fuel-mediated teratogenesis may be present whenever maternal metabolism is perturbed for any reason. Hales and colleagues have found that impaired growth *in utero* and in infancy is associated with impaired glucose tolerance and T2DM in adulthood. Thus, diabetes in pregnancy has merely served as a paradigm for a more general truism, and the broad ramifications for all of feto-maternal medicine extend far beyond the more parochial preoccupation with diabetes *per se*. To quote Freinkel and Metzger, "No single period in human development provides a greater potential (than pregnancy) for long-range 'pay-off' via a relatively short-range period of enlightened metabolic manipulation."

ACKNOWLEDGMENTS

The authors are grateful to their many collaborators in the Departments of Medicine, Obstetrics, and Pediatrics who have contributed to The Northwestern University Diabetes in Pregnancy Center studies that are cited in this chapter. This work has been supported in part by National Institutes of Health (NIH) research grants DK10699, HD11021, HD19070, HD62903, HD23141, and RR-48; by Training Grant DK07169 from the U.S. Public Health Service; and by a grant from the Ronald McDonald Foundation.

ADDITIONAL READINGS

Cornblath M, Schwartz R, Aynsley-Green A, et al: Hypoglycemia in infancy: The need for rational definition. *Pediatrics* 1990;85:834.

Freinkel N, Metzger BE: Pregnancy as a tissue culture experience: The critical implications of maternal metabolism for fetal development. In: Pregnancy Metabolism, Diabetes and the Fetus. CIBA Foundation Symposium No. 63. Excerpta Medica; 1979:3.

Kitzmiller JL, Gavin LA, Gin GD, et al: Preconception care of diabetes. Glycemic control prevents congenital anomalies. *JAMA* 1991;265:731.

Pettitt DJ, Nelson RG, Saad MF, et al: Diabetes and obesity in the offspring of Pima Indian women with diabetes during pregnancy. *Diabetes Care* 1993;16:310.

Silverman BL, Rizzo TA, Cho NH, et al: Long-term effects of the intrauterine environment: The Northwestern University Diabetes in Pregnancy Center. *Diabetes Care* 1998;21(Suppl 2):B142.

For a more detailed discussion of this topic and a bibliography, please see Porte *et al: Ellenberg & Rifkin's Diabetes Mellitus,* 6th ed., Chapter 39.

Diabetes and Surgery

Stephanie A. Amiel   K. George M. M. Alberti

A diabetic person has a 50% chance of having a surgical procedure during his or her lifetime. This chance is steadily increasing with the greater life expectancy of diabetic people and the greater proportion undergoing cardiovascular interventions. Surgery in diabetic patients is complicated by the need for metabolic control during surgery itself and in the postoperative period when feeding is reinstated. The chronic complications are also likely to complicate recovery, particularly with respect to autonomic nephropathy and macrovascular disease. A further challenge is offered by the greatly increased volume of (ambulatory) day surgery now performed.

Surgery and anesthesia have profound metabolic effects, which will be exacerbated in diabetes by insulin deficiency or hyposecretion and by insulin insensitivity. The poorly controlled diabetic will already be in a catabolic state, which will amplify the effects of surgery. There will be diminished phagocyte function, with impaired resistance to infection and delayed wound healing. Together with the chronic complications of diabetes, these factors will add to the morbidity and mortality of the surgical procedures themselves. The aim of treatment of the diabetic patient undergoing surgery must therefore be to control the metabolic scenario in such a way that the risks are no greater and the outcome no worse than for the nondiabetic person.

In this chapter, practical aspects of the pre-, peri-, and postoperative management of the diabetic patient will be reviewed.

METABOLIC EFFECTS OF ANESTHESIA AND SURGERY IN THE NORMAL AND DIABETIC STATES

Anesthesia

The impact of modern anesthetic agents on metabolic control is relatively small. Epidural anesthesia blocks catecholamine release and can reduce postoperative protein catabolism. Both locoregional and general anesthesia can be used safely. More important is the presence of autonomic neuropathy or cardiovascular disease in the recipient.

Surgery

By contrast, surgery induces a trauma-like stress state, and provides a classic hyperglycemic challenge. The stress response to both the condition for which the surgery is being performed and any associated anxiety includes adrenergic and sympathetic activation and elevations of circulating catecholamines, cortisol, and growth hormone. These may be sufficient to convert well-controlled diabetes into hyperglycemia—even ketoacidosis, particularly when the surgical condition is an acute one. Furthermore, immobility reduces muscle consumption of glucose and contributes to the hyperglycemia. Surgery is associated with a reduction in insulin sensitivity that persists for several weeks. Food deprivation further worsens the catabolic state. In health the small amounts of circulating insulin still present limit the extent of the catabolic processes. This does not pertain in surgery. The molecular mechanisms

231

of the insulin resistance of surgery remain to be elucidated, but a major effect on peripheral glucose utilization has been observed.

Neural effects are also important in the catabolic response. Epidural anesthesia, spinal blocks, and splanchnic nerve blocks have all been shown to ameliorate the endocrine and metabolic response.

Diabetes

The uncontrolled diabetic patient will already be in a catabolic state. Superimposition of the metabolic stress of surgery will result in a major worsening of this state. In order to minimize the adverse effects of these metabolic events on the diabetic patient, meticulous attention to metabolic control is required. The response of surgery relates to the severity of the surgery. Type 1 diabetic patients will require insulin replacement regardless, but type 2 diabetic patients will probably be able to mount an adequate insulin response to minor surgery and insulin therapy may not be required. By contrast, they usually do require insulin for major surgery.

Aims of Therapy

The main aim of therapy must be to avoid any excess morbidity and mortality when compared with the nondiabetic population. To achieve this, hypoglycemia, excessive hyperglycemia, increased protein catabolism, and undue electrolyte disturbances should be prevented. In addition, attention should be paid to cardiovascular status and to problems created by the long-term complications of diabetes. These goals are best achieved by controlling the metabolic status of the patient. In general, it is wise to aim for blood glucose levels at which resistance to infection and phagocyte function are not impaired and at which normal wound healing can take place. The threshold for these effects is probably around 200 mg/dL (11 mmol/L), so that to aim for glycemia in the range of 125–180 mg/dL (7–10 mmol/L) is reasonable. It should be noted that recent studies from critical care setting suggest that even more stringent targets reduce morbidity and mortality (i.e., blood glucose < 110 mg/dL) in postoperative patients.

Preoperative Management

All patients require a full preoperative assessment. The diabetic patient presenting for surgery is more likely to have co-morbidity than the patient without diabetes. Assessment of glycemic control and current therapeutic regimen is mandatory. The glycated hemoglobin will indicate the patient's habitual control. The random glucose is not useful until starting perioperative management.

Cardiovascular status should be assessed by history and resting EKG. Symptomatic autonomic neuropathy is uncommon in diabetes, but lesser degrees of cardiac denervation are not. The anesthetist should be aware of potential defects in the normal cardiovascular responses to hypotension in anesthesia induction. An exaggerated pressor response to intubation has been reported in patients presenting for vitreous surgery. All had some degree of autonomic dysfunction preoperatively, and all failed to show a heart rate increase when blood pressure fell. This is particularly important, as cardiorespiratory arrest is known to occur in patients with autonomic neuropathy and diabetic patients are more likely to have respiratory arrests postoperatively.

Hypertension coexisting with diabetes is common, and its management should be optimized prior to surgery. Clinical examination for peripheral vascular disease and peripheral neuropathy are vital. The patient with impalpable pedal pulses, especially if the feet are insensitive, is very vulnerable to pressure ulceration. Retinal status is unlikely to be adversely affected by surgery, although renal impairment is a common problem in long-duration diabetes and renal status must be assessed preoperatively.

Careful assessment of metabolic status is essential. In type 1 diabetic patients every effort should be made to achieve good glycemic control before admission. Patients should be on a combination of short- and intermediate-acting insulins. In type 2 diabetic patients, sulfonylureas should be stopped, because of the risk of hypoglycemia. Metformin should be stopped on the day of operation except in those with abnormal renal function, in whom it should be stopped forthwith. Thiazolidinediones may be continued, although it is probably prudent to withold them on the day of surgery. α-Glucosidase inhibitors are ineffective when the patient is fasting.

All these measures (Table 15-1) should be undertaken preadmission. Ideally, patients should be admitted 1 or 2 days before surgery to allow final assessment. However, this rarely occurs, making preadmission screening even more important.

Diabetes, particularly type 2, may be diagnosed for the first time when a patient is admitted for routine surgery. This is particularly true for elderly patients. Operation should be delayed until glycemic control has been achieved and the patient fully assessed. In general, one should aim for fasting glucose levels of <125 mg/dL (7 mmol/L) and postprandial levels of <180 mg/dL (10 mmol/L). For urgent surgery—e.g., for malignant disease—control

TABLE 15-1 Preoperative Assessment and Preparation
of the Diabetic Patient for Surgery

General measures
Cardiovascular assessment
History of angina, infarction
History of hypertension
EKG
Blood pressure
Full examination including peripheral pulses
Neurologic assessment
Peripheral neuropathy
Autonomic examination: R–R interval
Renal assessment
Proteinuria
Serum creatinine
Urine culture
Electrolytes (sodium, potassium)
Metabolic Assessment
Glycosylated hemoglobin
Home glucose control
T1DM: Stop long-acting insulin, substitute twice-daily split and mixed or tid regimens*
T2DM: Stop long-acting sulfonylureas (e.g,. glyburide), substitute short-acting agents; stop metformin and all other oral agents on day of surgery

*For outpatient surgery, omit or use half the dose of intermediate-acting insulin the evening before surgery.

can be rapidly established in hospital over days with insulin therapy; in less urgent situations, time can be taken to establish control conventionally with diet, exercise, and oral hypoglycemic agents.

Ideally, pre- and postoperative care should be under the joint management of the diabetes, anesthetic, and surgical teams.

Perioperative Management

In type 1 diabetic patients the need for continued insulin replacement is self-evident. In type 2 patients the indications are also clear. In a patient who is very well controlled on diet alone, management may be possible, especially for minor procedures, as with nondiabetic patients, with the exception that blood glucose should be monitored frequently, with the requirement to start insulin replacement should glucose levels rise above 200 mg/dL (11 mmol/L). With all other type 2 diabetic patients on any form of pharmacologic therapy to lower blood glucose, substitution of that therapy with monitored intravenous insulin therapy is generally required.

Ambulatory surgery offers special challenges, and is best avoided except in well-controlled type 2 diabetic patients. Operations under local anesthetic, such as for cataract, can then safely be undertaken with omission of therapy on the morning of the operation. It has been shown that cataract operations under local anesthesia cause relatively minor hormonal and metabolic disturbance compared with general anesthesia.

Blood Glucose Control

A glycemic aim should be determined for each patient. The risk of hypoglycemia is a concern, as the classic signs may be masked by anesthesia and may be absent in patients with long-standing diabetes who are taking insulin. A glycemic goal of 125–200 mg /dL (7–11 mmol/L) is therefore acceptable during operation and can be tightened up postoperatively. This will keep glucose levels below those that cause glycosuria and dehydration and also will not inhibit phagocyte function and wound healing.

Blood glucose should be measured at the bedside on the morning of surgery, 2-hourly until the patient is anesthetised, hourly during surgery, and then 2–4-hourly during the first 24 hours, depending on the severity of the procedure.

Type 1 Diabetic Patients

All type 1 diabetic patients should be treated with insulin during surgery involving general anesthesia, regardless of the severity of the operation (Table 15-2). Operations should be scheduled early in the day.

Insulin Therapy

Over the years a large number of different regimens have been advocated for glycemic management during surgery. These have ranged from giving no insulin at all to using a low-dose SC insulin infusion with no added glucose. The former has obvious unwanted catabolic sequelae, while the latter was only safe because patients were hyperglycemic preoperatively and therefore did not become hypoglycemic.

The main recommendations, however, are variants on two themes: (1) SC insulin with IV dextrose; and (2) IV infusion of glucose and insulin either separately or together, generally with added potassium.

TABLE 15-2 Outline Guide to Management of Diabetes during Surgery

| | Current diabetic treatment | | |
	Diet	Oral agents	Insulin
Minor surgery	Check BG preop. If <200 mg/dL, continue. If >200 mg/dL, start GIK.	Check BG preop. If <200 mg/dL, continue. If >200 mg/dL, start GIK. Delay oral agents on day of surgery until first meal.	Check BG preop. If <270 mg/dL, continue. If >270 mg/dL, stabilize on insulin infusion until BG <200 mg/dL and/or delay operation.
Major surgery	Use GIK as for T1DM. If BG >270 mg/dL, stabilize on insulin infusion until BG <200 mg/dL and/or delay operation.	Use GIK as for T1DM. If BG >270 mg/dL, stabilize on insulin infusion until BG <200 mg/dL and/or delay operation. Omit SUs.	As above.

For GIK patients, monitor BG preop, intraop (if operation >2 hours), immediately postop, then 2-hourly until BG stable. For others, check BG pre- and postop. Use test strips + meter for BG monitoring (see text for cautions). GIK: glucose/insulin/potassium or insulin (pump) + glucose:potassium infusion.

Subcutaneous (SC) Regimens

SC regimens allow little flexibility and insulin absorption, always variable, may be further compromized by changes in circulation and peripheral perfusion induced by anesthesia. There seems little rationale for their continued use, except perhaps for day surgery under local anesthesia.

Intravenous (IV) Regimens

A large number of different routines have been proposed for the use of IV insulin. Some give a fixed infusion rate of insulin, modifying the glucose infusion according to blood glucose levels, whereas the converse of keeping glucose infusion constant and varying insulin infusion rate has also been suggested. Others have varied the initial insulin dose according to preoperative blood glucose level or to previous insulin dose, while complex algorithms to determine the rate of insulin administration have also found favor.

Two main variants of insulin infusion protocols are now recommended. These are (1) combined insulin and glucose infusions with added potassium (GIK); and (2) insulin given by infusion pump with glucose (and potassium) given by separate infusion (IP/GK). In both cases potassium is necessary, as insulin infusion lowers plasma potassium levels. Both regimens have advantages, with GIK being safest, but the separate infusions are the gold standard for well-equipped, well-staffed centers.

Glucose, insulin, and potassium regimen: This system was originally designed for use in average general hospitals and needed to be simple, safe, and reproducible. Safety is ensured by glucose and insulin being in the same infusion so that they will speed up and slow down together. It remains essentially as described in 1979. The infusate comprised 10 U of regular insulin plus 10 mmol of potassium chloride in 500 mL of 10% dextrose given at 100 mL/h. Based on the original data, we subsequently increased the content of insulin to 15 U (0.30 U/g glucose). In one study, plasma glucose levels remained within the target range in 82% of cases and unexplained hypoglycemia and severe hyperglycemia were avoided. The amount of insulin required varies to some extent depending on the state of the patient and preexisting conditions (Table 15-3). These can be used as starting doses.

Some have recommended use of 5% rather than 10% dextrose. We prefer the latter, as it gives 240 g carbohydrate (960 kcal) per 24 hours, rather than 120 g (480 kcal). It has been suggested that at least 150 g carbohydrate per day plus insulin is needed to inhibit hepatic glucose production and protein catabolism, although this is somewhat arbitrary. Slower rates of administration of more concentrated solutions of glucose are appropriate when it is necessary to restrict fluid administration or when complex fluid replacement regimens are needed for other reasons. Thus 50 mL/h of 20% dextrose or 20 mL/h of 50% dextrose may be used, given through a central line.

TABLE 15-3 Insulin Requirements during Surgery

Condition	Insulin (U)/glucose (g)
Normal weight	0.25–0.35
Obesity	0.4
Liver disease	0.4–0.6
Steroid therapy	0.4–0.5
Grass sepsis	0.5–0.7
Cardiopulmonary bypass	0.9–1.2

There are some disadvantages to the GIK regimen. These include the need to change the whole infusate bag if a change of insulin dose is needed, although this is surprisingly infrequent for routine operations. More important perhaps is that insulin is absorbed on to IV fluid bags and giving sets. The problem can be diminished by flushing the infusate through the giving set. It is not a major problem in practice but is avoided by using a more concentrated insulin solution in a syringe pump.

Separate insulin and glucose regimens: Many centers, particularly in the United States, prefer to give insulin separately using an infusion pump. This gives more precise delivery of insulin and allows speedy change of dose or infusion rate as required. It has also been used extremely effectively in children and adolescents. It is probably the gold standard, being extremely flexible, although if not carefully monitored, there is a risk of giving glucose without insulin and vice versa. The same rules apply, however, regarding units of insulin per gram of glucose.

Practical Guidelines

Blood glucose and potassium should be checked on the morning of surgery. Glucose can be measured with a test strip and meter. A simultaneous sample should be sent to the laboratory as a later check. If blood glucose is greater than 270 mg/dL (15 mmol/L), surgery should be delayed, particularly if major surgery is planned. Either an attempt can be made to achieve control rapidly using the glucose-insulin-potassium (GIK) infusion with twice the usual insulin content (60 U/L 10% glucose) or surgery is delayed. Alternatively, insulin can be given at 4–6 U/h by syringe pump. If blood glucose is greater than 400 mg/dL (22.2 mmol/L), then delay and restabilization are mandatory.

The intravenous insulin and glucose infusion can be started when the surgical patient is due his or her first insulin dose after being made NPO. The patient scheduled for morning surgery who is normally controlled on intermittent insulin injection therapy does not need to start intravenous insulin (with its requirements for hourly blood glucose monitoring) until just before breakfast the day of the procedure, despite stopping eating after the evening meal the day before. This allows the patient a near-normal night's sleep. Plasma glucose should be checked at bedtime and at 3.00 A.M., as these are the times when the action of the evening's subcutaneous regular and intermediate-acting insulins, respectively, will be waning. Supplemental subcutaneous regular insulin (25–50% of the patient's usual premeal dose) can be prescribed for these times if the blood glucose is over 11 mmol/L to avoid starting the intravenous insulin in a hyperglycemic state. Similarly, the patient scheduled for afternoon surgery can be given a light breakfast with a suitably adjusted dose of regular insulin and intravenous insulinization started mid-morning.

The GIK regimen can be based on either 10% (preferably) or 5% dextrose (Table 15-4). Careful monitoring of the plasma glucose is key. The first check after the fasting sample should be at 2 hours or immediately preoperatively, whichever is first. Plasma glucose and potassium are measured again in the recovery room, and intraoperatively for long operations.

For the insulin pump regimen, it is usual to make a solution of regular insulin in saline of 1 U/mL, by putting 50 U of the insulin in a 50-mL syringe and making the solution up to 50 mL with the diluent. The dextrose is given as in the GIK regimen—preferably 10% solutions, 50–100 mL per hour, each liter containing 20 mmol potassium. The insulin infusion rate is set at slightly

TABLE 15-4 Glucose-Insulin-Potassium (GIK) Infusion Protocols

Plasma glucose	Protocol A*	Protocol B†
(mg/dL)	Insulin dose (U/l)	
<80	↓ 10	↓ 5
<120	↓ 5	↓ 3
120–180	Leave unchanged	
>180	↑ 5	↑ 3
>270	↑ 10	↑ 5

*A. 30 U regular insulin (human) + 20 mmol KCl in 1000 ml 20% dextrose. Give at 100 mL/h.
†B. 15 U regular insulin (human) + 20 mmol KCl in 1000 ml 5% dextrose. Give at 100 mL/h.

less than the patient's usual hourly requirement (total daily subcutaneous insulin doses divided by 24, or 0.3 U/g IV glucose for adults if not known) for the glucose level 120–180 mg/dL and adjusted up or down according to hourly plasma glucose measurements made at the bedside (see Table 15-5). The scale should be reviewed regularly and adjusted to maintain plasma glucose in the range 121–160 mg/dL.

Type 2 Diabetic Patients

All patients left on their usual hypoglycemic drugs risk hyperglycemia in response to the stress of surgery and hypoglycemia in response to the lack of food intake. Patients on metformin are unlikely to become hypoglycemic, but any fall in renal perfusion associated with the anesthesia or the surgery increases their risk of lactic acidosis. Sulfonylureas carry a risk of hypoglycemia, especially the longer-acting agents, such as glyburide (glibenclamide), which is likely to be both late in onset and prolonged. There are no data on surgery in patients on thiazolidenediones or meglitinides. In all cases

TABLE 15-5 An Example of the Separate Intravenous Glucose and Insulin Regimen*

Plasma glucose (mg/dL)	Insulin (U/h)	Insulin (mL/h)
<80	0.5	0.5
80–120	1.0	1.0
121–160†	2.0†	2.0†
161–200	3.0	3.0
201–250	4.0	4.0
251–300	5.0	5.0
>300	6.0	6.0

*Glucose: 10% dextrose containing 20 mmol KCl/L, 100 mL/h
Insulin: 50 U regular insulin made up to 50 mL in 0.9% saline = 1 U/mL
†The regimen should be personalized to the patient, such that this dose is calculated as the patient's usual total daily insulin dose (all regular and intermediate- or long-acting insulin doses taken in one normal day) divided by 24. The doses for measured plasma glucose outside this range are then increased or reduced by 1 U/h for each range above or below this target. The insulin scale can be rewritten if needed to keep plasma glucose in the 121–160-mg/dL range.

the drugs should not be taken on the day of surgery. This is especially true for the insulin secretagogues. Thiazolidinediones may be continued since, as monotherapy, they do not result in hypoglycemia; however, it may be prudent to withold them on the day of surgery. Despite previous recommendation, metformin too can just be withheld on the operative day.

The main determinants of therapy in the type 2 diabetic patient are (1) the magnitude of the intended surgical procedure; and (2) the metabolic state of the patient on the day of surgery. The exception is the insulin-treated type 2 diabetic patient, who should be treated like a type 1 diabetic patient.

The patient who is well controlled on diet alone or diet plus oral agents does not require any specific therapy for minor surgery. We have shown pre- and postoperative glucose values of 140–155 mg/dL in such patients, well within the desirable target range.

There is more argument as to how the poorly controlled type 2 diabetic patient should be treated for minor surgery. Some still advocate no specific therapy, but this seems unwise and a glucose/insulin infusion regimen would seem appropriate. A fasting plasma glucose of 200 mg/dL (11.1 mmol/L) seems an appropriate cutoff in that metabolic deterioration seems to occur with minor surgery only at higher levels.

Many different regimens have been suggested for metabolic control during major surgery in type 2 diabetic patients. It is logical and simple to use the same regimen as for type 1 diabetic patients. This does give similar results in terms of glycemic regulation.

Practical Guidelines—Minor Surgery

Control should be improved preoperatively, and long-acting sulfonylureas stopped if feasible. On the day of surgery, all oral agents are withheld and fasting plasma glucose is checked at the bedside. If plasma glucose is <200 mg/dL, surgery is carried out as planned. If plasma glucose is > 200 mg/dL, a standard GIK or IP/GK protocol is commenced and the patient treated like a type 1 diabetic patient. It should be noted that many type 2 diabetic patients are obese and may need 40 U insulin/L, 10% glucose, rather than the standard 30 U.

Major Surgery

Control should be optimized preoperatively, and short-acting insulin therapy used for the 24–48 hours before operation if control is not satisfactory. On the morning of surgery, sulfonylurea therapy is withheld, an infusion regimen is commenced, and the fasting plasma glucose level is checked. Thereafter management is as for the type 1 diabetic patient.

Postoperative Management

In all patients who have received GIK, plasma glucose should be checked every 1–2 hours following operation until stable glycemia is achieved, and then every 4 hours. Potassium should be checked 6 hours postoperatively and again on the following day, although it is rare to have to change the potassium content of the infusate. The GIK or separate insulin/glucose infusions are continued until the patient begins to eat again. At that time the usual pre-operative SC insulin dose is given. The GIK mixture should be continued for a further hour or so to allow absorption of some of the SC dose. If resumption of feeding is delayed, then parenteral nutrition can be instituted with insulin still given by the IV route. In this situation it should be given via a separate line using an infusion pump.

Good glycemic control postoperatively is paramount. It has been clearly shown that wound infections are fewer in better-controlled patients, although a precise threshold has not been established.

SPECIAL SITUATIONS

Day (Outpatient) Surgery

In recent years there has been a dramatic increase in outpatient surgery. It is certainly not necessary for all diabetic patients to be excluded from this trend.

Day surgery in type 2 diabetic patients is appropriate for all minor procedures. Preoperative assessment a few days before surgery is, however, a *sine qua non*. Patients should be treated as outlined above and scheduled for operation early in the day. Cataract surgery under local anesthesia in type 2 diabetic patients is entirely safe as an outpatient procedure.

Insulin-treated patients may present a greater problem, but with appropriate preoperative assessment, the availability of blood glucose monitoring equipment and insulin dose adjustment, together with a halving of intermediate insulin on the evening before surgery, they can also be treated as day patients. They should also be scheduled for early operation and should be given IV insulin as discussed above. Subcutaneous insulin is recommended as soon as possible postoperatively. This applies of course to minor surgery. Blood glucose levels should be checked at the bedside hourly.

Emergency Surgery

Emergency surgery is at least as likely in the diabetic as the nondiabetic subject. Management will depend to a large extent on the metabolic condition of the patient. Surgical emergencies, particularly if there is underlying infection, can cause rapid metabolic decompensation, with dehydration, hyperglycemia, and ketoacidosis. Uncontrolled diabetes may also be precipitated in patients not previously known to have diabetes. Diabetic ketoacidosis can also present with symptoms indistinguishable from an acute abdomen. In these patients the signs and symptoms resolve on metabolic correction. If such patients are less than 25 years old, the problem is likely to be metabolic, whereas if they are older, a genuine surgical emergency should be suspected. Such patients should be managed conservatively in the early stages, with correction of the metabolic derangement. If the problem is metabolic rather than surgical, it will resolve in the next 3–4 hours.

Practical Guidelines

In all cases, blood should be sent for immediate analysis of glucose, urea, and electrolytes, as well as arterial pH and gases if clinically warranted. Plasma, urine, or both should be checked for ketones. It should be noted that in DKA a raised white cell count does not necessarily indicate infection, but correlates with ketone levels.

If the patient is in early or established DKA, surgery should be delayed 3–4 hours if possible. This will put the patient in a better state to withstand the stress of surgery. Treatment comprises rapid saline infusion and insulin delivery via an infusion pump at 6 U/h. Potassium should be given in the saline (20 mmol/h), assuming adequate renal function. Glucose should be monitored hourly and electrolytes checked after 3–4 hours. Once blood glucose concentration has fallen below 270 mg/dL (15 mmol/L), a standard GIK insulin pump regimen is commenced, but with 40 U insulin/L 10% glucose because patients will be insulin-resistant. Blood glucose should be monitored hourly and the insulin content of the infusion increased if necessary.

In patients without severe metabolic disturbance, initial diabetic management is with a GIK or IP/GK protocol. Again a higher-than-usual insulin concentration is likely to be needed.

Cardiopulmonary Bypass Surgery

Coronary artery bypass grafting is common in people with diabetes. Morbidity and mortality are higher than in the nondiabetic patient, and it is possible that the intraoperative management of the diabetes contributes to this.

Cardiopulmonary bypass (CPB) surgery involves the use of large volumes of exogenous fluid, hypothermia, and adrenergic agents, all of which can affect metabolic homeostasis. CPB is known to be associated with severe insulin resistance. When GIK is used for glycemic control, insulin:glucose ratios of 1 to 1.6 are needed by contrast with 0.3 to 0.4 used for routine surgery. Good results may be achieved by infusing insulin alone with monitoring of plasma glucose every 15–30 minutes in the operating theater. Insulin requirements vary between 5 and 12 U/h. GIK is then introduced postoperatively. Clear indication of the benefits of using GIK therapy in diabetic patients undergoing coronary artery surgery has been reported.

Hyperglycemia may also be associated with poor outcomes in diabetic patients undergoing cardiovascular surgery, emphasizing the need for good glycemic control.

SUMMARY AND CONCLUSIONS

Surgery in the diabetic patient poses special problems. Not only the metabolic problems of diabetes, but also the proneness of the patient to cardiovascular disease, neuropathy, and infection put the patient at special risk. Surgical stress is accompanied by increased secretion of the counterregulatory hormones and cytokines with resultant insulin resistance, inhibition of insulin secretion, and hyperglycemia. In type 1 diabetic patients this will lead to metabolic deterioration. In type 2 diabetic patients there is already insulin resistance and metabolic worsening will also occur. The extent of the stress response to surgery depends, however, on the severity of the operation. Minor surgery leads to only minor metabolic derangement.

In the well-controlled type 2 diabetic patient, on diet alone or diet with oral agents, it is sufficient to withhold current therapy on the day of minor surgery. In the poorly controlled type 2 diabetic patient and in all type 1 diabetic subjects undergoing minor surgery and all diabetic patients having major surgery, insulin therapy is required. The simplest regimen is the combined glucose-insulin-potassium (GIK) infusion, which can be used from the morning of surgery until the patient is eating again. In better-staffed and -equipped centers, insulin can be given by separate infusion pump. Meticulous monitoring of plasma glucose is essential and appropriate "sliding scales" used.

With proper attention to preoperative assessment, outpatient surgery is safe for diabetic patients for minor operations. Emergency surgery is common in the diabetic subject. It is imperative that any severe metabolic disturbance be corrected before embarking on surgery. The GIK or insulin pump regimen is then used. Cardiopulmonary bypass surgery is also a particular problem in diabetes patients because of massive insulin resistance. Here insulin is given intraoperatively without accompanying glucose, standard IV insulin/glucose being reinstituted postoperatively.

With appropriate care, the outcome of surgery in the diabetic patient should be little worse than in the nondiabetic patient when matched for clinical status.

ADDITIONAL READINGS

Gill GV, Alberti KGMM: The care of the diabetic patient during surgery. In: Ferrannini E, Zimmet P, DeFronzo RA, Keen H, eds. *International Textbook of Diabetes Mellitus*. Chichester: Wiley; 2004:1741.

Glister BC, Vigersky RA: Perioperative management of type 1 diabetes mellitus. *Endocrinol Metab Clin North Am* 2003;32:411.

Hoogwerf BJ: Postoperative management of the diabetic patient. *Med Clin North Am* 2001;85:1213.

McAnulty GR, Robertshaw HJ, Hall GM: Anaesthetic management of patients with diabetes mellitus. *Br J Anaesth* 2000;85:80.

Lazar HL, Chipkin S, Philippides G, et al: Glucose-insulin-potassium solutions improve outcomes in diabetics who have coronary artery operations. *Ann Thorac Surg* 2000;70:145.

For a more detailed discussion of this topic and a bibliography, please see Porte *et al: Ellenberg & Rifkin's Diabetes Mellitus*, 6th ed., Chapter 37.

16 | Diabetic Ketoacidosis

Elizabeth Delionback Ennis   Robert A. Kreisberg

Diabetic ketoacidosis (DKA) is an important and serious complication of decompensated diabetes mellitus. Each year there are approximately 798,000 individuals with newly diagnosed diabetes mellitus (DM).

DKA is the presenting manifestation of type 1 diabetes mellitus (T1DM) in only 20–25% of cases, and most cases of DKA do not occur in individuals with new-onset diabetes mellitus. Eighty percent of DKA episodes occur in patients who are known to have diabetes mellitus.

DKA occurs with equal frequency in men and women; however, it does not occur with equal frequency in all races. African-Americans have an excess DKA burden, and data show that African-Americans had 2.3 times more hospital discharges for DKA than whites (15.7 episodes versus 6.8 episodes per 1000 diabetic population).

Ketoacidosis is generally thought to be a problem of young diabetics; however, the average age of patients with ketoacidosis is 43 years, and 50–85% of the episodes of DKA occur in adults. Some older patients have T1DM and are predisposed to the development of DKA, just as are younger patients. Many patients with DKA probably have type 2 diabetes mellitus (T2DM), since 19% of the patients in one series were obese.

PATHOGENESIS OF DIABETIC KETOACIDOSIS

Although DKA is a complex metabolic disturbance of glucose, fat, and protein metabolism, the signs and symptoms are primarily due to abnormalities in the metabolism of carbohydrate and fat.

Hyperglycemia and consequently hyperosmolality occur as a result of overproduction of glucose by the liver and underutilization of glucose by peripheral tissues. When the blood glucose concentration exceeds the threshold for renal tubular reabsorption of glucose, glucosuria occurs and, as a result of the osmotic diuresis, water is lost in excess of electrolyte. Glomerular filtration is initially increased as water moves from the intracellular to the extracellular compartment because of the increase in extracellular osmolality. With the development of marked hypovolemia, glomerular filtration and renal glucose losses diminish, resulting in more severe hyperglycemia.

Because of the tight metabolic coupling of hepatic gluconeogenesis to ketogenesis, ketone body production is activated in DKA; its magnitude usually parallels that of glucose production. Ketoacidosis is primarily due to the overproduction of ketoacids by the liver, although underutilization of ketones makes a minor contribution to the ketonemia. The increase in ketoacid production causes the loss of bicarbonate and other body buffers, resulting in the development of metabolic acidosis.

DKA develops as a consequence of a deficiency of insulin and an excess of the glucose counterregulatory hormones: catecholamines, cortisol, glucagon, and growth hormone. The insulin deficiency may be relative rather than absolute. The glucose counterregulatory hormones are increased in DKA, as a result of coexistent physical and emotional stress or illness, or simply as a con-

TABLE 16-1 Effects of Insulin and Insulin Counterregulatory Hormones

	Gluconeogenesis, liver	Ketogenesis, liver	Glucose utilization, muscle	Lipolysis, adipose tissue
Insulin	↓	↓	↑	↓
Glucagon	↑	↑	→	→
Epinephrine	↑	↑	↓	↑
Cortisol	↑	↑	↓	↑
Growth hormone	→	↑	↓	↑

sequence of insulin deficiency. In addition, the biologic response to a given concentration or dose of a glucose counterregulatory hormone is exaggerated in DKA.

Glucagon is of particular importance in the development of DKA, because it influences both gluconeogenesis and ketogenesis. In the setting of insulin deficiency, glucagon directly stimulates gluconeogenesis and ketogenesis. Free fatty acids (FFAs) provide the substrate necessary to support glucagon-stimulated hepatic ketogenesis. Glucagon can directly increase ketone body production in the absence of increased FFA release from adipose tissue by activating lipolysis of hepatic triglyceride. However, sustained production of ketone bodies requires an adequate supply of substrate FFAs. When insulin is withdrawn from diabetic patients, the major hormonal factors leading to DKA are probably insulin deficiency and glucagon excess.

The presence of increased concentrations of cortisol, epinephrine, growth hormone, and norepinephrine accentuates the impairment in peripheral glucose utilization and enhances lipolysis produced by insulin deficiency. In addition, epinephrine and cortisol are capable of increasing hepatic glucose production, through both glycogenolysis and gluconeogenesis (Table 16-1).

TABLE 16-2 Precipitating Factors for DKA

Acute Illness
   Infection, 30–40%
   Cerebrovascular accident
   Myocardial infarction
   Acute pancreatitis
New-onset DM, 20–25%
Insulin omission/CSII failure,* 15–20%
Menstruation
Gestational diabetes with glucocorticoid therapy
Other medical illness
Drugs
   α-Interferon (INF-α)
   Clozapine
   Cocaine
   Ecstasy followed by physical exertion
   Lithium
   Olanzapine
   Orlistat
   Protease inhibitor (indinavir, ?others)
   Terbutaline

*CSII, continuous subcutaneous insulin infusion (insulin pump therapy).

PRECIPITATING FACTORS

Intercurrent illness and discontinuation of insulin represent the two most readily identifiable factors that lead to the development of DKA. Other common precipitating factors are listed in Table 16-2.

An atypical form of ketoacidosis has been described in young, obese African-Americans but has recently also been seen in other races and ethnic groups. There is no history of preexistent diabetes mellitus and no obvious precipitating event. Their C-peptide levels are normal, and anti-islet cell antibodies are negative. Because of the absence of autoimmune markers and its lack of association with specific HLA alleles and increased insulin secretion, it appears to be a form of type 2 diabetes mellitus (T2DM). This is supported by the high prevalence of coexistent hypertension in these patients. Following control of DKA, these patients can often be initially managed with diet and low doses of sulfonylurea agents.

DIAGNOSIS (SEE TABLE 16-3)

Traditionally, DKA is defined by a glucose level $\geq$ 300 mg/dL, HCO_3^- $\leq$ 18 mEq/L with a pH $\leq$ 7.30. A pH less than 7.35 in a patient with ketonemia and a glucose concentration greater than 300 mg/dL identifies mild DKA. Because acute hyperventilation can lower the serum bicarbonate by as much as 5 mEq/L, the presence of a bicarbonate less than 18–19 mEq/L in a patient with appropriate hyperglycemia should also suggest this diagnosis. The blood glucose concentration used as a criterion for DKA is difficult to define because there are patients with blood glucose concentrations above 300 mg/dL who have no evidence of DKA and a substantial number of patients with established DKA whose blood glucose concentrations are less than 300 mg/dL. This emphasizes the variable expression of diabetic decompensation. Hyperglycemia need not be striking, and approximately 15% of patients with DKA have glucose concentrations of less than 350 mg/dL. Low glucose concentrations may be seen in settings where there may be inhibition of gluconeogenesis, such as with the use of alcohol, and in settings where glucose utilization is not completely insulin-dependent, such as in women who are pregnant in whom the fetoplacental unit uses glucose in the absence of insulin. Fasting may also be an important factor in the patient with DKA and mild hyperglycemia. Fasting in the setting of insulin deficiency is associated with less severe hyperglycemia and more severe ketoacidosis. It is important to realize that despite relative "euglycemia," patients may be critically ill as a result of severe metabolic acidosis.

TABLE 16-3 Diagnostic Features of Diabetic Ketoacidosis*

Glucose (mg/dL)	$\geq$300[†]
pH	$\leq$7.3
HCO_3^- (mEq/L)	$\leq$18
S_{osm} (mOsm/kg)	<320
Ketones[‡]	++ − +++
Dehydration	+ − ++

*HCO_3^-, bicarbonate; S_{osm}, serum osmolality; +, mild; ++, moderate; +++, severe.
[†]Excluding "euglycemic diabetic ketoacidosis."
[‡]Nitroprusside reaction method.

TABLE 16-4 Calculations

Anion gap = $[Na^+ - (Cl^- + HCO_3^-)]$	Normal = 8–14 mEq/L
	Average = 5–12 mEq/L

ΔGap = (anion gap – 12)
Primary gap acidosis = Δ anion gap/$HCO_3^- \geq 0.8$
Primary nongap acidosis = Δ anion gap/ $HCO_3^- \leq 0.4$
Na^+_{corr} = SNa^+ + 1.5 [(glucose – 150)/100]

The pH of a patient with DKA depends on the degree of respiratory compensation as well as the presence of coexistent acid–base disturbances. The metabolic acidosis that occurs in DKA is one in which there is an increase in the anion gap. The anion gap is calculated by subtracting the sum of the chloride and bicarbonate concentrations from the "uncorrected" sodium concentration $[Na^+ - (Cl^- + HCO_3^-)]$ (Table 16-4). This difference represents the unmeasured anions that are present in plasma, primarily albumin and phosphate. The normal range is from 8 to 14 mEq/L; a value of 12 mEq/L is usually used to determine whether the anion gap is increased. In DKA, the increase in the anion gap is usually equal to the reduction in the bicarbonate concentration. However, many patients with DKA may deviate from this pattern and demonstrate varying degrees of anion-gap and hyperchloremic metabolic acidosis. Wide variability in the type of metabolic acidosis will be detected if the increase in the anion gap is compared to the reduction in bicarbonate concentration (assuming that a normal baseline bicarbonate level existed before ketoacidosis developed) in DKA patients. At presentation ~46% of patients with DKA have a predominant anion-gap acidosis, 43% have a mixed anion-gap and hyperchloremic acidosis, and 11% have a predominantly hyperchloremic metabolic acidosis. (Table 16–5). Thus, in contrast to traditional thinking, at presentation approximately 54% of the patients have a hyperchloremic metabolic acidosis or a component of hyperchloremia. The variable degree of hyperchloremia in DKA correlates with the magnitude of the hypovolemia that exists in the patient. Patients with severe hypovolemia develop the typical reciprocal change in the anion gap and the bicarbonate concentration, due to retention of both the hydrogen ion and the ketoacid anion. In contrast, those patients who can maintain adequate volume and glomerular filtration while developing DKA excrete the ketoacid anions in the urine while reabsorbing chloride, which leads to hyperchloremia.

TABLE 16-5 Acid–Base Disturbances in DKA: At Admission and During Therapy

	Hyperchloremic acidosis	Mixed acidosis	Anion-gap acidosis
Gap/HCO_3^-*	<0.4	0.4–0.8	>0.8
Admission	11%	43%	46%
4 hours	46%	36%	17%
8 hours	72%	19%	9%

*Gap = calculated anion gap (mEq/L) – 12
ΔHCO_3^- = 24 mEq/L – measured HCO_3^-
Source: Reprinted with permission from Adrogue HJ, Wilson H, Boyd AE 3d, et al: N Engl J Med 1982; 307:1603–1610.

TABLE 16-6 Average Deficits of Water and Electrolytes in DKA

Parameter	DKA
Water (L)	6
Water (mL/kg)*	100
Na (mEq/kg)	7–10
Cl (mEq/kg)	3–5
K (mEq/kg)	3–5
Mg (mEq/kg)	1–2
PO_4 (mmol/kg)	1–1.5
Calcium (mEq/kg)	1–2

*Per kilogram of body weight.
Source: Reprinted with permission from Ennis ED, Stahl EJvB, Kreisberg RA: *Diabetes Rev* 1994; 1:115–126.

The coexistence of other acid–base disturbances—such as metabolic alkalosis from nausea and vomiting or diuretic use, respiratory alkalosis from fever, infection, sepsis, or pneumonia, and hyperchloremic metabolic acidosis from diarrhea—can confound the diagnosis of DKA. Thus, patients with coexistent medical problems may not have simple acid–base disturbances.

In an uncomplicated patient with DKA, the respiratory response may be capable of reducing the P_{CO_2} to 10 mm Hg, and the bicarbonate concentration may be as low as 5 mEq/L. More severe reductions in the bicarbonate concentration or less than optimum reduction in the P_{CO_2} indicates the coexistence of other acid–base disturbances.

The osmolal gap (difference between the measured and calculated serum osmolality) may be increased in DKA. This value is usually < 10 mOsm/L. When increased it suggests the presence of low-molecular-weight alcohols which also cause a "gap acidosis." The increase appears to be due in part to acetone and amino acids and in part to hemoconcentration.

LABORATORY AND WATER ABNORMALITIES

Substantial deficits of sodium, potassium, magnesium, phosphorus, and water can develop in patients with DKA (Table 16–6). However, despite these deficits, most patients have normal or elevated plasma concentrations of potassium, magnesium, and phosphorus at the time of presentation (Tables 16–7 and 16–8). The presence of normal or increased electrolyte concentra-

TABLE 16-7 Serum Electrolyte Levels at Entry and after Therapy in Patients with DKA

	Entry			12 Hours		
	% low	% normal	% high	% low	% normal	% high
Sodium	67	26	7	26	41	38
Chloride	33	45	22	11	41	48
Bicarbonate	100	0	0	46	50	4
Calcium	28	68	4	73	23	4
Potassium	18	43	39	63	33	4
Magnesium	7	25	68	55	24	21
Phosphate	11	18	71	90	10	0

Source: Reprinted with permission from Martin HE, Smith K, Wilson IL: *Am J Med* 1958; 20:376–388.

TABLE 16-8 Average Laboratory Findings in DKA

	Diabetic ketoacidosis
Glucose (mg/dL)	475
S_{osm} (mosm/kg)	309
Na^+ (mEq/L)	131
K^+ (mEq/L)	4.8
HCO_3^- (mEq/L)	9
BUN (mg/dL)	21
Anion gap (mEq/L)	29
ΔGap (anion gap − 12) (mEq/L)	17
pH	<7.3
Ketonuria	≥ 3+
Growth hormone (ng/mL)	7.9
Cortisol (μg/dL)	49
FFA (mmol/L)	2.26
Glucagon (pg/mL)	400–500
Lactate (mmol/L)	4.6
β-Hydroxybutyrate (mmol/L)	13.7
Catecholamines (ng/mL)	1.78 ± 4

Source: Reprinted with permission from Ennis ED, Stahl EJvB, Kreisberg RA: *Diabetes Rev* 1994; 1:115–126.

tions should not be interpreted to indicate that body stores of these elements are normal or increased. The deficit in potassium is the most important; recognition and treatment of potassium deficiency is of major therapeutic importance.

The deficit of potassium in patients with DKA is 3–5 mEq/kg. During the course of therapy, the serum potassium concentration rapidly decreases, reaching a nadir at approximately 4–12 hours after beginning insulin therapy. The deficit of potassium will become obvious during the course of therapy, particularly if potassium is not administered in adequate amounts. The hyperkalemia that exists in patients with DKA is usually attributed to a shift of hydrogen ion from the extracellular to the intracellular compartment and of potassium from the intracellular to the extracellular compartment. Other factors have been identified that may be more important determinants of the potassium concentration in DKA. The potassium concentration in patients with DKA correlates best with the severity and magnitude of the existing ketoacidosis and hyperglycemia. Insulin deficiency has been shown to be a major cause of the hyperkalemia that develops in patients with DKA. Finally, when volume contraction becomes sufficiently severe so as to reduce the glomerular filtration rate, decreased excretion of both potassium and glucose in the urine accentuates the hyperkalemia. Thus the tendency for the serum potassium concentration to decrease rapidly during therapy may be a reflection of the direct action of insulin on cellular potassium uptake, alterations in systemic pH, a reduction in the serum glucose concentration and associated hyperosmolality, and enhanced renal potassium excretion.

A deficit of phosphorus occurs during the development of DKA and may reach 1.0–1.5 mmol/kg of body weight. However, since total body phosphorus stores are 6000–8000 mmol, this represents a mild degree of phosphorus deficiency. The hyperphosphatemia that exists at diagnosis of DKA is attributed to the effects of metabolic acidosis on cellular function and the release of phosphate.

While hypophosphatemia often develops during the course of therapy, adverse effects are rare. Serious complications of hypophosphatemia are encountered only when the serum phosphate concentration falls to less than 1 mg/dL. Nonetheless, studies have shown that diaphragmatic and skeletal muscle function may be adversely affected by more modest reductions in the phosphate concentration, and that hypophosphatemia may lead to impaired myocardial contractility. The routine use of phosphate supplementation has not been demonstrated to alter morbidity or mortality and is not recommended.

Hyponatremia is seen in approximately two-thirds of patients with advanced DKA, despite an osmotic diuresis and loss of water in excess of electrolyte. The presence of hyponatremia is due to the effect of hyperglycemia and hyperosmolality on the distribution of water in the intra- and extracellular compartments. Hypernatremia would be expected because of the osmotic diuresis and excretion of water in excess of solute, but the hyperglycemia holds a relative excess of water in the extracellular compartment and contributes to the persistence of hyponatremia until the water deficit is extreme. Thus a disproportionate amount of body water exists in the extracellular compartment in the face of volume contraction (hypovolemia). The shift of water from the intracellular to the extracellular compartment would be expected to produce a predictable lowering in the serum sodium concentration if the water remained exclusively within the extracellular compartment; however, because it is excreted in the urine, this relationship is less precise. As a rule, a 1.6–1.8 mEq/L reduction in the serum sodium concentration can be expected for every 100 mg/dL increase in the glucose concentration (Table 16–4). Recently, it has been suggested that the serum sodium decreases by ~2.4 mEq/L for hyperglycemia $\leq$ 400 mg/dL and by 4.0 mEq/L for glucose concentrations > 400 mg/dL. These data suggest that the change in the serum sodium due to hyperglycemia is underestimated by using a factor of 1.6–1.8 mEq/L. This approximation is valuable because it allows identification of those patients whose degree of hyponatremia is excessive for the prevailing hyperglycemia. Serum sodium concentrations that are less than 120 mEq/L are uncommon and, when present, suggest the presence of hypertriglyceridemia or other disorders that are associated with hyponatremia. Serum sodium, potassium, and chloride levels are spuriously decreased in the presence of extremely elevated triglycerides. Similarly, "pseudonormoglycemia" has been reported. This occurs because electrolytes and glucose are present in the aqueous portion of plasma or serum, whereas concentrations are measured and reported per total volume of sample. It is essential that the laboratory report the presence of lipemia so that the spurious nature of unanticipated low concentrations of electrolytes and glucose can be appreciated.

Severe hyponatremia may be encountered in patients with end-stage renal disease in whom neither the glucose nor the water, which has shifted out of the cell, can be excreted. In such individuals, lowering the glucose concentration with insulin may be all that is necessary to correct the hyponatremia. When the serum sodium concentration is normal or increased in a patient with DKA, lowering the serum glucose concentration may be associated with the development of hypernatremia, particularly in those patients who receive large volumes of isotonic saline. This is due to loss of water from the extracellular to the intracellular compartment as the glucose concentration falls and to the increased renal tubular reabsorption of sodium induced by volume contraction.

Although magnesium deficiency develops in patients with DKA, the deficit is not usually significant. It is rarely associated with signs or symptoms, and generally corrects itself when a regular diet is resumed. Because magnesium deficiency impairs both the secretion and action of parathyroid hormone, patients may develop symptomatic hypocalcemia if they receive phosphate supplements. The phosphate reduces the plasma ionized-calcium concentration, which cannot be restored to normal because of magnesium deficiency. Such patients require calcium supplementation to acutely correct symptomatic hypocalcemia and magnesium replacement to maintain a normal serum calcium.

Hyperamylasemia may occur in patients with DKA. Because DKA is often associated with abdominal pain, the presence of hyperamylasemia is of considerable clinical importance. Isoenzyme studies indicate that the amylase in DKA patients is frequently nonpancreatic in origin. The presence of hyperamylasemia correlates poorly with abdominal complaints or physical findings in patients with DKA. In addition, hyperamylasemia may occur in 30% of patients with metabolic acidosis who do not have pancreatitis, indicating that it is specific neither for pancreatitis nor an intra-abdominal medical problem. Marked hyperlipasemia, in the absence of clinical or radiographic evidence of pancreatitis, has been demonstrated in patients with DKA. The clinical evaluation of the patient is important with regard to the possibility of an intra-abdominal problem or pancreatitis. At the outset, signs and symptoms suggesting an intra-abdominal problem should be pursued aggressively. If there is hyperamylasemia, or hyperlipasemia, but there are no physical findings to suggest another intra-abdominal process, the patient should be followed carefully. Abdominal pain commonly disappears in patients with DKA as the metabolic acidosis resolves.

BLOOD KETONES

In DKA, the plasma concentrations of β-hydroxybutyrate (B), acetoacetate (A), and acetone are increased. The ratio of B to A (B:A), representing the mitochondrial redox state, shows considerable interindividual variability; however, the mean value for the ratio is only mildly elevated when all patients with DKA are considered. Infrequently, the B:A ratio may be very high and the acidosis due almost exclusively to the production of β-hydroxybutyril, the acid of which results in increased β-hydroxybutyrate levels. This is an important diagnostic problem because quantitative plasma ketone measurements are not routinely available, whereas qualitative tests, which detect acetoacetate, may be negative or weakly positive in this situation. The tendency to a higher B:A ratio in DKA is attributed to the more reduced redox state of the cell that accompanies increased FFA metabolism. The increased B:A ratio may also reflect impairment of β-hydroxybutyrate conversion to acetoacetate and the reduced utilization of ketones that occurs with insulin deficiency. The B:A ratio is shifted toward β-hydroxybutyrate when a more reduced intracellular redox state exists, such as with lactic acidosis resulting from low flow and tissue hypoxia, or from the use of alcohol. Patients with alcoholic ketosis may have significant ketosis, but a negative or weakly positive plasma ketone test. The presence of a combined keto- and lactic acidosis could be overlooked under these circumstances.

Plasma acetone concentrations are markedly elevated in patients with DKA. Acetone, a water-soluble and freely diffusible compound, is distributed throughout total body water so that the acetone pool is markedly expanded. Acetone is of low toxicity, but in large concentrations may produce narcosis. It has been suggested that the drowsiness of some patients with DKA is due to high plasma acetone concentrations. The plasma acetone concentration may remain elevated for up to 48 hours, long after the glucose, β-hydroxybutyrate, and acetoacetate concentrations return to normal. This likely explains the ketonuria that has been observed for several days following successful therapy of DKA.

Plasma and urinary ketones are detected and semiquantitated by the use of the nitroprusside reaction. The nitroprusside reagent does not react with β-hydroxybutyrate, and on a molar basis is only one-twentieth as reactive with acetone as with acetoacetate. Thus, despite concentrations that are three- to fourfold greater than those of acetoacetate, acetone contributes only minimally to the color reaction. Acetoacetate, therefore, is the predominant determinant of the nitroprusside reaction. Thus, for a variety of reasons, this test correlates poorly with the degree of ketonemia. Additionally, several drugs have been associated with false-positive tests using the nitroprusside reaction. Drugs that contain a sulfhydryl group, such as captopril, dimercaprol, mesna, acetylcysteine, and penicillamine, may give a false-positive result. Additionally, very high intake of ascorbic acid may cause urinary acidification and result in a false-negative nitroprusside reaction. Routine monitoring of ketones during treatment of DKA has not been shown to provide significant additional data to that provided by measuring the anion gap and glucose.

TREATMENT OF DIABETIC KETOACIDOSIS

Successful treatment of DKA requires vigilant patient care as well as the use of effective doses of insulin, correction of volume deficits, and appropriate electrolyte supplementation. Adherence to these guidelines has resulted in a significant reduction in mortality from DKA (Table 16–9).

Most authorities recommend a loading dose of regular insulin, 0.1 U/KG body weight (5–10 U intravenously), followed by the use of low-dose insulin therapy wherein low doses of regular insulin, 0.1 U/kg/h (5–10 U/h, intramuscularly or intravenously), are used. Although the rate at which the glucose concentration decreases varies from patient to patient, it is fairly constant in any given patient. The average decline in the blood glucose concentration is 75–100 mg/dL/h and occurs at a predictable rate. Insulin can be administered either intramuscularly or intravenously, and at these doses produces plasma concentrations that are well within the maximum physiologic range (100–200 μU/mL). Although most patients respond to these doses of insulin, there are some who will not. Patients who are resistant to low doses of insulin cannot be identified prospectively by any clinical or laboratory parameter; consequently, blood glucose measurements should be obtained at hourly intervals. In the presence of infection, the rate of decrease in the blood glucose may be reduced by 50% to approximately 50 mg/dL/h.

During the course of therapy, the plasma glucose concentration reaches a target of 250–300 mg/dL in approximately 4–6 hours, whereas correction of the acidosis (pH ≥ 7.30 or a bicarbonate concentration of ≥ 18 mEq/L) requires approximately 8–12 hours.

The low-dose intravenous and intramuscular insulin regimens appear to be equally effective for resolving hyperglycemia and acidosis. However, intramuscular low-dose insulin administration is not recommended in the severely hypovolemic patient because of unpredictable absorption. Subcutaneous insulin administration should not be used.

The early decrease in plasma glucose concentrations will be largely a consequence of fluid administration, and therefore cannot be used as an indica-

TABLE 16-9 Therapy of DKA

Insulin

1. 0.1 U/kg body weight regular insulin as intravenous bolus followed by 0.1 U/kg/h (5–10 U/h) thereafter as a continuous infusion until glucose concentration is 250–300 mg/dL and pH $\geq$ 7.3 or HCO_3^- $\geq$ 18 mEq/L

OR

10 U of regular insulin intravenously as a loading dose followed by 5–10 U/h intramuscularly

2. Decrease administration to 2–3 U/h when the plasma glucose is 250–300 mg/dL *and* the HCO_3^- $\geq$ 18 mEq/L

Fluids

0–1 hour

1000–2000 mL 0.9% saline for prompt correction of hypotension/hypoperfusion

1–4 hour

750–1000 mL/h 0.9% saline or 0.45% saline based on intake, urinary output, clinical assessment of volume status, and laboratory measurements

Glucose

When the plasma glucose reaches 250–300 mg/dL, administer glucose at a rate of 5–10 g/h, either as a separate infusion or combined with saline.

Electrolye replacement*

Potassium (replace as the chloride or phosphate)[†]

Assure urinary output prior to potassium supplementation

Maintain K^+ between 4 and 5 mEq/L

K^+ > 5.0 mEq/L; no supplementation

K^+ = 4–5 mEq/L; 20 mEq/L of replacement fluid

K^+ = 3–4 mEq/L; 30–40 mEq/L of replacement fluid

K^+ $\leq$ 3.0 mEq/L; 40–60 mEq/L of replacement fluid

Phosphate

Not routinely recommended; if indicated, 30–60 mmol of phosphate as potassium phosphate (K_2PO_4) over 24 hours

Magnesium

If Mg^{2+} < 1.8 mEq/L or tetany present, give magnesium sulfate ($MgSO_4$), 5 g in 500 mL 0.45% saline over 5 hours

Calcium

For symptomatic hypocalcemia, give 10–20 mL of 10% calcium gluconate (100–200 mg elemental calcium as indicated)

Bicarbonate

Not routinely recommended in the treatment of DKA; consider if other indications present

Laboratory

Comprehensive admission profile

Arterial blood gases

Serum/urine ketone measurements

q1h glucose[‡]   q4h electrolytes[‡]   q4h Ca^{2+}, Mg^{2+}, phosphate

Cultures of blood, urine, sputum as indicated

General care

EKG prior to administration of supplemental potassium

Review urine output, vital signs, neurologic status, and laboratory data hourly

Frequent assessment of clinical status and repeat physical examination

Protection of the airway in the unconscious patient

Nasogastric suction as indicated for ileus, emesis, or obtundation with vulnerable airway

Chest radiograph and other imaging studies as needed

Consider CVP, Swan-Ganz catheterization in selected patients

Footnotes are on next page.

tion of the adequacy of the insulin dose. Adequate rehydration contributes significantly to the decrease in the blood glucose concentration, not only as a consequence of dilution of glucose in a larger volume and improved glomerular filtration rate (GFR), but because it may also diminish the stimulus to release glucose counterregulatory hormones. During the initial phases of therapy, rehydration alone and dilution of glucose in the glucose space may account for 30–50%, and perhaps as much as 50–75%, of the reduction in the glucose concentration that occurs. Glucosuria accounts for approximately 15–20% of the decrease in the glucose concentration when insulin and rehydration are used together. The actual effects of insulin on glucose metabolism during treatment of DKA are rather small and are due primarily to inhibition of hepatic glucose production (accounts for 75% of insulin's effect) and not to increased glucose utilization (accounts for 25% of insulin's effect).

Changes in systemic pH usually do not occur for at least 1–2 hours after the onset of therapy. If after 3–4 hours there has not been a substantial reduction in the glucose concentration and improvement in pH, larger doses of insulin should be used.

If fluid deficits are inadequately addressed, persistent hypovolemia continues to stimulate the release of counterregulatory hormones as well as impair glucose excretion in the urine. The sensitivity of patients with DKA to relatively low doses of insulin should not be interpreted to mean that these patients are insulin-sensitive and that no insulin resistance exists. Patients with DKA who receive 5–10 U/h of insulin are obviously insulin-resistant. In a normal subject, the infusion of insulin at a rate of approximately 8 U/h requires the concomitant administration of 40 g of glucose per hour to maintain a constant blood glucose concentration.

The mechanisms of the insulin resistance in DKA patients are poorly understood and multifactorial, including glucose counterregulatory hormones; hyperosmolality, which decreases insulin-mediated glucose utilization; acidemia (decreases receptor-mediated glucose metabolism); phosphate deficiency (produces a mild postbinding defect in glucose utilization); and ketoacids, which induce a postbinding abnormality in insulin action.

A rare cause of extreme insulin resistance in patients with DKA is the presence of anti-insulin antibodies that bind insulin. Since the maximum biologic response to insulin is significantly reduced in the postbinding type of insulin resistance, and because resistance resolves slowly, it is not clear how or why large doses of insulin overcome unusual insulin resistance within the brief period of treatment of DKA. Changes occur slowly (over 96 hours) in insulin sensitivity and in glucose metabolism following the achievement of euglycemia. This leads to the frequent clinical observation that it takes more insulin to get patients under control than to keep them in control.

The discrepancy between the rates of correction of hyperglycemia and acidemia has important clinical implications. Insulin administration must be continued despite relative euglycemia until the pH and bicarbonate targets have been achieved. Consequently, glucose must be administered to "buffer"

---

*Drug doses should be modified in the patient with significant renal impairment.

†Dosage suggested using KCL.

‡Modified as necessary depending on clinical assessment.

Source: Modified with permission from Ennis ED, Stahl EJvB, Kreisberg RA: *Diabetes Rev* 1994; 1:115–126.

a further decrease in the glucose concentration during the continued administration of insulin. Because glucose disposal is 5–10 g/h under these circumstances, glucose should be initially administered at these rates. If the glucose concentration increases, then the rate of glucose administration should be reduced; if the glucose concentration continues to decrease, additional glucose is needed. Occasionally, the plasma glucose concentration is less than 300 mg/dL at the initiation of therapy and glucose must be incorporated into the initial fluids used for correction of hypovolemia. Although there has been considerable discussion over whether hypotonic or isotonic fluid should be used in DKA, most would agree that hypovolemia should be corrected with isotonic saline, 2–4 L. Thereafter, the decision to use 0.45% or 0.9% saline solution should be guided by hemodynamic considerations, fluid balance, and the prevailing serum sodium and chloride concentrations. In adult patients without severe volume deficits, a lower rate of saline infusion is associated with more rapid recovery of the plasma bicarbonate.

ACID–BASE CHANGES DURING DKA THERAPY

Systemic pH is unchanged during the first 1–2 hours after starting therapy with insulin and fluids. Thereafter, the pH begins to increase, and by 6–12 hours it is usually between 7.25 and 7.35. After 24 hours the systemic pH is normal or near-normal, but arterial Pco_2 and bicarbonate are still reduced, a pattern consistent with compensated mild metabolic acidosis. It is unusual for the respiratory rate and therefore the Pco_2 to normalize during the first 24 hours, because the respiratory center continues to drive ventilation. Alkalosis should be avoided because it reduces cerebral blood flow and increases the affinity of hemoglobin for oxygen, thereby reducing oxygen delivery to tissues. It also predisposes to hypokalemia and hypophosphatemia.

There is some controversy concerning the routine use of bicarbonate in the treatment of DKA. Under normal circumstances, the pH of the intracellular compartment is substantially lower than that of the extracellular space and is relatively well protected against the adverse effects of acidemia in acute metabolic acidosis. Whereas bicarbonate equilibrates slowly across the cell membrane, CO_2 equilibrates rapidly. Thus when extracellular pH falls, respiration is stimulated and the Pco_2 decreases, minimizing intracellular pH changes. In fact, intracellular pH may actually increase acutely. While hepatic intracellular pH is markedly reduced in DKA owing to the production of metabolic acid at that site, other cells within the body are initially protected against the adverse effects of acidemia.

Because hemodynamic abnormalities begin to appear when the pH falls below 7.1–7.2, bicarbonate use may be considered in patients with acidemia of this severity. On the other hand, some investigators do not recommend bicarbonate supplements unless the pH is less than 7.0. Bicarbonate therapy has not been shown to favorably affect the correction of hyperglycemia, acidosis, or level of consciousness in DKA. It has been shown to prolong the clearance of ketones and lactate and increase supplemental potassium requirements in DKA. Patients treated with bicarbonate may require significantly more potassium supplementation. Thus the routine use of bicarbonate in DKA appears to offer no therapeutic advantage. It should be noted, however, that in those patients with a marked reduction of the bicarbonate concentration and maximal respiratory compensation, any further reduction in the bicarbonate concentration is associated with a drastic shift in pH.

Consequently, the use of small quantities of bicarbonate in individuals whose plasma bicarbonate is of the order of 5–10 mEq/L might be prudent.

Patients recovering from DKA commonly demonstrate hyperchloremia and develop a non-anion-gap metabolic acidosis. During the treatment of DKA, the anion-gap metabolic acidosis resolves quickly and is replaced by a mixed metabolic acidosis in which features of both an anion-gap and a hyperchloremic metabolic acidosis are present. The hyperchloremic metabolic acidosis begins to develop with therapy and evolves progressively until it becomes the dominant acid–base disturbance. During the course of recovery, patients with a hyperchloremic metabolic acidosis at presentation may have a lower final bicarbonate concentration than those who present with the typical anion-gap metabolic acidosis. The development of the hyperchloremic metabolic acidosis during the recovery phase is attributed to several factors: (1) the bicarbonate and buffer deficit in such patients is greater than is apparent from the reduction in the plasma bicarbonate concentration because buffer in bone and other tissues has also been lost; (2) the availability of substrate (ketones) for regeneration of bicarbonate is less than that required to stoichiometrically replace the buffer that has been lost because considerable quantities of ketones have already been lost in the urine; (3) rapid volume expansion further increases the excretion of ketones in the urine, accentuating the deficit in substrate availability required to regenerate bicarbonate; (4) increased proximal tubular chloride reabsorption occurs, owing to limited bicarbonate availability; and, perhaps, (5) if volume replacement is excessive, there is also decreased proximal tubular reabsorption of bicarbonate. Though persistence of acidemia in the early phases of the treatment of DKA is an indication for the continued administration of insulin, it is important to recognize that this recommendation does not hold for the hyperchloremic metabolic acidosis that emerges toward the end of active therapy when the other metabolic abnormalities have been corrected. When the hyperglycemia has been controlled, the pH has reached 7.3, the bicarbonate is ≥ 18 mEq/L, and the patient is feeling well without any signs or symptoms of DKA, the rate of insulin administration can be reduced. The acquired hyperchloremic metabolic acidosis will resolve over several days as the kidneys adjust acid secretion and bicarbonate is regenerated.

ALTERATIONS IN CENTRAL NERVOUS SYSTEM FUNCTION AND STRUCTURE

There has been great interest in the central nervous system of patients with DKA. This is a result of the infrequent but devastating development of cerebral edema in some patients recovering from DKA. Though rare, the syndrome of cerebral edema usually occurs during treatment of the first episode of ketoacidosis, but its mechanisms are poorly understood. Neither hyponatremia nor the rate of fluid administration appears to be a precipitating factor. Excessive lowering of the glucose concentration during therapy is probably not important, since it is less than 200 mg/dL in only approximately 25% of patients who develop this complication. An etiologic role for the rate at which the hyperglycemia is corrected cannot be demonstrated.

In patients with coexistent hyponatremia, the plasma osmolality may be normal or just modestly elevated despite the presence of severe hyperglycemia. Correction of hyperglycemia during therapy without simultaneous elevation of the plasma sodium concentration permits adverse osmolar gradients to be created that favor the shift of fluid into the intracellular compartment of the brain and the development of cerebral edema. Careful intake and output measurements indicate that simple fluid overload is unlikely to be responsible for this problem. Large doses of glucocorticoids or mannitol or both have been recommended as therapy, but there is little experience with the problem and it is difficult to know whether such an approach is beneficial. The theory that unfavorable osmotic gradients develop during DKA therapy is more strongly supported than any other at the present time.

Cerebral edema is often unpredictable; however, 50% of patients in one series had prodromal headache, confusion, incontinence, changes in arousal and behavior, pupillary changes, blood pressure changes, bradycardia, disturbed temperature regulation, or seizures. The development of headache or confusion during the course of therapy, particularly in a young patient or one being treated for the first episode of DKA, suggests incipient cerebral edema and the need for aggressive intervention. Thus, cerebral edema may be a common subclinical occurrence during the course or treatment of DKA. If this supposition is true, then the difference between those who do and those who do not develop symptomatic cerebral edema is quantitative and not qualitative. All patients may develop cerebral edema, but only those with the greatest degree of cerebral edema are likely to have clinical complications. The issue of cerebral edema has been recently reviewed, and its cause remains controversial and unresolved.

MISCELLANEOUS COMPLICATIONS

It is well known that the Po_2 of patients presenting with DKA is significantly elevated and may decrease dramatically during the course of therapy. Hypoxemia has been noted in 53% of patients during the treatment of DKA. In association with the marked reduction that occurs in plasma colloid oncotic pressure during therapy, the arterial Po_2 may decrease by a mean of 33 mm Hg and the Pao_2–Pao_2 gradient may indicate pulmonary dysfunction, of which pulmonary edema may be one of several causes. The development of noncardiac pulmonary edema as a complication of DKA treatment has been described. A reduction in plasma oncotic pressure in combination with reduced pleural pressure may predispose the patient to the development of pulmonary edema. Pulmonary edema has also been described in patients with chronic renal failure during therapy for DKA.

Aspiration of gastric contents with subsequent respiratory problems or death is a rare complication of the treatment of DKA. Gastric decompression may prevent this complication in selected patients.

The presence of hypothermia in patients with DKA is associated with a poor outcome. Despite hypothermia or absence of temperature elevation, a search for infection and consideration of concomitant endocrinopathy (i.e., myxedema) as a precipitating event for DKA are warranted. Mortality rates of 30–60% have been encountered in hypothermic patients. Fulminant malignant hyperthermia has also been associated with DKA and coma.

MORBIDITY AND MORTALITY

There is a common misconception that the mortality rate in DKA is low. Because a substantial number of patients with DKA are elderly, mortality is expected. Intercurrent illnesses are likely to be more serious in elderly patients with coexistent multisystem disease. In the elderly, the intercurrent illness is often the factor limiting survival, not the ketoacidosis.

Although the mortality rate of DKA has decreased, there remains an excess DKA burden in the African-American population, in whom there is a 2.3-fold increase in DKA. Educational and economic resources must be allocated to this segment of the population to improve the mortality rate from DKA. Above the age of 15 years, DKA mortality increases progressively, reaching 15–28% in patients over the age of 65 years.

Although coma is now infrequently encountered in patients with DKA, its presence is a bad prognostic sign and high mortality should be expected. Mortality may approach 45% when coma is present.

Prevention of DKA through improved recognition of precipitating factors, early diagnosis and therapy, and education should decrease the incidence of DKA and further improve its associated morbidity and mortality.

ADDITIONAL READINGS

American Diabetes Association: Hyperglycemic crises in patients with diabetes mellitus. *Diabetes Care* 2001;24:1988.

DeFronzo RA, Matsuda M, Barrett EJ: Diabetic ketoacisosis: A combined metabolic-nephrologic approach to therapy. *Diabetes Rev* 1994;2:209.

Ennis ED, Stahl EJvB, Kreisberg RA: The hyperosmolar hyperglycemic syndrome. *Diabetes Rev* 1994;2:115.

Kitabchi AC, Kreisberg RA, Umpierrez GE, et al: Management of Hyperglycemic Crises in Patients with Diabetes. *Diabetes Care* 2001;24:131.

Kreisberg RA. Diabetic ketoacidosis: new concepts and trends in pathogenesis and treatment. *Ann Intern Med* 1978;88:681.

For a more detailed discussion of this topic and a bibliography, please see Porte *et al: Ellenberg & Rifkin's Diabetes Mellitus,* 6th ed., Chapter 34.

17 | Hyperglycemic Hyperosmolar Syndrome

Robert Matz

DEFINITION

The term *hyperglycemic hyperosmolar syndrome* (HHS) was used by Ennis et al in 1994 to replace previous names such as hyperosmolar nonketotic coma (HONK). The entity is characterized by severe hyperglycemia (plasma glucose ≥ 600 mg/dL or ≥ 34 mmol/L), hyperosmolarity (effective osmolarity ≥ 320 mOsm/L), and dehydration in the absence of significant ketoacidosis (the presence of some ketonuria or mild ketonemia and an arterial pH as low as 7.3 or a serum bicarbonate as low as 15 mEq/L do not preclude the diagnosis) (Table 17-1). It occurs more frequently in the elderly, often mild, type 2 diabetic; develops more insidiously than diabetic ketoacidosis (DKA); is frequently associated with central nervous system dysfunction; is typically associated with severe fluid depletion and renal functional impairment; and has been claimed to have an extraordinarily high mortality. It is part of a clinical spectrum of severe hyperglycemic disorders that ranges from hyperglycemic hyperosmolarity without ketosis to full-blown DKA, with a significant degree of overlap in the middle. Thus 50–75% of uncontrolled diabetic patients warranting acute inpatient care will have hyperglycemic hyperosmolarity.

HYPERGLYCEMIC HYPEROSMOLAR NONACIDOTIC DIABETES

The common precipitants and contributory factors in HHS are similar to those in DKA (Table 17-2). While it has been called nonketotic and nonacidotic, this is incorrect because as many as half of the adults and most children with hyperglycemic hyperosmolarity exhibit some degree of metabolic acidosis, with an increased anion gap reflecting excess lactate, azotemia, or a mild degree of ketonemia.

The normal serum osmolarity is 290 ± 5 mOsm/L. A rough approximation of the actual value can be obtained as follows:

Serum osmolarity (mOsm/L) =

$$2[Na^+ \text{ (mEq/L)} + K^+\text{(mEq/L)}] + \frac{\text{plasma glucose (mg/dL)}}{18} + \frac{\text{BUN (mg/dL)}}{2.8}$$

In some calculations the serum K^+ is omitted. Because urea is freely diffusible across cell membranes, it contributes little to the effective serum osmolarity relative to the intracellular space, and it is the effective osmolarity that is the critical determinant in hyperosmolar states. While HHS is referred to as "hyperosmolar" diabetes, the distinction should be made between osmolarity, which is the concentration of an osmolar solution, and tonicity, which is the osmotic pressure of a solution. Tonicity more appropriately reflects what we refer to as the *effective osmolarity* or Eosm.

The effective serum osmolarity (Eosm) is calculated as follows:

$$Eosm = 2[Na^+ \ (mEq/L) + K^+(mg/dL)] + \frac{plasma \ glucose \ (mg/L)}{18}$$

When Eosm exceeds 320 mOsm/L, significant hyperosmolarity exists; when Eosm exceeds 350 mOsm/L, severe hyperosmolarity is present.

PATHOGENESIS (SEE TABLE 17-2 AND FIG. 17-1)

The critical initiating event is the development of a persistent glucosuric diuresis. Glucosuria develops when the amount of glucose presented to the proximal tubule exceeds the renal threshold for glucose (~225 mg/min). When the tubular load of glucose exceeds the tubular maximum for glucose reabsorption (TmG) of approximately 320 mg/min, almost all of the glucose reaching the tubules beyond this amount is lost in the urine. As long as fluid intake is adequate and intravascular volume and glomerular filtration rate (GFR) are maintained, loss of glucose above the threshold and TmG functions as a renal "safety valve" by preventing accumulation in the extracellular fluid of nondiffusible glucose and associated life-threatening hyperosmolarity. A normally perfused kidney will not permit marked hyperglycemia to be present even for short periods of time. Since most patients with HHS do not have renal failure after treatment, their GFR must be reduced by a reversible mechanism, namely, a marked contraction of the extracellular volume. It is failure to maintain adequate renal function due to primary kidney disease or secondary to intravascular volume depletion and the associated fall in GFR that results in remarkable elevations of the plasma glucose. During the course of the glucosuric osmotic diuresis, these patients have massive losses of water and electrolytes, but the loss of water accompanying glucose always exceeds the loss of electrolytes.

Patients may suffer from the "latent shock of dehydration" that can be made manifest by rapid correction of hyperglycemic hyperosmolarity without adequate volume replacement. If the plasma glucose concentration falls rapidly, the intracellular space, which is severely depleted of water and in osmotic equilibrium with the extracellular compartment, takes up water freed by the metabolism of glucose along an osmotic gradient favoring the movement of water from the extracellular to the intracellular space. This leaves behind a contracted intravascular space with concomitant hypotension and oliguria. Prevention is achieved by the infusion of larger volumes of crystalloid solutions early in therapy or at the first recognition of the complication.

There is an age-related reduction in renal-concentrating ability associated with a low-grade arginine vasopressin (ADH) resistance in the aged kidney. Additional changes that occur with aging include a 30–50% decrease in GFR,

TABLE 17-1 Hyperglycemic Hyperosmolar Syndrome

- Blood glucose ≥ 600 mg/dL or ≥ 34 mmol/L
- Eosm* ≥ 320 mosm/L
- Arterial pH ≥ 7.30
- SERUM BICARBONATE > 15 mEq/L

Some authors omit the serum K^+ when calculating the Eosm.

*Eosm = effective osmolarity = $2[Na^+ + K^+ \ (mEq/L)] + \dfrac{blood \ glucose \ (mg/dL)}{18}$

TABLE 17-2 Precipitating/Contributory Factors in HHS

Acute illness
    Infection (pneumonia, UTI, sepsis) ~25–30%
    Myocardial Infarction
    CNS (CVA, subdural hematoma)
    GI (acute pancreatitis, mesenteric thrombosis, intestinal obstruction, gastroenteritis)
    Renal failure
    Peritoneal dialysis
    Hypo- and hyperthermia
    Acute burns
    Endocrine (thyrotoxicosis, acromegaly, Cushing's syndrome)
Drugs
    Good evidence
        Thiazide diuretics
        Glucocorticoids
        β-Adrenergic agonists
        Loop diuretics (furosemide, ethacrynic acid)
        Pentamidine
        Diazoxide
        Cyclosporine
        L-Asparaginase
        Pentamidine
        Clozapine
        Olanzepine
        Didanosine (DDI)
        Dapsone
    Case reports
        Encainide
        Loxapine
        Cimetidine
        β-Adrenergic blockers
        Nalidixic acid
Other
    Omission or withdrawal of insulin in known diabetic
    New onset of diabetes mellitus (up to 25%)
    Nonadherence to therapy
    Social isolation, especially in the elderly diabetic (up to 25%)
    Nasogastric/PEG feedings of hypertonic solutions
    Failure of adequate free water intake in hospitalized/institutionalized diabetics (e.g., due to nausea, vomiting, restraints, siderails, extremes of age, excessive sedation, confusion, mental deficiency, impaired thirst response)
    Unrecognized uncontrolled glucosuric diuresis
    Unreplaced GI losses (e.g. vomiting, diarrhea, N-G suction)
    Impaired renal concentrating ability (decreased ability to respond to ADH; old age; renal insufficiency) resulting in inability to conserve free water
    Residence in a nursing home (neglect, failure to recognize symptoms or a change in mental state)
    Obesity in adolescents/young adults

renal blood flow (RBF), and kidney mass by age 70. The elderly also have a reduced total body water content. A young individual is approximately 70% water, whereas the elderly are 60% water by weight. This means that a 70-kg (155-lb) 30-year-old has 7–8 L more total body water than a 75-year-old of the same weight. The elderly have less total body water with which to buffer

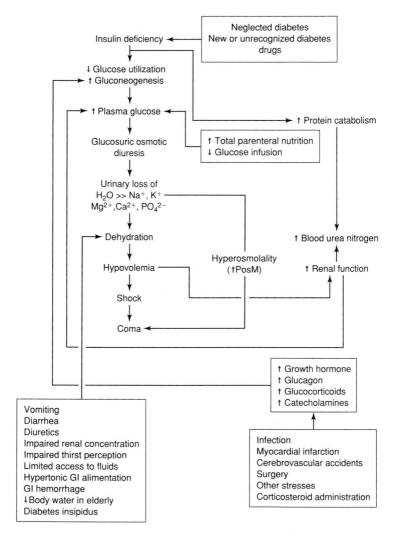

FIG.17–1   Pathogenesis of hyperglycemic hyperosmolar syndrome.

losses in water and changes in osmolarity, and a decreased sense of or response to thirst at serum osmolarities at which younger individuals are driven to drink, so they may not voluntarily drink water to correct significant hyperosmolarity and dehydration. Thus the elderly, for multiple reasons, are more vulnerable to and have limited ability to deal with an osmotic diuresis or any major loss of free water.

CLINICAL MANIFESTATIONS

Gluconeogenesis by the liver is primarily responsible for hyperglycemia, which causes a massive solute diuresis, total body water depletion, and intracellular dehydration resulting in the classic features of uncontrolled diabetes mellitus: polyuria and polydipsia leading to hypovolemia, hypotension, organ hypoperfusion, and tachycardia. The osmotic diuresis results in loss of glucose, water, and multiple electrolytes. In the hyperosmolar nonacidotic patient, the entire syndrome evolves over a longer period of time (usually days to weeks) as compared to classical DKA, and ketosis either does not supervene or is a minor part of the picture.

The typical patient is over 60 years old, but HHS is seen in infants, children, and young adults. As the current epidemic of obesity explodes worldwide, HHS is increasingly being seen (typically with ketonuria) in adolescents. Often the patient is not a previously known diabetic, or the disease is mild and managed by diet, an oral hypoglycemic agent, or a small amount of insulin. Presentation may include a depressed mental status, and 45% of the patients presenting with an Eosm > 350 mOsm/L may be comatose. The history is one of days to weeks of increasing thirst, polyuria, and frequently, in the background, a disease such as a stroke or renal insufficiency. Patients present with heavy glucosuria and minimal or no ketonuria or ketonemia. A history of weight loss, weakness, visual disturbances, and leg cramps during the preceding days or weeks may be elicited. Patients usually, but not invariably, appear severely ill. Physical examination demonstrates profound dehydration, poor tissue turgor, soft sunken eyeballs, cool extremities, and, at times, a rapid thready pulse. In contrast to DKA, respirations are not Kussmaul in nature, and the aroma of acetone cannot be appreciated on the breath.

Nausea, vomiting, and abdominal pain occur less frequently than in DKA, while constipation and anorexia are occasionally seen. Gastric stasis and ileus is less frequent than in classical DKA. Hyperglycemia (levels $\geq$ 250 mg/dL) slows gastric emptying and gastric motility, but cannot alone explain the nausea and vomiting seen. Mild gastrointestinal bleeding from hemorrhagic gastritis occurs in as many as 25% of patients. These findings are typically reversed by hydration and insulin. The occurrence of abdominal pain, tenderness, nausea and vomiting, lack of bowel sounds, and ileus in uncontrolled diabetes must not obscure possible intra-abdominal processes requiring urgent attention (e.g., mesenteric ischemia or cholecystitis). The response to therapy and the history are of critical importance. Findings secondary to uncontrolled diabetes usually improve dramatically following the rapid infusion of fluids and insulin, and their development follows the onset of the symptoms of uncontrolled diabetes rather than preceding them. Another cause of abdominal pain and tenderness in the uncontrolled diabetic is fatty infiltration of the liver resulting in distension of Glisson's capsule.

Hypothermia (rectal temperature $\leq$ 96.8°F or 36°C, or an oral temperature below 95°F or 35°C) or normothermia is the rule in DKA, and deep hypothermia is a poor prognostic sign in the presence of ketoacidosis. In HHS the average rectal temperature on admission in our series of 130 patients was 99.8°F (37.7°C), and in the fatal episodes 100.7°F (38.2°C).

The development of acute respiratory distress syndrome (ARDS) in uncontrolled diabetes has been fully described by Carroll and Matz, but is rarely seen in pure HHS. Nevertheless, 75% of the patients with this complication have had an Eosm exceeding 320 mOsm/L.

Few patients with HHS or DKA now present in true coma, and many have no clouding of consciousness. The depth of stupor parallels hyperglycemia and correlates better with the degree of hyperosmolarity and the rapidity with which it develops. Acidosis is poorly correlated with the development of an altered mental state. When the "effective osmality" or "tonicity" is calculated, patients with levels < 320 mOsm/L typically do not have altered mental status, while those with levels > 320 mOsm/L may and at Eosm levels > 340–3250 mOsm/L stupor or an altered mental status is common (over 45% in one series). The "take-home message" is that coma or an obtunded mental status in an uncontrolled diabetic is primarily the result of hyperosmolarity, not acidosis, once hypoglycemia is excluded. The absence of significant hyperosmolarity (at least > 320 mOsm/L) in a nonhypoglycemic obtunded diabetic suggests that the alteration in consciousness is not due to metabolic decompensation and mandates a search for another etiology.

A variety of neurologic abnormalities that are rare in DKA may be seen in HHS (Table 17-3) and are typically reversible after successful correction of HHS.

Hypotension may be present on admission or develop subsequently if body water and intravascular volume are not adequately repleted. This should be rare with early recognition of the syndrome and the more aggressive use of large-volume infusions.

Vascular occlusions have been reported as the most important complication of HHS. These include mesenteric artery occlusion, low-flow syndrome, and disseminated intravascular coagulation. Arterial thromboses are claimed to be responsible for 33% of the deaths in comatose diabetics, and there is speculation about the potential benefits of using anticoagulants and inhibitors of platelet function in these patients. Recommendations for low-dose heparin in elderly comatose patients or those with severe hyperosmolarity have been made. We have found the incidence of vascular occlusions to be low (2%), and these events occurred in the presence of severe hypotension, dehydration with associated hemoconcentration, and hyperviscosity associated with low flow in an already compromised circulation. Since platelet aggregation is increased in diabetic subjects, insulin-mediated vasodilation via endothelial release of nitric oxide is impaired in insulin-resistant states, and both type 2 diabetes and insulin resistance are associated with impaired fibrinolysis and elevated plasminogen activator inhibitor-1 (PAI-1) levels, the invocation of an additional coagulopathy in HHS is questioned. Heme-positive gastric con-

TABLE 17-3 Neurologic Manifestations of HHS

Grand mal/focal seizures
Transient hemiparesis
Extensor plantar reflexes [(+) Babinski]
Aphasia
Homonymous hemianopsia
Hemisensory deficits
Visual hallucinations
Muscle fasciculations
Opsoclonus–Myoclonus
Nystagmus
Acute (reversible) quadriplegia
Exacerbation of previous organic mental syndrome
Recrudescence of prior focal neurologic signs

Almost all of the above are reversible with correction of the metabolic abnormality.

tents are seen in up to 25% of uncontrolled diabetes. If full anticoagulation becomes routine, an increase in the incidence and severity of gastrointestinal hemorrhage might ensue. No prospective studies have demonstrated the safety or benefit of prophylactic full anticoagulation or of low-dose heparin. As in any acutely ill, bedridden, elderly patient with compromised circulatory status, underlying vascular disease, and a hypercoagulable state, low-dose heparin or low-molecular-weight heparin may be beneficial if there are no contraindications and the peripheral circulation is adequate to permit absorption. If there are specific indications for full anticoagulation, its use should be based on weighing the benefits versus the risks.

Rarely, pleural, pleuropericardial, and pericardial friction rubs and pain may occur in severely dehydrated patients with ketoacidosis, as well as in hyperglycemic hyperosmolar patients. Transient ST- and T-wave changes compatible with pericarditis may be seen in patients with HHS with DKA. These evanescent findings are typically seen on presentation and rapidly resolve with hydration..

LABORATORY FINDINGS

See Tables 17-4 and 17-5.

TREATMENT (TABLE 17-6)

Generally accepted aspects of therapy include searching for correctable precipitants, such as infection, and treating them promptly. In older patients and

TABLE 17-4 Fluid, Electrolyte, Mineral, and Vitamin Losses in HHS

Substance	Comments
H_2O	Avg. loss 100–200 mL/kg. Results in dehydration, hypovolemia, and hyperosmolarity. Losses are hypotonic with respect to electrolytes, so replacement initially should be with hypotonic balanced electrolyte solutions in large volumes early in treatment.
Na^+	Loss: 5–13 mEq/kg. Correction factor for serum Na^+ in hyperglycemic hyperosmolarity: For every 100 mg/dL increase in plasma glucose serum, Na^+ may decrease by 2.4 mEq/L.
Cl^-	Loss: 3–7 mEq/kg. Use of isotonic or half-normal saline (with Na^+ and Cl^- in 1:1 ratio) is unphysiologic and risks causing hyperchloremia (especially in DKA) due to excess Cl^-; delays restitution of bicarbonate in DKA/HHS.
K^+	Loss: 5–15 mEq/kg. Initial levels may be high even with total body depletion. Symptoms of hypokalemia include neuromuscular weakness, cardiac conduction abnormalities, rhabdomyolysis, cardiac arrest, respiratory muscle paralysis. Begin repletion with K^+ phosphate or K^+ acetate to avoid excess Cl^-. Objective of early K^+ replacement is not to correct the often-massive total body losses, but to maintain normokalemia.
Mg^{2+}	Loss: 50–100 mEq. Losses parallel those of K^+. Severe depletion interferes with K^+ repletion. Initial levels may be high. Symptoms of hypomagnesemia include lethargy, weakness, altered mental status, convulsions, stupor, coma, nausea, vomiting, refractory arrhythmias. Mg^{2+} is a key component of over 300 critical enzyme systems.

(continued)

TABLE 17-4 *(continued)* Fluid, Electrolyte, Mineral, and Vitamin Losses in HHS

Substance	Comments
Ca^{2+}	Loss: 50–150 mEq. Symptoms of hypocalcemia are rare. Include tetany, cramps, cardiac conduction abnormalities, mental status changes.
P	Loss: 70–140 mM. Initial serum levels usually high; may fall to low levels with insulin and glucose even if total body stores are normal. Symptoms of hypophosphatemia are never seen at levels > 2 mg/dL and significant morbidity is seen only with levels < 0.5 mg/dL. Symptoms: weakness, rhabdomyolysis, coma, convulsion, hyporeflexia, hemolysis. Phosphate is required as the anion accompanying Mg^{2+} and K^+ into the intracellular compartment as treatment progresses.
Thiamine	May be depleted in catabolic states in as little as 1 week. May lead to Wernicke's encephalopathy, cardiac dysfunction when made manifest by "refeeding" (i.e., restoration of anabolism with insulin/glucose). Rare. Preventable by giving thiamine.
B-complex vitamins	Also depleted in chronically catabolic states. May be replaced by IV route early in therapy.

Table 17-5 Laboratory Values in HHS

Plasma glucose	> 600 mg/dL (Avg. 998 mg/dL)
WBC	10,000–15,000/mm^3 (may exceed 50,000).
HCT	"Elevated" (a normal HCT on presentation may presage anemia after treatment); often ≥ 55%.
MCV	May be artificially elevated in Coulter technique, since diluting fluid is isotonic with normal serum and causes hypertonic RBCs to swell.
LFTs	Abnormal enzymes in 20–65%. May be due to hepatic steatosis. Reversible with treatment.
Thyroid	↓ T_3, T_4, TSH (euthyroid "sick").
Cholesterol	Typically elevated.
Triglycerides	Elevated. May be markedly elevated with lactescent serum ("lipemia retinalis" on funduscopy) and when Na^+ is determined volumetrically is responsible for "pseudohyponatremia."
Amylase/lipase	May be elevated in the absence of pancreatitis; reversible with treatment although lipase elevation may be prolonged.
Creatine kinase (CK)	Elevated (>1000 U) in up to 25%; reversible with treatment.
Na^+	Avg. 143 mEq/L, although where measured volumetrically may be artificially low in the presence of hypertriglyceridemia and low in the presence of very high glucose levels.
K^+	Avg. 5.0 mEq/L. May fall dramatically with insulin and fluid replacement. A low or low normal K^+ initially may reflect severe total body depletion and warrants replacement before insulin is given.

TABLE 17-6 Treatment of Hyperglycemic Hyperosmolar Syndrome

General
- Perform directed history and physical examination.
- Obtain plasma glucose, P, K^+, Ca^{2+}, Mg^{2+}, Bun, creatinine, electrolytes, CBC, urinalysis, chest X-ray, electrocardiogram, appropriate cultures, and ABGs.
- Aspirate stomach if patient is nauseated or vomiting, or if distension or bowel sounds are absent. Leave nasogastric tube in place on suction if large volume of gastric contents is obtained or if contents are guaiac-positive.
- Insert urinary catheter if unable to void or obtunded. Monitor urine output hourly.
- Administer thiamine and vitamin B complex IV.
- Administer antibiotics as appropriate for infection or suspected infection.
- Check for hypotension, state of consciousness (coma, stupor, or obtundation), hypothermia, or hyperthermia.
- Other directed studies as indicated (e.g., lumbar puncture if meningitis is suspected).
- Consider airway protection in obtunded or unconscious patients.

Fluids
- Administer 0.5 N electrolyte solution if Eosm > 320 mOsm/L, at a rate of 1500 mL/h (15–30 mL/kg/h) for first hour, 1000 mL/h for second and third hours, and 500–750 mL/h for fourth hour.
- When Eosm <320 mOsm/L, crystalloid fluid prescription should be changed to 1 N concentration (isotonic).
- If hypotensive, give 2000 mL/h of electrolyte solution (osmolarity dependent on Eosm as above).
- If hypotension is unresponsive to crystalloids, consider use of colloid and pressors.
- May require central venous pressure and/or pulmonary capillary wedge pressure monitoring to guide treatment. (In complicated cases, monitoring of cardiac output, peripheral resistance, and other parameters may be essential.)
- Add 5% D5W when plasma glucose is 250–300 mg/dL.
- Caution! Reduce fluid administration in presence of renal failure.

Insulin
- Give 15 U regular insulin bolus intravenously, followed by intravenous (or intramuscular or subcutaneous) infusion of regular insulin at a rate of 0.1 U/kg/h (5–10 U/h).
- Decrease dose to 2–3 U/h when plasma glucose is 250–300 mg/dL.
- If plasma glucose fails to decrease over 2–4 hours and urine output, fluid administration, and blood pressure are adequate, double insulin dose hourly.

Potassium
- Administer no K^+ if plasma K^+ >5.0 mEq/L.
- Administer 20 mEq/h of K^+ as one-half potassium acetate and one-half potassium phosphate if plasma K^+ is 4–5 mEq/L.
- Administer 40 mEq K^+/h two times if plasma K^+ is 3–4 mEq/L, then administer 20 mEq/h while rechecking K^+.
- Administer 60 mEq/h one time if plasma K^+ <3.0 mEq/L, and then 40 mEq/h one time while plasma K^+ is rechecked.
- Monitor ECG hourly (leads V_4 and V_5) for T waves to assist in guiding therapy between K^+ determinations.

Phosphate
- Administer 0.1 mmol/kg/h (5–10 mmol/h) to maximum of 80–120 mmol/24 h.

(continued)

TABLE 17-6 *(continued)* Treatment of Hyperglycemic Hyperosmolar Syndrome

- If serum P falls below 1.0 mg/dL, increase infusion to 0.15 mmol/kg/h (10–15 mmol/h).
- If tetany develops, stop phosphate infusion, administer Ca^{2+}/Mg^{2+}, and check Ca^{2+} and Mg^{2+} levels.
- Do not use in presence of renal failure.

Magnesium
- Utilize physiologic multielectrolyte solutions containing Mg^{2+} (3–5 mEq/L) as standard intravenous fluid vehicle.
- Administer 0.05–0.1 mL/kg of 20% $MgSo_4$ intramuscularly (or IV) (i.e., 4–8 mL of 20% $MgSo_4$ [0.08–0.16 mEq/kg]).
- If Mg^{2+} is low or tetany develops, administer 500 mL of 2% $MgSo_4$ solution intravenously over 4 hours plus additional IM doses of 6–12 mEq every 6–8 hours.
- Do not use in presence of renal failure.

Calcium
- If Ca^{2+} is low or tetany develops, administer 10 mEq as an intravenous bolus and repeat as indicated.

Comments
- Repeat K^+ hourly as indicated.
- Repeat Na^+, venous bicarbonate, BUN every 2–4 hours.
- Once plasma glucose is <600 mg/dL, utilize bedside fingerstick blood glucose testing hourly to monitor. Confirm with chemistry lab values every 2–4 hours.
- Monitor blood pressure, pulse rate, temperature, and respiratory rate hourly until stable for 2–4 hours.
- Repeat pertinent physical exam as necessary, with special concentration on neurologic (mental) status; repeat exam of lungs for evidence of pneumonia, CHF, or ARDS; perform abdominal exam if NG tube has been inserted.
- Monitor intake and output hourly for at least 8 hours or until stable.
- Repeat pertinent tests as clinically indicated; ABGs, Hb/Hct, Mg^{2+}, chest X-ray.
- In the absence of contraindications, consider prophylactic low-dose heparin or low-molecular-weight heparin.

those with cardiovascular disease, a central venous line capable of monitoring the central venous pressure or a Swan-Ganz catheter is often warranted. If the patient is alert and capable of voiding, an indwelling urinary catheter should be avoided; however, in obtunded patients an indwelling catheter is necessary until they can void on demand, and urine output should be continuously monitored.

Nasogastric intubation may be required because ileus, gastric distension, and mild gastrointestinal bleeding occur in a number of patients, and the obtunded patient is liable to vomit and aspirate gastric contents, further complicating therapy.

Neither body temperature nor white blood counts are reliable indicators of infection in these patients. Once appropriate cultures are obtained, if an infection is strongly suspected, conventional wisdom dictates antibiotic therapy.

If hypotension is present, large volumes of a crystalloid solution or a volume expander should be administered, and correction of hypoperfusion takes precedence over all other considerations. If necessary, pressors should be added to the regimen when the hypotension is refractory to volume replacement. When the hyperosmolar patient becomes hypotensive, there is no volume reserve to call upon since the hyperosmolar state has already effected maximum removal of water from the intracellular space to maintain the integrity of the intravascular compartment. This "autotransfusion" serves to preserve vascular volume and organ perfusion at the expense of intracellular volume. Therefore, when shock supervenes, water must be rapidly replaced to restore the integrity of the circulation. If hypotension persists after large-volume infusions and/or pressors, other causes must be considered (e.g., myocardial infarction, sepsis, pancreatitis, or gastrointestinal hemorrhage).

While insulin resistance is present in virtually every diabetic and although hyperosmolarity results in impairment of insulin-mediated glucose metabolism and reduced pancreatic insulin secretion, the large doses of insulin previously used to treat uncontrolled diabetes are unnecessary. If there is any question about the adequacy of peripheral perfusion, the intravenous route of insulin administration is most reliable. We recommend an intravenous bolus of approximately 10–15 U of regular insulin to provide a rapid blood level, followed by a continuous infusion of 0.1 U/kg/h (in the average adult, 5–10 U/h). With all reported regimens, the rate of plasma glucose decline is linear and predictable at between 75 and 150 mg/dL/h, provided no other complicating features are present. The amount of insulin required to treat HHS is comparable to that required in DKA.

Once intravenous insulin is discontinued and intermittent subcutaneous insulin begun, management typically defaults to "sliding-scale" insulin coverage. This method of treatment has never undergone objective scrutiny and violates what is known about the physiology of insulin action, which indicates that preemptive administration is needed to control hyperglycemia and repair the metabolic chaos of the uncontrolled diabetic state. It is intellectually, intuitively, and practically impossible to regulate blood glucose retroactively, and sliding-scale coverage delays the establishment of a suitable prospective treatment regimen and prolongs hospitalization. Therefore, the use of intermediate- or long-acting insulins, perhaps in *combination* with short-acting insulins, upon withdrawl of intravenous insulin is preferred by many.

Because of the "safety-valve" function of the normal kidney in the presence of plasma glucose concentrations exceeding the TmG, significant hyperglycemia can occur only if RBF and GFR are reduced. Early in treatment the primary mechanism for glucose disposal is urinary excretion rather than insulin-mediated enhancement of glucose utilization. Three mechanisms account for the early fall in plasma glucose in HHS. Dilution by infused fluids accounts for 24–34% of the total reduction, while glucosuria in those with a preserved GFR and the least reduced ECF accounts for most of the reduction (a 29–76% fall in the glucose pool). Raising the GFR in the presence of high plasma glucose results in excretion of larger amounts of glucose. The remaining early fall in blood glucose concentration is due to non-insulin-dependent glucose metabolism in organs such as the brain and kidney.

The fall in plasma glucose concentration during the early hours of treatment serves as an index of the adequacy of rehydration and the restoration of renal blood flow. Failure of the plasma glucose to fall implies either inadequate volume expansion or renal function impairment. Therefore, the clinician must be wary of patients with uncontrolled diabetes and renal failure. For hyperglycemia accompanying renal failure, therapy with insulin alone, often in high doses, is appropriate. Insulin will reduce elevated potassium levels and, as plasma glucose falls, the water freed will move out of the ECF into the intracellular space, thus decreasing the manifestations of circulatory congestion. Sudden loss of control of diabetes in the presence of advanced renal failure may cause pulmonary edema and life-threatening hyperkalemia, both reversible by the use of insulin alone.

The fluid lost in HHS is hypotonic with respect to electrolytes. Therefore, the losses should be replaced with a hypotonic electrolyte solution (0.45% NaCl or a 0.5 N balanced electrolyte solution). Half-normal balanced electrolyte solutions (e.g., Plasmalyte™, Isolyte S™, Normosol™, or lactated Ringer's) avoid the administration of excess chloride that occurs when saline is used to replace the lost free water. Isotonic solutions, while initially hypotonic to the patient's serum, provide excessive amounts of sodium, and in the case of saline, excess chloride, resulting in hypernatremia or hyperchloremia while aggravating the tendency toward insulin-induced edema (see Table 17-7).

The arguments against the use of hypotonic solutions in HHS include the concerns that there will be too rapid a fall in ECF osmolarity, that isotonic solutions are already hypotonic with respect to the hyperosmolar fluid compartment of the patient, and that isotonic saline provides a better means of maintaining adequate ECF volume. While isotonic saline initially lowers the osmolarity, it provides more sodium and chloride relative to water than the hypertonic patient needs. As the water freed from the osmotic hold of glucose pours into the hyperosmolar intracellular space, the osmotically active particles of glucose are replaced by equally osmotically active sodium, with resultant prolongation of the hyperosmolar state and development of hypernatremia.

Genuth suggests that the increase in serum Na^+ levels, sometimes to 160–170 mEq/L, during therapy of HHS and the occasional persistence of hypernatremia in the 150–155-mEq/L range for days after correction of hyperglycemia in some patients is associated with an elevated serum creatinine, high antidiuretic hormone (ADH) levels, and unresponsiveness to exogenous arginine vasopressin (AVP), all of which suggest temporary nephrogenic diabetes insipidus. In these patients, provision of additional free water in the form of hypotonic solutions may be essential to correct the elevated Na^+.

If hypotonic solutions are delayed until later in treatment, by the time they are administered the intracellular space may no longer be as hyperosmolar as it was initially, and it will no longer provide a sink for any excess infused fluids, paving the way for circulatory overload. Early in the therapy of the hyperosmolar dehydrated patient, the hypertonic intracellular space, which is huge in comparison to the ECF and intravascular space, acts like a sponge soaking up the fluid administered, thus preventing volume overload. This capacity progressively diminishes with fluid repletion, so that attempts to "catch up" and reduce persistently elevated serum osmolarities late in the course of treatment are hazardous. The first few hours of fluid replacement are key to rapidly replacing water and electrolyte losses in their proper proportion.

HHS typically develops over days to weeks, during which time the patient is catabolic and may demonstrate many of the features of protein-calorie undernutrition. When malnourished patients are first given nutritional support, they may develop what has been called the "refeeding syndrome." This term describes the sequelae of rapid refeeding, and includes hypophosphatemia (with associated rhabdomyolysis, hemolysis, neurologic dysfunction, and muscle weakness), hypokalemia, hypomagnesemia (which may contribute more to the clinical syndrome than hypophosphatemia or hypokalemia), vitamin deficiency (especially thiamine), congestive heart failure, and benign refeeding edema (which may share pathogenetic features with insulin edema). This syndrome is well described in chronically malnourished patients (e.g., concentration camp victims), chronic alcoholics, and in anorexia nervosa, but also develops after as few as 7–10 days of hypermetabolic stress with inadequate nutritional support (or its equivalent, the inability to anabolize nutrients). Uncontrolled diabetes, especially the hyperosmolar syndrome, and its subsequent treatment may be a common cause of the refeeding syndrome. It may go unrecognized when only parts of the biochemical (e.g., hypokalemia, hypophosphatemia, hypomagnesemia) or clinical (e.g., insulin edema, muscle weakness) picture are present, but prophylaxis is prudent. A sample of potential pitfalls which may occur during treatment of HHS and an approach to their analysis are provided in Table 17-7.

COMPLICATIONS

Cerebral edema occurring in patients dying of otherwise uncomplicated DKA is well described. Most of the patients with this syndrome are young and have DKA rather than HHS, which runs counter to expectations. This complication accounts for at least 50% of DKA-associated deaths and over 30% of all deaths in diabetic patients under 20 years of age. The overwhelming majority of diabetics who develop overt cerebral edema are young adults or children with DKA. The same is true of the rare patient with HHS who develops fatal cerebral edema. The cerebral atrophy that accompanies the aging process may allow cerebral edema in the elderly diabetic to remain clinically silent by accommodating excess cerebral water without significant damage. No one has ever demonstrated that slower correction of hyperosmolar hyperglycemia prevents cerebral edema. Many more patients die because of undertreatment than from overtreatment of uncontrolled diabetes. Thus any recommendation that would reduce the rate of correction of hyperglycemia risks increasing the mortality rate and should be viewed with alarm.

Other complications seen in HHS include thromboembolic events and possible disseminated intravascular coagulation, pulmonary aspiration of gastric contents in the presence of gastric stasis and obtundation, and the remarkably rare occurrence of renal failure and rhabdomyolysis.

Creatine kinase elevations of greater than 1000 IU/L have been described in over 25% of patients with HHS in the absence of stroke, myocardial infarction, or end-stage renal disease. Thus subclinical rhabdomyolysis is not uncommon in HHS, but clinical manifestations are mild or absent.

PROGNOSIS

The best prognostic indicator in uncontrolled diabetes is the age of the patient. In two large series of HHS, advanced age, a higher BUN, and a higher Na^{2+} concentration were predictors of a poor outcome. In these series the mortality for HHS was 10–17%.

PREVENTION

Improvement in the outcome of this potential metabolic disaster requires an effective preventive strategy. Patients with HHS are elderly, have type 2 diabetes, and often live alone, and social isolation is a precipitant in 25–30% of episodes. The availability of a knowledgeable significant other (friend, neighbor, or family member) who maintains daily contact with the elderly diabetic is essential. They should be educated to recognize alterations in the

TABLE 17-7 Potential Pitfalls during Therapy of Hyperglycemic Hyperosmolar Syndrome

Problem	Consider	Approach
1. Hypotension	(a) Myocardial infarct, sepsis, bleeding (b) Internal redistribution of fluid as hyperglycemia is corrected (c) Total body fluid depletion due to osmotic diuresis with inadequate volume replacement (d) Ongoing osmotic diuresis	(a) Std. work-up/specific therapy (b–d) Increase IV fluids
2. Worsening level of consciousness	(a) Meningitis, CVA, drugs, head trauma (b) Hypovolemia/hypoperfusion (c) Increasing Eosm (increasing Sna$^+$) (d) Cerebral edema (very rare in HHS) (e) Hypoglycemia (f) Wernicke's encephalopathy (refeeding syndrome) (g) $\downarrow$Mg^{2+}	(a) Std. work-up/specific therapy (b) Increase IV fluids (c) Give hypotonic fluids (d) Mannitol IV/steroids IV/$\downarrow$insulin (e) Give glucose; reduce insulin (f) Thiamine/B-complex vitamins (g) Give Mg^{2+}
3. Seizures	(a) CVA, prior seizure disorder, withdrawal, drugs, etc. (b) Early in HHS (Seen in ~19%) (c) Cerebral edema (very rare in HHS) (d) $\downarrow$P, $\downarrow$Mg^{2+}	(a) Std. work-up/specific therapy (avoid diphenylhydantoin) (b) Insulin/hypotonic IV fluids (c) Mannitol IV/steroids IV/$\downarrow$insulin (d) Replace P, Mg^{2+}
4. Tetany	(a) $\downarrow$Ca^{2+}, $\downarrow$Mg^{2+} (b) P infusion (causing $\downarrow$Ca^{2+}, Mg^{2+}); rare when Mg^{2+} is given routinely/proactively	(a) Replace Ca^{2+}, Mg^{2+} (b) Stop P: replace Ca^{2+}/Mg^{2+} (c) Proactive Mg^{2+} replacement

(continued)

TABLE 17-7 *(continued)* Potential Pitfalls during Therapy of Hyperglycemic Hyperosmolar Syndrome

Problem	Consider	Approach
5. Muscle weakness (may be associated with respiratory failure)	(a) $\downarrow K^+$, $\downarrow Mg^{2+}$, $\downarrow P$ (b) Rhabdomyolysis (commonly asymptomatic)	(a) Replace K^+, Mg^{2+}, P (b) Obtain creatine kinase (CK); if CK > 1000 watch for ATN/renal failure and maintain high urine output (c) Respiratory failure may require mechanical ventilation
6. Cardiac/ECG abnormalities	(a) Peaked precordial T waves, prolonged PR, Vfib: $\uparrow K^+$ (b) Ectopy, tachyarrhythmias, (+)U waves, flat T waves: $\downarrow K^+$ (c) Wide QRS: $\downarrow K^+$, $\downarrow Ca^{2+}$ (d) Short QT: $\uparrow Ca^{2+}$ (e) Prolonged QT^c: $\downarrow Ca^{2+}$, $\uparrow Mg^{2+}$ (f) Vtach: $\uparrow Mg^{2+}$ (g) Underlying heart disease (in presence of arrhythmias, CHF, etc.) (h) CVA (especially subarachnoid hemorrhage) with deeply inverted precordial T's. (i) ST segment elevation; friction rubs (underlying pericarditis vs. severe dehydration)	(a)–(f) Monitor ECG hourly, especially T waves. Measure K^+, Mg^{2+}, Ca^{2+}, correct as necessary; routinely administer K^+, Mg^{2+} unless levels are very high (g) Std. work-up/specific therapy (h) Std. work-up/specific therapy (i) If due to severe dehydration, especially with DKA, will rapidly resolve with fluid repletion
7. Persistent hyperglycemia	(a) Inadequate fluid infusion or oliguria (b) Renal failure (chronic or acute rhabcomyolysis) (c) Insulin resistance	(a) Increase fluids—hypotonic (b) May need to reduce fluids and increase insulin (c) Double insulin dose hourly

8. Persistent hyperosmolarity	(a) Persistent hyperglycemia	(a) See 7 above
	(b) Hypernatremia—unmasked as glucose falls or excess Na^+ in infused isotonic solutions or inadequate free water replacement	(b) Increase IV fluids; use hypotonic electrolyte solutions
	(c) Nephrogenic diabetes insipidus related to HHS (resistance to ADH)	(c) Maintain high-volume hypotonic fluid intake
9. Oligura	(a) Renal vascular occlusion or urinary obstruction or papillary necrosis	(a) Std. work-up/specific therapy
	(b) Chronic renal failure (CRF)	(b) History; reduce IV fluids; use caution in volume replacement; ↑ dose of insulin
	(c) Acute renal failure (ARF)	(c) Std. work-up; if trial of increased volume infusion fails, treat as CRF (above)
	(d) Hypovolemia: Internal fluid redistribution as hyperglycemia is corrected, inadequate volume replacement, ongoing osmotic diuresis, or a combination of these	(d) Increase IV fluid replacement
	(e) Rhabdomyolysis (↑↑CK)	(e) Check K^+, P, Mg^{++} and correct; adjust IV fluid volume to attempt to sustain high urine output
10. Edema	(a) Underlying cardiac, hepatic, renal, or GI disease	(a) History/std. work-up/specific therapy
	(b) Excess Na^+/H_2O administration (especially in elderly)	(b) Restrict Na^+ and/or H_2O; diuretics
	(c) "Insulin edema"	(c) If asymptomatic, recognize, reassure, and observe; if symptomatic, give diuretics and restrict Na^+

(continued)

TABLE 17-7 (continued) Potential Pitfalls during Therapy of Hyperglycemic Hyperosmolar Syndrome

Problem	Consider	Approach
11. Hyperchloremia	(a) Underlying renal disease; RTA (b) DKA with ketonuria resulting in Cl⁻ retention (c) Administration of excess Cl⁻ in treatment (e.g. use of NaCl and KCl⁻ solutions)	(a) History/std. work-up/specific therapy (b) Use physiologic (hypotonic if associated with HHS) electrolyte solutions; avoid use of NaCl and KCl (c) See (b) above. Use Plasmalyte, Isolyte, Normosol, lactated Ringer's, etc.; for K⁺ replacement use K acetate/K phosphate
12. Hypokalemia	(a) Typical of catabolic state of uncontrolled diabetes and unmasked as anabolism begins (b) Insulin (and refeeding syndrome) (c) Ongoing catabolism, osmotic diuretic losses and, in DKA, as cation accompanying ketoacids in urine (d) Hypomagnesemia (refractory hypokalemia) (e) Exogenous diuretic therapy (f) Bicarbonate administration	(a) Begine K⁺ repletion at outset of therapy unless hyperkalemia, ECG changes, or renal failure present (b) Proactive and therepeutic K⁺ replacement (c) Insulin plus K⁺ (d) Replace K⁺ plus Mg⁺⁺ (e) History; stop diuretic; replace K⁺ (f) Stop HCO₃⁻; replace K⁺
13. Hypophosphatemia	(a) Catabolic depletion (b) Internal redistribution (insulin/glucose) (c) As part of refeeding syndrome [see (a) & (b) above] (d) If severe, may cause hemolysis	(a)–(c) Give P; it is the necessary intracellular anion to enable K⁺ and Mg⁺⁺ to cross cell membranes and enter cell during anabolism; Cl⁻ does not cross cell membranes easily or facilitate translocation of K⁺ and Mg⁺⁺ to cell interior (d) Administer P

14. Hypomagnesemia	(a) Chronic catabolic deficiency state seen in >50% of poorly controlled diabetics (b) Osmotic diuretic loss (c) Internal redistribution (refeeding syndrome)	(a)–b) Replace Mg^{++}; it is a component of over 300 critical enzyme systems and of all energy generating systems in the body
15. Anemia	(a) Preexistent; may become manifest after rehydration (b) Hemolysis: (1) G-6-PD deficiency, (2) ↓P (c) Bleeding; may see "coffee grounds" gastric contents in up to 25% of DKA/HHS	(a) Std. work-up/specific therapy (b) (1) Primarily seen in African-Americans and persons of Mediterranean decent (2) Measure P and replace; usually not seen Unless P is <0.5 mg/dl (c) Std. work-up/specific treatment; hemorrhagic gastritis resolves with treatment; may require NGT drainage
16. Thrombotic events	(a) Hyperviscosity, low flow, hypotension (b) Hypercoagulable state (seen in diabetes mellitus in general) not necessarily specific to HHS	(a) Rapid large-volume crystalloid infusions; pressors if necessary, Mg^{++}; low-dose heparin prophylaxis (b) Consider anticoagulation as necessary, appropriate, and safe
17. Respiratory distress	(a) Pneumonia, CHF (b) Renal failure (c) Pneumothorax (iatrogenic due to central lines) (d) Pneumomediastinum or pneumothorax in DKA (e) ARDS (f) Rhabdomyolysis	(a) Std. work-up/specific therapy (b) History; reduce fluids if CRF and increase insulin may improve general circulatory and pulmonary fluid overload by redistribution of fluid to intracellular compartments (c) CXR; specific therapy (d) CXR; specific therapy (e) Central monitoring to exclude CHF or circulatory overlaod; supportive therapy and std. ICU monitoring; prognosis poor (f) Check CK; supportive therapy

(continued)

TABLE 17-7 *(continued)* Potential Pitfalls during Therapy of Hyperglycemic Hyperosmolar Syndrome

Problem	Consider	Approach
17. Respiratory distress *(continued)*	(g) $\downarrow$P, $\downarrow$K$^+$, $\downarrow$Mg^{++}	(g) Monitor serum levels and replace as necessary
	(h) Pulmonary embolism	(h) Std. work-up/specific therapy
18. Hypoxemia	(a) Pneumonia, pulmonary embolus, CHF	(a) Std. work-up/specific therapy
	(b) ARDS, especially with DKA	(b) Poor prognosis; monitor with PCWP to differentiate from CHF; supportive care
	(c) Pneumrothorax, spontaneous in DKA	(c) CXR; specific therapy
19. Hypothermia	(a) Sepsis/infection	(a) Std. work-up/specific therapy
	(b) Hypoglycemia	(b) Monitor plasma gluose, administer glucose
	(c) DKA	(c) Poor prognostic sign in DKA
20. Abdominal pain	(a) Acute surgical abdomen (e.g., appendicitis, pancreatitis, cholecystitis, mesenteric ischemia)	(a) Std. work-up/specifc therapy
	(b) Fatty liver	(b) Monitor LFTs; hydration plus insulin usually resolves this problem
	(c) DKA	(c) Especially in children may mimic acute surgical abdominal condition; rapidly responds to hydration and insulin
21. Hyperamylasemia/hyperlipasemia	(a) Pancreatitis, bowel infarction	(a) Std. work-up/specific therapy
	(b) DKA	(b) Responds to hydration/insulin
22. Leukocytosis	(a) Sepsis	(a) Std. work-up/specific therapy
	(b) DKA	(b) Resolves with hydration/insulin

patient's mental status and symptoms of loss of diabetic control, and to promptly report these to the physician. Public education about the presenting symptoms of diabetes will help reduce the one-quarter to one-third of patients who have HHS at presentation.

Residence in nursing homes predisposes to HHS, and nursing home residents are prone to develop dehydration and hyperosmolarity, so education of nursing home staff members in prevention and detection of this syndrome is essential. Prompt recognition and treatment of infections and the use of Pneumovax™ and annual influenza immunizations are important preventive measures in the elderly diabetic.

Providers should take into account the potential for medications prescribed for the elderly to cause or worsen glucose intolerance; aggressively apply home blood glucose monitoring in elderly diabetics; intensify efforts to improve blood glucose control; and reinforce education of patients and families regarding compliance with diet and hypoglycemic agents.

The current obesity pandemic in adolescents and young adults accompanied by a dramatic increase of type 2 diabetes in this cohort is paralleled by the development of HHS in a group in whom it was previously a rarity. This requires practitioners caring for this population to develop an awareness of the syndrome and its manifestations. Primary prevention depends on identification of high-risk individuals (e.g., the obese, Native Americans, African-Americans, Latinos, those with a history of familial type 2 diabetes, etc.) and an emphasis on appropriate dietary habits (most critically, avoidance of high-calorie cheap foods), counseling regarding the dangers of a sedentary lifestyle while encouraging regular aerobic exercises.

ADDITIONAL READINGS

Clement S, Braithwaite SS, Magee MF, et al: Management of diabetes and hyperglycemia in hospitals. *Diabetes Care* 2004;27:553.

Ennis D, Stahl EJvB, Kreisberg RA: The hyperosmolar hyperglycemic syndrome. *Diabetes Rev* 1994;2:115.

Genuth SM. Diabetic ketoacidosis and hyperglycemic hyperosmolar coma. *Curr Ther Endocrinol Metab* 1997;6:438.

Kitabchi AE, Umpierrez GE, Murphy MB, et al: Management of hyperglycemic crises in patients with diabetes (Technical Review). *Diabetes Care* 2001;24:131.

Matz R: Hyperosmolar nonacidotic diabetes [HNAD]. In Porte D, Sherwin RS, eds: *Ellenberg and Rifkin's Diabetes Mellitus: Theory and Practice*, 5th ed, Norwalk, CT: Appleton & Lange; 1987:845.

For a more detailed discussion of this topic and a bibliography, please see Porte *et al: Ellenberg & Rifkin's Diabetes Mellitus,* 6th ed., Chapter 35.

---

18 | Host Defense and Infections in Diabetes Mellitus

Brian P. Currie   Joan I. Casey

GENERAL PROBLEM OF INFECTION IN DIABETIC PATIENTS

Literature reviews examining the association of infections with diabetes mellitus are often difficult to interpret and fraught with contradictions. A major contributory factor is that diabetes mellitus is a heterogeneous disease and so study populations need to be carefully identified in order to allow comparisons between studies (e.g., type 1 versus type 2 diabetes, well-controlled disease versus poorly controlled disease). In addition, diabetes mellitus is a relatively common disease, and as a consequence, anecdotal reports of various infections in diabetic patients can lead to spurious associations. Nonetheless, it is well established that certain infections occur almost exclusively in diabetic patients and that diabetic patients have a worse prognosis than nondiabetic patients after acquiring certain infections, such as acute pyelonephritis complicated by papillary necrosis or emphysematous pyelonephritis.

A knowledge of the normal host defense mechanisms and of those that are abnormal in the diabetic individual may be helpful in understanding the unusual predilection for certain infectious diseases among diabetic patients.

NORMAL HOST DEFENSE MECHANISMS

Skin

Normal skin is impenetrable to most bacteria, and infection rarely occurs unless the skin is damaged. The normal bacterial flora of the skin maintains an environment that is hostile to most pathogenic bacteria. The nerve supply of the skin is important in maintaining the integrity of the mechanical barrier by warning of potential injury from prolonged pressure or penetration by foreign bodies.

Blood Supply

Maintenance of normal nutrition and oxygen tension to tissues, as well as delivery of the humoral and cellular components of the immune system, is dependent on an adequate blood supply.

Humoral Immunity

The two major components of humoral immunity are antibodies and the complement system. Antibodies may neutralize the effect of bacteria, bacterial toxins, or viral capsids by combining with the organisms and preventing their attachment to cell surfaces. Other antibodies act by agglutinating organisms, thereby increasing clearance by the reticuloendothelial system, or by lysing bacteria. Opsonins, antibodies that may be specific or nonspecific, coat bacteria and enhance phagocytosis. Most of these reactions require or are enhanced by the action of complement, through either the classic or the alternate (properdin) pathway.

Phagocytic Function

This component of the immune response is mainly related to polymorphonuclear cells and macrophages. The latter cells are either wandering (alveolar, peritoneal, and skin macrophages and tissue histiocytes) or fixed to vascular endothelium in the liver, spleen, and lymph nodes. Various functions of phagocytes have been recognized, including random migration, chemotaxis and attachment, ingestion, and intracellular killing of bacteria. After ingestion of bacteria by phagocytic cells, a vigorous burst of oxidative metabolism leads to the production of hydrogen peroxide, which combines with myeloperoxidase and halogen (iodide or chloride). This results in rapid killing of most pathogenic bacteria.

Lymphocytes

There is considerable information about the types and functions of lymphocytes and the substances elaborated by these cells when exposed to antigens or mitogens. There are at least three types of lymphocytes now recognized. These are the thymus-derived or T-lymphocytes, the bone marrow-derived or B-lymphocytes, and the non-B-, non-T-lymphocytes. The B-cells can transform into antibody-secreting or plasma cells, whereas the T-cells are regarded as the cells responsible for cell-mediated defense against viruses, fungi, and mycobacteria. T-cells may help or suppress the immune functions of other cells such as the B-lymphocytes, usually by the production of lymphokines.

ABNORMALITIES OF HOST DEFENSE IN DIABETES MELLITUS

Skin

Nasal and skin flora of diabetic patients have been studied frequently, with varying results. Some studies have suggested an increased prevalence of *Staphylococcus aureus* colonization among diabetics. Smith and coworkers found that 53% of type 1 diabetic adults were nasal carriers of *S. aureus,* compared with 34% of nondiabetic adults and 35% of type 2 diabetic adults. Of diabetic children, 76% were nasal carriers, compared with 44% of nondiabetic children.

Peripheral neuropathy in diabetic patients can permit undetected disruption of the dermal barrier, which can serve as a portal of entry for pathogens. This decreased sense of touch prevents warning of potential injury from prolonged pressure or penetration injuries. In addition, once dermal barrier disruption occurs and infection is established, this decreased sense of touch contributes to delayed recognition and treatment.

Blood Supply

Vascular problems in diabetic patients, secondary to both the microangiopathy of diabetes and the accelerated course of atherosclerosis in these patients, may predispose them to infection by disrupting normal nutrient and oxygen delivery, as well as disrupting normal immune function.

Decreased adherence of polymorphonuclear cells and decreased diapedesis have been described in diabetic subjects, and there is evidence that this activity is a function of blood vessel endothelial cells, as well as of the polymorphonuclear cell itself. In addition, poor metabolic control may result in increased vascular permeability, leading to increased diffusion of nutrients and edema formation. Finally, a reduction in blood supply can translate into a reduction in delivery of antibiotics when treating established infections in diabetic patients.

Humoral Immunity

Antibody production after exposure to a variety of bacterial antigens has been studied in diabetic patients. Decreased agglutinating antibodies to a number of pathogens have been reported in diabetics relative to nondiabetic persons. However, other studies, including those using pneumococcal polysaccharide, have shown that diabetic patients respond well to vaccines. Likewise, conflicting results have been reported when the bactericidal capacity of diabetic blood has been studied, and the majority of studies of serum complement in diabetic patients have found normal or elevated levels.

Baker and associates studied opsonization of group B streptococci in neonates, type 1 diabetic patients, and healthy adults using type II group B streptococci. They found that inefficient bactericidal activity occurred among neonatal and diabetic sera compared to normal sera. Only 6 of 15 diabetic patients had sera with efficient bactericidal activity for type II group B streptococci. While bactericidal activity was not dependent on the level of antibody, type-specific antibody did have the capacity to correct certain opsonophagocytic deficiencies.

Phagocytic Function

Phagocytosis of bacteria cannot occur in the absence of opsonization except in unusual circumstances. Indeed, many of the problems in interpreting the inconsistent data relating to phagocytic function in diabetic patients may be due to the fact that there are so many separate steps in this process.

Random migration of leukocytes, which is probably the first step in the process of phagocytosis, has been reported to be abnormal in type 1 diabetic persons. The ability of polymorphonuclear cells and macrophages to get to an area of infection also depends on their ability to adhere to and migrate through the endothelium of the capillary walls. As noted previously, this diapedesis of phagocytic cells could be dependent in part on the vessel wall. Migration and chemotaxis of cells have been tested by using the Rebuck skin window, and two studies have indicated a significant delay in response to skin abrasion in diabetic patients who were ketoacidotic. Brayton and colleagues tested both ketotic and nonketotic patients and found impaired responses in both groups. Chemotaxis of polymorphonuclear cells from diabetic and non-diabetic subjects was studied by Donovan and coworkers using time-lapse microcinematography and video techniques, which revealed that diabetic cells move at normal rates. However, other *in vitro* studies have reported delayed chemotaxis in both type 2 and type 1 diabetic patients.

Defects in phagocyte engulfment and intracellular killing of bacteria have been reported by several authors. In studies in which *S. aureus* was used, ingestion of organisms was found to be normal in the diabetic patients, except for those with ketoacidosis. Nolan and coworkers found impaired engulfment and intracellular killing of *S. aureus* among diabetic patients. They also noted that neutrophils from poorly controlled uninfected diabetic patients did not kill *S. aureus* as well as those from well-controlled diabetic patients or nondiabetic persons. Impairment of ingestion of *Streptococcus pneumoniae* has also been reported, and this defect was partially corrected by improved metabolic control of the diabetes. In a later study, Bagdade and associates suggested that the defect was related to serum factors, because it was partially corrected by serum from normal controls, whereas the diabetic serum caused impairment of phagocytic function in cells from nondiabetic controls. In contrast, Crosby and Allison were unable to demonstrate any impairment of ingestion of *S. pneumoniae* in diabetic patients who were not ketoacidotic.

Lymphocytes

Cell-mediated immunity, as measured by blast transformation of peripheral blood lymphocytes, has been measured in diabetic patients. When phytohemagglutinin stimulation was used, the response of diabetic patients in good metabolic control was normal, whereas that of hyperglycemic patients was depressed. Lymphocyte response to streptokinase-streptodornase stimulation has also been found to be impaired in diabetic subjects with poor glucose control, and this defect normalized with institution of metabolic control. When staphylococcal antigen was used in the blast transformation assay, the response of lymphocytes from both type 1 and type 2 diabetic subjects was less than that of nondiabetic subjects. This impaired response to staphylococcal antigen appeared to be unrelated to serum factors or metabolic control.

Summary

There is strong evidence suggesting multiple immune defects in subsets of diabetic patients, summarized in Table 18-1. The strongest evidence regarding an immune defect in diabetic patients is related to abnormalities of neutrophil function in patients with poor metabolic control (ketoacidosis or hyperglycemia). Studies using *in vitro* systems have documented impaired chemotactic responses and phagocytic activity of neutrophils in these subsets of diabetic patients. However, even among these patients, the mechanisms of the defects have not been identified, and the clinical significance of impaired neutrophil function remains to be determined.

In addition, it has become clear that there is a complex interaction among polymorphonuclear cells, endothelial cells, and serum factors that control neutrophil function.

TABLE 18-1 Summary of Potential Leukocyte Dysfunction Reported among Diabetic Patients

Neutrophils	↓ Leukocytosis
	↓ Chemotaxis
	↓ Phagocytosis
	↓ Intracellular killing
	↓ Metabolic burst
Lymphocytes	↓ Antibody function/opsonization
	↓ Chemotactic factor
	↓ Lymphokines

SERIOUS INFECTIONS CAUSING MORBIDITY AND MORTALITY IN DIABETES MELLITUS

Although the entire immune system is probably alerted to defend against microbial invasion, certain defects may be more directly associated with certain types of infections. Some of the infections to which diabetic patients seem particularly vulnerable may well be related to some or all of the previously described defects, whereas others are still unexplained. The relationships of these host defense deficits to disease syndromes are summarized in Table 18-2.

Skin and Soft Tissue Infections

Whether or not staphylococcal infections of the skin are more common in diabetic than nondiabetic persons is a controversy that has never been resolved. The increased skin and nasal carriage that is described in diabetic persons could lead to increased susceptibility to infection. Farrer and MacLeod found staphylococcal infections to be twice as common among diabetic as nondiabetic patients who had other severe debilitating diseases.

Candidal skin infections commonly occur in moist, warm areas around the breasts, thighs, and genitalia and are especially common in diabetic patients who are overweight or who have been on antibiotics.

Diabetic foot infections account for at least one-quarter of all diabetic hospital admissions and are the most common cause of partial or complete foot amputations. Most of these infections probably begin with unrecognized soft tissue injury, secondary to peripheral neuropathy. Subsequent tissue edema, inflammation, and necrosis disrupt the dermal barrier and allow a portal of entry for infection. Concomitant peripheral vascular disease contributes to reduced healing and the onset of chronic infections. The resulting infected diabetic foot ulcer frequently involves deeper tissues, and a chronic underlying osteomyelitis can be established. The infections are characteristically polymicrobial and include aerobic gram-positive or gram-negative organisms coupled with microaerophilic and anaerobic organisms. Peptostreptococci can be recovered from 32–80% of diabetic foot ulcers, and *P. magnus* is the most commonly isolated species. Krepel and coworkers demonstrated that 94% of *P. magnus* isolated from diabetic foot ulcers produced collagenase, as opposed to 18% of isolates from intra-abdominal infections, and suggested that collagenase production from *P. magnus* may be a significant pathogenic factor contributing to the establishment of infected diabetic foot ulcers.

TABLE 18-2 Relationship of Host Defense Deficit to Disease Syndrome in Diabetic Patients

Host defense deficit	Disease syndrome
Skin integrity	Erythrasma, cellulitis
Neuropathy	Infections secondary to trauma and ulceration; bladder infections
Blood supply	Peripheral vascular disease with ulcers, gangrene, and synergistic infections; invasion of vessels with bacteria and fungi resulting in malignant otitis or mucormycosis; possibly periodontal disease
Humoral immunity	Possibly bacterial infections due to *Pseudomonas* and group B *Streptococcus*

Serious and often life-threatening infections of the skin and underlying tissues can occur when aerobic gram-positive (e.g., *S. aureus* or streptococci) or gram-negative (e.g., Enterobacteriaceae or *Pseudomonas*) microorganisms act synergistically with microaerophilic or anaerobic gram-positive (e.g., peptococci or peptostreptococci) or gram-negative (e.g., *Bacteroides*) microorganisms to produce necrotizing infections of the skin or underlying soft tissues. This syndrome is probably related to the neuropathy and peripheral vascular disease that allows minor infections to become established; the aerobic organisms consume the already compromised oxygen supply and allow anaerobic organisms to thrive. In this situation, the disease is frequently persistent and destructive. The initial presentation may range from that of an indolent ulcer to a fulminant infection, causing marked systemic toxicity and death. Stone and Martin described 63 patients with necrotizing cellulites, of whom 47 were diabetic. The mortality rate was 85% for diabetic patients and 44% for nondiabetics.

These patients presented with high fever, toxicity, and skin ulcers draining thin serosanguineous pus. Variable amounts of skin necrosis were noted, but gangrene was not necessarily extensive. Exquisite local tenderness inconsistent with the amount of skin involvement is characteristic. Subcutaneous gas may or may not be present. Infection of muscle and fascia is common, and necrosis of skin occurs as the underlying vessels become thrombosed.

Such infections may begin in the perianal or pelvic regions, where anaerobic organisms are common, or in the extremities, where the vascular supply is compromised. When the infectious process involves the male genitalia and surrounding region it is known as Fournier's gangrene. Deep fascial planes of the neck may be infected from infected teeth or tonsils. Bessman and associates found that enterococci were more synergistic for the growth of *B. fragilis* than *E. coli*. In mixed infections, enterococci are sometimes regarded as nuisances rather than true pathogens, but this study clearly indicated that this is not the case.

Bessman and Wagner described 48 diabetic patients with nonclostridial gas gangrene of the lower extremities. Of the 83 organisms cultured from these patients, only three were anaerobic. This entity is much more common in the diabetic than is clostridial gas infection. It is important to make the distinction because the organisms are very different in their antibiotic sensitivities. *Clostridium perfringens* is sensitive to penicillin, whereas the anaerobes such as *Bacteroides* usually require metronidazole, clindamycin, cefoxitin, or possibly ticarcillin/clavulanic acid or imipenem. The Enterobacteriaceae may be sensitive to a variety of antibiotics such as aminoglycosides, third-generation cephalosporins, extended-spectrum penicillins, or imipenem. Extensive surgical debridement is usually necessary and should be done early in the course of these infections.

Goodman and coworkers described risk factors for complications among 172 diabetic patients undergoing local operations for diabetic gangrene. Increased severity of infection, as measured by temperature, total white cell count, and subcutaneous gas, was associated with failure. The authors suggest delay of surgical procedures until medical control of infection has occurred. However, it should be emphasized that medical control must be accomplished as rapidly as possible, because extensive surgical debridement is usually necessary and should be done as early as possible in the course of these infections.

Infections of the hands, although not as common as those of the lower extremities, nevertheless require comment because of the serious nature of the problem. Of 20 diabetic patients admitted to the hospital with hand infections, 6 required amputation to control infection and 1 because of impaired function of the extremity. Only 6 patients regained normal function. Most of these infections were synergistic.

Erythrasma is an unusual disease of the skin caused by *Corynebacterium minutissimum* (a gram-positive rod). In 19 patients with extensive erythrasma, 9 were known to be diabetic and 6 others had clinical evidence of diabetes.

Malignant Otitis Externa

This disease is well named because associated mortality is over 50%. Over 90% of cases have occurred in diabetic patients over 35 years of age. Swimming and use of a hearing aid are additional predisposing factors. *Pseudomonas aeruginosa* is the usual infecting agent, and only rarely are other organisms involved. The presenting manifestations are those of chronic ear infection (i.e., pain and purulent drainage). However, the presence of tenderness and swelling of the surrounding tissues, and in particular polyps or granulation tissue in the floor of the external canal, strongly suggest this diagnosis. The infection spreads via the clefts between cartilage and bone in the auditory canal to involve the deep soft tissues, parotid gland, the temporomandibular joint, the mastoid bone, and eventually the cranial nerves. Infection can also spread outward to involve the entire pinna. *P. aeruginosa* invades small blood vessels and produces an infectious vasculitis that compounds the microangiopathy of diabetes and makes this infection particularly virulent. Diagnosis is often delayed for 6–8 weeks because patients are misdiagnosed with noninvasive otitis externa. A high index of suspicion and early diagnosis are essential for successful treatment. Parenteral antibiotics (usually a beta-lactam with activity against *Pseudomonas* and an aminoglycoside), topical antipseudomonal ear drops, and surgical debridement are the mainstays of therapy.

Mucormycosis

Mucormycosis is another unusual but highly virulent infection that occurs most commonly in patients with diabetes, in particular those with ketoacidosis. The disease is caused by a variety of species of molds of the order Mucorales, with *Rhizopus* and *Rhizomucor* being the most commonly isolated agents. *Rhizopus* species are the ubiquitous gray-black molds found on bread and vegetables. The particular susceptibility of the diabetic for this infection may be related to decreased leukocyte mobilization. Artis and colleagues have also shown that ketoacidotic sera from diabetic patients have poor iron-binding capacity. They suggest that the free iron enhances growth of *Rhizopus oryzae* and that this may be a mechanism for the increased susceptibility of ketotic diabetic subjects to this fungus. It is also noteworthy that this organism is capable of invading blood vessels, and this combination of factors may explain why diabetic patients are particularly vulnerable to this infection.

The organism probably first colonizes the nose or paranasal sinuses and spreads by direct extension to the orbit and surrounding tissues. Invasion of the cribriform plate and cranial cavity may occur rapidly. The clinical presentation is usually acute, with periorbital pain, induration and discoloration of the lid, and bloody nasal discharge. Ischemic infarction of the lid and orbital contents may follow vessel invasion. Blindness and loss of sensation in the distribution of the ophthalmic division of the trigeminal nerve are diagnostic clues, because these are unusual with other orbital infections. Black necrotic tissue may be seen in the nose or posterior hard palate. The internal jugular vein or the cavernous sinus may become thrombosed, and chemosis, proptosis, and retinal hemorrhage may occur.

Although this disease resembles malignant otitis externa in that blood vessels are invaded and progressive infection occurs, extension to the meninges and brain is more common in mucormycosis. Morbidity and mortality from this infection are very high, and therapy may have to be started on the basis of clinical findings even in the absence of supporting laboratory evidence for mucormycosis. Biopsy of nasal turbinates or pharyngeal tissues must be done early for diagnostic purposes. Extensive surgical debridement is necessary. Amphotericin remains the antifungal therapy of choice, and even with early and optimal therapy the disease is extensively disfiguring.

Oral Infections

The problem of periodontal disease in diabetic patients has received significant attention in the dental literature, and it has been reported that this disorder was more common and more severe in diabetic than nondiabetic patients. Associated factors were the age of the patient, the duration of diabetes, the occurrence of complications, and the severity of hyperglycemia. In a study of patients with rapidly progressive periodontitis, 48% were found to have impaired leukotaxis. Manouchehr-Pour and associates also demonstrated significantly reduced chemotactic responses of polymorphonuclear cells from diabetic patients with severe periodontal disease relative to cells from diabetic and nondiabetic subjects with mild periodontal disease or nondiabetic patients with severe periodontal disease.

Oral candidiasis is a well-recognized problem in diabetic patients. Carriage rate and density of *Candida albicans* in the mouth have been reported to be higher in diabetic than nondiabetic patients.

Gastrointestinal Infections

Telzak and coworkers recently investigated the largest nosocomial foodborne outbreak of *Salmonella enteritides* ever described in the United States. Investigation of multiple potential risk factors indicated that diabetes (defined as a patient treated with insulin or an oral hypoglycemic agent) was the only independent risk factor identified for developing infection after exposure to a *Salmonella*-contaminated meal. While noting that diabetic patients may have granulocyte and T-cell function abnormalities, the authors suggest that diabetes-associated decreased gastric acid production and decreased bowel motility may be contributory factors. Even more recently, an association between *Campylobacter* gastroenteritis and diabetes has also been described.

Urinary Tract Infections

The data relating to urinary tract infections in diabetic patients have been examined in two authoritative reviews which reached contradictory conclusions. Wheat states that the majority of controlled studies noted a two- to fourfold higher incidence of bacteriuria in diabetic women, whereas Gocke and Grieco conclude that in well-controlled diabetes, urinary tract infections are no more likely in diabetics than in nondiabetic patients. Several studies support both views. In diabetic children, a prevalence rate similar to that of non-diabetic children is found, and the same appears to be true for diabetic men. Among patients with hospital-acquired urinary tract infections, diabetic patients are more susceptible than nondiabetic patients.

Thus, it appears that within populations in whom the prevalence of urinary tract infection is known to be high, the diabetic is even more likely than the nondiabetic to develop a urinary tract infection. Some of the reasons for this are that the diabetic patient may have a neurogenic bladder with urinary stasis, may be catheterized frequently, may have underlying renal disease, and may have impaired host defenses, all of which are predisposing factors for urinary tract infection.

There is universal agreement that urinary tract infections are more likely to cause serious complications for the diabetic patient than for others. Ooi and colleagues found that 63% of diabetic women with asymptomatic bacteriuria had upper tract involvement, whereas Forland and associates found 80% of such patients had upper tract involvement. However, a prospective study suggested that diabetic women with asymptomatic bacteriuria do not have an increased incidence of subsequent symptomatic urinary tract infection, including pyelonephritis.

Diabetic patients may experience higher complication rates when they do develop renal infections. In a series of 52 patients with perinephric abscesses, 36 were diabetic. The causative organisms are usually those associated with urinary tract infections, although *S. aureus* can cause cortical abscesses by the hematogenous route.

Gas-forming infections of the kidney, renal pelvis, ureter, or bladder are uncommon, but not rare, and most occur in diabetic patients. The severity of this disease is related to the site of infection. When gas is confined to the collecting system, survival rates are much better than when the renal parenchyma is involved. As with the other renal complications, this disease should be suspected in any diabetic patient not responding quickly to appropriate antibiotics, especially if nausea, vomiting, and diarrhea are present. Tenderness, a palpable mass, or rarely, crepitus, may be felt in the costovertebral angle. Diagnosis is made by abdominal CT scan or MRI, since plain radiographs identify gas in only one-third of patients. The pathogenesis of this disease is obscure but is thought to be related to the ability of organisms such as *E. coli* or *Klebsiella pneumoniae* to utilize glucose with subsequent formation of carbon dioxide and hydrogen. When infection with these organisms occurs in an area with vascular insufficiency, a severe necrotizing infection can occur. What is not clear is why it happens so infrequently, considering the frequent occurrence of urinary tract infections in diabetic patients with vascular disease and hyperglycemia.

Fungal infections of the urinary tract are not uncommon in diabetic patients. This may be a result of the use of antibiotics for bacterial infections and subsequent overgrowth of *Candida* species, or the fungus may spread from perineal candidal infection. Oral fluconazole is highly efficacious in the treatment of *Candida albicans* cystitis.

Pneumonia

Phagocytosis by the pulmonary macrophage is the major defense mechanism against inhaled bacteria, and this may well be defective in the diabetic patient. Acidosis impairs the bactericidal mechanisms of the lung, and this could be an added factor in the uncontrolled diabetic patient.

Infections with either *S. aureus* or aerobic gram-negative rods can produce severe, necrotizing pneumonias. Antibiotic therapy for 2–4 weeks is usually necessary, and the mortality rate may be as high as 40–50%.

There is no documented evidence that pneumococcal pneumonia is more common in diabetic than nondiabetic hosts; nevertheless, the serious nature of this disease in any patient with chronic disease warrants the use of pneumococcal vaccine in these patients, especially those in the older age groups.

Emphysematous Cholecystitis

Although it is difficult to document an increased incidence of cholecystitis among diabetic patients, a significant percentage of the more severe and fulminating infections involving gas-producing organisms occur among diabetics. In 136 cases of emphysematous cholecystitis, diabetes mellitus was found in 38%. This disease differs from emphysematous pyelonephritis in that *C. perfringens* is isolated in about one-half of the cases. In one series of 109 cases in which gall bladder bile was cultured, 95 were culture positive, with *Clostridia* spp. isolated from 46% and *E. coli* from 33%.

The clinical presentation of this disease resembles that of acute cholecystitis, but the outcome is radically different. Gall bladder perforation and gangrene are frequent, and the mortality rate is 3–10 times higher than in acute cholecystitis. The male-to-female ratio is about 3:1, the reverse of that seen in acute cholecystitis. Diabetic vascular disease is thought to be a factor in the pathogenesis of this unusual syndrome as it is with the other gas-forming infections. The diagnosis is made by finding radiographic evidence of gas in the gall bladder wall. Antibiotic coverage includes the triple combination of ampicillin (or an extended-spectrum penicillin such as piperacillin or mezlocillin), metronidazole, and an aminoglycoside. Imipenem may be useful for alternative antibiotic coverage because it is active against anaerobic bacteria and aerobic gram-negative rods. This drug does not have the nephro- or ototoxicity of the aminoglycosides, an important consideration in the diabetic patient. As with the other gas-forming infections, antibiotic coverage is useful only when used in association with early surgical therapy.

Bacteremia

While bloodstream invasion may result from infection with most bacterial pathogens, certain bacteria have been reported to pose a particular threat to diabetic patients.

Staphylococcal Bacteremia

It has long been suggested that diabetic patients are predisposed to staphylococcal bacteremia, but this has never been established by controlled studies. Diabetes has been recognized as an underlying disease in 8–36% of patients with staphylococcal bacteremia, but studies designed to specifically evaluate the frequency of staphylococcal bacteremia in diabetic and nondiabetic patients have yet to be performed.

Group B Streptococcal Bacteremia

Beta-hemolytic streptococci of the Lancefield group B have emerged as a leading cause of sepsis of neonates and pregnant women. However, in a population-based assessment of invasive disease due to group B streptococci,

Farley and colleagues found that 68% of cases occurred among adult men and nonpregnant women. Of these patients, 31% were diabetic. This striking predilection for diabetic patients confirmed previous reports of an association between these two diseases.

The carriage rate of group B streptococci was studied in a group of diabetic compared to nondiabetic subjects. No differences were found between the two groups. Studies by Baker and coworkers which document inefficient opsonization of group B streptococci in diabetic patients suggest at least one reason for an increased prevalence of these infections among diabetic patients.

The drug of choice for treatment of group B streptococcal infection is penicillin. The organism is less sensitive to penicillin than group A streptococci, and therefore higher doses may be required. In a patient who is allergic to penicillin, sensitivities must be obtained from the laboratory because several of the strains are resistant to clindamycin, erythromycin, and tetracycline. Cephalosporins could be used, but there is a 10% risk of cross-reaction in cases of penicillin allergy.

Gram-Negative Rod Bacteremia

Bacteremia with aerobic gram-negative rods usually results from urinary tract infection, gastrointestinal disease, gallbladder disease, or, in the hospitalized patient, intravenous catheters. In the diabetic patient, synergistic gangrene and gram-negative rod pneumonias are an additional hazard. Several studies document a high prevalence of diabetes among patients with gram-negative rod bacteremias, and the associated mortality rate among these patients was almost twice the overall mortality rate. Infection with gram-negative rods frequently requires the use of an aminoglycoside, and these antibiotics may be especially toxic in diabetic patients with compromised renal function. Dosage of these drugs should be carefully monitored, drug levels should be measured, and renal function tests should be done every day or every other day.

Tuberculosis

Diabetes has been suggested as a potential risk factor for reactivation of latent tuberculosis. A study comparing 5290 cases of tuberculosis to 37,366 controls identified diabetes mellitus as a risk factor for tuberculosis, especially among middle-aged Hispanics. This association awaits further confirmation.

SUMMARY

Despite advances in the knowledge of host defense in diabetes, there are numerous aspects of the complex host–pathogen interrelationship in diabetic subjects that remain unexplained. Why diabetic patients appear to have increased problems with pyogenic organisms such as *S. aureus* and group B streptococci and not with common pathogens such as pneumococci has not been elucidated. Despite numerous unanswered questions, there is clear evidence of increased morbidity and mortality from infectious agents in the diabetic population. A knowledge of these problems coupled with appropriate preventive and therapeutic measures may lessen the impact of these diseases in the diabetic host.

ADDITIONAL READINGS

Brodsky JW, Schneidler C: Diabetic foot infections. *Orthop Clin North Am* 1991;22:473.

Gocke TM: Infections complicating diabetes mellitus. In: Greieco MH, ed. *Infections in the Abnormal Host*. New York: Yorke Medical: 1980;585.

Huang J, Tseng C: Emphysematous pyelonephritis: clinicoradiological classification, management, prognosis and pathogenesis. *Arch Intern Med* 2000;160:797.

Joshi N, Caputo G, Weitekamp MR, et al: Infections in patients with diabetes mellitus. *N Engl J Med* 1999;341:1906.

Zaky DA, Bently DW, Lowy K, et al: Malignant external otitis: A severe form of otitis in diabetic patients. *Am J Med*. 1976;61:298.

For a more detailed discussion of this topic and a bibliography, please see Porte *et al: Ellenberg & Rifkin's Diabetes Mellitus,* 6th ed., Chapter 36.

19 | Relationship of Glycemic Control to Diabetic Complications

Jay S. Skyler

The most important issue facing clinicians who care for patients with diabetes is the extent to which the frequency or severity of chronic complications can be influenced by the degree to which glycemia is controlled. For many years, this was one of the most controversial questions in the field of diabetes. This was in spite of the fact that substantial accumulated evidence demonstrated that the frequency, severity, and progression of retinopathy, nephropathy, and neuropathy are related to the degree of hyperglycemia over time. That evidence came from epidemiologic, clinical, and pathologicl studies in human beings; from studies using animal models of diabetes; and from the elucidation of a number of biochemical mechanisms, putatively involved in the pathogenesis of these complications, that are influenced directly by hyperglycemia. Yet controversy on this subject continued, principally because longitudinal prospective randomized intervention studies were lacking. Now, however, it has been unequivocally established—by randomized controlled clinical trials—that careful control of glycemia can indeed lessen the risk of the microangiopathic and neurologic complications of diabetes. This has been demonstrated for type 1 diabetes in the landmark Diabetes Control and Complications Trial (DCCT), the Stockholm Diabetes Intervention Study (SDIS), and a number of smaller prospective intervention studies. It also has been demonstrated for type 2 diabetes by the United Kingdom Prospective Diabetes Study (UKPDS) and the smaller Kumamoto Study from Japan. Analyses from the Wisconsin Epidemiologic Study of Diabetic Retinopathy (WESDR) (which examined other complications as well as retinopathy) and other epidemiologic studies confirm a strong relationship between glycemia and diabetic microvascular and neurologic complications.

A growing number of epidemiologic studies also have shown that there is a relationship between degree of glycemia and the incidence and prevalence of macrovascular complications of diabetes, that is, cardiovascular disease, cerebrovascular disease, and peripheral vascular disease. Indeed, the relationship between glycemia and macrovascular disease extends throughout the range of glycemia, including nondiabetic individuals. However, the large randomized controlled clinical trials have failed to show convincingly that macrovascular disease is affected by glycemic control.

In this chapter the focus will be on the two large randomized controlled clinical trials: DCCT and UKPDS. However, because of their historical importance, the Brussels study and the WESDR study also are briefly discussed.

EPIDEMIOLOGIC AND OBSERVATIONAL STUDIES

Brussels Study

The Brussels Study, reported in 1978, represented a landmark in the study of the relationship between glycemia and diabetic complications. Between 1947 and 1973, Jean Pirart of Brussels, Belgium, personally followed 4400 patients for up to a quarter-century, and meticulously recorded observations on their glycemic control and the appearance of diabetic complications. He found that the frequency and severity of diabetic retinopathy, nephropathy, and neuropathy were related to both duration of disease and to cumulative glycemic control. Poor control assessed cumulatively over the years was associated with a higher prevalence and incidence of microangiopathy and neuropathy, especially severe retinopathy. However, Pirart did not randomly allocate patients *a priori* to either "good" or "poor" control. Thus, it was impossible to exclude the possibility that patients with mild diabetes achieved "good" control and escaped complications, whereas patients with more severe diabetes achieved "poor" control and suffered more complications. Moreover, the study was conducted in an era prior to the availability of glycated (glycosylated) hemoglobin determinations to assess glycemic control.

Wisconsin Study

The Wisconsin Epidemiologic Study of Diabetic Retinopathy (WESDR) is a population-based study which has reported on the evolution of diabetic complications, particularly retinopathy, among diabetic patients receiving community care in 11 counties in southern Wisconsin. WESDR included a younger-onset cohort—presumably mostly individuals with type 1 diabetes—and an older onset cohort which for many analyses is divided into those treated with insulin and those not treated with insulin, the latter group presumably with type 2 diabetes, while those treated with insulin are a mixed group with most probably having type 2 diabetes.

In all three cohorts (younger-onset, older-onset treated with insulin, older-onset not treated with insulin), at both 4- and 10-years' follow-up, and in the younger-onset cohort at 14-years follow-up, there was a statistically significant relationship between baseline HbA1 and (1) incidence of retinopathy, (2) progression of retinopathy by two or more steps on a 15-step scale, and (3) progression to proliferative retinopathy. The WESDR also found that there was a significant relationship between baseline HbA1 and 4-year incidence of gross proteinuria and microalbuminuria, and 10-year incidence of gross proteinuria. There also was a significant relationship between baseline HbA1 and incidence of lower-extremity amputation both at 10 years and 14 years.

In terms of mortality, in both younger and older cohorts, after controlling for other risk factors and considering underlying cause of death, HbA1 was significantly associated with 10-year mortality from all causes, from diabetes *per se,* and from ischemic heart disease, and in the older-onset cohort, from stroke.

The data from the Wisconsin study demonstrate a strong and consistent relationship between glycemia and the incidence and progression of microvascular (diabetic retinopathy, loss of vision, and nephropathy) and macrovascular (amputation and cardiovascular disease mortality) complications in people with both type 1 diabetes and type 2 diabetes. The relationship was such that the investigators could calculate the effect on risk of development of complications of a 1% increase in baseline glycosylated hemoglobin, as illustrated in Fig. 19-1.

INTERVENTION TRIALS

The major intervention trials exploring the relationship between glycemic control and diabetic complications are the Diabetes Control and Complications Trial (DCCT) and the United Kingdom Prospective Diabetes Study (UKPDS).

The Diabetes Control and Complications Trial (DCCT)

The DCCT examined whether intensive treatment with the goal of maintaining blood glucose concentrations close to the normal range could decrease the frequency and severity of diabetic microvascular and neurologic complications. A total of 1441 subjects with type 1 diabetes were enrolled. Of these,

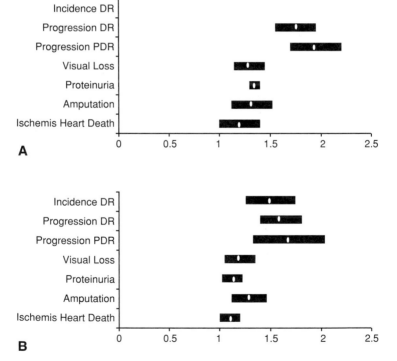

FIG. 19-1   The effect on risk of development of complications of a 1% increase in glycated hemoglobin at baseline in: (Panel A) the younger-onset group, and (Panel B) the older-onset group, in the Wisconsin Study. In each case the points are the estimate and the bars represent the 95% confidence interval of the estimate. DR, diabetic retinopathy; PDR, proliferative diabetic retinopathy. (*Adapted from Klein R:* Diabetes Care *1995; 18:258–268, with permission of the American Diabetes Association.*)

726 subjects were recruited within the first 5 years after developing diabetes (mean duration at entry 2.5 years) and had no evidence of diabetic retinopathy nor of microalbuminuria at baseline (the primary prevention cohort). Another 715 subjects were recruited within the first 15 years (mean duration at entry 8.8 years) after developing diabetes and had mild to moderate background diabetic retinopathy with either normoalbuminuria or microalbuminuria (the secondary intervention cohort). Subjects were randomly assigned either to intensive therapy (IT) or to conventional therapy (CT). They had to be willing to accept random allocation and maintain their treatment assignment for the duration of the study. IT involved insulin administered either by continuous subcutaneous insulin infusion (CSII) with an external insulin pump or by multiple daily insulin injections (MDI) (3 or more injections per day); guided by frequent self-monitoring of blood glucose (SMBG) 3–4 times daily, with additional specified samples including a weekly overnight sample; meticulous attention to diet; and monthly visits to the treating clinic. CT involved no more than 2 daily insulin injections; urine glucose monitoring or SMBG no more than twice daily; periodic diet review; and clinic visits every 2–3 months. Glycemia was assessed by quarterly measurements of A1C. Retinopathy was assessed by seven-field fundus photography every 6 months. Renal function was assessed by annual measurement of creatinine clearance and albumin excretion rate on timed 4-hour urine samples. Neuropathy was evaluated by clinical examination (neurologic history and physical examination), electrophysiology (peripheral nerve conduction velocities), and autonomic nerve testing, at baseline, 5 years, and study end. Subjects were followed for a minimum of 4 years and up to 9 years, with mean follow-up of 6.5 years, and a total of approximately 9300 patient years of observation. Of 1430 subjects alive at the end of the study, 1422 came for evaluation of outcomes. Throughout the study, 98–99% of data was collected.

The IT group achieved a median A1C throughout the study of 7.2% versus 9.1% in the CT group ($p < 0.001$) (Fig. 19-2). The upper limit of normal, and

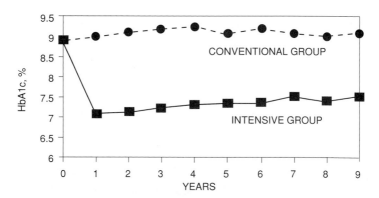

FIG. 19-2 Measurement of glycosylated hemoglobin (A1C) in DCCT patients with type 1 diabetes, assigned to intensive or conventional therapy. Median values are shown. Differences are statistically significant at all time points after baseline ($p < 0.001$). *(Adapted from The Diabetes Control and Complications Trial Research Group:* N Engl J Med *1993; 329:683–689, with permission of the New England Journal of Medicine.)*

treatment target in the intensive group, was 6.05%. Thus, even in the IT group, the goal of normalization of A1C was not achieved, yet the "glycemic separation," or difference between the two groups, was statistically significant throughout the study. The mean blood glucose, obtained on periodic glucose profiles, was 155 mg/dL (8.6 mmol/L) in the intensive group and 231 mg/dL (12.8 mmol/L) in the conventional group, whereas the corresponding value for nondiabetic individuals is 110 mg/dL (6.1 mmol/L).

Outcomes

The DCCT was planned to have the power to detect a 33.5% treatment effect for diabetic retinopathy. The results dramatically exceeded these projections. Cumulative 8.5-year rates of clinically important sustained progression of diabetic retinopathy, that is, three or more steps change on the quantitative grading scale sustained at two consecutive 6-month visits, were: 54.1% with CT and 11.5% with IT in the primary prevention cohort and 49.2% with CT and 17.1% with IT in the secondary intervention cohort (Fig. 19-3). Thus, retinopathy progression was significantly reduced, by 70.3% overall—by 78.5% for those in the primary prevention cohort and by 64.5% for those in the secondary intervention cohort. The analysis over time suggested that these beneficial effects may actually be underestimated, since event rates increased substantially in the CT group over time, while changing relatively little in the IT group.

In the secondary intervention cohort, progression to severe nonproliferative retinopathy or worse was reduced by 60.8%, and progression to neovascularization was reduced by 46.3%. The need for laser photocoagulation, an index of progression to sight-threatening retinopathy, was significantly reduced by 56% in the combined cohorts. In addition, the initial appearance of *any* retinopathy in the primary prevention cohort was significantly reduced by 27%.

The DCCT investigators noted that the slowing in progression of retinopathy was substantial in magnitude, increased with time, was consistent across all outcome measures assessed, and was present across the spectrum of retinopathy severity enrolled in the DCCT.

Diabetic nephropathy was also examined in the DCCT, and again dramatic improvements were observed, yet these effects were not evident in the first 3–5 years of time in the study. The incidence of microalbuminuria, a sign of early renal damage, defined as an albumin excretion rate (AER) greater than 28 μg/min (40 mg/24 hours), was significantly reduced by 39% in the combined cohorts, by 34% in the primary prevention cohort, and by 43% in the secondary intervention cohort (Fig. 19-4). The incidence of sustained microalbuminuria, that is, an AER ≥ 28 μg/min (40 mg/24 hours) on two consecutive annual evaluations was significantly reduced by 60% in the combined cohorts, by 56% in the primary prevention cohort, and by 61% in the secondary intervention cohort. Clinically significant renal damage, termed "clinical-grade albuminuria" and defined as an AER > 208 μg/min (300 mg/24 hours), was significantly reduced by 54% in the combined cohorts. This event was mostly confined to the secondary intervention cohort, where the reduction was by 56% (both for initial and sustained appearance) (Fig. 19-4). In the primary prevention cohort, there was a 44% reduction, but the event rate was so low that this did not achieve statistical significance (Fig. 19-4).

Marked improvement in neuropathic outcomes was also seen, despite the fact that most of these were only assessed at baseline, at 5 years, and at study end. (Autonomic nerve testing was done every 2 years.) Confirmed clinical

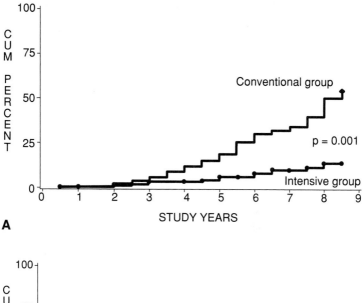

A

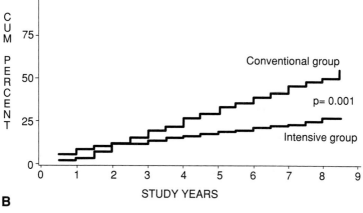

B

FIG. 19-3 Cumulative incidence in the DCCT of a sustained change in retinopathy (defined as a change in fundus photography of at least three grading-scale steps from baseline that was sustained for at least 6 months) in patients with type 1 diabetes receiving intensive or conventional therapy in: (Panel A) the primary prevention cohort, and (Panel B) the secondary intervention cohort. *(Adapted from The Diabetes Control and Complications Trial Research Group:* N Engl J Med *1993; 329:683–689, with permission of the New England Journal of Medicine.)*

neuropathy was defined as a history and/or physical examination consistent with clinical neuropathy, confirmed by either abnormal peripheral nerve conduction or autonomic nerve testing. The incidence of such confirmed clinical neuropathy in the combined cohorts after 5 years of follow-up was 13% with CT and 5% with intensive treatment. This corresponded to a risk reduction of

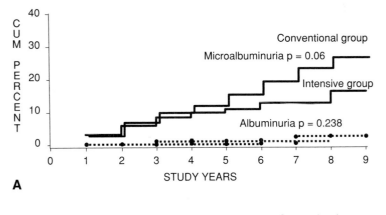

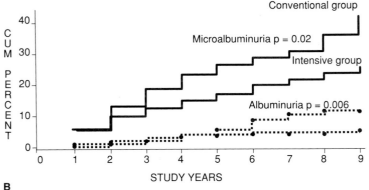

FIG. 19-4   Cumulative incidence in the DCCT of clinical nephropathy (urinary albumin excretion ≥ 300 mg/24 hours) (dashed lines) and microalbuminuria (urinary albumin excretion ≥ 40 mg/24 hours) (solid lines) in patients with type 1 diabetes receiving intensive or conventional therapy in: (Panel A) the primary prevention cohort, and (Panel B) the secondary intervention cohort. (Subjects with baseline urinary albumin excretion ≥ 40 mg/24 hours were excluded from the analysis of development of microalbuminuria.) *(Adapted from The Diabetes Control and Complications Trial Research Group:* N Engl J Med *1993; 329:683–689, with permission of the New England Journal of Medicine.)*

64% in the combined cohorts, by 71% for those in the primary prevention cohort, and by 61% for those in the secondary intervention cohort. The prevalence of abnormal autonomic nerve testing was reduced by 53% in the combined cohorts, by 56% in the primary prevention cohort, and by 51% in the secondary intervention cohort.

These beneficial effects of intensive therapy were not without associated risks. The chief adverse event associated with intensive therapy was a threefold increase in severe hypoglycemia, defined as those episodes requiring assistance of another person to recover. This included a threefold increased risk of coma or seizures consequent to hypoglycemia. Emergency room visits or hospitalization for hypoglycemia was increased 2.3-fold in the intensive therapy group. There were no deaths attributable to hypoglycemia among subjects in either treatment group, although a study patient was involved in a motor vehicle accident leading to the death of a non-study participant. Importantly, 53% of severe hypoglycemic episodes occurred during sleep, and 35% occurred without warning symptoms while awake. It was noted that 23% of severe hypoglycemic episodes were associated with missed meals.

Average weight gain was 10.1 pounds greater in the intensive group. This group had a 33% increased risk of becoming overweight, defined as in excess of 120% of ideal body weight

Macrovascular events, both cardiac and peripheral vascular, were not significantly reduced in the primary analysis, yet the outcome when episodes of cardiac and peripheral vascular events are combined showed a 41% risk reduction, which just missed statistical significance ($p = 0.06$). Certainly, there was no evidence, feared by some critics, of an increased rate of macrovascular events in the IT group.

In subsequent analyses, the DCCT investigators examined the relationship of glycemic exposure to the risk of development and progression of diabetic complications. Within each treatment group, the mean A1C during the trial was the dominant predictor of retinopathy progression (and the other outcome

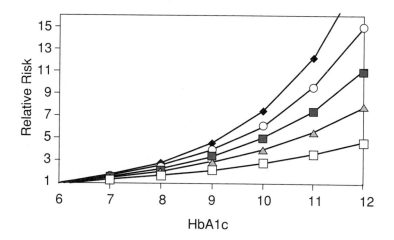

FIG. 19-5 Stylized relative risks for development of various complications as a function of mean A1C during follow-up in the DCCT. For the purposes of illustration, the relative risk of various complications is set to 1 at A1C of 6%. The lines depict a stylized relationship for risk of: (A) sustained progression of retinopathy (◆), (B) progression to clinical nephropathy (urinary albumin excretion ≥ 300 mg/24 hours) (O), (C) progression to severe nonproliferative or proliferative retinopathy (■), (D) progression to clinical neuropathy (▲), and (E) progression to microalbuminuria (urinary albumin excretion ≥ 40 mg/24 hours) (□). *(Adapted from Skyler JS: Diabetic complications. The importance of glucose control. Endocrinol Metab Clin N Am 1996; 25:243 with permission of the Medical Clinics of North America.)*

measures), with a continuous risk gradient without an apparent glycemic threshold. Figure 19-5 shows a stylized model of the kind of continuous risk gradients demonstrated by the DCCT results, in which the event rate for any outcome measure is set to "1" for a A1C of 6%.

At the end of the DCCT, the patients in the CT group were offered IT, the care of all patients was transferred to their own physicians, and most patients were enrolled in a long-term observational study—the Epidemiology of Diabetes Interventions and Complications (EDIC) study. Retinopathy was evaluated by fundus photography and nephropathy on the basis of urine specimens. The difference in the median A1C values between the CT and IT groups during the DCCT (average, 9.1% versus 7.2%) narrowed during follow-up (median during the first 4 years of follow-up, 8.2% versus 7.9%, $p < 0.001$), and by year 6 both groups had A1C levels of 8.1%. Nevertheless, during 8 years of EDIC follow-up, a smaller proportion of patients in the IT group than in the CT group had worsening of retinopathy or nephropathy. The EDIC follow-up demonstrated that the effects of any level of hyperglycemia increase exponentially over time, and continue even after the differences between groups narrow. They suggest that intensive therapy offers a prolonged benefit in terms of reduction in the risk of complications.

Thus, intensive therapy effectively delays the onset and slows the progression of diabetic retinopathy, diabetic nephropathy, and diabetic neuropathy in patients with type 1 diabetes. It results in increased life expectancy and a prolonged period free of complications. There may be beneficial effects on macrovascular disease, but these have yet to be convincingly demonstrated. The risks of intensive therapy are increased frequency of severe hypoglycemia, and greater weight gain. The benefits more than outweigh the risks in most patients with type 1 diabetes. Therefore, intensive therapy, with the goal of achieving glucose levels as close to the nondiabetic range as possible should be employed in most patients with type 1 diabetes.

The United Kingdom Prospective Diabetes Study (UKPDS)

The United Kingdom Prospective Diabetes Study (UKPDS), a randomized, multicenter controlled clinical trial, demonstrated that an intensive treatment policy in type 2 diabetes, with the goal of meticulous glycemic control, could decrease clinical diabetic complications. The UKPDS was conducted in 23 centers. Enrollment was between 1977 and 1991, and end-of-study evaluations were performed during 1997. UKPDS screened 7616 newly diagnosed patients who had the clinical phenotype of type 2 diabetes. Of these, 5102 were recruited and completed a 3-month vigorous dietary treatment run-in period. A total of 4209 individuals with newly diagnosed type 2 diabetes were randomized in the main protocol. At entry, they were 25–63 years of age (median 53 years).

Subjects were randomly assigned either to "intensive treatment policy" (ITP) (originally called "active treatment policy") or "conventional treatment policy" (CTP). ITP aimed at achieving fasting plasma glucose (FPG) of 108 mg/dL, using various pharmacologic agents. CTP attempted control with diet alone, adding pharmacologic therapy when symptoms developed or FPG exceeded 270 mg/dL. The randomization was not balanced, as there were several arms in the intervention group. These included insulin, sulfonylureas, and, among obese patients, metformin. However, it was a bit more complicated than that. In the first 15 (of the 23) centers, the sulfonylureas were either glyburide (glibenclamide) or chlorpropamide, and it was only in these 15 centers that obese patients could receive metformin. In the last 8 centers, the sulfonylureas were either glipizide or chlorpropamide. Moreover, in these 8 centers, the protocol was different and involved early addition of insulin if FPG could not be maintained less than 108 mg/dL. It is important to note that therapeutic additions (in contrast to dose titrations) could not otherwise be made unless FPG reached 270 mg/dL, with the exception of some subgroups to be discussed later.

The primary outcome measures in the UKPDS were three aggregate endpoints: "any diabetes-related endpoint" (sudden death, death from hyperglycemia or hypoglycemia, myocardial infarction, angina, heart failure, stroke, renal failure, amputation, vitreous hemorrhage, retinopathy requiring photocoagulation, blindness in one eye, or cataract extraction); "diabetes-related death" (death from myocardial infarction, stroke, peripheral vascular disease, renal disease, hyperglycemia or hypoglycemia, and sudden death); and all-cause mortality. Multiple other individual clinical and surrogate subclinical endpoints were also assessed. Additional clinical-endpoint aggregates were used: myocardial infarction (fatal and nonfatal) and sudden death; stroke (fatal and nonfatal); amputation or death due to peripheral vascular disease; and microvascular complications (retinopathy requiring photocoagulation, vitreous hemorrhage, and renal failure).

The primary analysis was based on the "intention to treat" principle—comparing subjects assigned ITP with those assigned CTP. Inexplicably, those obese subjects randomized to metformin were not included in the primary "intention to treat" analysis. Since these subjects were randomized with the other subjects, there appears to be no reason for them to have been excluded from analysis. Although the investigators claim they never intended to include them in the primary analysis, that might be inappropriate, since a major aspect of the "intention to treat" principle is to include all subjects randomized.

Secondary analyses of the effects of individual treatments also were reported. In one paper, the results of treatment with glyburide, chlorpropamide, or insulin, among subjects in the first 15 centers, were compared. In a second paper, the results of treatment with metformin, among obese subjects in the first 15 centers, also were considered.

The ITP group achieved a median A1C of 7.0% versus 7.9% in the CTP group ($p < 0.001$) (Fig. 19-6). Initially, with vigorous dietary therapy during the 3-month run-in period, there was a dramatic reduction of A1C, from ~9.0% to 7.08%, accompanied by a weight loss of ~5 kg (~11 lb). Over the first few years, the ITP group achieved A1C levels in the 6% range, while the CTP group maintained A1C levels in the 7% range. Subsequently, there was a progressive deterioration in glycemia over time. Nevertheless, approximately the same degree of glycemic separation was maintained for 6–20 years, with a median duration of follow-up of 11.1 years.

As noted, the primary outcome measures in the UKPDS were three aggregate endpoints: "any diabetes-related endpoint," "diabetes-related death," and all-cause mortality. Of these, only any diabetes-related endpoint was significantly affected: a 12% risk reduction. Other risk reductions are summarized in Table 19-1.

With sulfonylurea therapy, there was no evidence of deleterious effect on myocardial infarction, sudden death, or diabetes-related deaths. With insulin

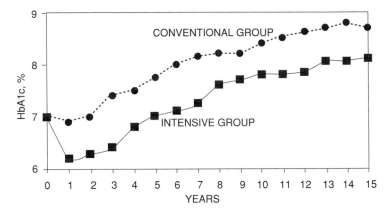

FIG. 19-6 Measurement of glycosylated hemoglobin (A1C) in UKPDS patients with type 2 diabetes, assigned to intensive treatment policy or to conventional treatment policy. Median values are shown. Differences over the course of the study are statistically significant ($p < 0.0001$). *(Adapted from UK Prospective Diabetes Study [UKPDS] Group:* Lancet *1998; 352:837–853, with permission of the Lancet.)*

therapy, there was no evidence of more atheroma-related disease. Thus, there was no evidence in the UKPDS of an adverse effect of insulin or insulin secretagogues on macrovascular disease, thus negating the erroneous (but widely held) belief that increasing insulin availability may in some way be detrimental to patients with diabetes.

In the substudy of metformin monotherapy in overweight patients embedded within the UKPDS, treatment with this insulin sensitizer was associated with significant reductions in any diabetes-related endpoint, diabetes-related deaths, all-cause mortality and myocardial infarction (see Table 19-1). These data suggest a beneficial effect on macrovascular disease endpoints from met-

TABLE 19-1 UKPDS Risk Reduction for Intensive Therapy
(versus Conventional Therapy)

Event	Main analysis	Metformin subgroup
Any diabetes-related endpoint	12%	32%
Diabetes-related deaths	NS	42%
All-cause mortality	NS	36%
Myocardial infarction	16% ($p = 0.52$)	39%
Microvascular endpoints	25%	NS
Fatal myocardial infarction	NS	50%
Laser photocoagulation	29%	NS
Cataract extraction	24%	NS
Retinopathy at 12 years	21%	NS
Microalbuminuria at 12 years	33%	NS

NS = not significant.

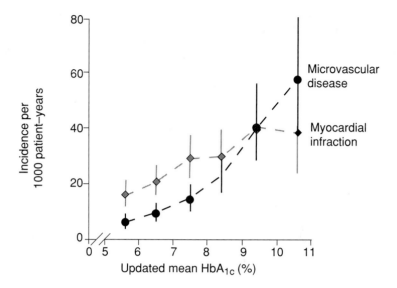

FIG. 19-7 UKPDS epidemiological analysis depicting the relationship between updated mean A1C (glycemic exposure) and incidence of microvascular disease (●) and of myocardial infarction (◆). *(Adapted from Stratton IM, Adler AI, Neil HAW, et al, on behalf of the UK Prospective Diabetes Study Group:* Br Med J *2000; 321:405–412, with permission of the British Medical Journal.)*

formin that may be more substantive than seen with sulfonylureas or insulin. In a subsequent analysis, performed across all UKPDS subjects, the relationship between exposure to glycemia over time and the risk of macrovascular or microvascular complications was determined. The incidence of clinical complications was significantly associated with glycemia. Each 1% reduction in updated mean A1C was associated with reductions in risk of 21% for any endpoint related to diabetes ($p < 0.0001$), 21% for deaths related to diabetes ($p < 0.0001$), 14% for myocardial infarction ($p < 0.0001$), 43% for peripheral vascular disease ($p < 0.0001$), and 37% for microvascular complications ($p < 0.0001$). No threshold of risk was observed for any endpoint. Figure 19-7 depicts the relationship between updated mean A1C (glycemic exposure) and incidence of microvascular disease and of myocardial infarction.

Thus, the UKPDS provides substantial evidence that glycemic control also affects type 2 diabetes. The continuous relationship of glycemic exposure to risk of complications, without a threshold, is similar to that seen in type 1 diabetes in the DCCT. Taken together, these findings suggest that the target for glycemic control should be an A1C level as close to normal as feasible.

CONCLUSIONS

There is no doubt that hyperglycemia is essential to the development of diabetic microangiopathy. Multiple randomized controlled intervention studies have convincingly demonstrated that. Particularly, the overall results reported by the DCCT dramatically exceeded all expectations. The benefits of intensive therapy include a slowing of the onset and progression of diabetic retinopathy, diabetic nephropathy, and diabetic neuropathy. The risks of intensive therapy are increased frequency of severe hypoglycemia, and greater weight gain. These risks clearly must be considered whenever intensive therapy is contemplated. However, although in the DCCT there was a threefold increased risk for hypoglycemia in the intensive therapy group, for coma or seizure this amounts to one episode every 6.25 patient-years of follow-up, versus one episode every 20 patient-years of follow-up in the conventional treatment group. This may very well be tolerable. Thus, the benefits of intensive therapy would seem to be worth the risks in most patients with type 1 diabetes mellitus. Therefore, intensive therapy, with the goal of achieving glucose levels as close to the nondiabetic range as possible, should be the standard management approach in most patients with type 1 diabetes.

The results of the UKPDS suggest that meticulous glycemic control also should be the therapeutic goal in type 2 diabetes. However, since the major morbidity and mortality in type 2 diabetes is a consequence of accelerated atherosclerosis, which is multifactorial in nature and not merely related to prevailing glycemia, attention also needs to be paid to other risk factors, such as blood pressure, lipids, and cigarette smoking.

There also is a general relationship between degree of hyperglycemia as manifested by mean level of A1C (or glycemia-years, analogous to pack-years of smoking) and the frequency, severity, and progression of micro-angiopathy. In both the UKPDS and the DCCT, the relationship between glycemic exposure and risk of development of complications was evident across the range of A1C and without evidence of a threshold. This supports the view that the least glycemic exposure, the less the risk of complications.

ADDITIONAL READINGS

The Diabetes Control and Complications Trial Research Group. The Effect of Intensive Treatment of Diabetes on the Development and Progression of Long-Term Complications in Insulin-Dependent Diabetes Mellitus. *N Engl J Med* 1993;329:683.

The Diabetes Control and Complications Trial/Epidemiology of Diabetes Interventions and Complications Research Group: Sustained effect of intensive treatment of type 1 diabetes mellitus on development and progression of diabetic nephropathy: The Epidemiology of Diabetes Interventions and Complications (EDIC) Study. *JAMA* 2003;290:2159.

Klein R: Hyperglycemia and Microvascular Disease in Diabetes. *Diabetes Care* 1995;18:258.

Skyler JS: Diabetic complications: The importance of glucose control. *Endocrinol Metab Clin North Am* 1996;25:243.

Stratton IM, Adler AI, Neil HAW, et al, on behalf of the UK Prospective Diabetes Study Group: Association of glycaemia with macrovascular and microvascular complications of type 2 diabetes (UKPDS 35): Prospective observational study. *BMJ* 2000; 321:405.

For a more detailed discussion of this topic and a bibliography, please see Porte *et al: Ellenberg & Rifkin's Diabetes Mellitus,* 6th ed., Chapter 54.

20 | Retinopathy and Other Ocular Complications in Diabetes

Ronald Klein

Diabetic retinopathy is an important cause of visual impairment in the United States. While its natural history has been described, its pathogenesis is not fully understood. Available data suggest that good glycemic and blood pressure control reduce the risk of the development and progression of retinopathy. Early identification and treatment of proliferative retinopathy or macular edema with photocoagulation may prevent or delay visual loss. This chapter describes current concepts of the natural history, pathogenesis, diagnosis, and management of retinopathy as well as other ocular complications of diabetes.

DIABETIC RETINOPATHY

Natural History

The earliest clinically apparent manifestations of diabetic retinopathy are classified as *nonproliferative*. During this phase a number of pathophysiologic changes associated with diabetes occur in the microvasculature, including occlusion, dilation, and increased permeability of the small retinal blood vessels. Usually the first changes seen with the ophthalmoscope are retinal microaneurysms, which appear as small (20–200-μm) circular red dots, typically arising in areas of capillary closure. Retinal microaneurysms generally appear 3 years or more after the diagnosis of diabetes. They were found in about 69% and 55% of patients with a 10-year history of type 1 and type 2 diabetes, respectively.

The number of retinal microaneurysms in an eye is an important predictor of progression of diabetic retinopathy. In the Wisconsin Epidemiologic Study of Diabetic Retinopathy (WESDR), there was an increased risk of progression of diabetic retinopathy over a 4-year period when four or more were present at baseline. Furthermore, the increase in the number of microaneurysms and the ratio of their number at the 4-year follow-up to the number at baseline were positively associated with the 10-year incidence of proliferative retinopathy or clinically significant macular edema. Because both hypertension and carotid artery disease are common in older-onset diabetic people, it may be difficult to determine whether diabetes or the presence of other systemic diseases is the cause of the microaneurysms when they are the only sign of retinopathy.

Retinal microaneurysms by themselves are usually not a threat to vision. However, as the disease progresses, retinal blot hemorrhages and hard exudates appear. Blot hemorrhages are round with blurred edges and result from an extravasation of blood from retinal capillaries or microaneurysms into the inner nuclear layer of the retina (Fig. 20-1). They usually disappear within 3–4 months. Retinal hard exudates are variable in size, sharply defined, and yellow; they may be scattered, aggregated, or ringlike in their distributions (Fig. 20-1). Hard exudates may last from months to years The exudates form

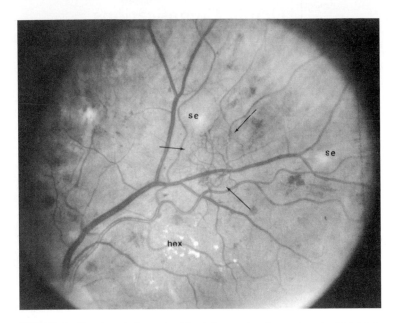

FIG. 20-1 Fundus photograph of the left eye, showing various lesions associated with nonproliferative and proliferative diabetic retinopathy in an area superior and temporal to the macula. Retinal hard exudates (hex) appear as white deposits with sharp margins. Soft exudates (se) or cotton-wool spots appear as grayish white areas with ill-defined edges. Retinal blot hemorrhages appear as spots of varying size with irregular margins and uneven densities. Retinal new vessels (long black arrows) are present.

preferentially in the posterior retina, especially temporal to the macula, and may extend into the macula, reducing visual acuity.

In the more advanced stages of nonproliferative retinopathy, closure of the retinal capillaries and arterioles occurs, causing decreased nutrition to the inner layers of the retina. These changes cause whitish or grayish swellings in the nerve fiber layer of the retina, termed "cotton-wool spots" or "soft exudates," which are infarcts of the nerve fiber layer (Figs. 20-1 and 20-2). They remain only a few weeks to months. After their disappearance, the retina may appear normal on ophthalmoscopy, but nonperfusion of retinal arterioles may be seen on fluorescein angiography. Late in the course of the disease, severe ischemia with thin-sheathed sclerotic (white "threadlike") arterioles may appear. Another manifestation of focal retinal ischemia is the presence of dilated capillaries (intraretinal microvascular abnormalities [IRMAs]) (Fig. 20-2).

Proliferative diabetic retinopathy is characterized by growth of abnormal blood vessels and fibrous tissue from the optic nerve head (Fig. 20-3) or from the inner retinal surface (usually near or from retinal veins) (Fig. 20-4). The vessels, which appear initially as fine tufts on the surface of the retina, subsequently grow into the outermost layer of the vitreous. Initially they consist of fine "naked" vessels, which are permeable to fluorescein. These vessels may hemorrhage into the vitreous. The mesenchymal cells responsible for the development of new blood vessels may also form fibrous tissue. Contraction of fibrovascular tissue may result in traction detachment of the retina.

Diabetic Macular Disease

Increased permeability of retinal capillaries and retinal microaneurysms results in accumulation of extracellular fluid and thickening of the normally compact retinal tissue. The leakage and resulting edema may be distributed around retinal microaneurysms or be diffuse. Focal leakage from retinal microaneurysms or capillaries is usually associated with the deposition of hard exudative material, in either small clumps, rings, or large deposits.

Macular edema appearing as diffuse thickening of the posterior retina is associated with retinal ischemia, and hard exudate is seldom present. Patients with diffuse edema have widespread extravasation of fluorescein dye from the capillaries to the retinal tissue during angiography. In the ETDRS study, clinically significant macular edema was associated with increased risk of loss of vision if left untreated by focal photocoagulation.

Classification

Most clinicians, using direct ophthalmoscopy, will classify retinopathy as either absent or present, or as absent, nonproliferative, or proliferative. More sensitive and reproducible diabetic retinopathy severity scales have been developed (example in Table 20-1). According to data from the ETDRS,

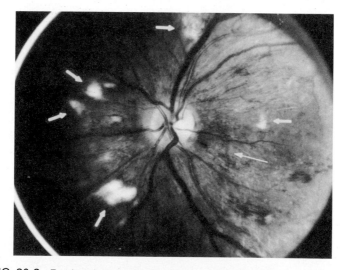

FIG. 20-2   Fundus photograph of the left eye with preproliferative retinopathy. Soft exudates or cotton-wool spots appear as grayish white areas with ill-defined edges (small thick white arrows); intraretinal microvascular abnormalities (thin white arrow), venous dilation, and retinal hemorrhages are present. *(Reprinted with permission from Klein R,: in Olefsky JM, Sherwin R, eds.:* Diabetes Mellitus: Management and Complications, *Churchill Livingstone 1985; 101.)*

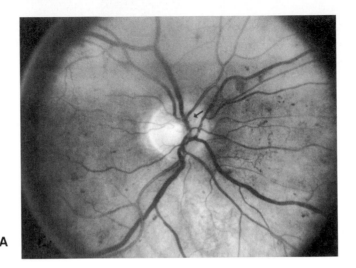

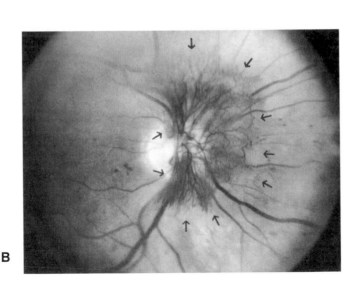

FIG. 20-3 Fundus photograph of the right eye. This sequence of photographs demonstrates progression from early proliferative retinopathy manifested initially as fine tufts of retinal new vessels on the optic disk (A, dated 2/75) (black arrows). There was further growth of retinal new vessels (B, dated 4/76) (black arrows). *(Reprinted with permission from Klein R,: in Olefsky JM, Sherwin R, eds.:* Diabetes Mellitus: Management and Complications, *Churchill Livingstone 1985; 101.)*

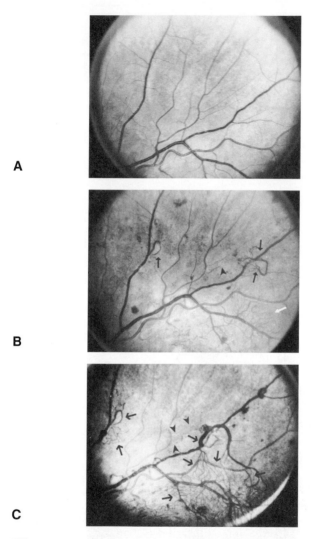

FIG. 20-4 Fundus photograph of the left eye showing progression from non-proliferative to proliferative diabetic retinopathy in an area superior and temporal to the macula. (A) When the patient was seen in 11/72 she was 25 years old and had a 14-year history of type 1 diabetic retinopathy. A few dilated capillaries and retinal microaneurysms are present here, and cotton-wool spots and blot hemorrhages were present in the macular area (not in photograph). The visual acuity was 20/15. (B) In 3/76, flat retinal new vessels (small black arrows) are present. An abrupt termination of a branch arteriole (black arrowhead), intraretinal microvascular abnormalities (white arrow), and venous beading are present. (C) By 10/76, there is an increase in the size of the retinal new vessels (black arrows) and the "feeder" vessel from the vein. The small arterioles above the vein are sheathed and appear white (small black arrowheads).

(continued)

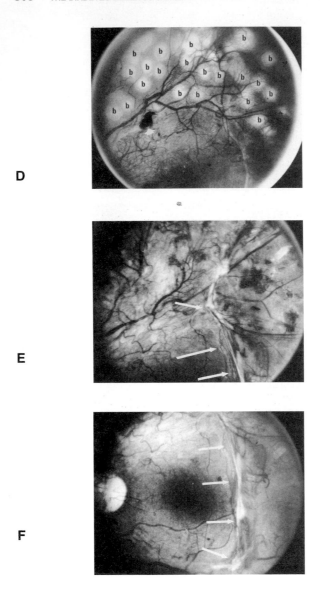

FIG. 20-4 *(continued)* (D) This picture was taken in 2/77, 2 hours after laser treatment; the photocoagulation burns appear white (b). A small preretinal hemorrhage, appearing black, is present (white arrowhead). (E, F) In 6/77 the visual acuity was 20/30. An area of fibrovascular proliferation with traction on the retina superior and temporal to the macula was present (white arrows). (G, H) On 7/15/77 further elevation of fibroproliferative tissue (white arrows) led to increased traction with detachment (det) of the area above the macula. The visual acuity had dropped to 20/70. (I) The macular area became detached,

G

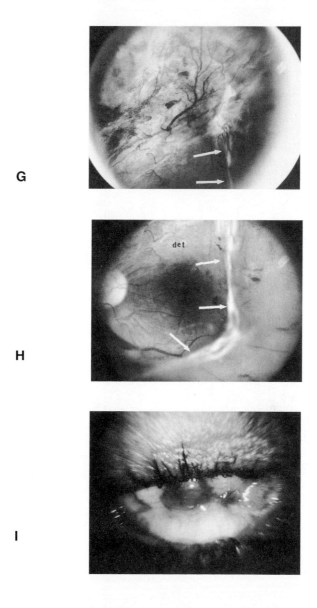

H

I

and she underwent a vitrectomy and scleral buckle on 7/28/77. Corneal edema and blood in the anterior chamber developed after surgery. Later the eye became phthisical, and she had no light perception when this photograph was taken in 10/78. Her other eye had been enucleated in 4/77 as a result of pain from rubeotic glaucoma, secondary to traction retinal detachment and vitreous hemorrhage. *(Courtesy of Dr. G. Bresnick, University of Wisconsin. Reprinted with permission from Klein R,: in Olefsky JM, Sherwin R, eds.:* Diabetes Mellitus: Management and Complications, *Churchill Livingstone 1985; 101.)*

TABLE 20-1 Modified Early Treatment Diabetic Retinopathy Severity Scale

Retinopathy	Level	Detailed descriptor
None	Level 10	No retinopathy
Nonproliferative	Level 21	Microaneurysms (Ma) only or retinal hemorrhages (H) or soft exudates (Se) in the absence of microaneurysms
	Level 31	Microaneurysms plus one or more of the following: Venous loops ≥ 31 μm; questionable Se, intraretinal microvascular abnormalities (IRMA), or venous beading; and retinal hemorrhage
	Level 37	Microaneurysms plus one or more of the following: hard exudate (hex) and Se
	Level 43	Microaneurysms plus one or more of the following: H/Ma ≥ standard photo (SP) #1 in 4–5 fields; H/Ma ≥ SP #2A in 1 field; and IRMA in 1–3 fields
	Level 47	Microaneurysms plus one or more of the following: Both IRMA and H/Ma characteristics from level 43; IRMA in 4–5 fields; H/Ma ≥ SP #2A in 2–3 fields; and venous beading in 1 field
Preproliferative	Level 53	Microaneurysms plus one or more of the following: Any 2–3 of level 47 characteristics; H/Ma ≥ SP #2A in 4–5 fields; IRMA ≥ SP #8A; venous beading in 2 or more fields
Proliferative without DRS high-risk characteristics for severe visual loss (DRS-HRC)	Level 60	Fibrous proliferations only
	Level 61	No evidence of levels 60 or 65 but scars of photocoagulation either in "scatter" or confluent patches, presumably directed at new vessels
	Level 65	Proliferative diabetic retinopathy less than Diabetic Retinopathy Study high-risk characteristics (DRS-HRC). Lesions as follows: New vessels elsewhere (NVE); new vessels on or within 1 disk diameter (NVD) of the disk graded less than SP #10A; and preretinal (PRH) or vitreous hemorrhage (VH) < disk area (DA)
Proliferative with DRS-HRC	Level 71	DRS-HRC, lesions as follows: Vh and/or PRH ≥ 1 DA; NVE ≥ one-half DA with VH and/or PRH; NVD < SP #10a with VH and/or PRH; and NVD ≥ SP #10A
	Level 75	Advanced PDR, lesions as follows: NVD ≥ SP #10A with VH and/or PRH
Proliferative with DRS-HRC and loss of vision	Level 85	End stage PDR, lesions as follows: Macula obscured by VH and/or PRH; retinal detachment at center of macula; phthisis bulbi; and enucleation secondary to complications of diabetic retinopathy

Source: Klein R, Klein BEK, Moss SE, et al: *Arch Ophthalmol* 1994; 112:1217.

each stepwise increase in the severity level of retinopathy was associated with an increased risk of progression to proliferative retinopathy 4 years later. In addition, in the WESDR, increasing severity of retinopathy as measured by the ETDRS severity scale at baseline was associated with increased risk of loss of vision over 10 years. A new international clinical classification system for diabetic retinopathy and diabetic macular edema has been proposed for use by ophthalmologists and other eye care providers, endocrinologists, diabetologists, and primary care physicians who care for patients with diabetes. Dilated ophthalmoscopy is required to use the scales. The retinopathy severity scale has five steps: (1) no apparent retinopathy, (2) mild nonproliferative diabetic retinopathy (microaneurysms only), (3) moderate nonproliferative diabetic retinopathy (more than just microaneurysms but less than severe nonproliferative diabetic retinopathy), (4) severe nonproliferative diabetic retinopathy (any of the following: more than 20 intraretinal blot hemorrhages in each of 4 quadrants; definite venous beading in 2+ quadrants; prominent intraretinal microvascular abnormalities in 1+ quadrant, and no signs of proliferative retinopathy), and (5) proliferative diabetic retinopathy (one or more of the following: neovascularization, vitreous/preretinal hemorrhage).

Microaneurysm counts from the grading of fundus photographs may provide a more sensitive measure of retinopathy severity in the earlier stages of disease. A number of studies have demonstrated that grading of stereoscopic fundus photographs is more sensitive than ophthalmoscopy in detecting retinopathy. Computer-assisted grading of digitized images has also been used to determine the presence and severity of diabetic retinopathy.

Pathogenesis

The exact pathogenesis of diabetic retinopathy is unknown. It is assumed that retinopathy is a consequence of hyperglycemia. This is supported by (1) the strong association of retinopathy with increasing duration of disease; (2) the finding of retinopathy in secondary diabetes; (3) the production of retinopathy in experimental diabetes in animal models; and (4) the results of the epidemiologic studies and clinical trials that show a strong relationship of glycemia to the incidence and progression of retinopathy. However, the actual mechanism by which high blood glucose levels lead to retinopathy is not known.

Epidemiology

Knowledge of the prevalence and incidence of diabetic retinopathy and various demographic, genetic, systemic, and intrinsic ocular factors associated with retinopathy is of great importance in (1) efforts to prevent or modify the course of retinopathy, (2) characterization of the high-risk patient, and (3) estimation of health service needs. A number of epidemiologic studies have provided data about the natural history of diabetic retinopathy and its risk factors. Data from one such study, the WESDR, a large geographically defined population of both type 1 and type 2 diabetic persons examined in 1980–1982, in 1984–1986, and again in 1990–1992, and type 1 diabetic persons in 1995–1996, are presented to provide information on the incidence and prevalence of retinopathy.

Prevalence of Retinopathy

In the baseline WESDR examination conducted in 1980–1982, the highest frequencies of any retinopathy (71%) and of proliferative retinopathy (23%) were found in the younger-onset group, diagnosed prior to age 30 years and taking insulin (n = 996), whereas the lowest frequencies of any retinopathy (39%) and proliferative retinopathy (3%) were present in the older-onset group not taking insulin who were diagnosed with diabetes at or after 30 years of age (n = 692). While the proportions of proliferative retinopathy and macular edema were highest in the WESDR younger-onset group, the largest number of people with proliferative retinopathy or macular edema had older-onset diabetes. Based on the WESDR data, it is estimated that in 1980–1982, approximately 700,000 people in the United States with diabetes had proliferative retinopathy, 130,000 of whom had Diabetic Retinopathy Study (DRS) high-risk characteristics for severe visual loss, and 325,000 of whom had clinically significant macular edema.

Data were recently published based on pooled analysis from two population-based studies (the WESDR and the New Jersey 725 Study) of persons with type 1 diabetes and eight population-based studies including the WESDR limited to persons 40 years of age and older with type 2 diabetes. In those with type 1 diabetes diagnosed prior to age 30 years (n = 889,000 in United States), 86% (n = 767,000) were estimated to have prevalent retinopathy with 42% (n = 376,000) having vision-threatening retinopathy (pre-proliferative or proliferative retinopathy or macular edema). In those with type 2 diabetes, the estimated prevalence of retinopathy was higher in the WESDR than in the seven other studies performed at least 10 or more years after the WESDR. The estimated crude prevalence of any retinopathy was 40% and the crude prevalence of vision-threatening retinopathy was 8%. It was estimated that in the United States in persons 40 years of age or older with type 2 diabetes, 4 million had retinopathy and 900,000 had vision-threatening retinopathy.

Incidence of Diabetic Retinopathy

The highest incidence and progression of retinopathy over the 10 years of the WESDR study were found in the younger-onset group, whereas the lowest incidence and progression were found in the older-onset group not taking insulin. In the younger-onset group, 89.3% without retinopathy and 29.8% without proliferative retinopathy at baseline developed retinopathy and proliferative retinopathy, respectively, by the time of the 10-year follow-up. The 10-year incidence of proliferative retinopathy was 10% in the older-onset group not taking insulin at baseline. The estimates of incident cases of proliferative retinopathy in the 10-year period are higher in the group with older onset than in the group with younger onset (387 versus 226). These data emphasize the need for timely referral and appropriate ophthalmologic care for older patients with type 2 diabetes (T2DM).

Despite marked changes in the management of type 1 diabetes (T1DM) over the 10-year follow-up period of the WESDR, there were few significant differences in the estimated annual incidence of proliferative diabetic retinopathy over the first 4 years of the study compared to the last 6 years of the study (Fig. 20-5). Based on the WESDR data, it was estimated that over the 10-year period, of the 5,800,000 Americans with known diabetes in 1980, 915,000 would have developed proliferative retinopathy, and 320,000 would have developed proliferative retinopathy with DRS high-risk characteristics.

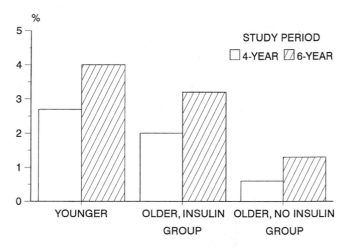

FIG. 20-5   Estimated annual incidence of proliferative retinopathy in the first 4 years and next 6 years in the younger-onset group taking insulin and the older-onset groups taking and not taking insulin in the Wisconsin Epidemiologic Study of Diabetic Retinopathy.

Risk Factors for Diabetic Retinopathy

Demographic Characteristics

While few differences in the prevalence or incidence of diabetes have been observed based on gender, recent data suggest differences among different racial and ethnic groups. Data from studies in Pima Indians and Oklahoma Indians with T2DM showed a higher risk of developing proliferative retinopathy than found in the non-Hispanic whites with T2DM in the WESDR. According to results of the Third National Health and Nutrition Examination Survey (NHANES III), the risk of retinopathy in non-Hispanic whites was comparable to that in non-Hispanic blacks and half that in Mexican-Americans. The prevalence of retinopathy in second-generation diabetic Japanese-Americans (12%) was significantly lower than that reported among patients in the diabetes clinic at Tokyo University Hospital (47–49%) and in diabetic white men not taking insulin reported in the WESDR (36%). Geographic and unmeasured factors may also result in variations within similar ethnic groups.

It is rare to find signs of diabetic retinopathy in children who are less than 10 years of age, regardless of the duration of T1DM. After this age, the frequency and severity of retinopathy begins to increase. Age has less of an effect on the prevalence or incidence of diabetic retinopathy in older-onset patients. In the WESDR, few people 75 years of age or older with T2DM developed proliferative retinopathy over the 10 years of follow-up.

Genetic Factors

The relationships of specific genetic factors to increased susceptibility to diabetic retinopathy are not clear. Support for a genetic relationship has come from studies that have shown similar severity and onset of retinopathy among concordant identical twins. In addition, an increased risk of severe retinopathy (odds ratio 3.1, 95% CI 1.2–7.8) has been observed among relatives of retinopathy-positive versus retinopathy-negative subjects with T1DM in the Diabetes Control and Complications Trial (DCCT).

Some studies have found relationships between retinopathy and various HLA antigens, while others have not. The reasons why specific HLA-DR antigens would increase the risk of developing more severe retinopathy are not apparent. Study of specific genetic factors associated with the pathogenesis of retinopathy, such as glycosylation, aldose reductase activity, collagen formation, endothelial dysfunction, inflammation, and platelet adhesiveness and aggregation may yield a better understanding of the possible causal relationships between genetic factors and diabetic retinopathy.

Duration of Diabetes

The frequency and severity of diabetic retinopathy, proliferative retinopathy, and macular edema increase with increasing duration of diabetes. For instance, the prevalence of retinopathy 3–4 years after diagnosis of diabetes in the WESDR younger-onset group with T1DM was 14.5% in males and 24% in females, and in all cases it was mild (Fig. 20-6). However, in persons with diabetes for 19–20 years, 50% of males and 33% of females had proliferative retinopathy. Early after the diagnosis of diabetes, retinopathy was more frequent in the older-onset group compared with the younger-onset group. In the first 3 years after diagnosis of diabetes, 23% of the older-onset group not taking insulin had retinopathy, and 2% had proliferative retinopathy (Fig. 20-7). However, after 20 years of diabetes, fewer older-onset persons not taking insulin had retinopathy (60% versus 99%) or proliferative retinopathy (5% versus 53%) than younger-onset people.

Data from the WESDR and other studies suggest that prior to puberty or within 5 years of diagnosis, younger-onset persons with T1DM do not need an ophthalmoscopic examination to detect proliferative retinopathy or macular edema.

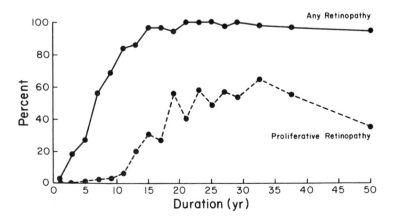

FIG. 20-6   The frequency of retinopathy or proliferative retinopathy by duration of diabetes in years in 995 insulin-taking persons diagnosed as having diabetes before 30 years of age who participated in the Wisconsin Epidemiologic Study of Diabetic Retinopathy. *(Reprinted with permission from Klein R, Klein BEK, Moss SE, et al: Arch Opthalmol 1984; 102:520.)*

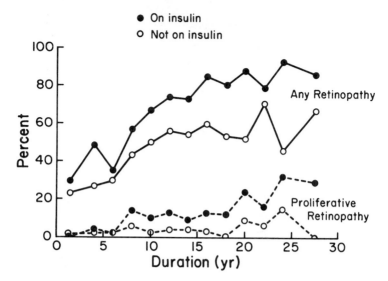

FIG. 20-7   The frequency of retinopathy or proliferative retinopathy by duration of diabetes in years in 673 insulin-taking and 697 non-insulin-taking persons diagnosed as having diabetes after 29 years of age who participated in the Wisconsin Epidemiologic Study of Diabetic Retinopathy. *(Reprinted with permission from Klein R, Klein BEK, Moss SE, et al:* Arch Opthalmol *1984; 102:520.)*

Age at Diagnosis

Age at diagnosis was not related to incidence or progression of diabetic retinopathy in any of the diabetes groups followed in the WESDR. However, after controlling for other risk factors in a cohort with T2DM in Rochester, Minnesota, the development of retinopathy was associated with younger age at diagnosis.

Control of Hyperglycemia

Review of the existing experimental literature using animal models leaves little doubt as to the strong relationship between good glycemic control and less retinopathy. Likewise, epidemiologic studies have consistently demonstrated an association between good glycemic control and the incidence and progression of diabetic retinopathy. The WESDR data demonstrated that lower blood sugar at any stage of retinopathy prior to the proliferative phase and at any duration of diabetes was associated with lower incidence and progression of retinopathy.

Results of the DCCT and UKPDS, randomized trials of metabolic control, showed that intensive glycemic control reduces the risk of retinopathy progression, incidence of macular edema, and the need for panretinal photocoagulation compared to conventional insulin treatment (Table 20-2 and Fig. 20-8).

Blood Pressure

Because high blood pressure *per se* can cause many of the lesions associated with diabetic retinopathy (e.g., cotton-wool spots, retinal hemorrhages, and

TABLE 20-2 Development and Progression of Long-Term Complications of Diabetes in the Study Cohorts and Reduction in Risk with Intensive as Compared with Conventional Therapy*

Complications	Primary prevention			Secondary intervention			Both cohorts†
	Conventional therapy (rate/100 patient-years)	Intensive therapy (rate/100 patient-years)	Risk reduction, % (95% CI)	Conventional therapy (rate/100 patient-years)	Intensive therapy (rate/100 patient-years)	Risk reduction, % (95% CI)	Risk reduction, % (95% CI)
≥ 3-Step sustained retinopathy	4.7	1.2	76 (62–85)‡	7.8	3.7	54 (39–66)‡	63 (52–71)‡
Macular edema§	—	—	—	3.0	2.0	23 (213–48)	26 (28–50)
Severe nonproliferative or proliferative retinopathy§	—	—	—	2.4	1.1	47 (14–67)¶	47 (15–67)¶
Laser Treatment¶ #	—	—	—	2.3	0.9	56 (26–74)‡	51 (21–70)¶

* Rates shown are absolute rates of the development and progression of complications per 100 patient-years. Risk reductions represent the comparison of intensive with conventional treatment, expressed as a percentage and calculated from the proportional-hazards model with adjustment for baseline values as noted, except in the case of neuropathy. CI denotes confidence interval.

† Stratified according to the primary-prevention and secondary-prevention cohorts.

‡ $p \leq 0.002$ by the two-tailed rank-sum test.

§ Too few events occurred in the primary-prevention cohort to allow meaningful analysis of this variable.

¶ $p < 0.04$ by the two-tailed rank-sum test.

# Denotes the first episode of laser therapy for macular edema of proliferative retinopathy.

Source: The DCCT Research Group: N Engl J Med 1993; 329:977.

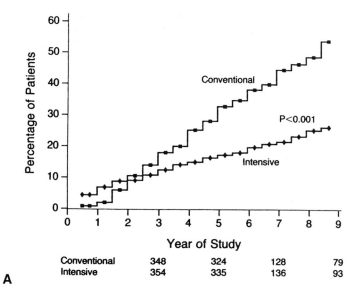

Conventional	348	324	128	79
Intensive	354	335	136	93

A

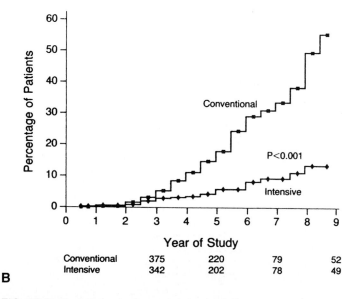

Conventional	375	220	79	52
Intensive	342	202	78	49

B

FIG. 20-8 Cumulative incidence of a sustained change in retinopathy in patients with T1DM receiving intensive or conventional therapy in (A) the primary prevention and (B) the secondary intervention arms of the Diabetes Control and Complications Trial. *(Reprinted with permission from the DCCT Research Group:* N Engl J Med *1993; 329:977.)*

microaneurysms), it is not unexpected that a positive association between blood pressure and severity of retinopathy and macular edema has been reported. Findings from controlled studies strongly support tight blood pressure control in people with T2DM as a means of preventing visual loss due to the progression of diabetic retinopathy.

Proteinuria and Diabetic Nephropathy

The prevalence and severity of diabetic retinopathy is associated with the presence of diabetic nephropathy, as manifest by microalbuminuria or gross proteinuria. WESDR data suggest that gross proteinuria is a risk indicator for proliferative retinopathy, and these patients might benefit from having more frequent ophthalmologic evaluation. Patients on dialysis or following renal transplantation usually experience a stabilization of visual function.

Serum Lipids

Information regarding the relationship of serum lipids to diabetic retinopathy is inconsistent. In the WESDR, higher total serum cholesterol was associated with higher prevalence of retinal hard exudates in patients using insulin. Randomized controlled clinical trials to investigate whether lipid lowering agents, such as the HMG CoA reductase inhibitors, prevent the incidence and progression of retinopathy and visual loss are underway.

Social History and Socioeconomic Status

The results of studies examining the relationship between smoking and alcohol consumption or socioeconomic status and diabetic retinopthy have been inconsistent.

Body Mass (Obesity)

The severity of retinopathy has been reported to be inversely correlated with body mass index in diabetic individuals not using insulin. This finding is compatible with the concept that obese, older-onset, non-insulin-taking patients have a milder form of the disease.

Pregnancy

Among women with diabetes, development of proliferative retinopathy or its progression is increased during pregnacy.

Current management recommendations include evaluation by an ophthalmologist of all type 1 diabetic patients considering pregnancy or those who have become pregnant. Those women with no or mild retinopathy, although at low risk of progression, should be followed by an ophthalmologist and seen more frequently than usual during gestation (perhaps every 2–3 months), especially if they develop complications (e.g., toxemia or progression of retinopathy). Because panretinal photocoagulation has been shown to cause significant regression of retinal new blood vessels and prevent serious reduction of vision, women with severe preproliferative or proliferative retinopathy should be referred for possible treatment.

Retinopathy, Comorbidity, and Mortality

Severe retinopathy is associated with cardiovascular disease risk factors such as increased fibrinogen, hyperglycemia, hypertension, and increased platelet aggregation. This probably explains in part why patients with diabetic retinopathy have a higher prevalence of coronary disease. In the WESDR, those with proliferative retinopathy were at increased risk of developing a heart attack, stroke, diabetic nephropathy, and amputation (Table 20-3). Aspirin usage does not prevent the incidence or progression of retinopathy. The risk of death also increases with increasing severity of retinopathy (Figs. 20-9 and 20-10), which is consistent with the association between severe retinopathy and incidences of cardiovascular disease and diabetic nephropathy. These data suggest that diabetic patients with retinopathy should be under close medical surveillance for diagnosis and treatment of cardiovascular disease.

Medical Therapy

Epidemiologic studies, the DCCT (for T1DM), and the UKPDS (for T2DM) have clearly demonstrated a significant reduction in the incidence and progression of diabetic retinopathy by reduction of hyperglycemia. The results of the UKPDS and from EUCLID clinical trials suggest that control of blood pressure may also reduce the progression of diabetic retinopathy, independent of glycemic control. Other drugs, however (e.g., anticoagulants; aldose-reductase inhibitors; and aspirin), have not prevented or decreased progression of diabetic retinopathy.

Surgical Therapy

Photocoagulation

The beneficial effects of photocoagulation were documented in the Diabetic Retinopathy Study (DRS) in 1972. A total of 1758 patients with proliferative retinopathy in at least one eye or severe nonproliferative or proliferative retinopathy in both eyes were randomly assigned to photocoagulation or conservative follow-up. The risk of severe visual loss in treated eyes was found to be less than one-half that in untreated control eyes (Fig. 20-11). The researchers concluded that in eyes with high-risk retinopathy characteristics, the risk of severe visual loss without treatment was 25% at 2 years, being reduced to 12% with treatment. The results of the ETDRS suggested that earlier panretinal treatment of eyes with high-risk proliferative retinopathy may result in a 90% decrease in the risk of severe loss of vision.

In eyes with early or moderate severe nonproliferative retinopathy (Levels 21–47; see Table 20-1), there is little or no reason to treat with panretinal photocoagulation because of the relatively low risk of progression to severe visual loss and the risk of complications associated with such treatment. However, in people in whom both eyes have bilateral severe preproliferative retinopathy or proliferative retinopathy without DRS high-risk complications (Level 53 or 65; see Table 20-1), the data suggest there may be some benefit in prompt initiation of panretinal photocoagulation in at least one eye. Photocoagulation may also improve macular edema.

Vitrectomy

Vitrectomy may be recommended if there has been no clearing of the vitreous hemorrhage after a few months in people with T1DM or after 6–12 months in people with T2DM. The procedure may be performed sooner if there is ultrasound or other evidence of a tractional retinal detachment threatening or involving the macular area. The major objectives of vitreous surgery

TABLE 20-3 Relative Risk for the Prevalence and Four-Year Incidence of Myocardial Infarction, Stroke, and Amputation of the Lower Extremities Associated with the Presence of Proliferative Retinopathy, Corrected for Age in the Wisconsin Epidemiologic Study of Diabetic Retinopathy

	Myocardial infarction		Stroke		Amputation of lower extremity	
	RR	95% CI	RR	95% CI	RR	95% CI
Younger-onset group						
Prevalence	3.5	1.5–7.9	2.6	0.7–9.7	7.1	2.6–19.7
Incidence	4.5	1.3–15.4	1.6	0.4–5.7	6.0	2.1–16.9
Older-onset group taking insulin						
Prevalence	0.8	0.4–1.4	1.2	0.6–2.4	4.2	2.3–7.9
Incidence	1.2	0.5–3.4	2.9	1.2–6.8	3.4	0.9–13.2
Older-onset group not taking insulin						
Prevalence	0.3	0–2.4	2.9	0.9–9.4	5.2	0.6–45.0
Incidence	1.5	0.2–12.5	6.0	1.1–32.6	7.0	0.8–64.4

CI, confidence interval; RR, relative risk.

Source: Reprinted with permission from Klein R, Klein BEK, Moss SE: *Diabetes Care* 1992; 15:1875.

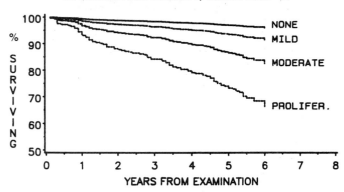

FIG. 20-9 Age- and sex-adjusted survival curves by diabetic retinopathy status at baseline examination in younger-onset persons participating in the Wisconsin Epidemiologic Study of Diabetic Retinopathy. *(Reprinted with permission from Klein R, Moss SE, Klein BEK, et al:* Arch Internal Med *1989; 149:266.)*

are to clear the optical axis of opacities and to release mechanical traction on the retina. In patient series, visual improvement following vitrectomy has been reported in 50–66% of operated eyes. There is a significant benefit in terms of restoring visual acuity by early vitrectomy (shortly after vitreous hemorrhage development) in those with T1DM.

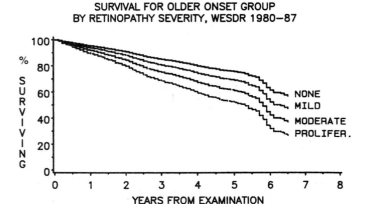

FIG. 20-10 Age- and sex-adjusted survival curves by diabetic retinopathy status at baseline examination in older-onset persons participating in the Wisconsin Epidemiologic Study of Diabetic Retinopathy. *(Reprinted with permission from Klein R, Moss SE, Klein BEK, et al:* Arch Internal Med *1989; 149:266.)*

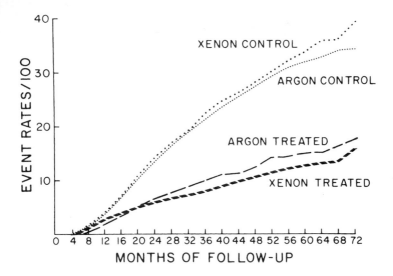

FIG. 20-11   Cumulative rates of severe visual loss (5/200 or less) in the Diabetic Retinopathy Study Group. *(Reprinted with permission from Diabetic Retinopathy Study Group:* Ophthalmology *1981: 88:583.)*

VISUAL IMPAIRMENT

Diabetes is an important cause of impaired vision. It accounts for an estimated 5000 new cases of legal blindness (visual acuity of 20/200 or worse in the better eye) in the United States each year. Blindness is 29 times more common in diabetic than in nondiabetic persons. Approximately 8% of people who were legally blind reported diabetes as the etiology of their blindness, and it is estimated that in the United States, more than 12% of new cases of blindness are attributable to diabetes.

More recent data from eight population-based studies (not including the WESDR) of persons 40 years of age or older that examined subjects over the past 20 years found diabetic retinopathy as a primary cause of legal blindness (best corrected visual acuity of poorer than 20/200 in the better eye) in 5.4% of whites, 7.3% of blacks, and 14.3% of Hispanics and visual impairment (best corrected visual acuity of poorer than 20/40 in the better eye) in 4.9% of whites, 14.5% of blacks, and 13.0% of Hispanics.

The prevalence of blindness in diabetic persons is related to current age and duration of diabetes in both younger- and older-onset groups. Eyes with more severe retinopathy are at higher risk of blindness. Other risk factors for impaired vision include age, duration of diabetes, severity of retinopathy, higher glycosylated hemoglobin, and gross proteinuria.

Diabetic patients as a group have poorer color vision than nondiabetic persons. With progression of maculopathy, further deterioration in color vision is found.

A frequent cause for sudden change in vision, especially in children and adolescents with diabetes, is related to a change in the refractive medium. In adults this may be one of the presenting symptoms at the time of diagnosis.

Reversible osmotic swelling of the lens due to rapid alterations in blood sugar has been postulated to be responsible for this phenomenon. With better control of the blood sugar, the refraction and acuity return to previous levels.

Cataracts may also often cause a decrease in vision in diabetic individuals. In the WESDR, multivariate analyses indicated that age and duration of diabetes were the most important risk factors for cataract presence. Severity of diabetic retinopathy was associated with a small but significant further increase in risk. Glycemic control in persons with T2DM may reduce the progression of cataracts. In the UKPDS, there was a 34% reduction in cataract extraction among patients in the intensive glycemic control group compared to the conventional treatment group.

Most reports also describe a higher prevalence of ocular hypertension and open-angle glaucoma in diabetic than in nondiabetic persons. Additionally, patients with open-angle glaucoma or ocular hypertension are reported to have a higher prevalence of diabetes. Because diabetic patients may be at increased risk of glaucoma, measurement of the intraocular pressure and ophthalmoscopic examination for changes of the cup-to-disk configuration and size is an important part of the ophthalmologic management of these patients. In patients who develop glaucoma, medical intervention is usually successful in preventing or retarding further visual loss.

OPHTHALMOLOGIC MANAGEMENT

Because it is possible in many cases to prevent visual loss with photocoagulation, and because proliferative retinopathy and clinically significant macular edema may be present before they affect vision, it is important to identify diabetic persons in need of ophthalmologic evaluation. The need for careful examination by ophthalmologists has been documented by Sussman and coworkers. They found that internists, diabetologists, and senior medical residents correctly diagnosed the presence of proliferative retinopathy in only 49% of patients they examined (under optimal conditions), whereas ophthalmologists and retinal specialists correctly diagnosed its presence in 96% of cases.

Guidelines have been developed and implemented that suggest that all diabetic patients be informed of the possible ocular complications and of the role of the ophthalmologist in the management (detection and prevention) of these complications (Table 20-4). Patients who are in poor glycemic control, are pregnant, or who have albuminuria should especially be examined by an ophthalmologist, as they may be at higher risk for progression of retinopathy.

REHABILITATION

Visual impairment in diabetes may range from minimal changes in color vision to total blindness and may include periods of rapid or slow progression with fluctuations in vision due to recurrent vitreous hemorrhage or macular edema. Visually impaired insulin-taking diabetic patients have unique problems with the management of their disease, including identifying the insulin type, determining the amount of insulin in the vial, measuring the dose, locating injection sites, monitoring glucose levels using blood test strips, and foot care. A number of low-vision aids, devices for insulin administration, and aids in glucose monitoring are available for the visually impaired diabetic patient. Depending on the degree of visual impairment, supportive rehabilitation services, including low-vision clinics, state vocational rehabilitation centers, and

TABLE 20-4 Recommendations for Eye Care for Diabetic Patients

Primary-care physician informs patient at time of diagnosis of diabetes that:
  Ocular complications are associated with diabetes and may threaten
    sight.
  Glycemic and blood pressure control reduces risk of developing
    retinopathy.
  Timely detection and treatment of retinopathy may reduce the risk of
    decreased vision.
Referral to an eye doctor competent in ophthalmoscopy:
  All patients 10–30 years of age who have ≥ 5 years of diabetes.
  All diabetic patients diagnosed after 30 years of age at the time of
    diagnosis or shortly thereafter.
Referral to an ophthalmologist:
  All women with type 1 diabetes mellitus planning pregnancy within
    12 months, in the first trimester, and thereafter at the discretion of
    the ophthalmologist.
  Patients found to have reduced corrected visual acuity, elevated
    intraocular pressure, and any other vision-threatening ocular
    abnormalities.

Source: Reprinted with permission from Klein R, Klein BEK, Moss SE: *Diabetes Metab Rev* 1989; 5:559.

schools for the blind, are available. Helping the patient accept the partial or complete visual loss is an essential step in planning living arrangements and in developing coping strategies.

ACKNOWLEDGMENTS

The author acknowledges the support of grant EY03083 from the National Eye Institute. He thanks Dr. Barbara E. K. Klein and Mr. Scot Moss for reviewing the manuscript, Gene Knutson and Michael Neider for preparing the photographs, and Colleen Comeau for secretarial assistance.

ADDITIONAL REFERENCES

The Eye Diseases Prevalence Research Group. Causes and prevalence of visual impairment among adults in the United States. *Arch Ophthalmol* 2004;122:477.

The Eye Diseases Prevalence Research Group. The prevalence of diabetic retinopathy among adults in the United States. *Arch Ophthalmol* 2004;122:552.

Klein R: Prevention of visual loss from diabetic retinopathy. *Surv Ophthalmol* 2002;47 (Suppl 2):S246.

Roy MS, Klein R, O'Colmain BJ, et al: The prevalence of diabetic retinopathy among adult type 1 diabetic persons in the United States. *Arch Ophthalmol* 2004;122:546.

Wilkinson CP, Ferris FL, Klein R, et al: Proposed international clinical diabetic retinopathy and diabetic macular edema disease severity scales. *Ophthalmology* 2003;11:1677.

For a more detailed discussion of this topic and a bibliography, please see Porte *et al: Ellenberg & Rifkin's Diabetes Mellitus,* 6th ed., Chapter 41.

21 | Diabetic Nephropathy

Ralph A. DeFronzo

INTRODUCTION

Renal disease is an all too common occurrence in individuals with diabetes mellitus. Of the approximately 1 million people in the United States with type 1 diabetes mellitus (T1DM), 30–40% eventually develop end-stage renal failure (Fig. 21-1). Unfortunately, there is little evidence that the incidence of diabetic nephropathy in patients with T1DM has changed within the last decade. The overall incidence of renal disease in type 2 diabetes mellitus (T2DM) is 5–10%; however, the incidence varies considerably among ethnic groups, being 3–4 times higher in blacks and Hispanics and 7 times higher in Native Americans compared to whites. In absolute terms, more patients with type 2 than type 1 diabetes eventually progress to end-stage renal failure. The magnitude of the problem can be readily appreciated when it is realized that every third patient who is started on dialysis has diabetes mellitus.

PATHOGENESIS OF DIABETIC NEPHROPATHY

Both acquired and genetic factors have been invoked to explain the development of diabetic renal disease. The acquired theory postulates that hyperglycemia sets in motion a number of metabolic and hemodynamic abnormalities leading to the histologic and clinical picture seen in patients with diabetic nephropathy (Fig. 21-2). The second theory argues that genetic factors are primarily responsible for the alterations in renal structure and function. The best synthesis of the available data indicates that metabolic derangements operate on a genetic background, which predisposes the kidney to the development of diabetic glomerulosclerosis in patients with poor glycemic control.

HISTOPATHOLOGIC CHANGES

Three major histopathologic alterations have been described in the diabetic kidney: glomerulosclerosis, vascular involvement, and tubulointerstitial disease.

Glomerulosclerosis

Involvement of the glomeruli is the most characteristic feature of diabetic nephropathy, with proteinuria and/or a reduction in glomerular filtration rate (GFR) the most common laboratory abnormalities, suggesting glomerular dysfunction. Of the distinctive glomerular lesions, glomerular basement membrane thickening represents an early and characteristic abnormality in patients with diabetic glomerulosclerosis (see Fig. 21-3a). Diffuse intercapillary glomerulosclerosis is the most common histologic abnormality. And, in 40–50% of patients, large acellular (Kimmelstiel-Wilson) nodules form at the center of peripheral glomerular lobules (see Fig. 21-3b). This nodular lesion invariably is associated with the diffuse lesion and is pathognomonic of diabetes mellitus, although it correlates poorly with the actual severity of clinical renal disease.

325

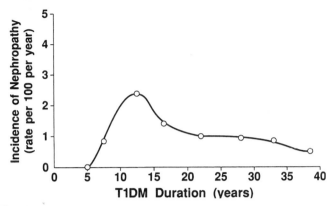

FIG. 21-1 Incidence of nephropathy according to the duration of type 1 diabetes mellitus. *(Adaped from Krolewski AS, Warram JH, Rand LI et al* N Engl J Med *1987; 317:1390.)*

Vascular Involvement

The kidneys of patients with established diabetic nephropathy commonly manifest accelerated renal arteriosclerosis and arteriolosclerosis (see Fig. 21-3b). In the larger arteries, atheromatous changes often are advanced and may contribute to renal failure by causing ischemic parenchymal atrophy. In the smaller renal arterioles, hyaline thickening involves the afferent and efferent vessels, and is believed to play an important role in the development of hypertension. Although arteriosclerosis and arteriolosclerosis may be extensive, neither process correlates with the severity of glomerular change.

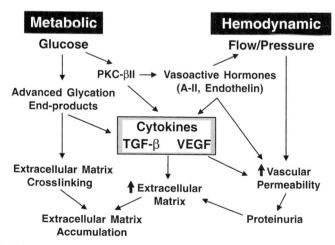

FIG. 21-2 Pathogenic schema depicting the contribution of metabolic and hemodynamic factors to the development of diabetic nephropathy. A-II, angiotensin II; PKC-βII, protein kinase C; VEGF, vascular endothelial growth factor.

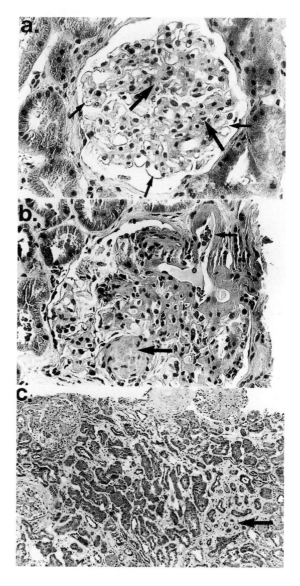

FIG. 21-3   (a) Diffuse diabetic glomerulosclerosis with marked mesangial matrix hyperplasia (thick arrows) and thickened glomerular basement membranes (thin arrows). No hypercellularity is evident. (b) Nodules (thick arrows) usually are observed in the peripheral capillary loops and rarely are seen without the diffuse lesion. Note the prominent arteriolosclerosis in the efferent and afferent arterioles. (c) Interstitial fibrosis, tubular atrophy (thick arrows), and thickening the the tubular basement membranes. *(Reproduced with permission from DeFronzo RA: in Olefsky JM, Sherwin RS, eds.* Diabetes Mellitus: Management and Complications. *Churchill Livingstone 1985; 161.)*

Tubulointerstitial Disease

Tubulointerstitial histologic changes (see Fig. 21-3c) are common in the diabetic kidney, and in advanced cases, there is marked tubular atrophy, thickening of the tubular basement membrane, and interstitial fibrosis. Tubular changes in diabetics also correlate poorly with the degree of vascular involvement and frequently occur in their absence.

Diabetes mellitus accounts for over half of all reported cases of a special type of interstitial lesion, *papillary necrosis.* Patients with papillary necrosis may present either with an acute fulminant illness, with fever, shock, flank pain, gross hematuria, pyuria, oliguria, and renal failure, or with a more subacute form of the disease that is characterized by microscopic hematuria, pyuria, and indolent renal failure. Because phenacetin has been associated with papillary necrosis, chronic use of this analgesic should be avoided in the diabetic population.

CLINICAL COURSE

The clinical course of renal dysfunction is characterized by hypertension, edema, severe albuminuria, and a progressive decline in GFR. Epidemiologic studies have documented that less than half of all patients with T1DM who have had their disease for 20–30 years develop clinically significant renal disease (Fig. 21-4). Unfortunately, at the time of diagnosis, there are no clinical or laboratory findings that predict which patients will progress to endstage renal failure.

Early Changes in Renal Function

Early in the course of diabetes (see Fig. 21-5) the GFR is characteristically increased and correlates with increased kidney weight and size, increased glomerular volume, and increased capillary luminal area per glomerulus.

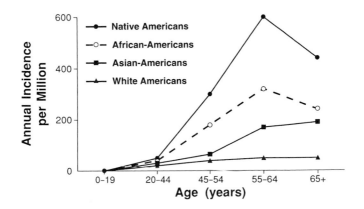

FIG. 21-4 The Medicare incidence of end-stage renal failure in Native Americans, African-Americans, Asian-Americans, and white Americans as a function of age. *(Adaped from Teusch S, Newman J, Eggers P:* Am J Kidney Dis *1989; 13:11.)*

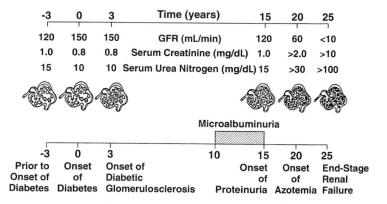

FIG. 21-5 Natural course of diabetic nephropathy. At the initial diagnosis, renal function and glomerular histology are normal. Within 2–3 years, increased mesangial matrix and basement membrane thickening are observed. Renal function remains normal until 15 years, when proteinuria develops. This is an ominous sign and usually indicates advanced diabetic glomerulosclerosis. Within 5 years after the onset of proteinuria, elevation of the serum urea nitrogen and creatinine levels are observed, and within 3–5 years after the development of azotemia, half of the patients have advanced to end-stage renal insufficiency. GFR, glomerular filtration rate. (Modified from DeFronzo RA: in Olefsky JM, Sherwin RS, eds. Diabetes Mellitus: Management and Complications. Churchill Livingstone 1985; 169.)

During this same period, renal biopsy has demonstrated the presence of increased mesangial matrix and basement membrane thickening. Institution of intensive, short-term (1–2 weeks) blood glucose control normalizes the GFR without any reduction in renal size, suggesting that the augmented GFR is not causally related to the renal hypertrophy. However, within 6 weeks after the start of intensive insulin therapy, a significant reduction in kidney size can be demonstrated in patients with T1DM. In early diabetes, the filtration fraction (GFR/RPF) is elevated, and renal plasma flow (RPF) is usually normal.

Late Changes in Renal Function

Patients who are destined to develop renal insufficiency follow a predictable clinical course, (see Fig. 21-5). After the onset of overt diabetes mellitus, there is a long (15–18 years) silent period, during which there is no laboratory evidence of renal dysfunction. However, if one were to perform a renal biopsy, a widespread increase in mesangial matrix material, capillary glomerular basement membrane (GBM) thickening, interstitial fibrosis, and arteriolosclerosis would be evident. In the advanced stages of diabetic nephropathy, encroachment of capillary lumina by the expanding mesangial matrix material contributes to the decline in GFR. However, nonstructural factors also must play an important role in the decay of renal function, because the severity of diabetic glomerulosclerosis in patients without clinically evident renal disease can be as marked as in patients with advanced renal insufficiency.

STAGING OF DIABETIC NEPHROPATHY

Microalbuminuria (defined as albumin excretion rate of 30–300 mg/day) is the earliest clinically detectable stage of diabetic nephropathy, and patients with microalbuminuria are sometimes said to have *incipient diabetic nephropathy* because of their increased risk of clinical nephropathy. T1DM patients with microalbuminuria have a 20-fold increased likelihood of developing clinical proteinuria (>300 mg/day of albumin) or a diminished GFR within a period of 10 years. Patients with high-grade microalbuminuria (>100 mg/day) are at particularly high risk of developing renal impairment. Microalbuminuria also precedes the development of diabetic nephropathy in patients with T2DM (fivefold increased risk of proteinuria over a 10-year period), although it is not as strong a predictor as in patients with T1DM. Microalbuminuria is also a very strong predictor of macrovascular complications (heart attacks, stroke) and death (Fig. 21-6) in all patients with diabetes.

When interpreting the results of microalbumin excretion, it is important to exercise some clinical judgement. Many factors (e.g., exercise, high blood pressure, urinary tract infection, and very poor diabetic control) elevate the urinary albumin excretion rate. If such confounding factors are present, the finding of microalbuminuria does not necessarily imply incipient diabetic nephropathy. In T1DM patients, microalbuminuria during the first 5 years is unlikely to have the same ominous prognostic significance as that occurring 10–15 years after the onset of diabetes. This statement is not applicable to T2DM patients, who may have had their disease for many years before the diagnosis of diabetes was established.

From the more routine laboratory standpoint, the earliest detectable manifestation of diabetic glomerulosclerosis is "dipstick-positive" proteinuria (positive at albumin excretion rate > 300 mg/day) (see Fig. 21-5), which begins about 15–18 years after the diagnosis of diabetes. At this time, the

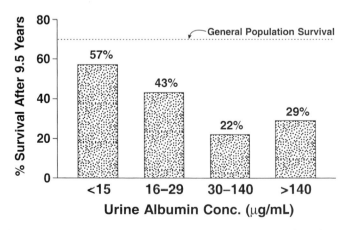

FIG. 21-6 Overall survival in 76 T2DM patients with varying degrees of microalbuminuria based on the urinary albumin concentration. Patients with microalbuminuria in the moderate to high range (two right bars) demonstrated a markedly shortened survival compared to an age-matched control population. *(Reproduced with permission from Mogensen CE:* N Engl J Med *1984; 310:356.)*

GFR may still be normal or even elevated, but within a mean of 5 years after the onset of this level of proteinuria, the GFR begins to decline, and the serum urea nitrogen and creatinine concentrations increase. Within ~3–5 years after an elevation in serum creatinine concentration is documented, about half of patients will have progressed to end-stage renal insufficiency. Severe proteinuria (> 3 g/day) and the nephrotic syndrome are common, occurring in over half of all diabetic patients who progress to end-stage renal failure.

LABORATORY ABNORMALITIES

Proteinuria

The earliest laboratory manifestation of diabetic renal disease is proteinuria. When the urine albumin excretion exceeds 300 mg/day (corresponding to a urine protein excretion of 500 mg/day), the patient is said to have *overt diabetic nephropathy.* The increased transglomerular flux of proteins has been shown to result from an augmented transglomerular ultrafiltration pressure gradient and an alteration in the molecular charge of the glomerular barrier, which results from the loss of anionic charges (heparin sulfate and sialic acid residues) from the GBM. At this stage, loss of barrier charge selectivity, without alteration of pore-size diameter, appears to be the primary factor that allows the escape of albumin without change in the clearance of other macromolecules, and improved glycemic control with intensive insulin therapy decreases the albumin excretion rate. Impaired tubular handling of albumin may also contribute in the development of microalbuminuria. With progressive proteinuria and the development of impaired renal function, glomerular charge- and size selectivity is lost, and there is an increase in pore size with the appearance of large-molecular-weight proteins in the urine.

Glomerular Filtration Rate

Prior to the onset of microalbuminuria, the GFR is increased as the result of increased intraglomerular pressure and increased glomerular capillary surface area (Fig. 21-7). The elevated GFR often persists even though marked renal

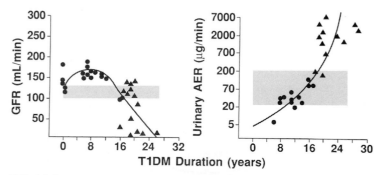

FIG. 21-7   Natural history of glomerular filtration rate (GFR) and urinary albumin excretion rate (AER) in 20 type 1 diabetic patients who progressed to overt diabetic nephropathy over a period of 12 ± 3 years. GFR and AER are shown at the time of initial examination (circles) and after varying periods of follow-up (triangles). Shaded areas show the normal range. *(Reproduced with permission from Mogensen CE:* Diabetes *1990; 39:761.)*

histologic changes are present. Thus a decline in GFR from elevated to normal values in the absence of an improvement in metabolic control represents an ominous finding (Fig. 21-7). Serum creatinine and serum urea nitrogen (SUN) concentrations are the most commonly used laboratory tests that provide an index of GFR. Since the GFR may decline by 40–50% before either test increases into the abnormal range, many nephrologists and diabetologists have advocated serial determinations of the creatinine clearance. The author advocates following the creatinine clearance in patients with diabetes with normal serum creatinine levels. Once the serum creatinine concentration becomes elevated, either the reciprocal of the serum creatinine (plot over time is linear) or the creatinine clearance can be followed.

Glucosuria

The maximum tubular reabsorptive capacity for glucose (Tm_G) varies inversely with the GFR in healthy individuals, as well as patients with new-onset T2DM. However, in patients with long-term diabetes with reduced GFR and diabetic glomerulosclerosis, the Tm_G is raised. Moreover, even in patients with diabetes without renal disease, glucosuria correlates relatively poorly with the plasma glucose concentration.

Hyperkalemia

The maintenance of normal potassium homeostasis depends on both renal and extrarenal mechanisms (Fig. 21-8). Many factors predispose the patient with diabetes to the development of hyperkalemia. Three hormones—insulin, epinephrine, and aldosterone—play a pivotal role in regulating the distribution of

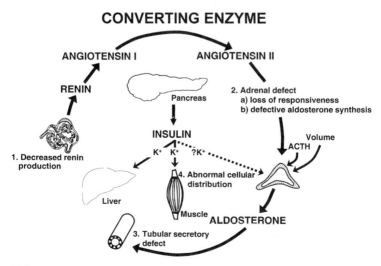

FIG. 21-8 Hyperkalemia and the renin–angiotensin–aldosterone system. *(Reproduced with permission from DeFronzo RA, Smith JD: in Arieff A, DeFronzo RA, eds.* Fluid, Electrolyte and Acid-Base Disorders. *Churchill Livingstone 1995; 319.)*

potassium between intracellular and extracellular compartments. In patients with long-standing diabetes mellitus, all three of these hormones may be deficient. Therefore, it is not surprising that hyperkalemia is a commonly encountered clinical problem in the diabetic population. Moreover, in poorly controlled patients the elevated plasma glucose concentration causes an osmotic shift of fluid and electrolytes, primarily potassium, out of cells. Metabolic acidemia, common in patients with diabetes, also predisposes to hyperkalemia.

Renal mechanisms also contribute to the development of hyperkalemia. When the GFR declines to less than 15–20 mL/min, the ability of the kidney to excrete potassium becomes impaired. Essentially, all of the filtered potassium is reabsorbed by the early to mid-distal tubule, and the potassium that appears in the final urine represents potassium that is secreted by the late distal tubule and collecting duct. Also, many patients with diabetes demonstrate a marked interstitial nephritis with prominent tubular atrophy and tubular basement membrane thickening. Because most urinary potassium is derived from distal and collecting tubular cell secretion, renal potassium excretion becomes further impaired.

Complex alterations in the renin–angiotensin axis in patients with diabetes lead to changes in renin and aldosterone secretion. Hypoaldosteronism is common in patients with diabetes, particularly in those with evidence of impaired renal function (Fig. 21-8). In most patients, the plasma renin level also is reduced and accounts for the hypoaldosteronism. Since aldosterone is a key regulator of potassium secretion by the distal tubule and collecting duct, aldosterone deficiency results in impaired potassium excretion.

A number of drugs have been shown to impair aldosterone secretion and, if prescribed for patients with diabetes, require close monitoring of the plasma potassium concentration. Of these medications, the β-blockers and angitensin-converting enzyme (ACE) inhibitors are the most widely known. The ACE inhibitors have been advocated for the treatment of diabetic nephropathy. These agents infrequently cause hyperkalemia, and this complication should be monitored closely at the start of therapy. Nonsteroidal anti-inflammatory prostaglandin inhibitors cause hyporeninemic hypoaldosteronism and hyperkalemia. Certain diuretics (e.g., spironolactone, triamterene, and amiloride) block potassium secretion by the renal tubular cell and also may result in hyperkalemia.

Metabolic Acidosis

Metabolic acidosis, both anion gap and hyperchloremic (nonanion gap), is commonly observed in patients with diabetes. There are three possible causes of an *anion gap acidosis:* renal insufficiency, ketoacidosis, and lactic acidosis, with all three potentially occurring in diabetic patients. In diabetic nephropathy, as in other causes of chronic renal disease, when the GFR declines to 20–25 mL/min, the ability of the kidney to excrete titratable acid becomes impaired, and the laboratory manifestation is an anion gap acidosis.

The causes of a *hyperchloremic* (or *non-anion gap*) *metabolic acidosis* are less appreciated. Hyporeninemic hypoaldosteronism, commonly observed in patients with diabetes, presents as hyperchloremic metabolic acidosis in over half of cases. Hyperchloremic metabolic acidosis is due to a primary renal tubular defect in hydrogen secretion in some patients, and due to widespread chronic interstitial nephritis and diffuse tubular injury, resulting in decreased ammonia production, in others. Hyperkalemia may also cause a hyperchloremic metabolic acidosis by inhibiting ammonia synthesis by the renal tubular cell.

CLINICAL CORRELATIONS

Diabetic nephropathy is unusual in the absence of retinopathy, neuropathy, and hypertension. However, recent reviews suggest a more variable association among the three microvascular complications.

Diabetic Retinopathy

Diabetic retinopathy (e.g., hemorrhages, exudates, proliferative retinopathy) is invariably present in patients with diabetes and end-stage renal failure who are admitted into dialysis or transplantation programs. However, when overt diabetic nephropathy is first diagnosed (i.e., documentation of persistent proteinuria or elevation of the serum creatinine concentration), 30–40% of patients do not have evidence of diabetic retinopathy by routine ophthalmologic examination, even though fluorescein angiography will demonstrate typical diabetic abnormalities in over 80–90% of patients. As the renal disease progresses, diabetic retinopathy appears to accelerate. A dissociation between retinopathy and nephropathy is evident if one examines patients with established retinopathy: After 15–20 years, over 80% of patients have evidence of diabetic retinopathy, but as many as 30–50% have no laboratory evidence of renal disease.

Diabetic Neuropathy

The association between diabetic nephropathy and neuropathy is much less striking than that between diabetic nephropathy and retinopathy. In patients with end-stage renal failure, the incidence of diabetic neuropathy varies from 50% to 90%. As with retinopathy, uremia appears to exacerbate the progression of diabetic neuropathy, which is often reversed by dialysis and transplantation. When diabetic nephropathy is first diagnosed, less than half of patients have clinically evident diabetic neuropathy.

Hypertension

The incidence of hypertension is very different in patients with T1DM and T2DM. In newly diagnosed type 2 patients, approximately 50–60% have hypertension, whereas the corresponding figure in T1DM patients is less than 10%. In both T1DM and T2DM patients, the incidence and severity of hypertension progress as proteinuria becomes more severe. When end-stage renal failure ensues, 70–80% of patients with diabetes are hypertensive. Patients with heavy proteinuria are particularly prone to develop hypertension. In most patients, the hypertension is volume dependent and becomes easier to control after dialysis is started and dry weight is attained.

Edema

In patients without renal disease or in those with mild–modest proteinuria (<0.5–1 g/day) and a normal GFR, edema is uncommon. However, when the urinary albumin excretion exceeds 1–2 g/day, and especially when the GFR begins to decline, the incidence of edema increases precipitously. When end-stage renal failure ensues, over 50–75% of patients have some evidence of edema.

TREATMENT OF DIABETIC NEPHROPATHY

The treatment of patients with *established* diabetic nephropathy is aimed at slowing the progressive decline in GFR (Table 21-1). Once overt albuminuria is present and the serum creatinine concentration begins to increase, the progression to end-stage renal disease is difficult to halt. If end-stage renal failure ensues, two options are available: dialysis or transplantation.

Hypertension

Hypertension, even in its mildest form, is associated with decreased survival in patients without diabetes, and this effect is magnified in patients with diabetes. Hypertension is the single most important factor that increases the progression of diabetic renal disease. Elevated blood pressure interacts synergistically with poor glycemic control, hypercholesterolemia, and microalbuminuria to accelerate the decline in GFR (Fig. 21-9). Treatment of hypertension, regardless of the agent employed, markedly slows the progression of renal insufficiency in patients with established renal disease. Therefore, it is essential that all patients with diabetes have their blood pressure normalized. The Seventh Report of the Joint National Committee recommends a blood pressure goal of 130/80 mm Hg in patients with diabetes. This is consistent with the recommendation of the American Diabetes Association. The Hypertension Optimal Treatment (HOT) trial, which compared the achievement of a diastolic blood pressure less than 80 mm Hg to higher levels, concluded that the optimal blood pressure in patients with diabetes in order to prevent macrovascular complications is less than 120–130/80 mm Hg. The National Kidney Foundation Hypertension and Diabetes Working Group also recommends a diastolic blood pressure of < 80–85 mm Hg in patients with diabetes (Fig. 21-10). In the author's opinion, the goal of antihypertensive therapy should be to reduce blood pressure to the level before the onset of hypertension or renal disease. In some cases, this may be lower than 120/80 mm Hg. If the patient's blood pressure before the onset of hypertension or renal impairment is not known, then the goal of 120/80 mm Hg is appropriate. Special care should be taken in normalizing the blood pressure in elderly patients, especially those with underlying cardiovascular disease.

Hypertension in patients with diabetes is very volume-sensitive. Therefore, a low-sodium diet should be used to initiate therapy. Diuretics would also appear to be a logical first-line choice. However, this class of drugs, particularly at higher doses, may aggravate insulin resistance, impair insulin secretion, and worsen dyslipidemia. Because of these adverse effects on glucose tolerance and plasma lipid levels, if thiazide diuretics are to be used as first-line agents in the treatment of the hypertensive diabetic, they should be used in low doses (i.e., less than 25 mg/day of hydrochlorothiazide), and plasma glucose and lipid levels should be monitored closely after institution of therapy. In patients with edema or renal insufficiency, a diuretic usually is required to normalize blood pressure. If the serum creatinine concentration is more than 2 mg/dL, the more potent loop diuretics will be required.

TABLE 21-1 Treatment of Diabetic Nephropathy

Hypertension—the single and most important factor shown to accelerate the progression of renal failure.
  a. Angiotensin converting enzyme (ACE) inhibitors, angiotensin receptor blockers, and calcium channel blockers are efficacious and relatively free of side effects. Hyperkalemia and decreased glomerular filtration rate (GFR) may occur with ACE inhibitors.
  b. Because of the development of dyslipidemia and insulin resistance, diuretics should not be considered as first-line agents unless used in very low doses; they are, however, indicated in hypertensive patients with evidence of excessive sodium retention, i.e., edema.
  c. Attempt to avoid propranolol and other β-adrenergic blockers (hyperkalemia, hypoglycemia, hyperglycemia).
Urinary tract infection—increased incidence, frequent cultures.
Neurogenic bladder—parasymphatetic/adrenergic drugs, voiding maneuvers.
Intravenous pyelography—increased incidence of acute renal failure, particularly if heavy proteinuria and renal impairment are present.
Blood glucose control
  a. Tight blood glucose control, if instituted before or during the phase of microalbuminuria, prevents the development of overt proteinuria and progressive renal failure
  b. There is little evidence that tight metabolic control prevents or ameliorates the progression of established renal disease (albumin excretion rate > 200–300 mg/day or elevated serum creatinine).
  c. Uremia is associated with insulin resistance and increased insulin requirements.
  d. With advanced uremia (GFR <15–20 mL/minute), decreased insulin requirements may be observed because kidney removal of secreted insulin is impaired and hepatic degradation of insulin is inhibited.
  e. After the institution of dialysis, the situation is complex. Insulin sensitivity improves (hypoglycemia), but the degradation of insulin is enhanced (hyperglycemia); however, most insulin-treated diabetics who are started on dialysis experience an increase in their daily insulin requirement.

(continued)

β-Adrenergic antagonists, especially the nonspecific β-blockers, should be used with caution in diabetic patients. They can impair insulin secretion and worsen glucose tolerance in patients with T2DM. In patients with T1DM, β-blockers may cause hypoglycemia by inhibiting hepatic glucose production and impairing the counterregulatory hormone response to hypoglycemia. β-Blockers may also mask the clinical symptoms of hypoglycemia, and they can aggravate diabetic dyslipidemia and underlying peripheral vascular disease in both type 1 and type 2 patients. Despite these concerns, the results of the UKPDS demonstrated that after 9 years, treatment with atenolol (a selective β_1-antagonist) was as effective as captopril in reducing overall mortality, macrovascular complications (myocardial infarction, stroke, peripheral vascular disease), and microvascular complications (primarily retinopathy).

ACE inhibitors have gained widespread acceptance as the drug of choice in the treatment of the hypertensive diabetic, especially if proteinuria or renal insufficiency is present. ACE inhibitors also have been shown to retard the progression of albuminuria and decline in GFR in type 1 (Fig. 21-11) and type 2 (Fig. 21-12) patients with microalbuminuria. In a long-term, randomized, double-blind, prospective study of 409 type 1 diabetic patients with estab-

TABLE 21-1 *(continued)* Treatment of Diabetic Nephropathy

Dialysis
a. One in every three patients beginning dialysis in the United States has diabetes.
b. Diabetic patients do significantly worse on dialysis than do nondiabetic patients.
c. The increased mortality in diabetic patients treated with dialysis is largely due to cardiovascular deaths resulting from myocardial infarction and stroke. Other complications include peripheral vascular disease, infections, psychiatric problems, and progressive retinopathy and neuropathy.
d. Diabetic patients treated with peritoneal dialysis appear to do as well as those treated with hemodialysis.

Transplantation
a. If a well-matched, living, related donor can be found, renal transplantation is the preferable mode of therapy in most people with diabetes.
b. Survival statistics with kidneys transplanted from a haplotype-identical relative or unrelated donor are similar to those obtained with hemodialysis.

Protein restriction
a. There are good data in animals that show that a low-protein diet slows the progression of diabetic renal disease.
b. In small uncontrolled studies in humans, a low-protein diet has been shown to slow the progression of established diabetic renal diease.
c. In a large, well-controlled, prospective study, a low-protein diet did not alter the rate of decline in GFR. In this study, the majority of patients were on an antihypertensive agent (ACE inhibitor or calcium channel blocker). It is likely that a low-protein diet has no added beneficial effect beyond that afforded by the ACE inhibitor or a calcium channel blocker.

Source: Modified from DeFronzo RA: in Olefsky JM, Shewin RS, eds. *Diabetes Mellitus: Management and Complications.* Churchill Livingstone 1985, 189.

lished nephropathy, it was demonstrated that antihypertensive therapy with captopril decreased the doubling time of serum creatinine by 48% and reduced by 50% the combined end points of death, dialysis, and renal transplantation (Table 21-2). Parving has demonstrated a sustained protective effect of captopril in patients with T1DM over a follow-up period of 10 years. In short-term studies the antiproteinuric effect of the ACE inhibitors (and angiotensin II receptor blockers [ARBs], described below) has been shown to be similar in patients with and without diabetes with renal disease. An added advantage of the ACE inhibitors is that they may improve insulin sensitivity and may have a beneficial effect on the plasma lipid profile.

Recently, two long-term prospective studies have demonstrated the effectiveness of the angiotensin II receptor blockers (ARBs) losartan and irbesartan in slowing the progression of renal failure in patients with T2DM (Fig. 21-13). Some authorities have suggested that the ARBs may be more effective than the ACE inhibitors, since the latter reduce only ACE-dependent angiotensin II production, whereas the receptor blockers inhibit the effect of angiotensin II from any source. However, the renal protective effects of losartan and irbesartan appear to be no greater than those of the ACE inhibitors. Moreover, there is experimental evidence to suggest that elevated kinins (not

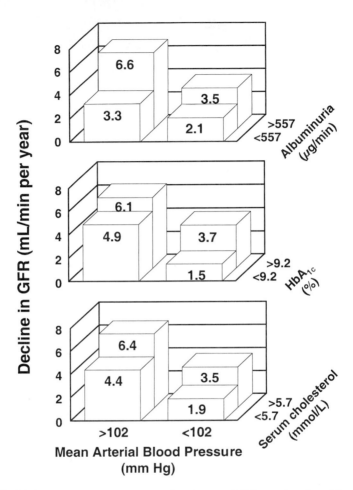

FIG. 21-9 The decline in glomerular filtration rate (GFR) as a function of the mean arterial blood pressure in 301 consecutive type 1 diabetic patients who were followed for 7 years (range 3–14 years). For any given blood pressure, elevated serum cholesterol and HbA₁c levels and an increased rate of urinary albumin excretion accelerated the decline in GFR. *(Reproduced with permission from Hovind P, Rossing P, Tarnow L, et al:* Kidney Int *2001; 59:702.)*

observed with the ARBs) may be responsible for some of the renal-protective effects of the ACE inhibitors. Although combination therapy with an ACE inhibitor and an ARB has been suggested, there are no long-term data in humans to support such an approach.

The calcium channel blockers and postsynaptic α_1-adrenergic blockers also effectively lower blood pressure in patients with diabetes, and have been shown to exert a beneficial effect on renal function in patients with proteinuria. Some evidence suggests that an ACE inhibitor plus a calcium channel

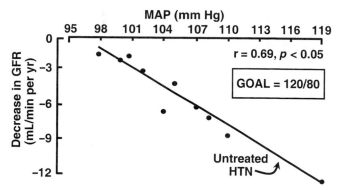

FIG. 21-10 Relationship between achieved mean arterial blood pressure (MAP) control and the decrease in glomerular filtration rate (GFR) in nine long-term, antihypertensive clinical trials of diabetic ($n = 6$) and nondiabetic ($n = 3$) renal disease. These trials suggest that to maximally preserve renal function, the blood pressure should be reduced to less than 130/85 mm Hg, and ideally to 120/80 mm Hg. *(Adapted from Bakris GL, Williams M, Dwprlom L et al: Am J Kidney Dis 2000; 36:646.)*

blocker may provide an additive effect in preventing the progression of renal disease. Moreover, when ACE inhibitors are used with calcium channel blockers, this combination has resulted in a reduction in cardiovascular events. The calcium channel blockers have no adverse effects on either glucose or lipid metabolism, while the β-blockers improve insulin insensitivity and promote a less atherogenic plasma lipid profile.

In summary, the ACE inhibitors or ARBs, along with the calcium channel antagonists and the β-blockers, should be considered the agents of choice in

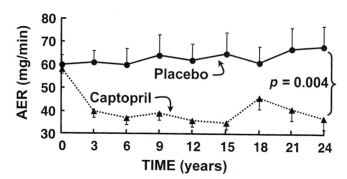

FIG. 21-11 Effect of captopril versus placebo therapy on albumin excretion rate (AER) in 225 type 1 diabetic subjects with microalbuminuria. Twenty-five of 114 (22%) placebo-treated and 8 of 111 (7/5) captopril-treated patients progressed to persistent clinical albuminuria over 2 years ($p < 0.01$). *(Reproduced with permission from The Microalbuminuria Captopril Study Group: Diabetologia 1996; 39:587.)*

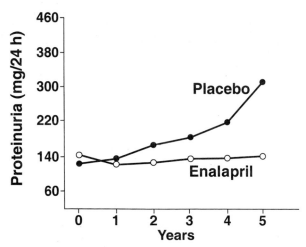

FIG. 21-12 Effect of enalapril treatment on the progression of microalbuminuria normotensive type 2 diabetic patients. *(Reproduced with permission from Ravid M, Savin H, Jutrin, et al:* Ann Intern Med *1998; 128:982.)*

treating the hypertensive diabetic patient. Since the treatment of hypertension is the single most important factor in preventing the progression of diabetic nephropathy, and since the ACE inhibitors appear to provide a modest additional benefit beyond their antihypertensive action by their effects on intrarenal hemodynamics and nonhemodynamic mechanisms, it is the author's opinion that the ACE inhibitors are the drugs of choice in treating hypertensive patients with diabetes and evidence of renal disease.

Microalbuminuria

Treatment of microalbuminuria with an ACE inhibitor has been shown to significantly reduce the rate of microalbumin excretion and retard the progression of microalbuminuria to clinical proteinuria in both type 1 and type 2 patients. ACE inhibitors also decrease the incidence of cardiovascular disease in both hypertensive and normotensive individuals with diabetes.

After quantitating the rate of microalbumin excretion, I recommend that a patient be started on the ACE inhibitor of choice (e.g., captopril, 12.5 mg

TABLE 21-2 Effect of Antihypertensive Treatment with Captopril on Renal Function and Outcome in Patients with Renal Insufficiency (Serum Creatinine <2.5 mg/dL) and Proteinuria (> 500 mg/day)

	Doubling time of serum creatinine (months)	Renal mortality, dialysis, or transplantation (no.)
Placebo	25	42
Captopril	43*	23*

*$p < 0.001$ versus placebo.
Source: Adapted from Lewis EJ, Hunsicker LG, Bain RP, et al: *N Engl J Med* 1993; 329:1456.

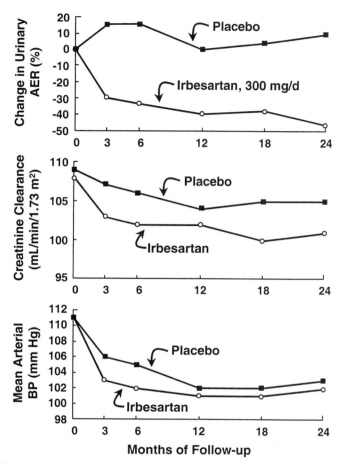

FIG. 21-13   Effect of irbesartan versus placebo therapy on albumin excretion rate (AER), creatine clearance, and mean arterial blood pressure in 395 hypertensive type 2 diabetic patients with microalbuminuria. Thirty of 201 (15%) placebo-treated and 10 of 194 (5%) irbesartan-treated patients progressed to persistent proteinuria over 2 years ($p < 0.001$). *(From Parving HH, Lehnert H, Brochner-Mortensen J, et al:* N Engl J Med *2001; 345:870.)*

three times a day; enalapril, 5 mg/day; monopril, 10 mg/day). Urine microalbumin excretion should be determined 6–8 weeks after initiation of therapy. If microalbuminuria is diminished but still present, the dose of the ACE inhibitor should be increased (e.g., captopril by 12.5 mg three times a day; enalapril by 5 mg/day; monopril by 10 mg/day) every 6–8 weeks until the microalbuminuria disappears or the microalbumin excretion rate remains unchanged over three successive dose titrations. The ACE inhibitors produce a maximum or near-maximum reduction in microalbumin excretion rate within 6–8 weeks. If a beneficial effect of the ACE inhibitor is observed, therapy should be continued for life, since withdrawal of the ACE inhibitor will lead to a return of the microalbuminuria.

TABLE 21-3 Definition of Microalbuminuria

	Urinary AER (mg/24 h)	Urinary AER (µg/min)	Urine albumin/ creatinine (mg/mg)
Normoalbuminuria*	<30	<20	<0.02
Microalbuminuria	30–300	20–200	0.02–0.20
Macroalbuminuria	>300	>200	>0.20

*The mean value for urinary albumin excretion rate (AER) in normal individuals is 10 ± 3 mg/day or 7 ± 2 µg/min.

All diabetic patients should have an annual test for microalbuminuria. This can be done using a timed urine collection (e.g., over 24 hours) or by checking the microalbumin:creatinine ratio or microalbumin concentration on a first-voided morning urine specimen. If microalbuminuria is detected, the author prefers to base future therapeutic interventions on the 24-hour microalbumin excretion rate or on the microalbumin:creatinine ratio (Table 21-3).

Urinary Tract Infection

The incidence of urinary tract infection is increased in patients with diabetes: Asymptomatic bacteriuria and pyelonephritis are twice as common in patients with diabetes, particularly women, than in patients without diabetes. This increased incidence of urinary tract infection results from a variety of factors, including impaired renal blood flow, bladder dysfunction, and interstitial scarring. Furthermore, high urine glucose concentrations provide an excellent culture medium for bacteria and inhibit white blood cell (WBC) function. Therefore, it is important that a urinalysis be performed periodically. If white blood cells or bacteriuria are noted, a urine culture should be done.

Intravenous Pyelography

Diabetic patients are at increased risk of developing acute renal failure after radiocontrast procedures (e.g., arteriography, intravenous and retrograde pyelography, computed tomographic scanning). This adverse event is observed less frequently with the newer nonionic contrast agents, but still remains a concern. Patients with impaired renal function (i.e., serum creatinine > 2 mg/dL) or heavy proteinuria are at greatest risk. With the judicious use of ultrasound, radionuclide studies, and computed tomographic scanning without contrast, most of the information necessary to ensure adequate diagnosis and treatment can be obtained. If patients with diabetes must receive radiocontrast dye, hydration with normal saline should be started 12–24 hours before the procedure.

Blood Glucose Control

Glycemic Control

Poor glycemic control is a major risk factor for diabetic nephropathy in both type 1 and type 2 patients, and diabetic nephropathy is uncommon when the glycosylated hemoglobin is maintained below 7.0%. In the Diabetes Control and Complications Trial, intensive glycemic control with insulin in type 1

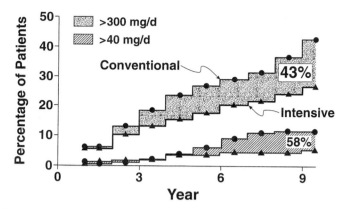

FIG. 21-14   Effect of intensive versus conventional glycemic control with insulin on the albumin excretion rate in T1DM patients. Tight glycemic control significantly reduced the risk of developing microalbuminuria (cross-hatched area) and macroalbuminuria (stippled area) in normoalbuminuric patients. *(Reproduced with permission from The Diabetes Control and Complications trial [DCCT] Research Group: N Engl J Med 1993; 329:977.)*

patients markedly decreased the risk of microvascular complications (Fig. 21-14). In type 2 patients, improved glycemic control with insulin or oral agents was equally effective in decreasing the risk of microalbuminuria, as well as other microvascular complications. Of note, the initiation of tight glycemic control after the onset of overt proteinuria or renal insufficiency generally has been ineffective in halting the relentless progression to end-stage renal failure, underscoring the need for early treatment (i.e., prior to or during the phase of microalbuminuria [see Fig. 21-5] and before the advanced histologic lesions of diabetic nephropathy have become well established). Combined pancreatic and renal transplantation has been shown to prevent the recurrence of diabetic nephropathy in the transplanted kidney as long as the pancreatic transplant functions normally.

Changes in Insulin Degradation and Insulin Sensitivity

A deterioration in glycemic control is observed with the onset of renal insufficiency in both type 1 and type 2 patients. However, when the GFR decreases to 15–20 mL/min, both the renal (loss of nephron mass) and hepatic (uremia inhibits insulin degradation by the liver) clearance of insulin become markedly reduced. At this stage, improvement in glucose tolerance is common because insulin, which normally would be cleared by the liver and kidneys, is returned to the systemic circulation. Some patients will require a reduction in their insulin (or sulfonylurea) dose to reduce hypoglycemia, and others will cease to require treatment entirely. The effect of dialysis on insulin requirements is difficult to predict. In general, most patients require an increase in insulin dose (by 50–100%) when dialysis is initiated.

Selection of oral hypoglycemic agents for treating patients with diabetes and impaired renal function requires special attention. The ideal oral agent should not enhance insulin secretion, and its metabolism should not be altered by diminished kidney function. In this context, the thiazolidinediones appear to be ideal candidates. Preliminary studies in human T2DM suggest that thiazolidinediones reduce microalbuminuria. Among the insulin secretagogues, Glipazide and Glimiperide are suitable for use in patients with chronic renal failure (CRF), whereas glyburide is not. Because all sulfonylureas stimulate insulin secretion, titration should be slow (every 2 weeks or more) in patients with CRF. Repaglinide and nateglinide, new nonsulfonylurea insulin secretagogues, are well suited for use in diabetic patients with impaired renal function. When prescribing insulin for patients with CRF, the physician must be mindful of the alterations in insulin metabolism discussed above. Acarbose is not approved for use in patients with diabetes and an elevated serum creatinine. Likewise, metformin, a biguanide insulin sensitizer, should not be used if the serum creatinine is greater than 1.4 mg/dL in females or 1.5 mg/dL in males, corresponding to a GFR of ~70 mL/minute. Accumulation of the biguanide in plasma and tissues may lead to lactic acidosis. Although HbA_{1c} levels may be slightly reduced in diabetic patients with advanced renal disease (because of shortened red blood cell survival), it remains the best tool for assessing glycemic control in diabetic patients.

Peritoneal Dialysis, Glucose Absorption, and Insulin Requirements

Standard hemodialysate solutions contain no glucose. In contrast, the dialysis fluid used for continuous ambulatory peritoneal dialysis (CAPD) contains hypertonic glucose, and severe hyperglycemia presents a significant problem with this mode of therapy. To prevent the development of excessive hyperglycemia, insulin may be added to the dialysis fluid (insulin requirements are usually increased two- to fourfold with CAPD), with intraperitoneal insulin administration effectively achieving excellent glucose control.

Protein Restriction

Low-protein diets have been advocated to slow the progression of chronic renal failure. Results of animal studies and a number of uncontrolled studies of humans (small number of patients, few of whom had diabetes) have consistently demonstrated that institution of a low-protein diet slowed the decline in GFR in those with advanced renal failure. More recently, a well-controlled prospective study involving 840 patients with renal disease of diverse etiology has been completed. Insulin-requiring patients with diabetes were not included in the study, and diet-treated and sulfonylurea-treated patients were not analyzed separately. After 3 years, no difference in the rate of decline in GFR was observed between the patients receiving the low-protein diet (0.58 g/kg) and those maintained on a normal protein intake (1.3 g/kg), although any beneficial effect of the low-protein diet was likely obscured by the concomitant use of antihypertensive medications (80% of patients) and the use of ACE inhibitors (44% of patients). Based on these results, it seems prudent to recommend modest protein restriction (~1.0 g/kg/day) in patients with diabetes who are taking an ACE inhibitor or calcium channel blocker, while reserving more severe protein restriction (0.6 g/kg/day) for patients who are not taking any antihypertensive medications. These severely restricted protein diets are associated with poor patient compliance and require close dietary supervision. A very-low-protein diet can lead to negative nitrogen balance and acceleration of muscle protein breakdown, with the development of clinically manifest myopathy.

Dyslipidemia

In patients with diabetes and renal insufficiency, the dyslipidemia of diabetes (hypertriglyceridemia, reduced high-density lipoprotein [HDL] cholesterol, small dense low-density lipoprotein [LDL] particles, and postprandial hyperlipidemia) is aggravated. Patients with diabetes and impaired renal function are at extremely high risk of developing heart attacks and stroke, and dyslipidemia represents a major risk factor for cardiovascular disease in this population. When patients are started on dialysis, the dyslipidemia usually worsens. Therefore, it is imperative that all patients with diabetes, whether they have normal renal function, impaired renal function, or are on dialysis, receive aggressive dietary and pharmacologic treatment for their dyslipidemia. The goal of therapy is to reduce the LDL cholesterol and triglycerides to less than 100 and 200 mg/dL, respectively. This can be achieved with diet, HMG-CoA reductase inhibitors, and fibric acid derivatives. The HDL cholesterol should be increased to at least 45 mg/dL. Exercise and the thiazolidinediones (although not approved for this indication) are particularly efficacious in increasing the plasma HDL cholesterol concentration.

Hyperlipidemia has also been implicated as a causative factor in the progression of diabetic nephropathy, and reduction of the plasma cholesterol concentration significantly slows the rate of GFR decline, regardless of the lipid-lowering agent that is used or the etiology of the renal disease. Thus patients with diabetes should receive aggressive antilipidemic therapy for the prevention of cardiovascular complications and possible protection against progressive renal deterioration.

Dialysis

Once end-stage renal failure occurs, the patient and physician must choose from one of four options: hemodialysis, peritoneal dialysis, CAPD, or renal transplantation. Vascular access and dialysis should be instituted earlier in patients with diabetes than in those without: Vascular access should be established when the serum creatinine reaches 4–5 mg/dL, and dialysis initiated at creatinine levels of 6–8 mg/dL. Although hemodialysis is the most frequently employed form of dialysis therapy in patients with end-stage renal failure, it does not appear to be superior to any other dialysis technique. Morbidity and mortality statistics are similar with intermittent peritoneal and chronic ambulatory peritoneal dialysis. Regardless of the type of dialysis chosen, survival in patients with diabetes is much worse than in patients without diabetes.

Renal Transplantation

Results from the United States Renal Data System indicate that patients with diabetes who are treated by kidney transplantation, especially if the kidney is donated by a living/human leukocyte antigen (HLA)-identical donor, have much better survival than those who are placed on dialysis. Although combined pancreatic/kidney transplantation is at an early stage, recent results suggest that this newer therapeutic option results in lower mortality than dialysis or kidney transplantation alone for patients with T1DM, and it may be beneficial in preventing the recurrence of diabetic nephropathy in the transplanted kidney. Newer immunosuppressive regimens may bring further improvements in patient survival after cadaveric renal transplantation.

ADDITIONAL READINGS

American Diabetes Association: Nephropathy in diabetes (Position Statement). *Diabetes Care* 2004;27(suppl. 1):579.

Gaede P, Vedel P, Larsen N, et al: Multifactorial intervention and cardiovascular disease in patients with type 2 diabetes. *N Engl J Med* 2003;348:1925.

Lewis EJ, Hunsicker LG, Clarke WR, et al; for the Collaborative Study Group: Reno-protective effect of the angiotensin-receptor antagonist irebesartan in patients with nephropathy due to type 2 diabetes. *N Engl J Med* 2001;345:870.

Molitch ME, DeFronzo RA, Franz MJ, et al; American Diabetes Association: Diabetic nephropathy. *Diabetes Care* 2003;26(suppl. 1):S94.

Parving H-H, Lehnert H, Brochner-Mortensen J, et al, for the Irebesartan in Patients with Type 2 Diabetes and Microalbuminuria Study Group: The effect of irebesartan on the development of diabetic nephropathy in patients with type 2 diabetes. *N Engl J Med* 2001;345:870.

Ravid M, Brosh D, Levi Z, et al: Use of enalapril to attenuate decline in renal function in normotensive, normoalbuminuric patients with type 2 diabetes mellitus. *Ann Intern Med* 1998;128:982.

Russo LM, Bakris GL, Comper WD. Renal handling of albumin: A critical review of basic concepts and perspective. *Am J Kidney Dis* 2002;39:899.

For a more detailed discussion of this topic and a bibliography, please see Porte *et al: Ellenberg & Rifkin's Diabetes Mellitus*, 6th ed., Chapter 43.

22 | Diabetic Autonomic Neuropathy

Aaron I. Vinik   Tomris Erbas
Michael A. Pfeifer   Eva L. Feldman
Martin J. Stevens   James W. Russell

Diabetic neuropathy is the most common and troublesome complication of diabetes mellitus, leading to great morbidity and mortality and an increase in the economic burden of public health. Diabetic neuropathy is a heterogeneous disorder that encompasses a wide range of abnormalities affecting both proximal and distal, peripheral sensory and motor, as well as the autonomic nervous system (ANS). The autonomic nervous system is primarily efferent, transmitting impulses from the central nervous system to peripheral organs. However, it also has an afferent component. Its two divisions—the parasympathetic and the sympathetic nervous systems—work in balanced opposition to control the heart rate, the force of cardiac contraction, the dilatation and constriction of blood vessels, the contraction and relaxation of smooth muscle in the digestive and urogenital systems, the secretions of glands, and pupillary size. Diabetes mellitus can cause dysfunction of any or every part of the autonomic nervous system, leading to a wide range of disorders. The organ systems that most often exhibit prominent clinical autonomic signs and symptoms in diabetes include the ocular pupil, sweat glands, genitourinary system, gastrointestinal tract system, adrenal medullary system, and the cardiovascular system (Table 22-1).

PREVALENCE

The reported prevalence of diabetic autonomic neuropathy (DAN) varies, with community-based studies finding lower rates than clinic-based and hospital-based studies, in which the prevalence may be as high as 100%. The main subgroups of autonomic disturbances recognized in diabetes mellitus include (1) subclinical DAN, determined by abnormalities in quantitative autonomic function tests and (2) clinical DAN, which presents with symptoms or signs. Symptomatic autonomic neuropathy, except for impotence, is rare and present in less than 5% of diabetic patients. Clinical symptoms generally do not develop for many years after the onset of diabetes. However, subclinical autonomic neuropathy can occur within a year of diagnosis in type 2 diabetic patients and within 2 years in the type 1 diabetic patients. The major confirmed risk factors are age, duration of diabetes, poor metabolic control, the presence of retinopathy, nephropathy, and cardiovascular disease.

DAN impairs the ability to conduct activities of daily living, lowers quality of life, and increases the risk of death. It also accounts for a large portion of the cost of care. Among the most troublesome and dangerous of the conditions linked to autonomic neuropathy are known or silent myocardial infarction, cardiac arrhythmias, foot ulceration, gangrene, nephropathy, and erectile dysfunction. Of patients with symptomatic autonomic dysfunction, 25–50% die within 5–10 years of diagnosis. The 5-year mortality rate in

347

TABLE 22-1 Clinical Manifestations of Autonomic Neuropathy

Cardiovascular
  Tachycardia, exercise intolerance
  Cardiac denervation
  Orthostatic hypotension
Gastrointestinal
  Esophageal dysfunction
  Gastroparesis diabeticorum
  Diarrhea
  Constipation
  Fecal incontinence
Genitourinary
  Erectile dysfunction
  Retrograde ejaculation
  Cystopathy
  Neurogenic bladder
Neurovascular
  Impaired skin blood flow
  Heat intolerance
  Gustatory sweating
  Dry skin
Metabolic
  Hypoglycemia unawareness
  Hypoglycemia unresponsiveness
  Hypoglycemia-associated autonomic failure
Pupillary
  Decreased diameter of dark-adapted pupil
  Argyll-Robertson-type pupil

patients with diabetic autonomic neuropathy is three times higher than in diabetic patients without autonomic involvement.

PATHOGENESIS

The pathogenesis of autonomic neuropathy is incompletely understood. There are metabolic, microvascular, and autonomic theories. Persistent hyperglycemia resulting in activation of the polyol pathway and tissue accumulation of sorbitol, fructose, and deficiency of myoinositol, disturbed phosphoinositide metabolism with consequently decreased nerve Na^+/K^+-ATPase activity, increased nonenzymatic glycation; decreased nitric oxide production leading to impaired endothelium-dependent vasodilation, and finally, deficiency in neurotrophic factors have all been proposed as pathogenetic mechanisms for DAN. An immunologic mechanism has also been suggested in the etiology of DAN. Autoantibodies to vagus nerve, sympathetic ganglia, and adrenal medulla are higher in patients with severe symptomatic DAN.

DIFFERENTIAL DIAGNOSIS

The diagnosis of DAN is one of exclusion, and many other causes of autonomic dysfunction should first be ruled out (Table 22-2). The clinician should take a careful history, asking about cancer, drug use, alcohol use, HIV exposure, and family history of familial amyloidosis. Patients should be asked whether they have traveled to South America, where they might have been exposed to *Trypanosoma cruzi,* the cause of Chagas disease.

TABLE 22-2 Differential Diagnosis of Autonomic Neuropathy

Idiopathic orthostatic hypotension
Shy-Drager syndrome *(orthostatic hypotension, pyramidal and cerebral signs including tremor, rigidity, hyperreflexia, ataxia, and urinary bowel dysfunction)*
Panhypopituitarism
Pheochromocytoma
Chagas disease
Amyloidosis
Hypovolemia due to diuretics
Congestive heart disease
Carcinoid syndrome
Other causes of diarrhea, constipation, and gastrointestinal dysfunction
Other causes of genitourinary and erectile dysfunction
Orthostatic hypotension caused by alcoholic neuropathy
The Argyll-Robertson pupil of syphilis
Medications (insulin, vasodilators, sympathetic blockers)
Hypoglycemia unresponsiveness and unawareness occurring with intensive glycemic control

CARDIOVASCULAR AUTONOMIC NEUROPATHY

Cardiovascular autonomic neuropathy (CAN) is a common form of autonomic neuropathy, embracing abnormalities in heart rate control and in central and peripheral vascular dynamics. CAN has been linked to postural hypotension, exercise intolerance, enhanced intraoperative cardiovascular lability, increased incidence of asymptomatic ischemia, myocardial infarction, and decreased likelihood of survival after myocardial infarction. The medical consequences of CAN in diabetes are dramatic: a meta-analysis of 11 studies of CAN among diabetic patients concluded that while diabetics without this complication have a mortality of 5% within 5.5 years, mortality among patients with CAN as determined by abnormal heart rate variability (HRV) tests jumps to 27% in that time period. CAN occurs in about 17% of patients with type 1 diabetes and in 22% of those with type 2. An additional 9% of type 1 patients and 12% of type 2 patients have borderline dysfunction. Lack of heart rate variability during deep breathing or exercise is a sign of autonomic neuropathy and is associated with a high risk of coronary heart disease in patients with or without diabetes. The Diabetes Control and Complications Trial (DCCT) found that 1.6% of patients with a 5-year history of diabetes had this sign. The rate rose to 6.2% of those with a 5- to 9-year history of diabetes, and to 12% in those who had had the disease for more than 9 years. Resting tachycardia is an early sign, as is loss of heart rate variation during deep breathing, whereas a heart rate that does not respond to mild exercise indicates nearly complete cardiac denervation. CAN leads to a reduced cardiac ejection fraction and systolic dysfunction, and decreased diastolic filling. Limited exercise tolerance is due to impaired sympathetic and parasympathetic responses that normally augment cardiac output and redirect peripheral blood flow to skeletal muscles. Exercise tolerance is also reduced by a reduced ejection fraction, systolic dysfunction, and decreased diastolic filling.

A prolonged corrected QT interval (QTc) and QT dispersion (the difference between the longest and shortest QT intervals) indicates an imbalance between right and left sympathetic innervation. Diabetic patients with a regional sympathetic imbalance and QT interval prolongation may be at greater risk for arrhythmias. Regional myocardial autonomic denervation and altered vascular responsiveness in DAN may predispose to malignant arrhythmogenesis and sudden cardiac death. In the resting state, the myocardium is well perfused in subjects with DAN, and thus circulatory deficiencies should not exacerbate arrhythmogenesis under resting conditions. During stress, relative regional ischemia in sympathetically innervated regions with diminished parasympathetic protection may be highly arrhythmogenic.

Diabetic patients have a high rate of coronary heart disease, which may be asymptomatic owing to autonomic neuropathy. Indeed, painless ischemia is significantly more frequent in patients with autonomic neuropathy than in those without it (38% versus 5%). In the Framingham study, 39% of patients with diabetes had had an asymptomatic myocardial infarction documented by electrocardiography. In nondiabetic patients, acute myocardial infarction has a circadian variation with a significant morning peak. The characteristic diurnal variation in the onset of myocardial infarction is altered in diabetic patients, demonstrating a lower morning peak and a higher percentage of infarction during evening hours. The blunted morning surge of incidence of myocardial infarction results from altered sympathovagal balance in patients with cardiac autonomic neuropathy. Chest pain in any location in a patient with diabetes should be considered of myocardial origin until proven otherwise. Other clues to a possible silent myocardial infarction include unexplained fatigue, confusion, edema, hemoptysis, nausea and vomiting, diaphoresis, arrhythmias, cough, and dyspnea.

The undetected autonomic dysfunction, when associated with nocturnal hypoglycemia, may predispose type 1 diabetic patients to fatal ventricular dysrhythmia constituiting the "dead-in-bed syndrome." Possible mechanisms of sudden death are silent ischemia, prolonged QT interval predisposing to ventricular arrhythmias, or abnormal central control of breathing.

Cardiac Function Testing of the Autonomic Nervous System

Tests of cardiovascular reflexes are sensitive, reproducible, simple, and noninvasive and allow extensive evaluation of cardiac autonomic neuropathy. These include measurements of the resting heart rate, beat-to-beat heart rate variation (HRV), Valsalva maneuver, heart rate and systolic blood pressure response to standing, diastolic blood pressure response to sustained exercise, and the QT interval (Table 22-3). Reduced 24-hour HRV, a newer measure of cardiac autonomic function, is believed to be a more sensitive measure of cardiac autonomic function and able to detect dysfunction earlier than standard reflex tests. Twenty-four-hour recording of HRV gives insights into abnormal patterns of circadian rhythms regulated by sympathovagal activity. In frequency-domain analysis, the very-low-frequency (VLF) heart rate fluctuations are thought to be mediated by the sympathetic system, the low-frequency (LF) heart rate fluctuations are under sympathetic control with vagal modulation, while the high-frequency (HF) fluctuations are under parasympathetic control. The balance between the sympathetic and parasympathetic components of autonomic nerve function can be assessed using the LF/HF ratio. The HF component is reduced in diabetic patients with vagal dysfunction. In diabetic patients with sympathetic dysfunction, the VLF and LF components are reduced. The VLF, LF, and HF components, and the LF/HF ratio, have been demonstrated to be reduced in diabetic patients with advanced stages of CAN.

TABLE 22-3 Diagnostic Tests of Cardiovascular Autonomic Neuropathy

- Resting heart rate
  100 beats/minute is abnormal.

- Beat-to-beat heart rate variation*
  With the patient at rest and supine (no overnight coffee or hypoglycemic episodes), breathing 6 breaths/min, heart rate monitored by EKG or ANSCORE device, a difference in heart rate of >15 beats/min is normal and <10 beats/min is abnormal, RR inspiration/R–R expiration >1.17. All indices of HRV are age-dependent.**

- Heart rate response to standing*
  During continuous EKG monitoring, the R–R interval is measured at beats 15 and 30 after standing. Normally, a tachycardia is followed by reflex bradycardia. The 30:15 ratio is > 1.03.

- Heart rate response to Valsalva maneuver*
  The subject forcibly exhales into the mouthpiece of a manometer to 40 mm Hg for 15 s during EKG monitoring. Healthy subjects develop tachycardia and peripheral vasoconstriction during strain and an overshoot bradycardia and rise in blood pressure with release. The ratio of longest R–R to shortest R–R should be > 1.2.

- Systolic blood pressure response to standing
  Systolic blood pressure is measured in the supine subject. The patient stands and the systolic blood pressure is measured after 2 minutes. Normal response is a fall of <10 mm Hg, borderline is a fall of 10–29 mm Hg, and abnormal is a fall of >30 mm Hg with symptoms.

- Diastolic blood pressure response to isometric exercise
  The subject squeezes a hand-grip dynamometer to establish a maximum. Grip is then squeezed at 30% maximum for 5 minutes. The normal response for diastolic blood pressure is a rise of >16 mm Hg in the other arm.

- EKG QT/QTc intervals
  The QTc should be <440 ms.

- Spectral analysis
VLF peak ↓	(sympathetic dysfunction)
LF peak ↓	(sympathetic dysfunction)
HF peak ↓	(parasympathetic dysfunction)
LF/HF ratio ↓	(sympathetic imbalance)

- Neurovascular flow
  Use noninvasive laser Doppler measures of peripheral sympathetic responses to nociception.

---

*These can now be performed quickly (<15 minutes) in the practitioners office, with a central reference laboratory providing quality control and normative values.
**Lowest normal value of E/I ratio: Age 20–24, 1.17; 25–29, 1.15; 30–34, 1.13; 35–40, 1.12; 40–44, 1.10; 45–49, 1.08; 50–54, 1.07; 55–59, 1.06; 60–64, 1.04; 65–69, 1.03; 70–75, 1.02.

Sympathetic innervation of the heart can be visualized and quantified by single-photon emission-computed tomography with ^{123}I-meta-iodobenzyl-guanidine (MIBG). Diabetic CAN has been directly characterized by reduced or absent myocardial MIBG uptake. The sympathetic innervation of the heart can also be visualized with positron emission (PET) imaging using carbon-11 hydroxyephedrine. Defects in carbon-11 hydroxyephedrine uptake have been correlated with CAN and impaired vasodilator response of coronary resistance vessels.

Treatment

Intensive glycemic control is critical to preventing the onset of diabetic autonomic neuropathy and slowing its progression. The Diabetes Complications and Control Trial (DCCT) demonstrated that DAN was reduced by 53% in patients with very intensive glycemic control. Intensive glycemic control can reserve deterioration in HRV in as little as 1 year of therapy. However, the response to improved glycemic control depends on the degree of autonomic dysfunction at baseline. In a study of diabetic patients with microalbuminuria, the stepwise implementation of intensified multifactorial treatment allowed the progression to autonomic neuropathy. Angiotensin-converting enzyme (ACE) inhibition increased heart rate variation and decreased mortality in patients with mild microalbuminuria. β-Blockers that are cardioselective or lipophilic might modulate the effects of autonomic dysfunction in diabetes, either centrally or peripherally by opposing the sympathetic stimulus, and thereby restore the parasympathetic–sympathetic balance. In addition, a survey of evidence from clinical trials showed that early identification of autonomic neuropathy permits timely initiation of therapy with the powerful antioxidant α-lipoic acid, which slows or reverses progression of CAN. Aldose reductase inhibitors may also reserve the progression of diabetic autonomic neuropathy. These drugs reduce the flux of glucose through the polyol pathway, inhibiting tissue accumulation of sorbitol and fructose. However, they are not currently approved for clinical use in the United States; the only patients receiving them are participants in clinical trials.

ORTHOSTATIC HYPOTENSION

Orthostatic hypotension, another sign of autonomic neuropathy, is a fall in systolic blood pressure of greater than 30 mm Hg upon standing. The cause is damaged vasoconstrictor fibers, impaired baroreceptor function, and poor cardiovascular reactivity. Orthostatic hypotension may be accompanied by symptoms of dizziness, weakness, faintness, visual impairment, pain in the back of the head, and loss of consciousness (Fig. 22-1).

Two pathophysiologic states cause orthostatic hypotension: autonomic insufficiency and intravascular volume depletion. Physical examination and history should easily rule out volume depletion. Factors that may aggravate orthostatic hypotension in diabetic autonomic neuropathy and should be looked for include volume depletion due to diuretics, excessive sweating, diarrhea, or polyuria. Medications that may contribute to the problem include antihypertensives, β-blockers, and tricyclic antidepressants and phenothiazines. Many people with this condition abruptly become hypotensive when eating or within 10–15 minutes of an insulin injection. The symptoms are similar to those of hypoglycemia and are often incorrectly ascribed to the hypoglycemic action of insulin.

Treatment

Orthostatic hypotension in the patient with DAN can present a difficult management problem. Elevating the blood pressure in the standing position must

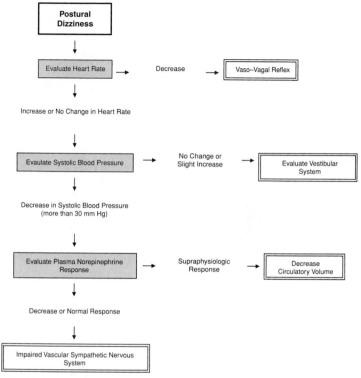

FIG. 22-1   Evaluation of postural dizziness in diabetic patients.

be balanced against preventing hypertension in the supine position. Whenever possible, attempts should be made to increase venous return from the periphery using total body stockings. Patients should be instructed to put them on while lying down and not to remove them until returning to the supine position. Fluorohydrocortisone and supplementary salt may benefit some patients with orthostatic hypotension. Unfortunately, these agents do not improve symptoms until edema develops, which carries a risk of causing congestive heart failure and hypertension. A α_2-adrenergic receptor deficiency may be treated with clonidine, which in this setting paradoxically may increase blood pressure. If the preceding measures fail, midodrine, a α_1-adrenergic agonist, may help. Octreotide may help some patients who experience particularly refractory orthostatic hypotension after eating.

IMPAIRED SKIN BLOOD FLOW

Microvascular skin flow is regulated by both the central and peripheral components of the autonomic nervous system and can thus be deranged by diabetic autonomic neuropathy. This derangement can disrupt the maintenance of regional and whole-body temperature through the apical or glabrous skin, which is the smooth skin on the palm of the hand, the sole of the foot, and the

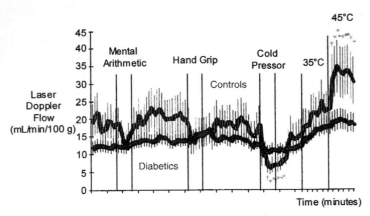

FIG. 22-2 Impaired skin blood flow in diabetic patients. *(Reproduced with permission from Stansberry KB, Shapiro SA, Hill MA, et al: Diabetes Care 1997; 20:1711.)*

face. Apical skin contains a large number of arteriovenous shunts for thermoregulation. Arteriovenous shunts provide a potential low-resistance pathway by which blood flow can be diverted from the arteriolar to venular circulations, bypassing the capillary bed. The shunts are maintained in a constricted state by sympathetic tone. Loss of this tone due to neuropathy causes the shunts to open, thus deviating blood flow from the skin. Increased venular oxygen levels, apparent ischemic lesions despite the presence of palpable pulses, and raised skin temperatures in the distal extremities are consistent with arteriovenous shunting. Unmyelinated C-fibers, which constitute the central reflex pathway, are assumed to be damaged in diabetic neuropathy, contributing to abnormalities in skin blood flow (Fig. 22-2). In type 2 diabetes, the predominant abnormality in skin blood flow is the loss of the active neurogenic vasodilative mechanism in nonapical or hairy skin (Fig. 22-3). Defective neurogenic vasodilation coexists with elements of the metabolic syndrome, elevated insulin resistance, hypertension, and dyslipidemia. Microvascular blood flow can be measured noninvasively using laser Doppler flowmetry under basal and stimulated conditions. The treatment of insulin-resistant type 2 diabetic patients with glitazones and regular exercise enhances skin blood flow. A prostaglandin analog, cilostazol, may benefit some people.

The factors that contribute to the development of foot ulceration include loss of cutaneous sensitivity to pain and warm thermal stimulation, impairment of sweating with dryness and cracking of the skin, and defective autonomic function with a decrease in blood flow, which compromises nerve function as well as impairing nutritive supply of essential nutrients and tissue perfusion. This constellation engenders the perfect milieu for developing foot ulcerations and gangrene. Charcot foot may present acutely with severe pain, a warm to hot foot with increased blood flow (despite decreased warm sen-

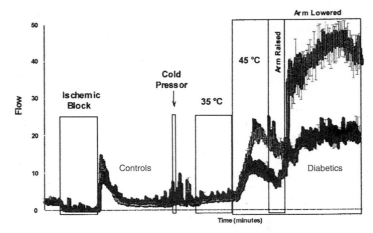

FIG. 22-3   Abnormal blood flow on dorsum of hand in patients with diabetes. *(Reproduced with permission from Stansberry KB, Peppard HR, Babyak LM, et al:* Diabetes Care *1999; 22:1549.)*

sory perception and vibration detection), and clear evidence of acute osteopenia. The repetitive trauma in the Charcot foot increases osteoclastic activity coupled with increased blood flow and consequently osteopenia. The osteopenia predisposes the small bones of the foot to small fractures with minimal provocation, especially with the development of equines.

Treatment

Drying between the toes after bathing and application of softening creams are critical measures for the prevention of foot ulcers. Daily inspection of the feet is paramount, and patients must be taught proper toenail-cutting techniques.

GASTROINTESTINAL AUTONOMIC NEUROPATHY

Autonomic neuropathy can affect every part of the gastrointestinal tract, i.e., the esophagus, stomach, small intestine, and colon. Thus, the gastrointestinal manifestations are quite variable and include dysphagia, abdominal pain, nausea, vomiting, malabsorption, fecal incontinence, diarrhea, and constipation. Diabetic patients may present with a spectrum of manifestations from mild gastrointestinal symptoms to severe clinical disease. The prevalence of symptoms caused by gastrointestinal dysfunction may reach 76% in a nonselected population of diabetic outpatients.

Esophageal Dysfunction

Esophageal dysmotility symptoms such as dysphagia, retrosternal discomfort, and heartburn are not uncommon in diabetes. Motor abnormalities include impairment of peristaltic activity with double-peak and tertiary contractions or impaired peristalsis and diminished lower esophageal sphincteric pressures. These factors may further predispose to gastroesophageal reflux disease, particularly in the setting of impaired gastric emptying. Esophageal dysfunction is detectable through esophageal motility testing and esophageal scintigraphy in diabetic patients. Clinicians should monitor patients who use drugs associated with esophageal erosion and perforation, such as the oral bisphosphonates.

Gastroparesis Diabeticorum

Diabetic autonomic neuropathy can impair both gastric acid secretion and gastrointestinal motility, causing gastroparesis diabeticorum, which can be detected in 25% of patients with diabetes. It is most often clinically silent, but the severe form is one of the most debilitating gastrointestinal complications of diabetes. The exact pathophysiology of gastric motor disturbances is not certain. It is clear that vagal parasympathetic function disturbances may occur. The release of the peptide motilin, which regulates gastrointestinal motility, is under vagal control. Motilin stimulates the initiation of phase 3 motor activity of the migrating motor complex of the stomach in patients with gastroparesis. Hyperglycemia itself may cause delayed gastric emptying in both diabetic and healthy individuals.

The typical symptoms of diabetic gastroparesis are early satiety, nausea, vomiting, abdominal bloating, epigastric pain, and anorexia. Patients with gastroparesis have emesis of undigested food consumed many hours or even days previously. Episodes of nausea and vomiting may last days to months or may occur in cycles. Upper gastrointestinal symptoms should not be attributed to gastroparesis until conditions such as gastric ulcer, duodenal ulcer, gastritis, and gastric cancer have been excluded. Even with mild symptoms, gastroparesis interferes with nutrient delivery to the small bowel and therefore disrupts the relationship between glucose absorption and exogenous insulin administration. This may result in wide swings of glucose levels and unexpected episodes of postprandial hypoglycemia and apparent "brittle diabetes." Gastroparesis should therefore always be suspected in patients with erratic glucose control.

Gastric emptying can be visualized by scintigraphic imaging after the patient consumes radionuclide-labeled food, but the scintigraphic results do not always correlate with the severity of the symptoms. The measurement of gastric emptying of solids is more sensitive than that of liquids (Table 22-4). Hyperglycemia exerts a major influence on gastric motor function in that it slows gastric emptying in diabetic patients. The [^{13}C]-octanoic acid breath

TABLE 22-4 Evaluation of the Patient with Suspected Diabetic Gastroparesis

Assessment of glycemic control

Medication history, including the use of ganglion blockers and psychotropic drugs

Gastroduodenoscopy to exclude pyloric or other mechanical obstruction

Manometery to detect antral hypomotility and/or pylorospasm

Double-isotope scintigraphy to measure solid- and liquid-phase gastric emptying; this requires techniques that require ingestion of a liquid or solid labeled with radionuclides.

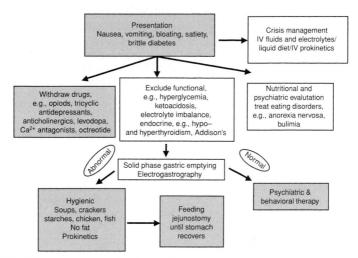

FIG. 22-4   Evaluation of patients with gastroparesis diabeticorum.

test represents a suitable measure of delayed gastric emptying in diabetic patients, which is associated with the severity of gastric symptoms but not affected by the blood glucose level. Gastroduedonal manometry may be helpful in patients with symptoms but apparently normal emptying, because it can help identify pylorospasm or incoordinate gastric and duedonal motility.

Treatment

Initial treatment of diabetic gastroparesis should focus on blood glucose control, which improves gastric motor dysfunction (Fig. 22-4). In addition, patients should be advised to eat multiple small meals (4–6 per day) and to reduce the fat content of their diet to less than 40 g/day. They should also restrict their fiber intake to prevent the formation of bezoars.

Prokinetic agents used to treat diabetic gastropathy are metoclopramide, domperidone, and erythromycin. Levosulpiride is a cholinergic and antidopaminergic agent with central antiemetic activity. Central nervous system side effects such as tremor, restlessness, tardive dyskinesia, and drowsiness limit use of metoclopramide. Other side effects observed with metoclopramide are galactorrhea and hyperprolactinemia. The recommended dosage is 10 mg four times a day, 30–60 minutes before meals and at bedtime. Metoclopramide may be given intravenously or as a liquid or suppository. Unfortunately, tachyphylaxis develops and it become progressively less effective. Periodic withdrawal restores responsiveness and should be tried in apparently refractory cases.

Domperidone is a peripherally acting dopamine 2-receptor antagonist without cholinergic activity. Domperidone has direct antiemetic activity. Central nervous side effects are observed less frequently with domperidone than with metoclopramide. The oral dose of domperidone for the treatment of gastroparesis is 20–40 mg, four times a daily, taken 30 minutes before meals, and, if necessary, at bedtime.

Erythromycin exerts its effect by stimulation of motilin receptors. Erythromycin and its derivatives improve gastric emptying of solids and liquids and increase antral contraction. Erythromycin may cause nausea, abdominal cramps and diarrhea, rash, and allergic manifestations. The oral dose of erythromycin is 250 mg three times a day, taken 30 minutes before meals. Intravenous erythromycin (3 mg/kg every 8 hours by infusion) is a useful drug for clearance of gastric bezoars.

Levosulpiride is a new prokinetic drug that is a selective antagonist for D_2-dopamine receptors. Recent studies have suggested that this medication, given at a dosage of 25 mg three times per day orally, maintained improvement in gastric emptying and improved glycemic control in diabetic subjects with gastroparesis.

If medications fail and severe gastroparesis persists, jejunostomy placement into normally functioning bowel may be needed. Satisfactory relief of intractable vomiting from diabetic gastroparesis is achieved by a percutaneous endoscopic gastrotomy or novel radical surgical procedure.

Diabetic Diarrhea

Diarrhea may be evident in 20% of diabetic patients, particularly those with known autonomic neuropathy. Autonomic neuropathy-associated diarrhea can be sudden, explosive, nocturnal, and paroxysmal. It is characterized by stool volumes greater than 300 g/day and up to 10–20 bowel movements per day. Fecal incontinence may be associated with severe diabetic diarrhea or constitute an independent disorder of anorectal dysfunction. Incontinent diabetics have decreased basal sphincteric tone, suggesting abnormal internal and external anal sphincter function. A number of factors may contribute to the diarrhea, including stasis of bowel contents with bacterial overgrowth, bile acid-induced intestinal hurry and malabsorption, and a diminution in pancreatic exocrine secretions, presumably due to the need for insulin to maintain exocrine pancreatic function and the vagal pancreatic neuropathy.

Drug-related diarrhea from agents such as metformin and acarbose should be excluded, as should lactose intolerance. Diarrhea that resolves with fasting may be osmotic, caused by ingested substances. In contrast, diarrhea that continues when the patient is not eating, such as nocturnal diarrhea, suggests that the cause is a secretory process, and neuroendocrine causes should be pursued (Table 22-5).

Treatment

Initial therapy of diabetic diarrhea should be directed toward correcting electrolyte and fluid disturbances and improving nutrition. As with all types of diabetic autonomic dysfunction, good control of glucose levels is also helpful. Antidiarrheal agents (loperamide and diphenoxylate) can reduce the number of stools, but they may also be associated with toxic megacolon and so should be used with extreme care. A broad-spectrum antibiotic (doxycyline or metronidazole) is usually the treatment of choice for bacterial overgrowth. Retention of bile sometimes occurs, which may be an irritant to the gut, and chelation of bile salts with 4 g cholestyramine four times a day, mixed with fluid and given orally, may be of considerable help. Clonidine may restore adrenergic nerve dysfunction and improve diarrhea. Initial treatment should begin with 0.1 mg twice a day. Clonidine may cause orthostatic hypotension. Octreotide slows

TABLE 22-5 Evaluation of Diarrhea in Patients with Diabetes Mellitus

---

History to rule out diarrhea secondary to ingestion of lactose, nonabsorbable hexitols, or medication (especially biguanides, α-glucosidase inhibitors and tetrahydrolipostatin).

Patients with large-volume diarrhea or fecal fat should be further studied with a 72-hour fecal fat collection: the d-xylose test is an appropriate screen for small-bowel malabsorptive disorders.

Travel and sexual histories and questioning regarding similar illnesses among both household members and coworkers.

History of prior ethanol consumption.

History of pancreatitis and biliary stone diseases.

Stools tested for occult blood, which, if present, requires follow-up upper and lower GI endoscopy.

If Crohn's disease is suspected, upper GI barium examination with dedicated small-bowel follow-through.

If history and examination suggest small-bowel disease, hydrogen breath test and Schillings test are required.
- Positive breath means lactose intolerance and/or bacterial
- Overgrowth
- Positive Schillings test may be diagnostic of bacterial overgrowth

If celiac disease is suspected, upper GI endoscopy with small bowel biopsy required

If significant steatorrhea is detected, assess pancreatic calcification with plain film of abdomen and perform formal pancreatic function tests.

Enteric pathogens and ova and parasites.

Measurement of vitamin B_{12} and folate.

---

motility and inhibits the release of gastroenteropancreatic endocrine peptides, which may be pathogenetic factors responsible for diarrhea and electrolyte imbalance in diabetic patients. Octreotide has been shown to be effective in improving diarrhea at a dose of 50–75 μg sc twice a day.

Constipation

The most common problem associated with diabetic gastrointestinal dysfunction is constipation, affecting nearly 60% of diabetic patients. Severe constipation may be complicated by perforation and fecal impaction. Before attributing constipation to diabetic autonomic neuropathy, the clinician should rule out other causes such as hypothyroidism, side effects of drugs such as calcium channel blockers or amitryptyline, and colonic carcinoma. All patients should have a careful digital rectal examination, and women should have a bimanual pelvic examination. Three stool specimens should be tested for occult blood. Anorectal manometry may be used to assess the rectal anal inhibitory reflex, which can distinguish rectosigmoid dysfunction and outlet-obstructive symptoms from colonic hypomotility.

Treatment

Treatment for constipation should begin with emphasis on good bowel habits, which include regular exercise and maintenance of adequate hydration and fiber consumption. Sorbitol and lactulose may be helpful. The intermittent use of saline or osmotic laxatives may be required for patients with more severe symptoms.

GENITOURINARY AUTONOMIC NEUROPATHY

Erectile Dysfunction

The prevalence of erectile or sexual dysfunction is about 50% in men with diabetes. Erectile dysfunction may be the presenting symptom of diabetes, and more than 50% of men with diabetes notice the onset of erectile dysfunction within 10 years of onset of the diabetes. In men, neuropathy can cause loss of penile erection, retrograde ejaculation, or both, without affecting libido, potency, or orgasmic function. Early symptoms include decreased rigidity and incomplete tumescence. Morning erections are lost, and impotence progresses gradually over a period of 6 months to 2 years. In contrast, a sudden loss of erections with a particular partner, while maintaining morning erections and nocturnal penile tumescence, suggests a psychological cause. However, psychogenic factors may be superimposed on organic dysfunction in diabetes. Importantly, erectile dysfunction is a marker for the development of generalized vascular disease and for premature death from a myocardial infarct. It may also presage a future cardiovascular event. Thus, physicians should perform cardiovascular evaluations in all diabetic patients with erectile dysfunction.

The etiology of erectile dysfunction is multifactorial. In addition to neuropathy, contributing factors include vascular disease, metabolic control, nutritional deficiencies, endocrine disorders, psychogenic factors, and drugs used in the treatment of diabetes and its complications. In diabetes, the development of autonomic neuropathy is partly responsible for the loss of cholinergic activation of the erectile process. In the penis, acetylcholine acts on the vascular endothelium to release NO and prostacylin, both of which are defective in diabetes. There is also evidence that nonadrenergic/noncholinergic nerve function is hampered, with decreased content of vasoactive intestinal polypeptide, substance P, and other vasodilatator neurotransmitters.

A thorough workup for impotence should include a medical and sexual history; physical and psycohologic evaluations; a blood test for diabetes; assays for testosterone, prolactin, and thyroid hormones; a test for nocturnal erections; tests to assess penile, pelvic, and spinal nerve function; and assessments of penile blood supply and blood pressure (Table 22-6). Physical examination must include an evaluation of the autonomic nervous system, vascular supply,

---

TABLE 22-6 Evaluation of Diabetic Patients with Erectile Dysfunction (ED)

Sexual function history (libido, erectile function, ejaculatory function, fertility)
Medication history
Assessment of glycemic control
Measurement of nocturnal penile tumescence with snap gauge
Measurement of penile blood pressure with Doppler probe; penile-brachial pressure index < 0.7 is suggestive of penile vascular disease
Sacral outflow (S2, S3, and S4) assessment which represent the sacral parasympathetic divisions (anal sphincter tone, perianal sensation)
Autonomic neuropathy testing (e.g., HRV)
Intracavernosal injection of vasoactive compound (e.g., papaverine, PGE_1), with a response of about 65–70% of the time reflecting predominantly neurogenic cause of ED and compatible with a significant arterial component.
Hormonal evaluation (luteinizing hormone, testosterone, free testosterone, prolactin)
Psychological evaluation (MMPI)

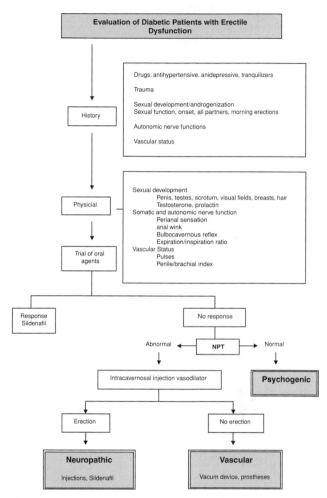

FIG. 22-5   Evaluation of diabetic patients with erectile dysfunction.

and the hypothalamic–pituitary–gonadal axis. Autonomic neuropathy that causes erectile dysfunction is usually accompanied by loss of ankle jerks and absence or reduction of vibration sense over the large toes. To determine the integrity of sacral parasympathetic divisions, the physician should assess perianal sensation, sphincter tone, and the bulbocavernous reflex. Vascular disease is usually manifested by buttock claudication but may be due to stenosis of the internal pudendal artery. A penile/brachial index of < 0.7 indicates diminished blood supply. A venous leak manifests as unresponsiveness to vasodilators and must be evaluated by penile Doppler sonography. To distinguish psychogenic from organic erectile dysfunction, nocturnal penile tumescence may be assessed. Patients with normal nocturnal penile tumescence are considered to have psyhogenic erectile dysfunction (Fig. 22-5).

TABLE 22-7 Drugs Known to Cause Erectile Dysfunction and Commonly
Used in Diabetic Patients

Antihypertensive agents
β-Blockers
Thiazide diuretics
Spironolactone
Methyldopa
Reserpine
Agents acting on the central nervous system
Phenothiazines
Haloperidol
Tricyclic antidepressants
Drugs acting on the endocrine system
Estrogens
Antiandrogens
Gonadotropin antagonist
Spironolactone
Cimetidine
Metoclopramide
Fibric acid derivatives
Alcohol
Marijuana

Treatment

Initially, the patient should be urged to forego alcoholic drinks and smoking, cease taking medications known to cause erectile dysfunction, and optimize metabolic glucose control (Table 22-7). For many men, direct injection of prostacyclin into the corpus cavernosum will produce satisfactory erections. Surgically implanted penile prostheses are also available.

Sildenafil is a GMP type-5 phospodiesterase inhibitor that enhances blood flow to the corpora cavernosae with sexual stimulation. A 50-mg tablet taken orally, 1 hour before sexual activity, is the usual starting dose. Lower doses should be considered in patients with renal failure and hepatic dysfunction. The duration of the drug effect is 4 hours. Side effects include facial flushing, headache, and dyspepsia. It is not recommended for patients with ischemic heart disease and is absolutely contraindicated in patients being treated with nitroglycerine or other nitrate-containing drugs. Severe hypotension and fatal cardiac events can occur. Tadalafil (20 mg) and Vardenafil (20 mg) are also effective in more than 60% of diabetic patients with erectile dysfunction.

Retrograde Ejaculation

Retrograde ejaculation is caused by damage to efferent sympathetic nerves that coordinate the simultaneous closure of the internal vesicle sphincter and relaxation of the external vesicle sphincter during ejaculation. Absence of spermatozoa in the semen and presence of motile sperm in a postcoital specimen of urine confirm the diagnosis. Clinically, retrograde ejeculation is of little significance unless it prevents a patient from fathering children. In that case, the patient needs to pursue assisted reproduction whereby the sperm are retrieved from the bladder for artificial insemination.

Female Sexual Dysfunction

Women may experience decreased sexual arousal or inadequate lubrication and pain during sexual intercourse. There are no guidelines for diagnosis of female sexual dysfunction, as there are for diagnosing erectile dysfunction. Some researchers have used vaginal plethysmography to measure lubrication and vaginal flushing, but the technique is not well established. Treatment usually requires application of vaginal lubricants, including topical estrogen creams. Current studies are being done on transdermal sildenafil to enhance blood flow.

Cystopathy

In diabetic autonomic neuropathy, the motor function of the bladder is unimpaired, but afferent fiber damage results in diminished bladder sensation. The bladder can become enlarged to more than three times its normal size, but the loss of sensation means that the distension causes no discomfort. Voiding frequency is diminished, and the patient is no longer able to void completely. Dribbling and overflow incontinence are common effects. A postvoiding residual volume of more than 150 mL is diagnostic of cystopathy. Cystopathy may put the patient at risk for urinary infections. More than two urinary tract infections per year should alert the physician to possible cystopathy and elicit appropriate diagnostic procedures. Postvoiding sonography can accurately and noninvasively evaluate the residual urine retained within the bladder. Postvoiding catheterization is invasive and may produce bacteriuria. Cystometrogram is the procedure of choice for evaluating both afferent and efferent bladder function (Table 22-8).

Treatment

The principal aim of the treatment should be to improve bladder emptying and to reduce the risk of urinary tract infection. Patients with cystopathy should be instructed to palpate their bladder and, if they are unable to initiate micturition when their bladders are full, to use Crede's maneuver to start the flow of urine every 4 hours. Parasympathomimetics such as bethanechol (10–30 mg three times a day) are sometimes helpful, although frequently they do not help to fully empty the bladder. Extended sphincter relaxation can be achieved with a α_1-blocker, such as doxazosin. Self-catheterization can be particularly useful in this setting, with the risk of infection generally being low. If α_1-blockade fails in males, bladder-neck surgery may help to relieve spasm of the internal sphincter. Because the somatic supply of the external sphincter remains intact, continence is preserved.

TABLE 22–8 Evaluation of Diabetic Patients with Bladder Dysfunction

Assessment of renal function
Urinary culture
Postvoid ultrasound to assess residual volume and upper urinary tract
    dilation
Cystometry and voiding cystometrogram to measure bladder sensation and
    volume pressure changes associated with bladder filling with known
    volumes of water and voiding

SUDOMOTOR DYSFUNCTION

Hyperhydrosis of the upper body and anhydrosis of the lower body is a characteristic feature of autonomic neuropathy. Hyperhydrosis associated with eating, known as gustatory sweating, may be linked with certain foods, particularly spicy foods, and cheeses. The loss of lower-body sweating can cause dry, brittle skin that cracks easily, predisposing the patient to ulcer formation that can lead to loss of the limb. For such patients, special attention must be paid to foot care.

Treatment

Glycopyrrolate (an antimuscarinic compound) may benefit diabetic patients with gustatory sweating. Intradermal injection of botulinum toxin A is also effective treatment for excessive sweating.

HYPOGLYCEMIA UNAWARENESS

The counterregulatory hormone responses and awareness of hypoglycemia are reduced in patients with diabetes mellitus. Unawareness of hypoglycemia and unresponsiveness to it are serious problems that hamper the patient's ability to manage his or her diabetes. Both are caused by impairments of the sympathetic and parasympathetic nervous systems. In most diabetic patients, catecholamine release, triggered by low glucose levels, produces noticeable symptoms such as tremulousness and cold sweat, which alert the patients to eat and take other measures to prevent coma. Diabetic autonomic neuropathy impairs catecolamine release and prevents the warning signs of hypoglycemia, leaving the patient unaware of it.

The related problem of glycemic unresponsiveness to hypoglycemia occurs when impaired autonomic responses derange glucose counterregulation during fasting or periods of increased insulin activity. In healthy people and in patients with early-stage diabetes, these autonomic responses result in the release of glucagons and epinephrine for short-term glucose counterregulation, and of growth hormone and cortisol for long-term regulation. Failure in glucose counterregulation can be confirmed by the absence of glucagons and epinephrine responses to hypoglycemia induced by a controlled dose of insulin. The glucagons response becomes impaired after 1–5 years of type 1 diabetes. After 15–30 years, the glucagons response is almost undetectable, and it is absent in patients with autonomic neuropathy.

Patients with hypoglycemia unawareness and unresponsiveness pose a significant management problem for the physician. Although autonomic neuropathy may improve with intensive therapy and normalization of blood glucose, there is a risk to the patient, who may become hypoglycemic without being aware of it and who therefore does not mount a counterregulatory response. It is our recommendation that if a pump is used, boluses of smaller than calculated amounts should be used, and if intensive conventional therapy is used, long-acting insulin in very small boluses should be given. One should not aim for normal glucose and HbA_{1c} levels in these patients, to avoid the possibility of hypoglycemia. A remarkable reduction in the frequency of severe hypoglycemia can be achieved with hypoglycemia awareness training.

PUPILLARY ABNORMALITIES

The pupillary iris is dually innervated by parasympathetic and sympathetic fibers. Patients with diabetic autonomic neuropathy show delayed or absent reflex response to light and diminished hippus, accounted for by decreased sympathetic activity and a reduced resting pupillary diameter. Autonomic neuropathy of the pupil is often apparent on routine eye examination but can be confirmed by more sophisticated testing using a pupillometer. The pupillary abnormalities do not tend to produce any significant functional defect, however, unless associated with failure of dark adaptation and difficulty with driving at night. Patients should be warned about driving at night.

RESPIRATORY DYSFUNCTION

Respiratory reflexes and ventilatory responses to hypoxia and hypercapnia are impaired in diabetic patients with autonomic neuropathy. Parasympathetic dysfunction can cause reduced airways tone. Obstructive sleep apnea is more prevalent in diabetic patients with autonomic neuropathy than in those without it. Nasal continuous positive airway pressure is an effective therapy for obstructive sleep apnea syndrome. A temporal relationship between sudden cardiac arrest and interference with normal respiration by hypoxia, drugs, or anesthesia has been reported. Sudden cardiopulmonary arrest in diabetic patients with cardiac autonomic neuropathy may be of respiratory origin due to loss of hypoxic respiratory drive.

ADDITIONAL READINGS

Spallone V, Menzinger G, Ziegler D. Diabetic autonomic neuropathy, cardiovascular system. In: Gries FA, Cameron NE, Low PA, et al (eds.). *Textbook of Diabetic Neuropathy.* New York, Thieme, 2003:225.

Vinik AI, Erbas T, Park TS, et al. Dermal neurovascular dysfunction in type 2 diabetes. *Diabetes Care* 2001;24:1468.

Vinik AI, Freeman R, Erbas T. Diabetic autonomic neuropathy. *Semin Neurol* 2003;23:365.

Vinik AI, Maser RE, Mitchell BD, et al. Diabetic autonomic neuropathy. *Diabetes Care* 2003;26:1553.

Vinik AI, Erbas T. Neurological disease and diabetes, autonomic. In: Luciano Martini (ed.). *Encyclopedia of Endocrine Diseases.* New York, Elsevier 2004:334.

For a more detailed discussion of this topic and a bibliography, please see Porte *et al: Ellenberg & Rifkin's Diabetes Mellitus,* 6th ed., Chapter 46.

23 | Somatosensory Neuropathy

Eva L. Feldman   Martin J. Stevens
James W. Russell   Amanda Peltier

Diabetic neuropathy, first identified as a clinical entity more than 200 years ago, is now the most common neuropathy in the Western world. Diabetic neuropathy is actually composed of several distinct syndromes with differing anatomic distributions, clinical courses, and possibly underlying pathogenetic mechanisms. The overall prevalence of diabetic neuropathy is approximately 50%, with a clinical course that parallels the duration and severity of hyperglycemia.

There are three general therapeutic approaches to the treatment of diabetic neuropathy. Preventive management strategies, e.g., education and hygiene, are designed to deal with potential risk factors for the development of neuropathy. Palliative management strategies are designed to alleviate specific symptoms of diabetic neuropathy, e.g., pain, foot deformities, or ulcers. Definitive therapeutic strategies are targeted against specific pathogenetic components of diabetic neuropathy. Currently, glycemic control is the only effective definitive therapy. The development of future adjunct therapies to prevent and potentially reverse the neurologic damage that underlies the clinical manifestations of diabetic neuropathy awaits clearer understanding of the pathogenetic mechanisms responsible.

EPIDEMIOLOGY, IMPACT, AND SCOPE OF DIABETIC NEUROPATHY

Estimates of the impact and frequency of diabetic neuropathy are dependent on the choice of terminology, diagnostic criteria, and study populations. In a frequently cited prospective study of over 4400 diabetic outpatients, Pirart reported an overall 12% prevalence rate of diabetic neuropathy in patients with newly diagnosed diabetes. The incidence of neuropathy increased with the duration of diabetes and, after 25 years of diabetes, over 50% of patients had diabetic neuropathy. Several cross-sectional multicenter studies of a mixed group of type 1 and 2 diabetic patients have yielded similar results. In the United Kingdom, 6487 diabetic patients were examined for the presence of neuropathy by a simple assessment of ankle reflexes, vibration, pinprick, and temperature sensation coupled with a 9-point symptoms score. The reported prevalence of neuropathy was 5% in the 20- to 29-year-old group and increased with age, reaching 44.2% in patients between 70 and 79 years of age. A simple screening tool examining ankle reflexes and great toe sensation was administered to 8757 diabetic patients, and 32.3% had abnormalities consistent with diabetic neuropathy. In the population-based Rochester Diabetic Neuropathy Study, which began in 1986, 54% of insulin-dependent and 45% of non-insulin-dependent diabetic patients had polyneuropathy, defined as two or more abnormalities, from quantitative assessment of symptoms, signs, sensation, autonomic function, and nerve conduction studies. Thus certain generalizations are clear from the available data: specifically, neuropathy is a frequent complication of diabetes, and estimated prevalence rates are on average 50% and rise with advancing age.

This high prevalence of diabetic neuropathy is associated with significant morbidity, including recurrent foot infections, ulcers, and amputations. On average, 15% of patients with diabetic neuropathy require an amputation, making diabetic neuropathy the most common cause of nontraumatic amputations in the Western world. Thus, diabetic neuropathy is generally conceded to be an extraordinarily common complication of diabetes, causing significant morbidity and related financial burden.

CLASSIFICATION OF DIABETIC NEUROPATHY

Diabetic neuropathy can be classified into two stages or classes, *subclinical* (class I) and *clinical* (class II) (Table 23-1). *Subclinical diabetic neuropathy* consists of evidence of peripheral nerve dysfunction such as slowed motor and sensory nerve conduction, elevated sensory perception thresholds that occur in the absence of clinical signs, and/or symptoms of diabetic neuropathy. *Clinical diabetic neuropathy* consists of the superposition of symptoms and/or clinically detectable neurologic deficits (Table 23-1). Clinically overt diabetic neuropathy manifests itself as the presence of one or more of the individual *clinical syndromes,* representing either *diffuse* or *focal* neuropathy. Although each syndrome has a characteristic presentation and clinical course, they frequently coexist in the same patient, often making classification of individual cases difficult.

Diffuse clinical diabetic neuropathy refers to distal symmetric sensorimotor polyneuropathy and autonomic neuropathy. *Distal symmetric polyneuropathy* is the most commonly recognized form of diabetic neuropathy and features sensory deficits and symptoms that overshadow motor involvement. Sensory deficits initially appear in the most distal portions of the extremities and progress proximally in a "stocking-glove" distribution, in the most advanced cases forming vertical bands on the chest as distal portions of truncal nerves become involved. The signs, symptoms, and neurologic deficits of distal symmetric polyneuropathy vary depending on the classes of nerve fibers. Loss of large sensory and motor fibers leads to a loss of light touch and proprioception and produces muscle weakness, while loss of small fibers diminishes pain and temperature perception and produces paresthesias, dysesthesias, and/or neuropathic pain. The other diffuse form of clinical diabetic neuropathy is *diabetic autonomic neuropathy.* This often but not always accompanies distal symmetric polyneuropathy and can impair virtually any sympathetic or parasympathetic autonomic function. This is fully discussed in Chapter 22.

The *focal forms of diabetic neuropathy* correspond to the distribution of single or multiple peripheral nerves ("mononeuropathy" and "mononeuropathy multiplex"), cranial nerves, regions of the brachial or lumbosacral plexuses ("plexopathy"), or the nerve roots ("radiculopathy"). With the exception of peripheral nerve mononeuropathies, these focal forms of diabetic neuropathy are relatively uncommon. In addition, they tend to be sudden in onset and generally self-limited. Among cranial nerves, the third cranial nerve is often affected, presenting with unilateral pain, diplopia, and ptosis with pupillary sparing in a syndrome termed "diabetic ophthalmoplegia." Diabetic ophthalmoplegia may occur in the absence of other manifestations of diabetic neuropathy, and may be bilateral, recurrent, or both. "Femoral neuropathy," typically seen in older male non-insulin-dependent diabetic patients, often involves motor and sensory deficits at the level of the lumbar plexus or lum-

TABLE 23-1 Classification and Staging of Diabetic Neuropathy

Class I: Subclinical Neuropathy*
 A. Abnormal electrodiagnostic tests (EDX)
  1. Decreased nerve conduction velocity
  2. Decreased amplitude of evoked muscle or nerve action potential
 B. Abnormal quantitative sensory testing (QST)
  1. Vibratory/tactile
  2. Thermal warming/cooling
  3. Other
 C. Abnormal autonomic function tests (AFT)
  1. Diminished sinus arrhythmia (beat-to-beat heart rate variation)
  2. Diminished sudomotor function
  3. Increased pupillary latency

Class II: Clinical Neuropathy
 A. Diffuse neuropathy
  1. Distal symmetric sensorimotor polyneuropathy
   a. Primarily small fiber neuropathy
   b. Primarily large fiber neuropathy
   c. Mixed
  2. Autonomic neuropathy (see Chapter 22)
   a. Abnormal pupillary function
   b. Sudomotor dysfunction
   c. Genitourinary autonomic neuropathy
    (1) Bladder dysfunction
    (2) Sexual dysfunction
   d. Gastrointestinal autonomic neuropathy
    (1) Gastric atony
    (2) Gall bladder atony
    (3) Diabetic diarrhea
    (4) Hypoglycemia unawareness (adrenal medullary neuropathy)
   e. Cardiovascular autonomic neuropathy
   f. Hypoglycemic unawareness
 B. Focal neuropathy
  1. Mononeuropathy
  2. Mononeuropathy multiplex
  3. Plexopathy
  4. Radiculopathy
  5. Cranial neuropathy

*Neurologic function tests are abnormal but no neurologic symptoms or clinically detectable neurologic deficits indicative of a diffuse or focal neuropathy are present. Class I, subclinical neuropathy, is further subdivided into class Ia if an AFT or QST abnormality is present, class Ib if EDX or AFT and QST abnormalities are present, and class Ic if an EDX and either AFT or QST abnormalities or both are present.

Source: Reprinted with permission from American Diabetes Association: *Diabetes,* 1988;37:1000.

bar roots as well as the femoral nerve, with the relative excess of motor versus sensory involvement differentiating diabetic "femoral neuropathy" from that seen in other conditions. Thoracic radiculopathies present as bandlike thoracic or abdominal pain that is often misdiagnosed as an acute intrathoracic or intra-abdominal emergency. The more common mononeuropathies mimic the compression neuropathies seen in nondiabetic individuals such as carpal tunnel syndrome or ulnar neuropathy. These various forms of diabetic neuropathy are listed in Table 23-2.

TABLE 23-2 Diabetes Mellitus: Potential Peripheral Nervous System Complications

---

A. Mononeuropathy or mononeuritis multiplex
   1. Isolated cranial or peripheral nerve involvement (e.g., cranial nerve III, ulnar, median [carpal tunnel syndrome], femoral, or peroneal)
   2. If confluent, may resemble polyneuropathy
B. Radiculopathy, polyradiculopathy, or plexopathy
   1. Thoracic
   2. Lumbosacral
   3. Diabetic amyotrophy
   4. Lumbosacral plexopathy
C. Autonomic neuropathy (see Chapter 22)
D. Polyneuropathy
   1. Diffuse sensorimotor
   2. Painful sensory

DIAGNOSIS AND STAGING OF DIABETIC NEUROPATHY

There are three recent areas of active investigation aimed at improving the diagnosis and classification of diabetic neuropathy: (1) the use of quantitative sensory testing and electrodiagnostic studies to quantify neural damage, (2) the use of standardized criteria to diagnose and monitor neuropathy, and (3) the development of simple neuropathy screening tools for use in outpatient clinics. This section discusses each area and presents an outpatient program for the diagnosis of neuropathy in the practitioner's office.

Quantitative Sensory Tests

Quantitative tests of nerve function are valuable in evaluating the extent, severity, natural history, and prevalence of diabetic neuropathy. They may also identify patients with unrecognized subclinical or asymptomatic clinical (e.g., signs alone) diabetic neuropathy. Vibratory perception threshold measures large nerve fiber integrity and perception and is normally poorer in the lower extremity than the upper extremity. It may be abnormal in the absence of clinical symptoms or deficits and may therefore indicate subclinical neuropathy. More frequently, abnormalities of vibration perception are associated with the loss or reduction of the Achilles tendon reflex. Abnormal vibratory perception threshold is more common than abnormal touch pressure and temperature threshold in diabetic individuals, and it may therefore be a more sensitive index of subclinical neuropathy. Patients with impaired vibratory sensation are more prone to develop foot ulceration, lending clinical significance to the impairment of vibratory perception. Thus, vibratory perception threshold is a sensitive and clinically significant index of large nerve fiber involvement in patients with diabetes.

Thermal perception threshold reflects small nerve fiber integrity. Because diminished temperature perception predisposes to accidental burns in diabetic individuals, it has important clinical implications. Both warming and cooling can be used to measure thermal perception, although the warming method may have a higher degree of sensitivity than cooling. Both methodologies have been well validated and are easy to perform.

Electrodiagnostic Studies

Nerve conduction studies are well accepted for the evaluation of diabetic neuropathy, including recent use in sequential studies to evaluate disease progression or response to treatment. These are sensitive measures, able to detect abnormalities in diabetic patients that may not be clinically apparent.

Nerve conduction studies are used to evaluate sensory and motor nerves. In these studies, measures of sensory nerve action potential (SNAP) or compound muscle action potential (CMAP) amplitude, distal latency, and conduction velocity are recorded. Amplitude measures are important in the evaluation of peripheral neuropathy, reflecting in part the size and number of nerve or muscle fibers. Conduction velocity, as used in conventional electrodiagnostic studies, reflects transmission time in the largest myelinated nerve fibers.

Electrodiagnostic Evaluation of Diabetic Neuropathy

The electrodiagnostic examination of diabetic patients must be thorough because a variety of diabetes-related peripheral abnormalities exist, including mononeuropathy, mononeuritis multiplex, plexopathy, polyradiculopathy, and sensorimotor polyneuropathy (Table 23-2). A complete evaluation allows detection and quantification of the peripheral disorder, as well as identifying the predominant pathophysiology. A standard evaluation can be outlined, (Table 23-3), although the strategy differs depending on the severity of the disorder. When symptoms or signs are minimal, evaluation is directed toward the most sensitive or susceptible nerves. In diabetic neuropathy, distal lower-extremity studies are more likely to be abnormal than upper-extremity studies, and sensory abnormalities are more common than motor abnormalities. Absent lower-extremity responses cannot be used to document subsequent progression and therefore it is important to study less involved nerves.

The needle examination is used in several ways. As a sensitive indicator of axonal degeneration, it may demonstrate the only abnormality in an early diabetic neuropathy. The electromyographer also can use needle electromyography to examine muscles inaccessible or poorly accessible to nerve conduction studies, including paraspinal, abdominal, and proximal extremity muscles. Abnormal findings in such muscles may provide evidence of polyradiculopathy (symptomatic or asymptomatic), amyotrophy, or other focal disorder. The subjective interpretation of the results of needle electromyography also allows differentiation of acute, subacute, and chronic peripheral disorders. This may be useful in identifying evidence of residual abnormalities, independent of diabetic neuropathy.

Summary

Electrodiagnostic studies are a valuable component of the overall evaluation of patients with known or suspected diabetes. Often abnormal in asymptomatic, clinically intact diabetic patients, these studies almost invariably are abnormal in the presence of clinically evident diabetic neuropathy. A normal electrodiagnostic examination makes the diagnosis of diabetic neuropathy unlikely, even in predominantly small-fiber disease. When used properly, nerve conduction studies and needle electromyography can suggest the underlying pathophysiology, monitor disease progression or improvement, or identify peripheral disorders other than neuropathy that may be causing diagnostic confusion. The use of electrodiagnostic studies in clinical trials is similarly important, although the trials must be sufficiently long to permit physiologic improvement or deterioration.

TABLE 23-3 Polyneuropathy Protocol

I. Conduction studies*
  A. General
    1. Test most involved site if mild or moderate, least involved if severe.
    2. Warm limb if temperature is < 32°C; monitor and maintain temperature throughout study.
    3. Use reproducible recording and stimulation sites (either fixed distances or standard landmarks).
    4. Use supramaximal percutaneous stimulation.
  B. Motor studies
    1. Peroneal motor (extensor digitorum brevis); stimulate at ankle and knee. Record F-wave latency following distal antidromic stimulation.
    2. If abnormal, tibial motor (abductor hallucis); stimulate at ankle; record F-wave latency.
    3. If no responses: peroneal motor (anterior tibial); stimulate at fibula.
    4. Ulnar motor (hypothenar); stimulate below wrist and elbow. Record F-wave latency.
    5. Median motor (thenar); stimulate wrist and anticubital fossa. Record F-wave latency.
  C. Sensory studies
    1. Sural sensory (ankle); may occasionally require:
      a. Needle recording
      b. Response averaging
    2. Median sensory (index); stimulate wrist and elbow. If antidromic response absent or focal entrapment suspected, record (wrist) stimulating palm.
    3. Ulnar sensory (fifth digit); stimulate wrist. If antidromic response absent or superimposed on motor artifact, perform orthodromic study.
  D. Autonomic studies
    1. Skin potential responses (palmar and plantar surfaces of hand and foot, respectively); stimulate contralateral median nerve.
  E. Additional
    1. Additional motor or sensory nerves can be evaluated if findings equivocal. Definite abnormalities should result in:
      a. Evaluation of opposite extremity
      b. Proceed to evaluation of specific suspected abnormality
II. Needle examination
  A. Representative muscles
    1. Anterior tibial, medial gastrocnemius, first dorsal interosseous (hand), and lumbar paraspinal muscles.
    2. If normal, intrinsic foot muscles should be examined.
    3. Any abnormalities should be confirmed by examination of at least one contralateral muscle.
  B. Grading
    1. Abnormal spontaneous activity should be graded subjectively (02 to 41) using conventional criteria.
    2. Motor unit action potential amplitude, duration, configuration, and recruitment graded subjectively.

*Recording sites indicated by ( ).

Standardized Criteria to Diagnose and Monitor Neuropathy

The diagnosis of *subclinical diabetic neuropathy* (Table 23-1, class I) requires the demonstration in a diabetic patient of objective measurement of peripheral neural impairment not attributable to a nondiabetic etiology in the absence of detectable clinical signs or symptoms of neuropathy. The diagnosis of *clinical diabetic neuropathy* (Table 23-1, class II) requires the demonstration in a diabetic patient of symptoms or signs plus objective measurement of peripheral neural impairment not attributable to a nondiabetic etiology. Since there are no distinguishing features unique to diabetic neuropathy, all other likely causes of peripheral neuropathy or disorders that mimic peripheral neuropathy must be excluded by careful history and physical examination and appropriate diagnostic tests (Table 23-4). Neuropathy must also accompany currently accepted diagnostic criteria for diabetes. Since neuropathic symptoms are often vague and nonspecific, confirmatory clinical signs or objective measurements of peripheral nerve dysfunction (somatic or autonomic) must be present.

OUTPATIENT DIAGNOSIS OF NEUROPATHY

The Michigan Neuropathy Program is a two-part assessment developed to diagnose and stage diabetic neuropathy in an outpatient setting. In part one, a simple 8-point clinical examination, designated the Michigan Neuropathy Screening Instrument (MNSI), is administered by a health professional (Fig. 23-1). An MNSI score of >2 indicates the presence of neuropathy with a high specificity (95%) and sensitivity (80%). The severity of neuropathy is determined in the second part of the Michigan Neuropathy Program. A focused 46-point neurologic examination is administered by a health professional (Fig. 23-2), followed by routine nerve conduction studies (sural, peroneal motor, median sensory, and motor and ulnar sensory). The severity of neuropathy is graded in each patient by a composite score consisting of the number of abnormal nerve conductions and total points from the clinical examination (Fig. 23-3). This program has been used successfully in diabetic outpatient clinics for the screening and simple staging of diabetic neuropathy.

The Semmes-Weinstein 5.07 (10-g) monofilament provides a simple screening tool for diabetic neuropathy and is recommended for this use by the International Diabetes Federation and the World Health Organization European St. Vincent Declaration. The monofilament buckles when a 10-g force is applied. In some office settings, patients are tested for the ability to sense the monofilament at 10 sites on the foot. Inability to perceive the filament correlates with an insensate foot and diabetic neuropathy. A recent study examined the variation and sensitivity of the 10 different sites and found that examining only 2 sites can provide useful information: these are sites 3 and 4, the plantar aspect of the first and fifth metatarsal heads. If a patient cannot feel the monofilament in these locations, there is a high sensitivity and specificity (80% and 86%, respectively) that the patient has diabetic neuropathy.

CLINICAL SYNDROMES OF DIABETIC NEUROPATHY

Focal Neuropathies

Focal and multifocal diabetic neuropathies with neurologic deficits confined to the distribution of single or multiple peripheral nerves are termed "diabetic mononeuropathy" and "diabetic mononeuropathy multiplex," respectively. The appearance of neurologic deficits in the distribution of focal lesions at the level of the bracial or lumbosacral plexes is termed "diabetic plexopathy," whereas those conforming to deficits at the level of nerve roots are termed "diabetic radiculopathy." When diabetic mononeuropathy or mononeuropathy multiplex involves cranial nerves, it is then termed "diabetic cranial neuropathy."

TABLE 23-4 The Differential Diagnosis of Diabetic Neuropathy

I. Distal symmetric polyneuropathy
  A. Metabolic
    1. Diabetes mellitus
    2. Uremia
    3. Folic acid/cyanocobalamin deficiency
    4. Hypothyroidism
    5. Acute intermittent porphyria
  B. Toxic
    1. Alcohol
    2. Heavy metals (lead, mercury, arsenic)
    3. Industrial hydrocarbons
    4. Various drugs
  C. Infectious or inflammatory
    1. Sarcoidosis
    2. Leprosy
    3. Periarteritis nodosa
    4. Other connective-tissue diseases (eg, systemic lupus
      erythematosus)
  D. Other
    1. Dysproteinemias and paraproteinemias
    2. Paraneoplastic syndrome
    3. Leukemias and lymphomas
    4. Amyloidosis
    5. Hereditary neuropathies
II. Pains and paresthesias without neurologic deficit
  A. Early small-fiber sensory neuropathy
  B. Psychophysiologic disorder (e.g., severe depression, hysteria)
III. Autonomic neuropathy without somatic component
  A. Shy-Drager syndrome (progressive autonomic failure)
  B. Diabetic neuropathy with mild somatic involvement
  C. Riley-Day syndrome
  D. Idiopathic orthostatic hypotension
IV. Diffuse motor neuropathy without sensory deficit
  A. Guillain-Barré syndrome
  B. Primary myopathies
  C. Myasthenia gravis
  D. Heavy-metal toxicity
V. Femoral neuropathy (sacral plexopathy)
  A. Degenerative spinal-disk disease (e.g., Paget's disease of the spine)
  B. Intrinsic spinal cord mass lesion
  C. Equina cauda lesions
  D. Coagulopathies
VI. Cranial neuropathy
  A. Carotid aneurysm
  B. Intracranial mass
  C. Elevated intracranial pressure
VII. Mononeuropathy multiplex
  A. Vasculidites
  B. Amyloidosis
  C. Hypothyroidism
  D. Acromegaly
  E. Coagulopathies

			Yes (0)	No (1)
Appearance of feet	Right	Normal	_____	_____
		If no, check all that apply:		
		_____ Deformed		
		_____ Dry skin		
		_____ Infection		
		_____ Ulceration (1)		

			Yes (0)	No (1)
	Left	Normal	_____	_____
		If no, check all that apply:		
		_____ Deformed		
		_____ Dry skin		
		_____ Infection		
		_____ Ulceration (1)		

		Present (0)	Present/reinforcement (0.5)	Absent (1)
Ankle reflexes	Right	_____	_____	_____
	Left	_____	_____	_____

		Present (0)	Decreased (0.5)	Absent (1)
Vibration perception at great toe	Right	_____	_____	_____
	Left	_____	_____	_____
		TOTAL	_____/8 pts.	

FIG. 23-1 Neuropathy screening instrument. *(Reprinted with permission from Feldman EL, Stevens MJ, Thomas PK, et al:* Diabetes Care *1994; 17: 1281.)*

Cranial Neuropathies

Isolated cranial neuropathies occur frequently in diabetic patients, especially the aged (but also rarely in diabetic children). Signs and symptoms of more generalized diabetic neuropathy may be absent, though the cranial palsies may be recurrent or bilateral. The third cranial nerve is most commonly involved, characteristically with pupillary sparing (in contrast to vascular oculomotor compression palsy, where pupillary dilatation is usually an early feature). Patients classically present with unilateral ophthalmoplegia, sparing lateral eye movement, and headache. The accompanying pain is typically intense and referred above or behind the eye, but may be mild or absent in 50% of cases. The nocioceptors responsible are thought to be either perineurial or in the adjacent first and second divisions of the trigeminal nerve, since the third nerve is essentially purely motor. Progressive diminution of pain and return of oculomotor function is the rule, even in elderly patients. Differential diagnosis includes lesions of the midbrain or posterior orbit, aneurysm of the internal carotid, cavernous sinus lesions, and tumors of the base of the brain.

Other cranial nerves that are less commonly involved in diabetic neuropathy include the sixth, the fourth (usually in combination with other cranial

Sensory Impairment

Right	Normal		Decreased		Absent
Vibration at big toe	0		1		2
10 gr filament	0		1		2
Pin prick on dorsum of great toe	Painful 0		Not Painful 2		

Left	Normal		Decreased		Absent
Vibration at big toe	0		1		2
10 gr filament	0		1		2
Pin prick on dorsum of great toe	Painful 0		Not Painful 2		

Muscle Strength Testing

Right	Normal	Mild to Moderate	Severe	Absent
Finger spread	0	1	2	3
Great toe extension	0	1	2	3
Ankle dorsiflexion	0	1	2	3

Left	Normal	Mild to Moderate	Severe	Absent
Finger spread	0	1	2	3
Great toe extension	0	1	2	3
Ankle dorsiflexion	0	1	2	3

Reflexes

Right	Present	Present with Reinforcement	Absent
Biceps brachii	0	1	2
Triceps brachii	0	1	2
Quadriceps femoris	0	1	2
Achilles	0	1	2

Left	Present	Present with Reinforcement	Absent
Biceps brachii	0	1	2
Triceps brachii	0	1	2
Quadriceps femoris	0	1	2
Achilles	0	1	2

Total: 146 points

FIG. 23-2 Diabetic neuropathy score used by the Michigan Neuropathy Program for Neurologic Examination. *(Reprinted with permission from Feldman EL, Stevens MJ, Thomas PK, et al: Diabetes Care 1994; 17:1281.)*

nerves rather than alone), and the seventh cranial nerves, presumably also on a vascular basis. Other than the third and sixth cranial nerves, there is little evidence to suggest that cranial nerve palsies occur more frequently in diabetic individuals.

VISIT		Date ___	Date ___	Date ___	Date ___	Date ___	
Abnormal Nerves	Clinical Points	Score ___	Score ___	Score ___	Score ___	Score ___	CLASS
0–1	0–6 (0,1,2,3,4,5,6)						0 no neuropathy
	>6						
	<7						
2	7–12 (7,8,9,10,11,12)						1 mild neuropathy
	>12						
	<13						
3–4	13–29 (13,14,15,16,17,18,19,20,21,22,23,24,25,26,27,28,29)						2 moderate neuropathy
	>29						
	<30						
5	30–45 (30,31,32,33,34,35,36,37,38,39,40,41,42,43,44,45)						3 severe neuropathy

FIG. 23-3   Michigan Diabetic Neuropathy Score Sheet. *(Reprinted with permission from Feldman EL, Stevens MJ, Thomas PK, et al: Diabetes Care 1994; 17:1281.)*

Mononeuropathy or Mononeuropathy Multiplex

Isolated peripheral nerve palsies occur more commonly in diabetics, but the causal and coincidental relationships are difficult to differentiate. However, 40% of unselected patients with clinically overt diffuse diabetic neuropathy have either electrophysiologic or clinical evidence of superimposed focal nerve damage at common entrapment or compression sites (e.g., median nerve at wrist and palm [carpal tunnel syndrome], radial nerve in upper arm, ulnar nerve at elbow, lateral cutaneous nerve of the thigh, and peroneal nerve at fibular head), suggesting that diffuse diabetic neuropathy predisposes to focal nerve damage. This contention is further supported by evidence that the risk of developing carpal tunnel syndrome is more than doubled in diabetic subjects. Nerves that are not commonly exposed to compression or entrapment damage occasionally demonstrate focal impairment in patients with diabetes, but this may simply reflect coincidental occurrence of diabetes and compression neuropathy.

Diagnosis of mononeuropathy or mononeuropathy multiplex should be confirmed by electrodiagnostic studies. Other nondiabetic causes of mononeuropathy, mononeuropathy multiplex, or both, should be excluded, such as vasculitides, acromegaly, coagulopathies, and hypothyroidism. Compression and entrapment palsies in diabetic patients respond to standard conservative or surgical management, that is, protection against additional mechanical trauma or surgical release procedures. Treatment of other mononeuropathies is the same as for nondiabetic mononeuropathy and is essentially supportive. Improved glucose control has been suggested, but there are no controlled data to suggest that it is specifically helpful.

Thoracic Radiculopathy (Intercostal Neuropathy, Truncal Neuropathy)

Diabetic thoracic radiculopathy presents with dermatomal pain and loss of cutaneous sensation. The syndrome may involve multiple dermatomal levels and may be bilateral in some cases. Hypesthesia or paraesthesia usually develops during the course of the disorder. Symptoms frequently are attributed to a compressive lesion such as a herniated nucleus pulposus, but radiographic studies and myelography are negative. When pain is prominent, truncal radiculopathy is frequently misdiagnosed as an acute intrathoracic or intra-abdominal visceral emergency, for example, myocardial infarction, cholecystitis, peptic ulcer, or appendicitis, with multiple fruitless diagnostic and/or exploratory surgical procedures before the correct diagnosis is recognized. Electrodiagnostic studies of the paraspinal muscles are usually diagnostic. Signs of diffuse distal symmetric polyneuropathy are often present. Spontaneous resolution of both symptoms and signs is the rule, usually within 6–24 months.

Diabetic Polyradiculopathy

In 1953, Garland and Taverner described a syndrome of pain and proximal limb weakness in diabetics, which was later called asymmetric (motor) proximal neuropathy. Among diabetic neuropathies, this syndrome, also known as diabetic amyotrophy, is second only to polyneuropathy in frequency. The pathogenesis of this syndrome is controversial and has been ascribed to lesions of the anterior horn cell, lumbar roots, lumbar plexus, or femoral nerve. Bastron and Thomas attempted to unify the diverse concepts surrounding diabetic amyotrophy by proposing that the syndrome represented a diabetic polyradiculopathy that preferentially involved the high lumbar roots L_2, L_3, and L_4. A recent study by Dyck suggests that ischemic injury secondary to microscopic vasculitis of lumbrosacral roots, plexus, and nerves underlies the disease process in both diabetic and nondiabetic patients.

In diabetics, the syndrome occurs spontaneously, with pain and sensory impairment with disabling weakness of thigh flexion and knee extension. Pain classically extends from the hip to the anterior and lateral surface of the thigh. The pain may develop insidiously or episodically, and may be worse at night. Muscle weakness most often involves the iliopsoas, quadriceps, and adductor muscles, but usually spares the hip extensors and hamstrings. The anterolateral muscles in the calf may also be involved, mimicking an "anterior compartment syndrome." Distal symmetric polyneuropathy is almost always present. Nearly complete recovery is the rule though not universal, and the syndrome may persist for several years or recur.

The syndrome may be distinguished from sciatic neuropathy by a normal straight leg-raising test. Because of the similarities between diabetic polyradiculopathy and that which occurs in association with other conditions, diabetic polyradiculopathy remains a diagnosis of exclusion: space-occupying lesions, trauma, nondiabetic vasculopathies, and skeletal abnormalities must be carefully excluded. Treatment for high-lumbar diabetic polyradiculopathy syndrome is supportive pending spontaneous recovery, although several investigators suggest that treatment with intravenous gammaglobulin may speed recovery. The beneficial effect of improved "diabetic control," though often commented on, remains unsupported.

POLYNEUROPATHY

Distal symmetric polyneuropathy is the most widely recognized form of diabetic peripheral neuropathy. The neurologic deficit is classically distributed over all sensorimotor nerves but demonstrates a distinct predilection for the most distal innervated sites in a more or less symmetric fashion. Similar distributions are shared by other "metabolic" neuropathies, including uremic and various nutritional neuropathies. Neurologic impairment begins in the most distal portions of the peripheral nervous system, usually the feet or toes, and extends proximally in both the upper and lower extremities. With continued progression, a coexisting vertical anterior chest band of sensory deficit develops as the tips of the shorter truncal nerves become involved (Fig. 23-4). Because the signs and symptoms of diabetic distal symmetric polyneuropathy are identical to those that occur in distal symmetric neuropathies of other etiologies (Table 23-4), the clinical diagnosis is one of exclusion.

Clinical Signs and Symptoms of Distal Symmetric Polyneuropathy

Usually both large and small sensory fibers are involved in the neuropathic process to a similar degree, producing a mixed sensorimotor peripheral polyneuropathy. Motor weakness is usually not marked, primarily involving the most distal intrinsic muscles of the hands and feet as a rather late feature. However, diminished deep-tendon reflexes, especially the Achilles tendon reflex, are often an early feature.

Some patients, with more selective fiber damage, present as variations of this general theme. If large fiber sensory loss predominates, patients present with impaired balance, diminished proprioception and position sense, and absent or reduced vibration sensation. Subjective symptoms of pain, paresthesia, or numbness are usually absent, and the neuropathy may present only via a late neuropathic complication such as a Charcot joint or a neuropathic ulceration (see below). With severe large fiber involvement, loss of position

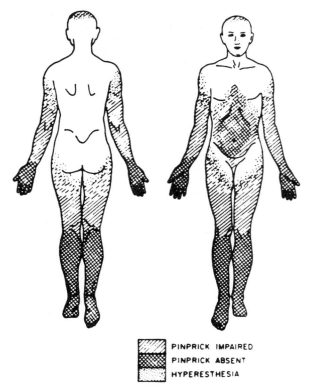

PINPRICK IMPAIRED
PINPRICK ABSENT
HYPERESTHESIA

FIG. 23-4   Sensory deficits in distal symmetric polyneuropathy. *(Reprinted with permission from Low PA, Tuck RR, Takeuchi M: in Diabetic Neuropathy, Saunders 1987:266.)*

sense may result in a sensory ataxia, which is referred to as a "pseudotabetic" form of diabetic neuropathy. In this variant, nerve conduction slowing is usually clearly demonstrable due to the involvement of the large, rapidly conducting fiber population. If the neuropathy primarily involves small sensory fibers, then the patient may present with undetected trauma of the extremities (burns of the fingers from cigarettes, or burns of the feet from stepping into hot bath water; acute abrasions and ulcerations of the feet from small objects retained inside the shoe that go undetected for prolonged periods due to insensitivity to pain, etc.). Alternatively, patients with small sensory fiber involvement may present with subjective symptoms of numbness or feelings of "cold feet" or "dead feet."

Several kinds of spontaneous pain may be associated with small fiber damage in diabetic neuropathy. Most commonly, the patients experience typical neuropathic distal paresthesias (spontaneously occurring uncomfortable sensations) or dysesthesias (contact paresthesias). Some patients complain of exquisite cutaneous contact hypersensitivity to light touch. At times the pain is described as superficial and burning, shooting or stabbing, or bone-deep and aching or tearing. Often the pains are more noticed at night, producing insomnia. At times, pain can become an overriding and disabling feature of diabetic neuropathy. Muscle cramps, which begin distally and slowly ascend, are similar to those reported in other muscle denervation disorders. Because disease involvement in these patients may be primarily confined to the small myelinated nerve fibers, conduction velocity may not be dramatically impaired, vibration sensation may be intact, motor weakness may be absent, and, if the patient's symptoms bring him or her to the physician's attention early in the course of the disease, sensory loss may not be striking. The presence of painful symptoms in the absence of striking neurologic deficit appears somewhat paradoxical, but pain may reflect increased fiber regeneration, which may commence before degeneration is sufficiently severe to present marked sensory deficit.

Complications of Distal Symmetric Polyneuropathy

The mechanical and traumatic consequences of distal symmetric polyneuropathy are largely preventable, and as such, represent a failure of medical management when they occur. Moreover, they constitute a significant risk to the neuropathic patient. Their prophylaxis is a major target of standard diabetes patient education, especially that dealing with foot care and hygiene.

Neuropathic Foot Ulceration

Traumatic damage to the skin and soft tissues of the foot occurs with great frequency in most sensory neuropathies, including diabetic distal symmetric polyneuropathy. Central to all forms of diabetic foot ulceration is insensitivity to pain, although diminished proprioception and muscle strength as well as vascular factors may play contributing roles. In the classic plantar ulcer, neurogenic atrophy of the intrinsic foot muscles, which normally tonically counterbalance the more proximal foot flexors and extensors, results in chronic flexion of the metatarsal-phalangeal joints, thereby drawing the toes into a cocked-up position (claw-toe deformity). Weight bearing is then shifted to the now uncovered metatarsal heads, leading to thinning and atrophy of the normal fat pad. In the absence of pain, thick calluses form over the exposed metatarsal bony prominences and protrude from the plantar surface of the foot, further shifting weight bearing to the metatarsal heads (Fig. 23-5). The calluses first thicken and then undergo liquefaction. The dry overlying skin breaks down, possibly reflecting in part the diminished lubrication secondary to decreased sudomotor activity of the generally accompanying autonomic neuropathy. The resulting central ulcerations may remain unnoticed in the absence of pain sensation even when secondary infection develops. Plantar ulcers, which develop when abnormal foot architecture transfers body weight onto normally non-weight-bearing areas of the foot, are usually located at callused sites of maximal walking pressure. With further architectural deformity due to neuroarthropathy or amputation, plantar ulcers may develop at alternative weight-bearing sites.

Neuropathic foot ulcers also develop at other locations in the absence of callus formation through other mechanisms. The deformed neuropathic foot does not conform well to the shape of the standard shoe, leading to pressure lesions and/or abrasions at locations other than weight-bearing sites. The generally thin dorsal dermis of the foot may be abraded within hours, so that repeated self-examinations are mandatory with new footwear or with prolonged walking or weight bearing in the absence of pain sensation.

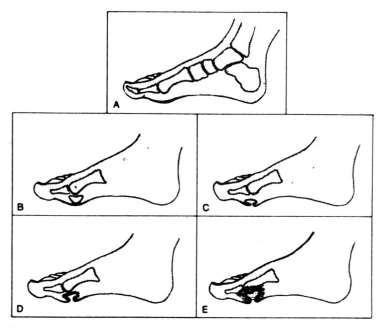

FIG. 23-5 The pathogenesis of diabetic ulcers. *(Reprinted with permission from Kwasnik E: Surg. Clin. N Am 1986: 66:305.)*

Prophylactic treatment of diabetic foot ulcers is through reinforcement of foot care education in patients with distal symmetric polyneuropathy, identification of abnormal weight bearing and/or callus formation before ulceration occurs, and prescription of appropriate behavioral and mechanical measures to reduce weight bearing. This is further reviewed in Chapter 28.

Neuroarthropathy (Charcot's Joint)

Neuroarthropathy can occur in any nervous system disease that leaves motor function relatively intact but impairs sensation. Unhealed painless fractures are often evident radiographically, and a recent history of painless trauma is frequently but not always illicited. In later stages, the disorder presents as gross architectural distortion of the foot, with shortening and widening of the joint. In its most advanced stage, there are multiple painless fractures accompanied by extensive bone demineralization and reabsorption, so that the foot appears to the examiner as "a bag of bones." As with other forms of neuroarthropathy, the pathogenetic mechanism is presumed to be multiple recurrent traumatic insults to the joint and surrounding bony structures that are not noticed by the patient because of insensitivity to pain. Increased bone blood flow due to arterio-venous shunting may also serve to weaken the bone, predisposing the foot to fractures. Prophylactic measures include reinforced education in patients with diminished pain and proprioceptive sensation, especially the avoidance of prolonged weight bearing, the wearing of cushioned shoes, avoidance of strenuous weight-bearing exercise or athletic activities, ambulating only over well-lighted smooth terrain, in well-fitting footwear. Therapy is directed at removal of continued trauma, by removing the involved extremity from weight bearing, either by decreasing ambulation or by providing other means of weight bearing, for example, a cane, crutches, or wheelchair.

TREATMENT OF NEUROPATHY

Initial treatment strategies in diabetic neuropathy consist of optimal glucose control and foot care. The Diabetes Control and Complications Trial (DCCT) provided direct evidence that optimal glucose control in insulin-dependent diabetic patients can decrease neuropathy frequency, with a reported 60% reduction in the incidence of clinical neuropathy in the combined primary- and secondary-prevention cohorts. Optimal glucose control must occur in the setting of rigorous foot care. On a nightly basis, patients are required to carefully inspect their feet for the presence of dry or cracking skin, fissures, plantar callus formation, and signs of early infection in between the toes and the toenails.

A stepwise, systematic treatment plan constitutes the best approach to a patient with painful diabetic neuropathy and has recently been reviewed in detail. Categorization of painful symptoms by duration and potential precipitating causes provides helpful prognostic indicators. Patients with symptoms of less than 6 months' duration associated with alterations in glycemic control have a good prognosis when compared to patients with chronic symptoms lasting longer than 6 months. Table 23-5 lists currently available drugs reported to have therapeutic benefits in the treatment of diabetic neuropathy. Nonsteroidal anti-inflammatory drugs can offer pain relief, especially in patients with musculoskeletal or joint abnormalities secondary to long-standing neuropathy. In this group of patients, joint deformities may actually be the primary source of pain. A double-blind, placebo-controlled, fixed-dose study revealed that both ibuprofen (600 mg four times daily) and sulindac (200 mg twice daily) provided substantial pain relief in patients with diabetic neuropathy.

The tricyclic antidepressants are the most commonly used drugs in the treatment of painful neuropathy. They act by blocking the reuptake of norep-

---

TABLE 23-5 Drugs Used in the Treatment of Painful Diabetic Neuropathy

1. Nonsteroidal drugs
   - Ibuprofen 600 mg QID
   - Sulindac 200 mg BID
2. Antidepressant drugs
   - Amitriptyline 50–150 mg at night
   - Nortriptyline 50–150 mg at night
   - Imipramine 100 mg QID
   - Paroxetine 40 mg QID
   - Trazadone 50–150 mg TID
3. Antiepileptic drugs
   - Gabapentin 600–1200 mg TID
   - Carbamazepine 200 mg QID
4. Others
   - Ultram 50–100 mg BID
   - Mexiletine 150–450 mg/QID
   - Capsacin 0.075% QID
   - Transcutaneous nerve stimulation

inephrine and serotonin, potentiating the inhibitory effect of these neuro-transmitters on nociceptive pathways. Double-blind, placebo-controlled trials have reported that both amitriptyline and imipramine relieve neuropathic pain. After 6 weeks of amitriptyline treatment, patients reported significant pain relief, independent of mood but correlating with increasing drug dosage. The side effects of amitriptyline, secondary to its strong anticholinergic proper-ties, include sedation, urinary retention, orthostatic hypotension, and cardiac arrhythmias. If side effects become intolerable, nortriptyline, which is less sedating, can be substituted for amitriptyline. Urinary retention may occur with either amitriptyline or nortriptyline, mandating a change to imipramine therapy. Two double-blind crossover studies have independently reported that imipramine improves neuropathic pain and nocturnal exacerbation of symp-toms. Additional support for the use of tricyclics for the treatment of neuro-pathic pain is provided by a recent meta-analysis of 21 trials. In patients with a significant cardiac history, amitriptyline or nortriptyline is contraindicated, and therapeutic regimens include either doxepin, the least cardiotoxic tri-cyclic antidepressant, or desipramine. The topical cream capsaicin can be added to the patient's therapeutic regimen if neuropathic pain persists in spite of treatment with maximally tolerated doses of antidepressant medication. In an outpatient setting, approximately two-thirds of diabetic patients treated with a combination of antidepressant medication and capsaicin cream experi-enced substantial relief of neuropathic pain.

Serotonin reuptake inhibitors may also alleviate neuropathic pain, but the evidence for this is less convincing than that for tricyclic antidepressants. In a randomized, double-blind, crossover study, 40 mg per day of paroxetine reduced neuropathic symptoms compared to placebo. In a double-blind, placebo-controlled study, 40 mg per day of fluoxetine was no more effective than placebo except in diabetic patients with depression superimposed on neuropathy. Open-label sertraline and trazodone are often used empirically, suggesting the possibility that these drugs may have some efficacy in treating painful diabetic neuropathy, but there are no controlled studies.

The anticonvulsants gabapentin has recently emerged as the therapy of choice for many clinicians. Gabapentin is more effective than placebo when used in doses ranging from 900 to 3600 mg per day, although the lower end of this dosage range (900 mg) may be relatively ineffective. Side effects of gabapentin therapy include dizziness, somnolence, headache, diarrhea, con-fusion, and nausea. A randomized double-blind study comparing the efficacy of gabapentin with anitryptyline found that both drugs provided equal pain relief, with no difference between mean pain score and global pain score.

In patients who experience continued pain on combination therapy (i.e., tri-cyclic or gabapentin with capsacicin), carbamazepine can be considered and added as a third drug. Dizziness, nausea, and a truncal skin rash are the com-mon side effects of this drug, although reports of leukopenia mandate that a patient have a complete blood count with differential weekly for the first month upon beginning carbamazepine therapy, and monthly for the next 3 months. Phenytoin has been used as an alternative to carbamazepine, although a double-blind, crossover study reported that phenytoin provides no significant relief of neuropathic pain in patients with diabetic neuropathy. In patients who experience continued pain on antidepressant medication or neu-rontin, capsacain cream, and carbamazepine, the carbamazepine can be dis-continued and a different third drug added to the therapeutic regimen. Choices include oral mexiletine or intravenous lidocaine, both of which are reported to improve neuropathic pain, but whose use requires clearance from a cardiologist and, in the case of lidocaine, an inpatient hospitalization with cardiac monitoring. Levodopa, γ-linolenic acid, and dextromethorphan also have reported efficacy. If neuropathic pain persists despite the outlined treatment regimen, addition of a transcutaneous electrical nerve stimulation (TENS) unit, acupuncture, or a series of local nerve blocks may be helpful, although the prognosis for pain relief in these patients is poor.

ACKNOWLEDGMENTS

The authors would like to thank Ms. Judith Boldt for excellent secretarial assistance. This work was supported by National Institutes of Health (NIH) grant RO1 NS36778 (EF), NIH grant RO1 NS38849 (EF), the Juvenile Diabetes Research Foundation Center for the Study of Complications in Diabetes (EF, MS, JR), and the Program for Understanding Neurological Diseases (PFUND).

ADDITIONAL READINGS

Arezzo JC, Zotova E: Electrophysiologic measures of diabetic neuropathy: Mechanism and meaning. *Int Rev Neurobiol* 2002;50:229.
Boulton AJ, Malik RA, Arezzo JC, et al: Diabetic somatic neuropathies. *Diabetes Care* 2004;27:1458.
Simmons Z, Feldman EL: Update on diabetic neuropathy. *Curr Opin Neurol* 2002; 15:595.
Singleton JR, Smith AG, Russell JW, et al: Microvascular complications of impaired glucose tolerance. *Diabetes* 2003;52:2867.
Vincent AM, Feldman EL: New insights into the mechanisms of diabetic neuropathy. *Rev Endo Metab Dis* 2004;5:227.

For a more detailed discussion of this topic and a bibliography, please see Porte *et al: Ellenberg & Rifkin's Diabetes Mellitus,* 6th ed., Chapter 45.

24 | Diabetic Dyslipidemia

Clay F. Semenkovich

For people with both type 1 and type 2 diabetes mellitus (T1DM and T2DM), the risk of premature death due to atherosclerosis is considerable. Atherosclerosis and its complications account for about 80% of mortality in diabetes. Dyslipidemia is common in diabetic patients and is probably a major contributor to the initiation and propagation of atherosclerotic lesions in these patients. Because of poorly understood interactions between the diabetic state and dyslipidemia, the effects of disturbances in circulating lipid levels are amplified in diabetes. Even modest abnormalities of circulating lipoproteins in diabetics disproportionately increase vascular risk. Since diabetic patients without known coronary artery disease appear to have the same risk for myocardial infarction as nondiabetic patients with previous myocardial infarction, an aggressive approach to lipid management should be considered in every patient with diabetes.

EPIDEMIOLOGY

In poorly controlled T1DM and T2DM, patients have elevated levels of triglycerides, low levels of high-density lipoprotein (HDL) cholesterol, and changes in the composition of low-density lipoprotein (LDL) cholesterol that may substantially enhance the atherogenic potential of this particle.

Regardless of the type of diabetes, the hallmark of diabetic dyslipidemia is hypertriglyceridemia. Triglyceride levels may better predict vascular risk than total or LDL cholesterol in diabetes. Triglyceride levels increase and HDL cholesterol levels decrease continuously as glucose intolerance increases in nondiabetic cohorts, suggesting that dyslipidemia predating the development of overt T2DM contributes to the high frequency of coronary heart disease present in these patients at the time of initial diagnosis.

Multiple studies indicate that the protective effect of being female with respect to heart disease is negated by diabetes. Over the past 30 years, coronary heart disease mortality in the United States has declined for the general population, but not for women with diabetes. This may be explained in part by the effects of diabetes on dyslipidemia in women. Diabetic women are more likely than diabetic men to manifest dyslipidemia, especially low HDL cholesterol.

The composition of LDL particles is frequently abnormal in people with diabetes. The most commonly described abnormality is small, dense LDL, a particle that may be particularly atherogenic. Lipoprotein particle size can be determined using specialized technology, but the utility of this testing in practice is uncertain since no prospective data show that such testing alters clinical outcomes.

Although LDL cholesterol levels are frequently not classified as elevated in people with diabetes, these "normal" LDL cholesterol levels should be considered elevated given the effects of modest hyperlipidemia in the setting of diabetes. Even at low levels, LDL cholesterol is a significant independent predictor of vascular disease, with risk increasing linearly from an LDL cholesterol concentration of 70 mg/dL.

GLYCEMIC CONTROL AND DYSLIPIDEMIA

Poor glucose control clearly exacerbates dyslipidemia. Improved glycemic control in both T1DM and T2DM improves dyslipidemia. However, most of the improvement in lipid levels occurs after early routine measures to improve diabetic control rather than later after intensive adjustment of hypoglycemic medications.

Glucose promotes hepatic lipogenesis. Since the flux of glucose through the liver is increased in T2DM, glucose alone can increase lipid content and promote dyslipidemia. Glucose can also modify lipoproteins. Like hemoglobin, which becomes glycosylated to form a marker for chronic glycemic control, components of lipoproteins such as apoB can become glycosylated. Advanced glycation end products are also found in lipoproteins from people with diabetes. These compositional changes interfere with the clearance of LDL by the LDL receptor and prolong its residence time in the circulation. Glycoxidation of LDL in the vessel wall may contribute to atherogenesis.

Type 1 Diabetes Mellitus

In a typical population of 212 people with T1DM treated with conventional therapy, a 1% decrease in glycosylated hemoglobin was associated with an 8% decrease in triglycerides. Intensive therapy of patients with T1DM (multiple daily injections or the use of an insulin pump) lowers triglycerides with near normalization of glucose levels. Changes in LDL and HDL levels are more variable.

In the Diabetes Control and Complications Trial (DCCT), intensive diabetes therapy was associated with a decrease in the incidence of retinopathy, nephropathy, and neuropathy. Triglyceride levels as well as LDL cholesterol levels were lower with intensive therapy, but HDL cholesterol did not increase. Weight gain was more common in the intensive therapy group and was associated with more small, dense LDL and lower concentrations of HDL cholesterol. Despite these potentially adverse effects on lipids, carotid intima-media thickness (a marker of atherosclerosis) showed less progression in the intensive therapy group 6 years after the completion of the trial. These data suggest that intensive insulin therapy may have beneficial effects on the vasculature that cannot be predicted by lipid levels.

Type 2 Diabetes Mellitus

Evaluating the effects of glycemic control on plasma lipoproteins in patients with T2DM is difficult because of the heterogeneous therapeutic approaches to this disease. Substantial effects on dyslipidemia are usually seen when therapy is initiated, regardless of the type of therapy. In previously treated patients for whom new therapies are added, lipoprotein effects are more modest.

Weight loss (as little as 5 kg in some studies) achieved by diet and exercise improves dyslipidemia in patients with T2DM and impaired glucose tolerance. T2DM patients gain weight when either sulfonylurea or insulin therapy is initiated. Despite this weight gain, triglycerides decrease and HDL cholesterol increases as glucose levels fall.

Metformin, an insulin sensitizer, has been available for use in the United States since 1995. It decreases hepatic glucose output and promotes insulin-mediated glucose disposal, reflecting improved insulin sensitivity. Metformin decreases triglycerides and may increase HDL cholesterol. Unlike insulin, sulfonylureas, and thiazolidenediones, metformin causes these improvements in dyslipidemia without causing weight gain. Adipose mass may actually decrease in some patients.

Thiazolidenediones are insulin sensitizers that include rosiglitazone and pioglitazone. These drugs are ligands for peroxisome proliferator-activated receptor (PPAR) gamma, a nuclear receptor that activates gene transcription, particularly in adipose tissue and macrophages. Effects of these agents on lipid metabolism are variable. One disadvantage of these compounds is that they may cause weight gain and edema.

PATHOPHYSIOLOGY

The mechanisms underlying lipoprotein abnormalities in diabetes are complex. However, many of the same mechanisms contribute to metabolic profiles in both T1DM and T2DM. In simplest terms, dyslipidemia in diabetes is caused by the lack of appropriate insulin signaling. In untreated T1DM, the defect is caused by insulin deficiency. In T2DM, the defect is caused by the combination of relative insulin deficiency and the inability of the insulin receptor to transmit its signal appropriately.

Type 1 Diabetes Mellitus

Diabetic ketoacidosis usually causes mild to moderate hypertriglyceridemia. Decreased expression of the enzyme lipoprotein lipase (LPL) appears to be mainly responsible. LPL catalyzes the rate-limiting step in triglyceride metabolism from its site at the capillary endothelium. In the setting of ketoacidosis, LPL activity is very low, leading to hypertriglyceridemia. Triglyceride levels improve rapidly with institution of appropriate insulin therapy, but mild dyslipidemia can persist for months after a bout of ketoacidosis. Insulin rapidly activates available LPL in tissues, but restoration of normal LPL expression requires chronic insulin treatment.

Although the degree of hypertriglyceridemia in diabetic ketoacidosis (DKA) is usually moderate, severe dyslipidemia can occur rarely with triglycerides exceeding 20,000 mg/dL. In this setting, triglyceride elevations may complicate initial management due to artifactual decreases in glucose and sodium.

Type 2 Diabetes Mellitus

T2DM is usually associated with obesity and insulin resistance. Insulin resistance has multiple effects on lipid metabolism, many of which are also relevant to well-controlled patients with T1DM who may have gained weight due to intensive insulin therapy:

- *Increased release of free fatty acids from fat.* The hydrolysis of triglycerides in adipocytes is mediated by hormone-sensitive lipase (HSL). HSL activity is stimulated by catecholamines, causing the release of fatty acids into the plasma. In insulin resistance caused by obesity, insulin does not suppress HSL, lipolysis occurs unchecked, and fatty acid levels are elevated.

- *Increased production of very-low-density lipoprotein (VLDL) by the liver.* VLDL is the major carrier of triglycerides. Fatty acids from the plasma are reesterified into triglycerides in the liver. Increased VLDL production driven by the synthesis of triglycerides from circulating fatty acids is probably the most important reason for dyslipidema in T2DM.
- *Decreased VLDL clearance.* LPL activity is usually normal in people with T2DM, but VLDL clearance tends to be decreased in these patients due to the increased production of VLDL. LPL becomes saturated at triglyceride levels between 150 and 250 mg/dL, preventing appropriate clearance of VLDL.
- *Increased levels of IDLs (intermediate-density lipoproteins or "remnants") and small, dense LDL.* IDLs are metabolized by hepatic lipase to LDL. Hepatic lipase activity is increased in T2DM and probably participates in the conversion of LDL to small, dense LDL.
- *Excessive modification of atherogenic lipoproteins in the vessel wall.* Oxidation of lipoproteins promotes their uptake by macrophages, leading to foam cell development. People with diabetes may be more likely to generate oxidized lipoproteins. Oxidized lipoproteins may increase vessel wall matrix components such as proteoglycans. Vascular calcification is associated with accelerated mortality in diabetes, and diabetic dyslipidemia activates osteogenic gene expression in diabetic vasculature. Oxidized lipoproteins appear to initiate an inflammatory cascade associated with the released of cytokines and the recruitment of new cells, including smooth muscle cells.
- *Abnormal postprandial lipoprotein metabolism.* After a fatty meal, chylomicrons are generated by the intestine and rapidly metabolized to chylomicron remnants (similar in composition to IDL) that are cleared by the liver. Chylomicron remnants are increased in diabetes, suggesting that atherosclerosis may in part be a postprandial phenomenon.

LIPID GOALS AND THE METABOLIC SYNDROME

Insulin resistance underlies many of the features of dyslipidemia in T2DM and may also account for some of the lipid disorders seen in treated T1DM. Several conditions associated with insulin resistance increase cardiovascular risk. When these occur together, they constitute the metabolic syndrome, a disorder that affects at least one-fourth of people in the United States. The Adult Treatment Panel III ATP (III) of the National Cholesterol Education Program has established criteria for this Syndrome (Table 24-1). Classifications for triglyceride and cholesterol levels relevant to people with diabetes are shown in Table 24-2. ATP III defines LDL cholesterol goals based on the 10-year risk for coronary events. The goal for diabetes is an LDL cholesterol less than 100 mg/dL, the same as for people with known vascular disease, because diabetics have a similarly high risk. Recent clinical data suggest that statin therapy should be considered for all diabetics, even those who present with LDL cholesterol of under 100 mg/dL (see the next page).

TREATMENT

The Chylomicronemia Syndrome

Extreme elevations of triglycerides (usually >2000 mg/dL) can cause a discrete clinical syndrome due to the presence of high concentrations of chylomicrons. The presentation can include pancreatitis, eruptive xanthomas,

TABLE 24-1 Metabolic Syndrome Diagnostic Criteria
(≥ three positive values required for diagnosis)

Risk factor	Positive value
Fasting glucose	≥ 110 mg/dL
Waist circumference	> 40 in in men > 35 in in women
Triglycerides	≥ 150 mg/dL
HDL cholesterol	< 40 mg/dL in men < 50 mg/dL in women
Blood pressure	> 130 mm Hg systolic ≥ 85 mm Hg diastolic

lipemia retinalis (the appearance of white arterioles and venules at fundoscopy), dyspnea, hepatosplenomegaly, and neurologic defects such as memory loss and carpal tunnel syndrome.

Most patients with the chylomicronemia syndrome have diabetes, but only a small percentage of people with diabetes develop this syndrome. People with diabetes and an underlying genetic hyperlipidemia are most likely to be affected. Familial combined hyperlipidemia (FCH) is a common contributor. FCH, present in about 1–2% of Western populations, is characterized by the overproduction of hepatic lipoproteins. Other common antecedents of chylomicronemia are obesity, ethanol, oral estrogens, hypothyroidism, thiazide diuretics, some β-adrenergic-blocking agents, gluococorticoids, and retinoids.

In patients with the chylomicronemia syndrome, conservative therapy for the routine management of pancreatitis is indicated. The cessation of oral intake, the use of intravenous hydration, and treatment of hyperglycemia with insulin usually result in striking decreases in triglycerides within days.

Clinical Trials Supporting the Use of Lipid-Lowering Medications in Diabetes

Several trials support the use of lipid lowering to decrease vascular risk in people with diabetes (Table 24-3). It was not until 2002 that results from the first lipid-lowering clinical trial directly relevant to diabetes became avail-

TABLE 24-2 Adult Treatment Panel III Triglyceride Classifications and Lipid Goals for Patients with Diabetes

Triglycerides
- Very high triglycerides   > 500 mg/dL
- High triglycerides   200–499 mg/dL
- Borderline high triglycerides   150–199 mg/dL
- Normal triglycerides   < 150 mg/dL

Lipid goals
- LDL cholesterol goal is < 100 mg/day
- Calculate non-HDL cholesterol (total cholesterol minus HDL cholesterol) in patients with high triglycerides; non-HDL cholesterol goal is < 130 mg/dL
- No specific target for HDL cholesterol

TABLE 24-3 Summary of Major Lipid-Lowering Clinical Trials Including Patients with Diabetes

Trial	Medication	Subjects with diabetes	Baseline lipid values for diabetics	Lipid outcomes	Clinical outcome compared with placebo group
MRC/BHF Heart Protection Study	Simvastatin (HMG-CoA reductase inhibitor)	5963 (70% men), 2912 with no known vascular disease	LDL: 124 mg/dL Triglycerides: 204 mg/dL HDL: 41	LDL ↓ 28% Triglycerides ↓ 13% HDL ↑1%	27% ↓ in first MI or coronary death 24% ↓ in first nonfatal or fatal stroke
Scandinavian Simvastatin Survival Study (4S)	Simvastatin	202 men and women (plus 281 with undiagnosed diabetes at entry), all with known vascular disease	LDL: 176 mg/dL Triglycerides: 153 mg/dL HDL: 42	LDL ↓ 36% Triglycerides ↓ 11% HDL ↑7%	37% ↓ in vascular events in diabetics; trend favoring lower total mortality in treated diabetics
Cholesterol After Recurrent Events (CARE) Trial	Pravastatin	586 men and women with known vascular disease	LDL: 136 mg/dL Triglycerides: 164 mg/dL HDL: 38	LDL ↓ 27% Triglycerides ↓ 13% HDL ↑4%	25% ↓ in coronary events in diabetics
Veterans Affairs HDL-Intervention Trial (VA-HIT)	Gemfibrozil (fibrate)	630 men with known vascular disease	LDL: 111 mg/dL Triglycerides: 161 mg/dL HDL: 32 (for entire study group)	LDL no change Triglycerides ↓ 31% HDL ↑ 6%	24% ↓ in coronary death or stroke in diabetics

able. The MRC/BHF Heart Protection Study enrolled people with diabetes, preexisting coronary disease, or preexisting peripheral arterial disease to take 40 mg simvastatin, an HMG-CoA reductase inhibitor, or placebo. Ninety percent of the 5963 diabetics in the study had type 2 diabetes and 2912 had no known vascular disease. Simvastatin therapy was safe and well tolerated. Its use substantially decreased the risk of coronary events, stroke, and revascularization. Substantial benefits were seen in diabetics of both sexes, those without known coronary disease at the beginning of the trial, and in those with low LDL cholesterol levels. These data strongly suggest that statin therapy should be considered for all people with diabetes, even in those with an LDL < 100 mg/dL. The issue of whether the LDL cholesterol goal should be even lower than 100 mg/dL is currently being addressed in clinical trials.

Post-hoc analyses of other trials that included subsets of diabetic subjects also support the use of lipid lowering to decrease vascular risk in people with diabetes (Table 24-3). Some of the major trials include the following.

• The Scandinavian Simvastatin Survival Study (4S). This study enrolled individuals with known vascular disease. The trial included 202 men and women with known diabetes, an additional 281 individuals who did not carry a diagnosis of diabetes but had fasting glucose levels consistent with that diagnosis, and 678 patients with impaired fasting glucose. There were substantial clinical benefits for patients with diabetes and abnormal glucose metabolism, and an economic analysis of the trial showed that simvastatin caused the greatest decrease in cardiovascular disease-related hospital days in people with diabetes.
• The Cholesterol and Recurrent Events (CARE) Trial also showed beneficial effects of using an HMG-CoA reductase inhibitor, pravastatin, in both men and women diabetics with known vascular disease.
• The Veterans Affairs HDL Intervention Trial (VA-HIT) used gemfibrozil, a fibrate drug, in men with vascular disease and low levels of HDL. There was no effect of drug treatment on LDL cholesterol levels, but HDL levels increased and triglyceride levels decreased, and coronary death as well as stroke decreased in those treated with gemfibrozil.

Dyslipidemia Management

The results of the UK Prospective Diabetes Study (UKPDS) indicated that glycemic control has clear beneficial effects on microvascular disease but marginal effects on macrovascular disease. One explanation is that some interventions lower glucose without affecting insulin resistance, a proatherogenic condition. Metformin-treated patients tend not to gain weight and have a reduction in insulin resistance as well as lower levels of triglycerides, making metformin a useful agent for glucose lowering in dyslipidemic T2DM patients with normal serum creatinine. In addition, a small subset in the UKPDS had a reduction in cardiovascular endpoints.

Diet and exercise counseling are indicated for every person with diabetes. Exercise is generally required for sustained weight loss. It improves dyslipidemia and is known to increase the expression of LPL in human muscle. A graded exercise test is appropriate for sedentary diabetics over the age of 35 before beginning an exercise program. Lower-extremity-protective sensation should be assessed, and non-weight-bearing exercises such as cycling, rowing, or swimming recommended for those with sensory defects. It may be helpful to keep a record of physical activity analogous to recording home blood glucose results. Lifestyle interventions show that diet and exercise are superior to metformin at reversing disorders associated with insulin resistance.

Dyslipidemia frequently persists even with excellent glycemic control. Given the risk of coronary events in diabetics, including those with no history of vascular disease, treating dyslipidemia with medications should be considered in every person with diabetes soon after diagnosis.

Very High Triglycerides: > 500 mg/dL

These patients are at risk for pancreatitis. Restriction of dietary fat in consultation with a dietician is indicated. Insulin is recommended to lower glucose levels.

Fibric acid derivatives such as gemfibrozil (600 mg twice a day taken 30 minutes before meals) or fenofibrate (160 mg once a day with meals) are indicated.

Fish oil capsules (containing *n*-3 polyunsaturated fatty acids) can be helpful. Fish oil (supplied as 1-g capsules containing at least 300–500 mg of docosahexanoic acid and eicosapentanoic acid) should be administered as 1 capsule twice a day with food and gradually increased to a total of 6–10 capsules a day. Gastrointestinal side effects are common.

Niacin (see below) may also be useful.

It is unlikely that these patients will achieve normal triglyceride levels in the absence of striking changes such as considerable weight loss.

High Triglycerides: 200–499 mg/dL

Fibrates (gemfibrozil or fenofibrate; see above for doses) are appropriate. These drugs are ligands for the nuclear receptor PPARalpha. They lower triglycerides and increase HDL cholesterol. LDL cholesterol may increase modestly with fibric acid therapy. These agents increase the lithogenicity of bile and should be used cautiously in patients with gallstones. Gastrointestinal side effects and erectile dysfunction can occur. The drugs displace warfarin from its binding sites; clotting parameters must be monitored closely, and most patients will require a reduction in warfarin dose. Hepatic dysfunction and myositis can occur, especially when fibrates are used in combination with other lipid-lowering agents.

In the patient already being treated with insulin, extended release niacin is an alternative. Niacin appears to work by decreasing the release of fatty acids from adipocytes, thereby decreasing VLDL synthesis. It is the most potent agent for increasing HDL cholesterol. Niacin increases glucose, which can be treated by increasing the insulin dose. Flushing is common but not serious for most patients. It can be minimized by taking aspirin before each dose, taking the medication with a small snack before bedtime, and by avoiding alcohol, spicy foods, and hot beverages. More serious side effects include hyperuricemia, hepatitis, and myositis. A once-nightly extended-release form of niacin (Niaspan) appears to be tolerated well. Doses should be gradually increased to 1500–2000 mg a day at bedtime. Niacin is contraindicated in gout and liver disease.

Statins (see below) may be an option, but the effects on triglycerides are variable in this group.

Borderline High Triglycerides: 150–199 mg/dL

Statin drugs (HMG-CoA reductase inhibitors) are the drugs of choice for this group, particularly in those patients who have not achieved their LDL cholesterol goal (see Table 24-2). Indeed, based on Heart Protection Study data, it is reasonable to consider statin therapy in all patients with diabetes, regardless of LDL cholesterol concentrations and barring any contraindications. These drugs inhibit the synthesis of cholesterol, causing the induction of LDL receptors in the liver and increased clearance of lipoproteins. At higher doses, all statins also lower triglycerides. The mechanism may be a combination of enhanced clearance of VLDL particles through the LDL receptor and inhibition of VLDL secretion. Statins also modestly elevate HDL levels.

Simvastatin at 40 mg (given with food in the evening), atorvastatin 20 mg (given with food at any time during the day), and pravastatin 40 mg (taken at bedtime on an empty stomach) may be effective. Rosuvastatin, recently approved for use in the United States, may be useful in some patients. The starting dose is 10 mg, but clinical experience is limited. Patients may complain of sleep disturbances or difficulty concentrating with some statins; pravastatin does not penetrate the central nervous system and may be an option for these individuals. Muscle aches with completely normal muscle enzymes (CPK and aldolase) are common with statin use. The etiology of this effect is unknown. Some patients improve when a different statin drug is used.

Statins rarely cause significant liver dysfunction and myositis. Risk increases with concomitant use of erythromycin, cyclosporine, antifungal agents, and protease inhibitors used to treat HIV infection. The risk is also increased in patients treated with statins in addition to other lipid-lowering medications such as fibrates or niacin.

Patients with dyslipidemia and established coronary heart disease are at high risk for subsequent vascular events. Many experts use combinations of lipid-lowering drugs to reach therapeutic goals. The combination of a statin with niacin may be considered in the patient at very high risk for coronary events who is taking insulin for glucose control. Some experts combine a fibrate such as fenofibrate at 160 mg in the morning with simvastatin at 20 mg in the evening. High doses of statins should be avoided in combination regimens. With combination therapy, liver function tests should be followed regularly, and patients should be warned about the symptoms of myositis and hepatitis. Combination therapy should not be used in patients with significant renal dysfunction or in those taking cyclosporine. Combination therapy with the fibrate gemfibrozil and the statin cerivastatin recently caused a high rate of rhabdomyolysis and caused cerivastatin to be withdrawn from the market.

Normal Triglycerides: <150 mg/dL

Statins are the drugs of choice in this group, particularly in those patients who are not at target LDL. As mentioned above, statin therapy regardless of lipid levels is now a reasonable approach in all patients with diabetes. Bile acid sequestrants are available, but they can increase triglyceride levels, are not as potent as statins for lowering cholesterol, and are not tolerated as well as statins.

In those who are statin-intolerant, ezetimibe at 10 mg a day is an option. This agent inhibits the absorption of dietary cholesterol. It was approved for use in combination with statins, and it may lower triglycerides in addition to LDL in this setting. Use with fibrates is not currently recommended.

Summary of Treatment Recommendations

Diabetics are at high risk for atherosclerotic complications. Treating dyslipidemia decreases the risk of these complications. Decreasing vascular risk requires a multifaceted approach (Table 24-4). Current data indicate that for most people with diabetes, treatment should include a statin regardless of cholesterol level.

TABLE 24-4 Methods to Decrease Vascular Risk in Patients with Diabetes

Statin therapy regardless of initial cholesterol*
Angiotensin-converting enzyme (ACE) inhibitor or angiotensin II receptor
   blocker (ARB)*
Smoking cessation
Identification of realistic goal for weight loss
Diet
Exercise, daily if possible
Optimized glycemic control
Aspirin*
β-Adrenergic receptor blocker in those with known coronary disease*

*For most patients in the absence of specific contraindications.

ACKNOWLEDGMENTS

This work was supported in part by National Institutes of Health grant HL58427.

ADDITIONAL READINGS

Executive summary of the third report of the National Cholesterol Education Program (NCEP) Expert Panel on Detection, Evaluation, and Treatment of High Blood Cholesterol in Adults (Adult Treatment Panel III). *JAMA* 2001;285:2486.

Knopp RH: Drug treatment of lipid disorders. *N Engl J Med* 1999;341:498.

MRC/BHF Heart Protection Study of cholesterol-lowering with simvastatin in 5963 people with diabetes: A randomized placebo-controlled trial. *Lancet* 2003;361:2005.

Nathan DM, Lachin J, Cleary P, et al: Intensive diabetes therapy and carotid intima-media thickness in type 1 diabetes mellitus. *N Engl J Med* 2003;348:2294.

UK Prospective Diabetes Study (UKPDS) Group: Effect of intensive blood-glucose control with metformin on complications in overweight patients with type 2 diabetes (UKPDS 34). *Lancet* 1998;352:854.

For a more detailed discussion of this topic and a bibliography, please see Porte *et al: Ellenberg & Rifkin's Diabetes Mellitus,* 6th ed., Chapter 47.

25 | Hypertension and Diabetes

Norman M. Kaplan

Hypertension and diabetes frequently coexist, in large part due to underlying obesity. Hypertension is found in over 70% of all patients with diabetes. Also, the risk for developing diabetes is almost doubled by the presence of hypertension, even among nonobese people with blood pressure > 130/85 mm Hg. When diabetes and hypertension coexist, cardiovascular–renal complications occur at a much higher rate—at least twofold overall and manyfold for nephropathy.

There may be an obvious explanation for some of the increased prevalence of hypertension, nephropathy, and diabetes: hyperglycemia during pregnancy reduces nephrogenesis in the fetus. Therefore, infants of women with abnormal glucose tolerance or overt diabetes might then be susceptible to more hypertension, diabetes, and nephropathy later in life.

Beyond the possible contribution of impaired fetal development, there are a number of other reasons for the increasing prevalence of diabetes and hypertension. These include:

- Advancing age of the population
- Rapid growth of more susceptible populations, including Hispanics and African-Americans
- Prolonged survival of type 1 diabetics
- Expanding reach of medical care
- Increasing prevalence of obesity due to decreased physical inactivity and increased caloric intake

THE PREDOMINANT ROLE OF OBESITY

The current U.S. population is likely the most obese of all time. Obesity, defined as a body mass index (BMI) > 30 kg/m^2, increased from 12% of U.S. adults in 1991 to 30% in 2000. The increase occurred in virtually every part of the population, among men and women, from the teens to old age, in all races and socioeconomic strata. With increasing BMI, type 2 diabetes increases markedly. A 5-kg weight gain doubles the risk for diabetes, and the risk increases with the duration of excess weight. Not surprisingly, cardiovascular mortality correlates with increasing BMI, with about 300,000 annual deaths attributable to obesity in the United States.

The problem begins in early childhood, when increasing weight is associated with hyperinsulinemia and increasing blood pressure and dyslipidemia, particularly in those with greater central (visceral or abdominal) adiposity.

Prevention of weight gain in adults is difficult; it may be easier in children if they can be kept physically active. Meanwhile, greater attention must be given to those who are both diabetic and hypertensive. Moreover, with tighter control of the hyperglycemia of both type 1 and type 2 diabetes, the associated weight gain may increase both blood pressure and dyslipidemia.

Recently published guidelines have emphasized the need both for earlier intervention at even lower levels of blood pressure for hypertensives with diabetes and for more intensive therapy. Therapy should be started when the blood pressure (BP) exceeds 130/80, and BP should be reduced to below this target.

ASSESSMENT OF BLOOD PRESSURE

Before therapy is begun, the presence of usually elevated blood pressure must be carefully ascertained. Such ascertainment should include out-of-the-office readings.

Out-of-Office Measurements

As with all patients, out-of-the-office measurements are needed both to establish the diagnosis and to monitor the management. White-coat hypertension is common, particularly among young type 1 diabetics, and if not recognized, may lead to misdiagnosis.

Ambulatory monitoring (ABPM) is best but likely will remain unavailable because third-party payers reimburse poorly or not at all. With ABPM, the common lack of nocturnal "dipping" in BP in patients with diabetes can be recognized and should lead to more intensive control of the blood pressure.

Recognition of Postural Hypotension

All patients with diabetes, particularly if over age 60, should have their blood pressure measured supine and standing, since postural and postprandial hypotension is common in this population and carries with it certain hazards. In 204 subjects with type 2 diabetes, average age 58, postural hypotension was found in 28.4% and postural dizziness in 22.5%.

If it is present, postural and postprandial hypotension must be managed before supine and seated hypertension is treated (Fig. 25-1).

NONPHARMACOLOGIC THERAPY

Therapy for all hypertension should begin and continue with lifestyle modifications, even more so in the typically obese patient with type 2 diabetes (Table 25-1). Despite the obvious attraction of lifestyle changes, they are difficult to accomplish and may not be as protective as drug therapy. The high cardiovascular risk of even mild type 2 diabetes almost mandates early and intensive antihypertensive drug therapy.

Weight Loss

Weight loss lowers blood pressure at least in part by improving insulin sensitivity.

Exercise

Those who are sedentary and unfit develop more diabetes, whether lean or obese. Just walking, without more vigorous activity, reduces the risk for diabetes and will lower blood pressure. The manner by which exercise helps both diabetes and hypertension goes beyond a decrease in body weight. Exercise increases glucose uptake into skeletal muscles, by making them more insulin-sensitive. The additional benefits of exercise in patients with diabetes include improvement in glycemic control, lowering of blood pressure, reduction in levels of triglyceride-rich very-low-density lipoprotein (VLDL), probable improvement in fibrinolytic activity, and reduction in overall cardiovascular disease risk.

CASUAL FACTOR	PATHOPHYSIOLOGY	THERAPY
Rapid rising	Pooling blood in lower body	Slow rising, particularly from sleep
Vasodilation	Venous pooling Splanchnic poolin Sympatholytic drugs	Supporttive pantyhose Avoid large meals Avoid such agents
Volume depletion	Low cardiac output • Diuretic • Very low sodium intake	Maintain intravascular volume by avoiding overdiuresis and sleeping with head of bed elevated
Baroreflex dysfunction	Loss of normal vasoconstriction by sympathetic stimulation	Drinking 16 oz of water before arising Various drugs: • Sympathomimetics • Volume expanders Isometric exercise
Cerebrovascular disease	Low cerebral prefusion	Avoid overtreatment of hypertension Correct dyslipedemia Stop smoking

FIG. 25-1 Summary of the pathophysiologic events that occur during the development of symptoms of postural hypertension *(middle column)* and the interaction of exacerbating factors *(left column)* and remedial measures *(right column)* with these events.

Moderate Sodium Reduction

Moderate sodium reduction is both safe and effective, perhaps even more in those diabetic patients whose hypertension is related to volume expansion from the renal impairment of nephropathy. Moreover, the antiproteinuric effect of angiotensin-converting enzyme (ACE) inhibitors is markedly enhanced by a lower sodium intake. Even without nephropathy, it is prudent for all patients with diabetes to reduce their sodium intake, since insulin-resistant subjects have an impaired natriuretic response to high sodium intake.

TABLE 25-1 Lifestyle Modifications for Hypertension Prevention and Management

Weight loss if overweight
Increase in aerobic physical activity
Reduction of sodium intake to no more than 100 mEq/day
Maintaining adequate dietary potassium and magnesium intake
Smoking cessation
Reduction in dietary saturated fat and cholesterol

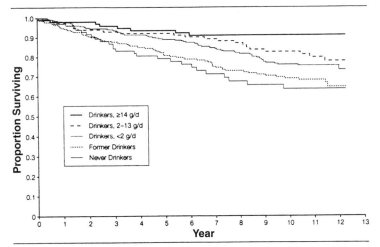

FIG. 25-2 Survival curves for coronary heart disease mortality over 13 years according to alcohol intake in 983 older-onset diabetic persons in the Wisconsin Endemiologic Study of Diabetic Retinopathy. *(Reprinted with permission from Valmadrid CT, Klein R, Moss SE, et al: JAMA 1999; 282:239.)*

Moderate Alcohol Consumption

Diabetic patients have been found to enjoy a protective effect against coronary artery disease by regular, moderate alcohol consumption (no more than 2 drinks a day), similar to that seen in other groups of individuals (Fig. 25-2). In addition to multiple other mechanisms for cardioprotection provided by alcohol, insulin sensitivity may be improved.

The type of alcoholic beverage is likely irrelevant: wine drinkers have the lowest risk for coronary disease, likely because of their healthier lifestyles; red wine drinkers have no greater protection than white wine drinkers.

Cessation of Smoking

As the most important lifestyle feature to be addressed, smoking may markedly aggravate insulin resistance in type 2 diabetics.

Dietary Fiber

Increased dietary fiber intake has been associated with lower body weight, lower waist-to-hip ratio, lower fasting insulin, lower blood pressure, and better lipid profiles.

ANTIHYPERTENSIVE DRUG THERAPY

The best documentation of the need to lower diastolic blood pressure in diabetics to or below 80 mm Hg comes from the Hypertension Optimal Treatment (HOT) trial. Among the 19,000 participants in the trial, the only significant

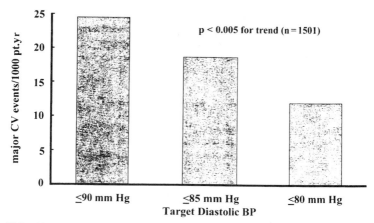

FIG. 25-3 The risk for major cardiovascular events in the 1501 diabetic patients in the HOT study according to the fertile of the target diastolic blood pressure level. *(Adapted from Hansson L, Zanchetti A, Carruthers SG, et al: Lancet 1998; 351:1755.)*

benefit of reducing diastolic blood pressure to near 80 mm Hg was seen among the 1501 diabetic hypertensives. They achieved a greater than 50% reduction in major cardiovascular events (Fig. 25-3). As in the HOT trial, to achieve the necessary goal of blood pressure < 130/80 mm Hg will typically require two or more antihypertensive drugs.

In the population of 3642 patients with newly diagnosed type 2 diabetes screened for the United Kingdom Prospective Diabetes Study (UKPDS) but not entered into the trial, a progressive reduction in major cardiovascular events was seen with progressive reduction of systolic blood pressure from over 160 mm Hg to 110 mm Hg accomplished by various antihypertensive drugs.

To properly address concomitant risk factors, multiple nondrug and drug therapies will be needed. The benefits of such intensive therapy are impressive. In one trial, 160 diabetics were randomly assigned to standard or more intensive therapy, the latter requiring a blood pressure below 140/85, HbA1c below 6.5%, total cholesterol below 5 mmol/L, and the use of ACE inhibitors, aspirin, plus multiple lifestyle modifications. At the end of the 7.8 years mean follow-up, those on intensive therapy achieved major benefits (Fig. 25-4). Such intensive therapies, though costly, not only reduce morbidity and mortality but also lower lifetime medical costs.

Antihypertensive Drugs

For those diabetic hypertensives without proteinuria, a low-dose diuretic may be the appropriate first choice, with an ACEI or angiotensin II-receptor blocker (ARB) as second drug and a long-acting calcium antagonist (CA) as third. Both β-blockers and α-blockers may also be indicated. Rarely, central α_2-agonists may be useful. For those with proteinuria, addressed further in Chapter 21, an ACE inhibitor or an ARB is mandatory.

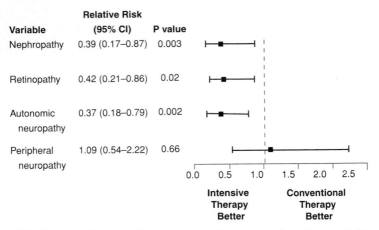

FIG. 25-4 Relative risk of the development or progression of nephropathy, retinopathy, and autonomic and peripheral neuropathy during the average follow-up of 7.8 years in the intensive-therapy group, as compared with the conventional-therapy group. *(Adapted from Gæde P, Vedel P, Larsen N, et al:* N Engl J Med *2003; 348:383.)*

Diuretics

Low doses, i.e., 12.5 mg of hydrochlorothiazide, are effective and safe in diabetes, as shown in the SHEP trial. A thiazide diuretic should be almost always included in the regimen, and loop diuretics should be given to those with serum creatinine above 1.5 mg/dL.

β-Blockers

Despite their potential to aggravate diabetes in various ways, β-blockers are mandatory for those who survive a myocardial infarction and those who have severe heart failure.

α-Blockers

In addition to their ability to relieve the symptoms of prostatism, α-blockers have the advantage over other classes of reducing insulin resistance and improving dyslipidemia.

Calcium Antagonists

Despite prior concerns about the safety of CAs, particularly the dihydropyridines (DHPs) and particularly in diabetic hypertensives, these drugs have now been proven to be both safe and effective as second and third agents in the treatment of both type 1 and type 2 diabetes, either with or without nephropathy (Table 25-2). As one example, in the Irbesartan Diabetic Nephropathy Trial, the ARB provided better renal outcomes but amlodipine was equal to the ARB in overall cardiovascular protection (Fig. 25-5).

As to their putative effect to increase coronary disease risk, the problem appears to be unique to large doses of short-acting agents and does not apply to long-acting agents. The safety of long-acting CAs in patients with coronary disease was further documented in a 1-year follow-up of over 51,000 patients who were prescribed one of these agents after surviving an acute myocardial infarction. Their relative likelihood of 1-year mortality was no different than among those not prescribed a long-acting CA.

Further evidence for the efficacy and safety of DHP CAs is provided by the excellent protection found in the Syst-Eur study with nitrendipine, which was greater than that found in a similar group of hypertensive diabetic patients given a diuretic in the SHEP trial (Fig. 25-6). The comparability of the two groups of diabetic hypertensives is shown by the similar rates of various cardiovascular events in the placebo groups of each study, shown on the right in the figure. In those who were treated, the nitrendipine-based regimen in Syst-Eur provided even better protection than did the chlorthalidone-based SHEP regimen.

In addition, there was a significant reduction in cardiovascular events in the 1501 patients with diabetes given felodipine-based therapy in the HOT trial (see Fig. 25-3). Perhaps most impressively, in the massive ALLHAT trial with over 15,000 diabetics enrolled, the results showed: "For the important diabetic population, lisinopril appeared to have no special advantage and amlodipine no particular detrimental effect for most CVD [cardiovascular disease] and renal outcomes when compared to chlorthalidone."

The data now available in diabetics without nephropathy provide no clear evidence that one class of drug is superior, although calcium channel blocker (CCB)-based therapy has been associated with fewer events than either diuretic- or angiotensin-converting-enzyme inhibitor (ACEI)-based therapy. Indeed, either DHP CAs or non-DHP CAs are frequently needed to control the hypertension in most diabetic patients, particularly to prevent the progression of renal damage. These agents may confer a renoprotective effect even if they do not reduce proteinuria as well as other drugs.

Angiotensin-Converting-Enzyme Inhibitors

An ACEI should always be used for those with proteinuria, including normotensive diabetics with microalbuminuria, because of increasing evidence that such therapy slows the development of nephropathy. Whether an ACEI should also be the routine first drug for all diabetics without microalbuminuria is less certain but has been proposed by many authorities.

The renin–angiotensin system may be set inappropriately higher in patients with type 2 diabetes and less suppressed by high sodium intake. Therefore, there is a theoretical reason to use ACEIs. Certainly, ACEIs have been found to be protective in diabetic patients who have survived a myocardial infarction. In the Heart Outcomes Prevention Evaluation (HOPE) trial, the 9297 patients with known cardiovascular disease included 38% with diabetes; over the 4–6-year follow-up, a 17% risk reduction for diabetic complications was reported for those given the ACEI ramipril compared to those assigned to placebo.

As attractive as they are, ACEIs are not without risk. They interfere with useful actions of angiotensin II such as vasodilator responses in skeletal muscle arterioles, may lead to hyperkalemia and worsen renal function in patients with overt diabetic nephropathy, and are frequently associated with a troublesome cough. Rarely these agents may also result in angioedema.

TABLE 25-2 Relationship between Blood Pressure Lowering and Risk of Cardiovascular Disease in Patients with Diabetes

Trial	No. of patients	Blood pressure control		Initial therapy	Outcome	Risk reduction (%)
		Less tight	Tight			
SHEP, 1996	583	155/72*	143/68*	Chlorthalidone	Stroke	NS
					CVD events	34
					CHD	56
Syst-Eur, 1999	492	162/82	153/78	Nitrendipine	Stroke	69
					CV events	62
HOT, 1998	1501	144/85	140/81	Felodipine	CV events	51
					MI	50
					Stroke	NS
					CV mortality	67
UKPDS, 1999	1148	154/87	144/82	Captopril or atenolol	Diabetes-related endpoints	34
					Deaths	37
					Strokes	44
					Microvascular endpoints	37
Micro-Hope, 2000	3577	Changes in systolic (2.4 mm Hg) and diastolic (1.0 mm Hg)		Ramipril vs placebo	CV events	25
					CV mortality	37
					MI	22
					Stroke	33
					New-onset diabetes	34
CAPP, 2001	572	155/89 vs 153/88		Captopril vs diuretics or β-blockers	Fatal + NFMI + stroke + CV deaths	41
IDNT, 2001, 2003	1715	≤135/85		Irbesartan vs amlodipine or placebo	Doubling of serum creatinine + end-stage renal disease + death from any cause	23 (vs amlodipine) 20 (vs placebo)

			CV events	10 (vs amlodipine) 10 (vs placebo)
IRMA, 2001	590	144/83 143/83 141/83	Irbesartan 150 mg or 300 mg vs placebo	Onset of diabetic nephropathy	35 (150 mg) 65 (300 mg)
RENAAL, 2001	1513	152/82 vs 153/82	Losartan vs placebo in addition to conventional therapy	Doubling of serum creatinine End-stage renal disease Death	25 28 NS
LIFE, 2002	1195	146/79 vs 148/79	Losartan vs atenolol	CV events Total mortality in diabetics New-onset diabetes	22 39 25

SHEP, Systolic Hypertension in the Elderly Program; Syst-Eur, Systolic Hypertension in Europe; HOT, Hypertension Optimal Treatment; CAPP, Captopril Prevention Project; IDNT, Irbesartan Diabetic Nephropathy Trial; IRMA, Irbesartan Microalbuminuria in type 2 diabetes; RENAAL, Reduction in End Points in NIDDM with Angiotensin II Antagonist Losartan; CVD, cardiovascular disease; CHD, coronary heart disease; CV, cardiovascular; MI, myocardial infarction; NFMI, nonfatal myocardial infarction; and NS, not significant.

*Blood pressure in diabetic + nondiabetic population because blood pressure not reported for diabetic patients alone.

Source: Data derived from Sowers JR, Haffner S: *Hypertension* 2002; 40:781.

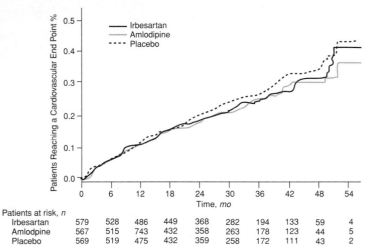

FIG. 25-5   Time to first cardiovascular event in the diabetic hypertensives enrolled in the Irbesartan Diabetic Nephropathy Trial who received irbesartan, amlodipine, or placebo in addition to other classes of antihypertensive drugs. *(Adapted from Berl T, Hunsicker LG, Lewis JB, et al: Ann Intern Med 2003; 138:542.)*

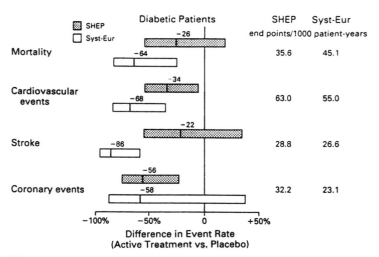

FIG. 25-6   Outcomes in the diabetic hypertensives enrolled in the Systolic Hypertension in the Elderly Program (SHEP) or the Syst-Eur trial. The two right-hand columns show the number of events per 1000 patient-years in the placebo groups in the two trials. The bars indicate the 95% confidence intervals. The numbers above the bars indicate the benefit of active treatments compared to placebo. *(Reprinted with permission from Tuomilehto J, Rastenyte D, Birkenhager WH, et al: N Engl J Med 1999; 340:677.)*

Angiotensin II-Receptor Blockers

Initially, angiotensin II-receptor blockers (ARBs) were recommended mainly as an alternative for the 10% of patients given an ACEI who develop cough. Their more widespread usage is now recommended based on trials in type 2 diabetic patients with nephropathy and recent evidence that they provide additional benefits when added to presumably maximal doses of an ACEI.

These agents are in many ways similar to ACEIs, but the renin–angiotensin system has three features that may give rise to differences in the benefits of ARBs versus ACEIs (Fig. 25-7).

1. *Non-ACE alternative pathways* for generation of angiotensin II have been recognized. In particular the chymotrypsin-like serine protease *chymase* has been found in heart tissue and shown to have the ability to convert AI to AII even in the presence of natural protease inhibitors.
2. *Beneficial effects of the increased levels of bradykinin* that accompany ACEIs but not ARBs have been observed. These include:
   a. Adding to the antihypertensive effect of ACEIs
   b. Providing an important vasodilation that is NO-mediated
   c. Inhibiting vascular smooth muscle cell growth
3. *Activation of the AT_2 receptors:* Most of the adverse effects of the renin–angiotensin system are mediated through the AT_1 receptor, but increasing evidence supports beneficial effects mediated through the AT_2 receptor, as shown in Fig. 25-7. Initial concerns that the increased levels of AII that circulate when the AT_1 receptor is blocked could induce deleterious effects have been largely replaced with evidence that AT_2 receptor stimulation is likely beneficial. For example, overexpression of AT_2 receptor activates the vascular kinin system and causes vasodilation.

Clinical Effects of ARBs

The multiple ARBs now available seem equipotent and equally free of side effects, although angioedema has rarely been observed. Losartan appears to be unique in having a modest uricosuric effect.

OTHER DRUGS FOR HYPERTENSIVE DIABETICS

Antihyperglycemic Agents

In addition to chronic effects, hyperglycemia will acutely raise blood pressure, probably by activating the renin system. As noted elsewhere in this book, to achieve adequate glycemic control, most patients will require multiple therapies. There may be special vasodilatory effects of thiazolidinediones mediated through increased NO synthesis. Any therapy that improves insulin sensitivity or lowers insulinemia may confer long-term vascular protective effects.

Aldosterone Blockers

The currently available spironolactone has been joined by a more specific agent, eplerenone, providing the full benefits of blockade of aldosterone's multiple pro-fibrotic effects with virtually none of the side effects caused by nonspecific effects of spironolactone on sex hormones. Eplerenone reduces proteinuria even in patients receiving ACEI therapy. Despite a potential for hyperkalemia in those with renal damage, eplerenone will likely be widely used in diabetic hypertensives.

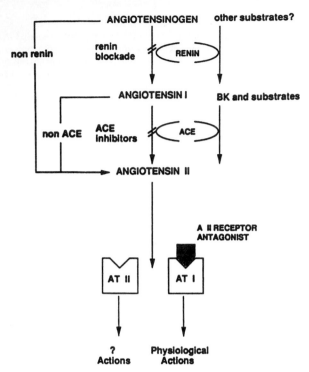

FIG. 25-7   The renin–angiotensin system with the sites of action of ACE inhibition and AT$_1$ receptor blockade.

Statins

Statin drugs have quickly established their value in prevention of atherosclerotic vascular diseases. Among the 2532 diabetic hypertensives enrolled in the ASCOT trial, the degree of protection against myocardial infarction was somewhat less in them than in the 7773 nondiabetics. Nonetheless, a statin is indicated in all patients at high risk for cardiovascular disease, obviously including diabetic hypertensives.

Aspirin

In the HOT trial, aspirin (75 mg/day) reduced major cardiovascular events by 15%, all myocardial infarction by 36%, and had no effect on stroke. There were more bleeding episodes in the ASA group, but no more fatal bleeds.

CONCLUSION

Hypertension and diabetes commonly coexist and pose a serious threat. Fortunately, significant protection can be provided, although the benefits may be difficult to achieve. Health care professionals must be more vigorous in applying more intensive therapy to this rapidly expanding, highly vulnerable population.

ADDITIONAL READINGS

The ALLHAT Officers and Coordinators for the ALLHAT Collaborative Research Group. Major outcomes in high-risk hypertensive patients randomized to angiotensin-converting enzyme inhibitor or calcium channel blocker vs diuretic: the Antihypertensive and Lipid-Lowering Treatment to Prevent Heart Attack Trial (ALLHAT). *JAMA.* 2002;288:2981–2997.

American Diabetes Association. Treatment of hypertension in adults with diabetes. *Diabetes Care.* 2003;26:S80–82.

Chobanian AV, Bakris GL, Black HR, et al. Seventh report of the Joint National Committee on Prevention, Detection, Evaluation, and Treatment of High Blood Pressure: the JNC 7 (Express) Report. *JAMA.* 2003;289:2560–2572. Also available at: http://www.nhlbi.nih.gov/guidelines/hypertension/jncintro.htm. Accessed May 25, 2004.

Lewis EJ, Hunsicker LG, Clarke WR, et al. Renoprotective effect of the angiotensive-receptor antagonist irbesartan in patients with nephropathy due to type 2 diabetes *N Engl J Med.* 2001;345:851–860.

Whelton PK, He J, Appel LJ, et al. Primary prevention of hypertension. Clinical and public health advisory from the national high blood pressure education program. *JAMA.* 2002;288:1882–1888.

For a more detailed discussion of this topic and a bibliography, please see Porte *et al: Ellenberg & Rifkin's Diabetes Mellitus,* 6th ed., Chapter 48.

26 Heart Disease in Patients with Diabetes

Lawrence H. Young   Deborah A. Chyun

Cardiovascular disease is the leading cause of mortality and a major cause of morbidity in patients with diabetes. The most common manifestations of cardiovascular disease are acute myocardial infarction, angina, heart failure, and sudden death. Cardiovascular disease results in large part from the sequelae of atherosclerotic coronary artery disease (CAD) and hypertension, which are highly prevalent in patients with type 2 diabetes. However, the course of cardiovascular disease in patients with diabetes is further complicated by additional abnormalities in cardiac contractile function, thrombosis, and autonomic function, which need to be appreciated in order to provide them optimal care.

CORONARY ARTERY DISEASE

Epidemiology

The high cardiovascular risk associated with diabetes has become well appreciated as the result of large epidemiologic trials. In the Framingham Study, the risk of cardiovascular disease was 2–3 times greater in otherwise healthy patients with diabetes. In the United Kingdom Prospective Diabetes Study, the overall incidence of myocardial infarction, stroke, angina and heart failure was over 20% during a 10-year follow-up period after the new diagnosis of type 2 diabetes. While diabetes predisposes to cardiovascular disease in both men and women, it affects certain groups in a particularly aggressive fashion. In particular, young women lose their protection against cardiovascular disease as the result of diabetes and are among the unusual group of women who present with myocardial infarction prior to menopause.

Diabetes clearly predisposes patients to the development of cardiovascular disease. In patients with type 1 diabetes, cardiovascular disease does not become clinically evident until patients have had diabetes for many years. In contrast, type 2 diabetes may be diagnosed for the first time when patients present to the hospital with acute medical problems, including myocardial infarction, heart failure, or stroke. In part, this difference relates to the fact that type 2 diabetes, as opposed to type 1 diabetes, may go undiagnosed for a number of years. However, the coincidental presentation of both disorders also is due to the fact that many of the same factors which predispose patients to type 2 diabetes are also involved in the development of atherosclerosis. These include genetic predisposition, physical inactivity, obesity, insulin resistance, hypertension, and dyslipidemia.

Etiology

Accelerated atherosclerosis in patients with type 2 diabetes is attributable to the presence of traditional cardiac risk factors as well as recently recognized physiologic abnormalities. Patients with type 2 diabetes often have multiple conventional cardiac risk factors, including dyslipidemia, hypertension, and

TABLE 26-1 Factors Associated with CAD in Diabetes

Traditional cardiac risk factors
Hypertension
Lipid abnormalities
• Reduction in high-density lipoproteins (HDL-C)
• Increased triglyceride (TG) levels
• Presence of oxidized and small, dense, low-density lipoproteins (LDL-C)
Obesity
Physical inactivity
Cigarette smoking

Nontraditional risk markers
Microalbuminuria
Homocysteine
Hemostatic abnormalities
• Factor VIII
• von Willebrand factor
• Plasminogen activator inhibitor-1
• Platelet reactivity
Inflammatory markers
• C -reactive protein
• Fibrinogen
• Soluble cell adhesion molecules

---

obesity, which are also associated with insulin resistance and the metabolic syndrome (Table 26-1). Alterations in lipids, such as low high-density lipoprotein (HDL) cholesterol, high triglycerides, and smaller, dense, more atherogenic, low-density lipoprotein (LDL) cholesterol, are common in these patients and play an important role in the pathogenesis of atherosclerosis.

Additional physiologic abnormalities, which are not part of routine clinical testing, contribute to both the development of atherosclerosis and the clinical manifestations of cardiovascular disease in type 2 diabetes. Increased oxidative stress and vascular inflammation are important mechanisms in atherosclerosis and render existing plaque vulnerable to rupture. Plaque vulnerability is particularly problematic in patients with diabetes due to their increased tendency toward thrombosis. Accentuated platelet aggregation promotes thrombosis, while elevated plasminogen activator inhibitor-1 impairs endogenous fibrinolysis and blood clot dissolution. These pathophysiologic mechanisms predispose the diabetic patient to acute coronary syndromes, myocardial infarction, and sudden death.

Pathology

By the time patients with diabetes have cardiac symptoms or a myocardial infarction, prompting cardiac catheterization and coronary angiography, CAD may be widespread. Significant stenoses in multiple coronary arteries are often detected, and it is not uncommon to find more than one obstructive lesion within each vessel. Potentially dangerous obstruction of the left main coronary artery is more common in patients with diabetes. In addition, diffuse atherosclerotic disease, involving long segments and/or the distal aspects of the arteries, may be present. Unfortunately, such diffuse disease adversely affects the suitability of the vessels for either percutaneous intervention with balloon angioplasty and stent placement or surgical revascularization. In such cases, patients may best be treated with anti-ischemic medication. While the gradual development of a severe stenosis in a coronary artery often stimulates compensatory collateral blood vessel development, patients with diabetes tend to respond with less collateral vessels, which leaves them more prone to ischemia.

Coronary atherosclerosis primarily affects the large and medium-size arteries of the heart which are visualized by coronary angiography. However, in patients with diabetes, there may be additional small-vessel disease. Although not evident on coronary angiography, the small arteries and arterioles of the diabetic heart may have pathologic abnormalities that are thought to sometimes produce myocardial ischemia. Endothelial dysfunction is frequently present in patients with diabetes, limiting their ability to vasodilate and augment blood flow during exercise or periods of hemodynamic stress.

Prevention

Since cardiovascular disease is the result of numerous factors in patients with diabetes, its prevention requires a multifaceted approach to risk reduction. The American Diabetes Association has provided treatment targets for lipid, blood pressure, and glycemic control, and has made exercise recommendations that are summarized in Table 26-2. Although this approach requires intensive and often expensive treatments, recent evidence emphasizes that a comprehensive approach of multiple-risk-factor modification prevents cardiac events in type 2 diabetes.

Important measures to prevent CAD complications in diabetes include aggressive lipid management, hypertension treatment, prevention of vascular thrombosis with aspirin, and control of blood glucose. There are numerous effective therapies for dyslipidemia and hypertension, which are reviewed in Chapters 24 and 25. Primary prevention of CVD in patients with diabetes should include the use of daily aspirin. Although there is somewhat limited evidence to date that intensive blood glucose treatment prevents CAD in patients with diabetes, there is still a strong rationale to achieve optimal glycemic control. Maintaining normal blood glucose is highly effective in preventing the microvascular complications of diabetes, i.e., retinopathy, nephropathy, and neuropathy. Normalizing hyperglycemia also improves the dyslipidemia of diabetes, by reducing triglycerides. Thus, both the American Diabetes Association (ADA) and the American Heart Association (AHA) recommend that physicians treat diabetes aggressively to reduce and maintain HbA1c concentrations below 7%.

An important and often neglected aspect of promoting cardiac risk reduction in diabetes management is exercise, which has beneficial effects on glycemic control, lipids, weight, and blood pressure. Exercise should be encouraged in all patients with diabetes. However, individualized recommendations are required to ensure safety in patients with neuropathy, severe retinopathy, or CAD. Sedentary individuals should always initiate exercise programs at a low level and gradually increase their intensity of exercise. All patients should be educated that the symptoms of myocardial ischemia include not only chest pain, but also pressure, tightness, heaviness, or constriction. They should understand that significant shortness of breath, lightheadedness, fatigue, or sweating during exercise should also be discussed

TABLE 26-2 Primary Prevention of Cardiovascular Disease
in Diabetic Patients

Goal	Strategies to achieve goal
Blood pressure	
< 130/80	Measured at each visit
	Lifestyle modification
	Medication
Lipids	
LDL < 100 mg/dL	Tested annually or every 2 years if low-risk
HDL > 45 mg/dL in men;	Medical nutrition therapy
> 55 mg/dL in women	Daily fat intake: < 7–10% saturated fat and
Triglycerides < 150 mg/dL	< 200–300 mg cholesterol
	Regular physical activity
	Weight control
	Glycemic control
	Medication
HbA1c	
< 7%	Tested 2–3 times annually if meeting goal; 4 times annually if above goal or therapy changed
	Medical nutrition therapy
	Weight control
	Regular physical activity
	Self-monitoring of blood glucose
	Education in self-management and problem solving
Physical activity	
Regularly 3–4 times per week for 30 minutes	Routinely assess physical activity and exercise status
	Moderate aerobic regimen
	Increase in daily activities
	With multiple CAD risk factors, complications or long duration of diabetes, consider screening for CAD
	Individualization of prescription
	Caution with peripheral neuropathy or cardiac autonomic neuropathy or proliferative retinopathy
Weight	
BMI 21–25 kg/m^2	Height, weight, BMI, and waist
Waist circumference	circumference at each visit
< 102 cm in men and	Weight control
< 88 cm in women	Regular physical activity
Smoking	
Complete cessation	Assess smoking status
	Counseling on prevention and cessation
	Provide counseling, problem solving, or coping skills training, and pharmacotherapy
Aspirin therapy	
	Consider enteric-coated aspirin 75–325 mg/day if age ≥ 40 years and 1 or more additional CAD risk factors

BMI, body mass index; CAD, coronary artery disease; HDL, high-density lipoproteins; LDL, low-density lipoproteins.

with their physician. Because individuals with type 2 diabetes may have unrecognized CAD without symptoms indicative of myocardial ischemia, high-intensity exercise regimens should generally be avoided. Running, strenuous aerobics or heavy weight lifting should be avoided without prior evaluation to exclude the presence of underlying ischemia. This is particularly the case for patients with a long duration of diabetes, multiple CAD risk factors, or known diabetic complications.

Asymptomatic Ischemia

Asymptomatic or "silent" ischemia occurs frequently in patients with diabetes and CAD who also have symptomatic ischemia with angina or dyspnea on exertion. However, as many as 1 out of 5 completely asymptomatic individuals with type 2 diabetes may have inducible myocardial ischemia. The significance of asymptomatic ischemia depends on the extent of myocardium which is compromised, with some patients having only minor regions of ischemia and others having major areas of ischemia. Of particular concern is when asymptomatic ischemia has caused prior myocardial infarction (MI), decreased left ventricular function, heart failure, or ventricular arrhythmias. These patients are at high risk for subsequent cardiac events and therefore require complete evaluation, usually including coronary angiography.

Patients with diabetes can have autonomic neuropathy involving the heart, as well as other organs. Cardiac autonomic neuropathy may play a role in decreasing ischemia awareness. Abnormalities in cardiac autonomic function serve as a risk marker for those patients with diabetes with underlying asymptomatic myocardial ischemia. In patients with cardiac autonomic neuropathy, the heart rate responses to deep breathing and the Valsalva maneuver are blunted. In advanced cases, orthostatic hypotension is present, with a drop in systolic blood pressure of more than 15–20 mm Hg, when the patient rises to the standing position.

Which asymptomatic patients with diabetes should be considered for specialized cardiac testing to exclude the presence of significant inducible ischemia? Exercise testing with myocardial perfusion imaging or echocardiography is recommended for risk stratification in any patient whose electrocardiogram shows evidence of ischemia or myocardial infarction, including significant Q waves or deep T-wave inversions. Left bundle branch block in patients with diabetes should also raise the possibility of a prior myocardial infarction. Screening for inducible ischemia is also considered in the completely asymptomatic patient with diabetes, with peripheral or carotid occlusive disease, cardiovascular autonomic neuropathy, or multiple (two or more, including microalbuminuria) cardiac risk factors in addition to diabetes. However, the risk for CAD appears to be widespread in patients with diabetes, and even those with fewer risk factors may have asymptomatic ischemia. Predictors of inducible ischemia include increasing age, higher cholesterol level, male gender, proteinuria, cardiac autonomic dysfunction, and ST-T wave abnormalities on resting electrocardiogram.

The identification of asymptomatic CAD has clear implications for the care of the patient with diabetes. It strongly reinforces the need to aggressively reduce modifiable cardiovascular risk factors, motivating the patient to take multiple medications when required to optimally treat dyslipidemia and hypertension. In some patients it may lead to the initiation or intensification of lipid-lowering therapy. A heightened concern for CAD can motivate efforts at smoking cessation and weight reduction, which otherwise may be difficult to accomplish. Once CAD is identified, providers are more apt to assure the patient's compliance with daily aspirin treatment and to consider the use of β-blockers to prevent ischemia. Recommendations for regular exercise are reinforced, with limitations placed on strenuous activity which might place the patient at risk for a cardiac event.

Medical Treatment of CAD

The treatment of symptomatic CAD in patients with diabetes needs to be comprehensive to reduce their substantial cardiac risk. It requires intensive lifestyle and dietary changes, aggressive treatment of dyslipidemia and hypertension, prevention of thrombosis, and β-blockers to prevent myocardial ischemia. The goals of intensive therapy in patients with diabetes are to slow the progression of coronary atherosclerosis, prevent ischemic symptoms, and decrease the likelihood of myocardial infarction and death.

Treatment of patients with diabetes requires careful consideration with an awareness of the benefits and potential side effects unique to these patients. Specific therapy in diabetic patients should include the following.

- β-Blockers have benefit in diabetic patients with either symptomatic CAD or heart failure. This benefit outweighs their minor potential for worsening glycemic control and for masking hypoglycemia in patients treated with sulfonylureas or insulin. As in all patients, they should be used with caution in the presence of bronchospastic lung disease, decompensated heart failure, and sinus or atrial-ventricular node conduction system disease
- Angiotensin-converting enzyme (ACE) inhibitors have benefit in the prevention of CAD, in the treatment of heart failure and hypertension, and in preventing heart failure in patients with either hypertension or decreased left ventricular function. Angiotensin receptor blockers are an alternative, and though more expensive, should be considered when a patient is intolerant to ACE inhibitors or has renal disease, for which they appear to have additional benefit.
- Nitrates have benefit for the symptomatic relief and prevention of angina. They should be used with caution in patients with diabetes who also have autonomic neuropathy, as they may develop symptomatic orthostatic hypotension due to reduction in preload.
- Calcium channel blockers have an important role in controlling blood pressure in hypertensive individuals with diabetes. They are helpful in the treatment of angina. However, they should be used with caution in patients with heart failure.
- Statins are critical to lowering LDL cholesterol and reducing CAD risk in most patients with diabetes. They also reduce inflammation, as evidenced by reduction in C-reactive protein levels, and thereby may attenuate the risk of cardiac events through mechanisms other than cholesterol lowering. Vascular inflammation is increased in insulin-resistant patients with type 2 diabetes and is thought to play an important role in their developing atherosclerosis and cardiac events.
- Fibrates are useful in patients with type 2 diabetes and the insulin resistance or metabolic syndromes, who typically have low HDL cholesterol and elevated triglycerides, but relatively normal LDL cholesterol. They are used with caution together with statins because of an increased incidence of rhabdomyolysis with combination therapy.

- Niacin is also useful in patients with type 2 diabetes with low HDL cholesterol and elevated triglycerides, when LDL cholesterol is normal. It causes flushing which many patients are unable to tolerate. Niacin also has a minor hyperglycemic effect which generally does not preclude its use in patients with low HDL cholesterol.
- Aspirin is indicated in all patients with type 2 diabetes without significant peptic ulcer disease or aspirin allergy. Current recommendations are for daily low-dose (81-mg) aspirin, although some patients with diabetes have increased platelet aggregation and daily adult-strength (325-mg) aspirin should be considered.
- Clopidogrel is an antithrombotic agent which inhibits platelets through a mechanism distinct from aspirin (ADP-induced aggregation). In patients who are allergic to or unable to take aspirin, or who have had recurrent symptoms on aspirin, clopidegrel is prescribed. After intra-coronary stent placement, the combination of aspirin and clopidigrel is generally used for 3–6 months, followed by indefinite aspirin therapy.

Revascularization

The clinical presentation, coronary anatomy, and overall medical condition are considered when deciding whether and by what means a patient with diabetes should undergo coronary intervention or revascularization. Patients with acute coronary syndromes, including unstable angina and myocardial infarction, or ischemic pulmonary edema are among those with highest risk. The number, location, morphology, and extent of coronary stenoses determine the feasibility of percutaneous intervention or coronary artery bypass grafting (CABG). The surgical risk is increased by additional noncardiac morbidities, including renal insufficiency, cerebral or peripheral vascular disease, lung disease, and generalized immobility.

Percutaneous coronary intervention with intracoronary stent placement has assumed an important role in the treatment of CAD in patients with diabetes. The outcomes of initial stent placement in patients with diabetes are favorable, particularly with the use of intensive antiplatelet therapy including glycoprotein IIb/IIIa inhibitors in the setting of acute coronary syndromes. In-stent restenosis is potentially a problem in patients with diabetes over the next 6 months, due to their increased tendency for intimal proliferation. However, the use of biologically coated coronary stents has reduced the incidence of restenosis from 40–50% to less than 10–20% in patients with diabetes. This has revolutionized the treatment of patients with diabetes who have relatively focal CAD, making the strategy of percutaneous intervention more attractive in these patients.

Advanced CAD is frequently found during angiography in patients with diabetes. Left main coronary artery stenoses, severe multivessel disease, or very complex calcified lesions favor the use of CABG. This assumes that the distal vessels have good distal runoff and are suitable targets for the surgeon, and that the patient does not have excessive co-morbidities. In a small number of patients with diabetes, coronary angiography reveals multivessel disease, which is technically suitable for either percutaneous intervention or CABG. In this case the lower initial morbidity of percutaneous intervention is weighed against the greater prevalence of recurrent ischemia and need for future revascularization.

Myocardial Infarction

Patients with diabetes represent 20–30% of patients who present to the hospital with acute myocardial infarction. In many cases, myocardial infarction may occur without the warning of prior angina. In addition, patients with diabetes may have atypical symptoms that delay their pursuing medical attention. In some cases, these patients succumb to ischemic arrhythmias and never reach the hospital.

Overall, there is a consistent twofold higher mortality and increased morbidity associated with myocardial infarction in patients with diabetes. Although early coronary reperfusion, aspirin, β-blockers, ACE inhibitors, lipid-lowering agents, and coronary revascularization have dramatically improved the survival of diabetic patients with MI, these patients still have a higher risk of complications, including:

- Heart failure and cardiogenic shock
- Postinfarct angina and recurrent MI
- Heart block
- Atrial arrhythmias
- Renal insufficiency

Patients with diabetes require careful management to prevent these complications. Those patients with ST-segment elevation often have coronary artery thrombosis and benefit from prompt opening of the occluded artery with either thrombolytic therapy or percutaneous intervention. However, patients with diabetes have several factors that may lead to less than optimal thrombolysis and predispose to reocclusion. They often have more extensive CAD and an increased tendency to thrombosis at the site of plaque rupture, due to increased plasminogen activator inhibitor (PAI-1) and fibrinogen, platelet hyperreactivity, and endothelial dysfunction.

Primary intracoronary stent placement has emerged as the preferred treatment for ST-segment elevation myocardial infarction in patients with diabetes. This approach has several advantages in that it provides more effective reperfusion, definitive information on the extent of CAD, and avoids the hemorrhagic complications associated with thrombolytic agents. Adjuvant antithrombotic treatment with clopidegrel and glycoprotein IIb/IIIa inhibitors is an essential part of this approach to prevent thrombosis in patients with diabetes. Thus, patients with diabetes and ST-segment elevation who are within 12 hours of the onset of symptoms should be considered for primary angioplasty with stent placement, particularly when there is evidence of heart failure or hemodynamic instability, where the establishment of secure vessel patency may be critical.

Multivessel disease is often identified in patients with diabetes at the time of primary angioplasty and presents a management challenge. Stent placement in the occluded vessel responsible for the infarction, referred to as the "culprit" lesion, is preferable for initial treatment in most cases. However, a small number (~5%) of patients with diabetes require urgent surgical revascularization due to inaccessibility of the lesion or the presence of left main coronary artery disease. In addition, when stent placement to the "culprit" lesion leaves the patient with significant residual obstructive CAD, careful evaluation of the need for additional revascularization should be made.

After initial revascularization, aggressive medical therapy of patients with diabetes is required after myocardial infarction. Treatment to reduce cardiac risk factors is essential (see Table 26-2). In addition, patients should be discharged from the hospital on the following medications:

- β-Blockers. Regardless of whether thrombolysis or primary stent placement was performed, patients with diabetes are at higher risk for recurrent ischemia and in most cases should be discharged on β-blockers. While patients with diabetes more often have heart failure during MI, once the pulmonary congestion has been treated with diuretics, β-blockers should be slowly initiated and carefully monitored.
- ACE inhibitors. Because of the increased incidence of heart failure in the acute setting as well as postmyocardial infarction, due to adverse myocardial remodeling in diabetes, ACE inhibitors should be prescribed for these patients as soon as possible during myocardial infarction. In addition to decreasing heart failure and mortality following MI, they may prevent progression of atherosclerosis.

In some cases relative hypotension will limit the amount of these medications that can be tolerated by the patient. Therapy should then be individualized, priority given to β-blockers in the diabetic patient with recurrent ischemia or severe multivessel disease, and priority given to ACE inhibitors when heart failure is the primary residual problem.

Intensive Diabetes Treatment

Hyperglycemia is a frequent occurrence in the setting of acute myocardial infarction in patients with diabetes. Optimization of glycemic control during hospitalization and following discharge may prevent recurrent events. In the hospital, patients should be carefully monitored and treated with insulin as needed to prevent significant hyperglycemia. The role of intensive glucose control during hospitalizations for acute myocardial infarction is now under intense investigation, and many coronary care units now have intravenous insulin protocols. The Diabetes Insulin Glucose Infusion in Acute Myocardial Infarction (DIGAMI) study suggested important benefits of intravenous insulin infusion during the coronary care unit stay to lower blood glucose levels to less than 200 mg/dL. More recently, studies in other critical care settings support even more rigid glucose criteria, although benefits specifically in the patient with myocardial infarction have not yet been demonstrated. Careful monitoring is needed to avoid the development of hypoglycemia. Hypoglycemia can trigger sympathetic activation and catecholamine release that may increase myocardial oxygen demand or potentially trigger arrhythmias. However, with careful monitoring, hypoglycemia should be an infrequent event and should not preclude intensive glycemic treatment. Current data indicate that any risk is outweighed by the benefits of such an approach.

Acute Coronary Syndromes

Unstable angina and non-ST-segment MI are now considered part of a spectrum of acute coronary syndromes which place the patient at increased risk for subsequent MI and death. These syndromes are normally characterized by progressive or prolonged anginal symptoms, but in patients with diabetes the symptoms may be atypical or the patient might present with new or worsening heart failure. Diabetes is an independent risk factor for death, progression to acute ST-segment elevation myocardial infarction, and readmission for unstable angina within the next year.

Like patients with diabetes and myocardial infarction, those with acute coronary syndromes have more extensive CAD, often involving a greater number and longer segments of vessels. Once again, angiography is more likely to show some degree of left main disease than in a patient without diabetes. Patients with diabetes also have an increased risk of saphenous vein closure after CABG, and those presenting with acute coronary syndromes often have imminent closure of a heavily diseased saphenous vein graft. These patients pose particular challenges, although percutaneous intervention with filter wires to prevent distal embolization of debris has improved the management of saphenous vein graft disease.

The initial therapy of acute coronary syndromes includes the administration of β-blockers and nitrates to prevent ischemia. The approach to antithrombotic therapy depends on whether coronary intervention is under consideration. Aspirin should be administered to all patients; in most in combination with clopidogrel, which, as mentioned previously, has a synergistic effect to inhibit platelets. Heparin should be administered either intravenously in the unfractionated form or as subcutaneous low-molecular-weight heparin. When patients are unstable and coronary intervention is planned, glycoprotein IIb/IIIa inhibitors should be given, as they improve interventional outcomes in this setting.

In patients with acute coronary syndromes who respond to initial medical therapy, the decision as to whether to pursue invasive evaluation or noninvasive imaging needs to be individualized, but generally, patients with diabetes are considered for cardiac catheterization and angiography. The risk of invasive evaluation is increased in patients with diabetes who have severe peripheral vascular disease or renal insufficiency. A noninvasive approach utilizing adenosine myocardial perfusion imaging or stress echocardiography may be helpful for initial risk stratification in these patients and those with other major co-morbidities. However, an invasive strategy is usually preferable when high-risk features are present, including elevated troponin levels, resting ST-segment depression, prior MI, poor left ventricular function, or heart failure.

HEART FAILURE

Epidemiology and Etiology

Heart failure causes substantial morbidity in patients with diabetes. The Framingham Study demonstrated that the risk of heart failure was increased 2.4-fold in men and 5.1-fold in women with diabetes. The diagnosis of diabetic cardiomyopathy is sometimes invoked as an explanation for heart failure in patients with diabetes without apparent cause. However, patients with diabetes alone do not develop overt dilated cardiomyopathy and usually do not develop symptomatic heart failure. On the other hand, symptomatic heart failure is common in patients with diabetes who have coexisting CAD (recognized or not) and/or hypertension. Indeed, unexplained heart failure in a patient with diabetes should always prompt evaluation for CAD, in most cases including cardiac catheterization, even in the absence of angina. Hypertension is present in approximately 40–60% of patients with type 2 diabetes, and the combination of hypertension and diabetes clearly predisposes the patient to symptomatic heart failure.

Why, then, are patients with diabetes predisposed to heart failure? Patients with both type 1 and type 2 diabetes may have alterations in left ventricular diastolic function due to interstitial fibrosis and myocardial collagen deposition, which may decrease left ventricular compliance. Patients with diabetes also have a reduced ability to increase left ventricle contractility during exercise. Diastolic abnormalities may be present at an early stage of disease.

Prognosis and Response to Therapy

Heart failure is an important cause of morbidity and mortality in patients with diabetes, particularly after myocardial infarction or coronary revascularization. Diabetes almost doubles the risk of morbidity and mortality in patients with heart failure, with female sex and longer duration of diabetes further predicting an elevated risk.

The prevention and treatment of heart failure in diabetic patients requires optimal management of coexisting hypertension, CAD, and left ventricular dysfunction. Specific aspects of the treatment of patients with diabetes and heart failure warrant attention.

- *ACE inhibitors.* ACE-inhibition plays an essential role in the prevention and treatment of heart failure in these patients. ACE inhibitors prevent heart failure in patients with diabetes, particularly when they are hypertensive. In symptomatic heart failure, these agents reduce left ventricular afterload, decrease the neurohumoral responses, and reduce left ventricular mass, which may improve diastolic dysfunction. These drugs should be part of the standard treatment of heart failure in patients with diabetes, unless they develop a contraindication, such as angioedema, severe cough, worsening renal function, or significant hyperkalemia. In the case of angioedema or cough, an angiotensin receptor blocker should be used.
- *Diuretics.* Loop diuretics have an essential role in alleviating pulmonary congestion and edema in patients with diabetes and symptomatic heart failure. The aldosterone antagonist spironolactone (25 mg/day) has additive benefit in the treatment of advanced symptomatic heart failure in patients with diabetes, but potassium levels need to be carefully monitored when renal insufficiency is present, because of an increased risk of hyperkalemia.
- *β-Adrenergic receptor blockers.* β-Blockers improve left ventricular function, prevent heart failure symptoms, and increase survival in patients with diabetes who have symptomatic heart failure. It is important that β-blockers be initiated only after the patient has been stabilized on a combination of ACE inhibitors, diuretics, and digoxin, but they are contraindicated when overt pulmonary congestion or hypotension is present. They rarely may worsen glycemic control in type 2 patients and, in certain circumstances, may mask the adrenergic symptoms of hypoglycemia in patients receiving insulin or sulfonylureas. While the care provider and patient should be aware of these potential side effects, they are usually minor, and the risk–benefit ratio favors use of these agents for patients with diabetes and heart failure.
- *Calcium channel blockers.* Patients with diabetes often have diastolic dysfunction that theoretically might be improved by calcium blockers. However, in most cases, these agents have little benefit, and diltiazem and verapamil are contraindicated in patients with systolic dysfunction. The primary approaches to treat heart failure due to diastolic dysfunction include intensive treatment of hypertension (to reduce afterload and left ventricular mass) and diuretics (to prevent volume overload). Calcium channel blockers are sometimes extremely useful in treating hypertension in type 2

patients with diabetes. In patients who remain hypertensive despite treatment with an ACE inhibitor or angiotensin receptor blocker, β-blocker, and diuretic, long-acting dihydropyridine antagonists are often helpful.

- *Mechanical assist and transplantation.* When conventional heart failure treatment fails in patients with diabetes who have cardiomyopathy and symptomatic heart failure, advanced measures are considered. However, the presence of significant end-organ disease, especially nephropathy, increases the risk of such interventions. Diabetes increases the risk of infection with left ventricular assist devices. After cardiac transplantation, diabetes also increases the risk of infection and renal insufficiency. Patients with diabetes may require high doses of insulin or oral hypoglycemic agents when receiving corticosteroids for immunosuppression. Following transplantation, diabetes increases the risk for transplant coronary vasculopathy. Thus, there are a number of issues related to diabetes that warrant careful attention in evaluating patients prior to cardiac transplantation.

- *Metformin and thiazolidinediones.* The presence of heart failure also complicates the use of commonly used oral hypoglycemic agents in patients with type 2 diabetes. Metformin is generally contraindicated because of the risk of renal hypoperfusion, decreasing drug clearance which can cause the development of severe lactic acidosis. Thiazolidinediones tend to promote weight gain and fluid retention and can worsen heart failure. They are contraindicated in patients with moderate-to-severe heart failure, but can be used with caution in patients who are asymptomatic or minimally symptomatic after treatment. In this case, the dose should be gradually titrated and patients should be carefully monitored for excessive weight gain, worsening edema, or shortness of breath. In some cases, these symptoms can be managed by increasing diuretic therapy or decreasing the dose of the drug, but other cases require discontinuation of medication.

CARDIAC AUTONOMIC NEUROPATHY

Cardiac autonomic neuropathy develops over time in approximately one-quarter of individuals with diabetes. Autonomic neuropathy may involve the parasympathetic and sympathetic innervation of the heart and peripheral vasculature, leading to a spectrum of manifestations. In its mildest form, cardiac neuropathy involves the parasympathetic innervation of the heart and may lead to a slightly increased resting heart rate. In advanced cases, autonomic neuropathy causes severe orthostatic hypotension with recurrent lightheadedness, unsteadiness, or even frank syncope.

Cardiac autonomic neuropathy should be considered in patients with diabetes who have peripheral neuropathy or other forms of autonomic neuropathy. A simple bedside test is to evaluate the patient for orthostatic blood pressure changes. A drop in systolic pressure > 15 mm Hg in the absence of acute hypovolemia is suggestive and > 20 mm Hg is fairly diagnostic of advanced autonomic dysfunction. Patients with diabetes and autonomic neuropathy also have blunted changes in heart rate during deep breathing, standing, and Valsalva maneuvers, along with diminished blood pressure responses to hand grip and standing. These are more sensitive measures of cardiac autonomic neuropathy, but are typically available only using specialized devices. On the other hand, an electrocardiographic rhythm strip which shows obvious sinus arrhythmia generally indicates that cardiac autonomic function is healthy in a patient with diabetes.

Patients with diabetes who have cardiac autonomic neuropathy have a high cardiovascular risk, with cardiovascular mortality approaching 25–40% over 5 years. The specific mechanisms through which this occurs remain incompletely understood. As discussed earlier, cardiac autonomic neuropathy may have a role in the pathogenesis of silent ischemia in patients with diabetes. Cardiac autonomic neuropathy may also contribute to abnormalities in left ventricular function, compromising exercise capacity and left ventricular contractile reserve. It may also cause repolarization abnormalities and potentially predisposing to sudden death in patients with diabetes. In addition, cardiac autonomic neuropathy is found in high-risk patients who have established severe CAD, renal disease, poor glycemic control, and dyslipidemia.

CONCLUSION

The association between diabetes and heart disease has been recognized for over one hundred years. In contrast to the overall population, progress in reducing heart disease morbidity and mortality has lagged behind in patients with diabetes. With this recognition, there have been recent efforts to better define the pathophysiology and treatment of heart disease in patients with diabetes. Ongoing research studies promise to answer key clinical questions related to how best to identify and treat CVD in patients with diabetes.

ADDITIONAL READINGS

Gaede P, Vedel P, Larson N, et al. Multifactorial intervention and cardiovascular disease in patients with type 2 diabetes. *N Engl J Med* 2003;348:383.

Heart Outcomes Prevention Evaluation (HOPE) Study Investigators. Effect of ramipril on cardiovascular and microvascular outcomes in people with diabetes mellitus: results of the HOPE study and MICRO-HOPE substudy. *Lancet* 2000;355:253.

Malmberg K. Prospective randomised study of intensive insulin treatment on long term survival after acute myocardial infarction in patients with diabetes mellitus. DIGAMI (Diabetes Mellitus, Insulin Glucose Infusion in Acute Myocardial Infarction) Study Group [see comments]. *British Medical Journal* 1997;314:1512.

Vinik AI, Mitchell BD, Maser RE, et al. Diabetic autonomic neuropathy. *Diabetes Care* 2003;26:1553.

Wackers FJT, Young LH, Inzucchi SE, et al. Detection of silent myocardial ischemia in asymptomatic diabetic subjects: The DIAD study. *Diabetes Care* 2004;27:1954.

For a more detailed discussion of this topic and a bibliography, please see Porte *et al: Ellenberg & Rifkin's Diabetes Mellitus,* 6th ed., Chapter 49.

Peripheral Vascular Disease in the Person with Diabetes

Cameron M. Akbari   Frank W. LoGerfo

PATHOPHYSIOLOGY OF VASCULAR DISEASE IN DIABETES MELLITUS

The complications of diabetes may best be characterized as alterations in vascular structure and function, with subsequent end-organ damage and death. Specifically, two types of vascular disease are seen in patients with diabetes: a nonocclusive microcirculatory impairment involving the capillaries and arterioles of the kidneys, retina, and peripheral nerves, and a macroangiopathy characterized by atherosclerotic lesions of the coronary and peripheral arterial circulation. The former is relatively unique to diabetes, whereas the latter lesions are morphologically and functionally similar in both nondiabetic and diabetic patients.

The so-called small-vessel disease of diabetes is an inaccurate term, since it suggests an untreatable occlusive lesion in the microcirculation. Prospective anatomic and physiologic studies have demonstrated that there is no such microvascular occlusive disease. Dispelling the notion of "small-vessel disease" is fundamental to the principles of limb salvage in patients with diabetes, since arterial reconstruction is almost always possible and successful in these patients.

Although there is no occlusive lesion in the diabetic microcirculation, diabetes is characterized by a microvascular dysfunction, with increased vascular permeability and impaired autoregulation of blood flow and vascular tone. The characteristic microvascular complications of diabetes are retinopathy, nephropathy, and neuropathy, and population-based studies have identified a correlation between their development and the duration of diabetes. Glycemic control affects both the severity and development of these complications, as noted from the Diabetes Control and Complications Trial (DCCT).

Although multiple theories have been postulated as to the etiology of accelerated microangiopathy, it is likely that several biochemical derangements work synergistically at multiple areas within the arteriolar and capillary level, including the basement membrane, smooth muscle cell, and the endothelial cell. Thickening of the capillary basement membrane is the dominant structural change in both neuropathy and retinopathy, and alterations of the basement membrane likely contribute to albuminuria and the progression of diabetic nephropathy. In the diabetic foot, capillary basement membrane thickening may theoretically impair the migration of leukocytes and the hyperemic response following injury, thereby increasing the susceptibility of the diabetic foot to infection. However, these changes do not lead to narrowing of the capillary lumen, and arteriolar blood flow may be normal or even increased despite these changes.

A variety of other microvascular abnormalities may be demonstrated in the diabetic foot. Both capillary blood flow and the maximal hyperemic response to stimuli are reduced in the diabetic foot, suggesting that a *functional* microvascular impairment is a major contributing factor for diabetic foot problems.

Furthermore, diabetes also affects the axon reflex (neurogenic vasodilatation), which further impairs the ability of the diabetic foot to achieve maximal blood flow following injury.

In the coronary and cerebral circulation, reduced coronary flow reserve and impaired coronary reactivity has been observed in diabetic patients with angiographically normal coronary arteries and no other detectable microvascular complications, suggesting an early endothelial dysfunction. Similarly, impaired cerebrovascular reserve is also noted in patients with diabetes, particularly among those patients with other microvascular complications.

Endothelial function is abnormal in patients with both insulin-dependent and non-insulin-dependent diabetes mellitus, and a variety of mechanisms responsible for vascular dysfunction have been proposed, principally abnormalities in the nitric oxide pathway, abnormal production of vasoconstrictor prostanoids, intracellular signaling, reduction in Na^+-K^+-ATPase activity, and advanced glycosylated end products. Several lines of evidence have indicated that the microcirculation is also implicated in the pathogenesis of diabetic neuropathy, and the etiology of diabetic neuropathy may be a complex interplay between metabolic and microvascular defects involving aldose reductase, Na^+-K^+-ATPase activity, and nitric oxide.

In contrast to the microcirculatory abnormalities, the macroangiopathy of diabetes is similar to that occurring in the nondiabetic population, and is due to atherosclerotic occlusive disease. The Framingham Study of over 5000 subjects demonstrated that diabetes is a powerful risk factor for atherosclerotic coronary and peripheral arterial disease, independent of other atherogenic risk factors. Within the coronary and extracranial carotid vessels, the risk of coronary ischemic events and stroke are increased between two- and fourfold over that of the nondiabetic population, and the presence of diabetes is equivalent to three other risk factors for cardiovascular death.

Lower-extremity arterial disease is more common among patients with diabetes. The presence of diabetes is associated with a two- to threefold excess risk of intermittent claudication compared with its absence. Despite significant advances in the prevention and treatment of peripheral vascular disease, diabetes continues to be the single strongest cardiovascular risk factor for the development of critical leg ischemia and limb loss. As noted earlier, the cause of lower-extremity occlusive disease is the same in both diabetic and nondiabetic patients; however, the major difference between these two populations of patients is the pattern and location of the occlusive lesions. Whereas occlusive lesions of the superficial femoral and popliteal segment are commonly found in nondiabetic patients with limb ischemia, diabetic patients commonly have occlusive disease involving the infrageniculate, or tibial, arteries. However, the foot arteries are almost invariably patent, which allows for successful distal arterial reconstruction despite extensive, more proximal tibial arterial disease.

DIABETES AND CEREBROVASCULAR DISEASE

As noted earlier, the incidence of ischemic stroke is at least 2.5-fold higher in diabetic patients, and the mortality and severity of stroke is higher among patients with diabetes. The relative risk of stroke increases even further among diabetic patients with established retinopathy, neuropathy, or nephropathy, thus suggesting that the presence of diabetes introduces additional microvascular and cerebrovascular pathophysiology which may increase the frequency and severity of stroke in these patients.

Elevated blood glucose is toxic to infarcted brain tissue, and stroke severity is greater in patients with hyperglycemia. Among patients with diabetes, poor glycemic control doubles the risk of ischemic stroke, even after adjustment for other variables. Abnormal cerebral blood flow may be seen in experimental diabetes, and among patients with diabetes and no history of cerebrovascular disease, single-photon emission tomography (SPET) scanning has demonstrated multiple subclinical alterations in cerebral blood flow. Hyperglycemia alone causes both a decrease in cerebral blood flow and an impaired cerebral vasodilatory response, and may impair the autoregulation of cerebral blood flow. As noted previously, altered cerebral vascular reactivity occurs among patients with long-standing diabetes and may reflect a generalized cerebrovascular microangiopathy involving the brain resistance arterioles.

Because of the worse prognosis of stroke in patients with diabetes, efforts should be directed toward reducing the risk of stroke in these patients, including reduction or elimination of concomitant risk factors. In addition, among selected symptomatic and asymptomatic patients with a high-grade internal carotid artery stenosis, carotid endarterectomy has been shown to reduce the risk of stroke. Although the safety of carotid endarterectomy in patients with diabetes may be questioned, morbidity and mortality rates of carotid endarterectomy are comparable with those of the nondiabetic population.

THE DIABETIC FOOT

Problems of the diabetic foot are the most common cause for hospitalization in diabetic patients, with an annual health care cost of over $1 billion. Diabetes is a contributing factor in half of all lower-extremity amputations in the United States, and the relative risk for amputation is 40 times greater in people with diabetes. Along with neuropathy and infection, ischemia from peripheral vascular disease is a fundamental consideration in the pathogenesis and treatment of diabetic foot disease.

Peripheral neuropathy is a common complication of diabetes, and may be broadly classified as sensorimotor or autonomic. Sensorimotor neuropathy initially involves the distal lower extremities, progresses centrally, and is typically symmetric. Sensory nerve fiber involvement leads to loss of the protective sensation of pain, whereas motor fiber destruction results in small-muscle atrophy in the foot. Consequently, the metatarsals are flexed, with metatarsal head prominence and "clawing" of the toes. This causes abnormal pressure points to develop on the bony prominences without sensation, with subsequent callus formation, cracking, erosion, and ulceration. Meanwhile, autonomic neuropathy in the foot causes loss of sympathetic tone, which results in increased arteriovenous shunting and inefficient nutrient flow. Autonomic denervation of oil and sweat glands leads to cracking of dry skin, which further predisposes the diabetic foot to skin breakdown and ulceration.

The spectrum of infection in diabetic foot disease ranges from superficial ulceration to extensive gangrene with fulminant sepsis. The majority of infections are polymicrobic, with the most common pathogens being staphylococci and streptococci; more complicated ulcers may harbor anaerobes and gram-negative bacilli. Potential sources of diabetic foot infection include a simple puncture wound or ulcer, the nail plate, and the interdigital web space. Untreated infection can lead to bacterial spread along tendon sheaths and fascial planes, destruction of the interosseous fascia, and spread to the foot dorsum. Edema in the foot elevates compartmental pressures, with resultant capillary thrombosis and further impairment of nutrient blood flow.

Classical signs of infection may not always be present in the infected diabetic foot due to the consequences of neuropathy, alterations in the foot microcirculation, and leukocyte abnormalities. Fever, chills, and leukocytosis may be absent in up to two-thirds of diabetic patients with extensive foot infections, and hyperglycemia is often the sole presenting sign. Therefore a complete examination of the infected areas is mandatory, and the wound should be thoroughly inspected, including unroofing of all encrusted areas, to determine the extent of involvement. Infections should be adequately drained, as diabetic patients simply cannot tolerate undrained pus or infection. Because most infections are polymicrobic, cultures should be obtained from the base or depths of the wound after debridement so that appropriate antibiotic treatment may ensue. Deep ulcers should be gently explored with a sterile probe, since the diagnosis of osteomyelitis may be made if bone is palpated.

A critical step for limb salvage in patients with diabetic foot ulceration is a thorough evaluation for ischemia. The complex milieu of motor and sensory neuropathy, capillary basement thickening, loss of the neurogenic inflammatory response, and the wide spectrum of microcirculatory and endothelial abnormalities result in a biologically compromised foot. Even moderate ischemia may lead to ulceration under these circumstances. Thus the concept of ischemia must be modified in making decisions about arterial reconstruction in the diabetic foot, since the biologically compromised foot requires *maximum circulation* to heal an ulcer. This leads to three significant principals: (1) All diabetic foot ulcers should be evaluated for an ischemic component. (2) Correction of a moderate degree of ischemia will improve healing in the biologically compromised diabetic foot. (3) Whenever possible, the arterial reconstruction should be designed to restore normal arterial pressure to the target area. Ultimately, all limb salvage efforts will fail unless ischemia is recognized and corrected.

Treatment of the diabetic foot should assume an orderly approach, with the first priority being prompt control of infection. Subsequently, the presence of ischemia should be evaluated, followed by prompt arterial reconstruction once active infection has resolved. Finally, secondary procedures, such as further debridement, toe amputations, local flaps, and even free flaps, may then be carried out separately in the fully vascularized foot.

EVALUATION OF LOWER-EXTREMITY VASCULAR DISEASE IN THE PATIENT WITH DIABETES

As with any other disease process, evaluation should begin with a detailed history and physical exam. In the patient with a diabetic foot ulcer, it is helpful to consider the duration of the ulcer, the type of treatments utilized, and any past history of foot ulceration and treatment. The history of the foot problem itself can give valuable insight as to the potential for healing, the presence of coexisting infection or arterial occlusive disease, and the need for further treatment. Any patient presenting with a foot ulceration or gangrene should immediately arouse suspicion of underlying arterial insufficiency, even if neuropathy or infection is present. Although nocturnal rest pain in the foot is strongly suggestive of lower-extremity arterial disease in the nondiabetic patient, the variable effects of neuropathy make pain more difficult to evaluate in the diabetic limb. Similarly, claudication symptoms may be entirely absent in the patient with an ischemic diabetic foot ulcer. Long-standing foot ulceration, coexisting cardiac disease (such as angina or heart failure), and sensorimotor neuropathy may all limit the ability to ambulate sufficiently to manifest claudication symptoms.

The duration of the ulcer also provides important clues, insofar as a long-standing, nonhealing ulcer is strongly suggestive of ischemia. Certainly, an ulcer or gangrenous area that has been present for several months is unlikely to heal without some type of further additional treatment, whether it be off-loading of weight-bearing areas, treatment of infection, or, most commonly, correction of arterial insufficiency. A history of previous leg revascularization (including percutaneous therapies) also provides an important clue as to underlying arterial insufficiency. Because of the predilection for mirror-image-type atherosclerotic occlusive disease, the contralateral leg need also be considered, in that previous revascularization in the opposite leg may suggest arterial insufficiency on the affected side. The history of other cardiovascular risk factors, such as cigarette smoking or hyperlipidemia, is also important, as their presence increases the likelihood that ischemia is contributing to the present foot problem.

In the presence of ischemia, all limb salvage efforts will fail, and therefore the physical exam must include a systematic approach to the assessment of arterial insufficiency. In the patient with foot ulceration, noting the location of the ulcer may be helpful, in that purely ischemic lesions typically occur in the most distal parts of the foot, such as the toes, forefoot, or heel, in contrast to the neuropathic ulcers seen on the weight-bearing areas. Multiple ulcerations or gangrenous areas on the foot, absence of granulation tissue, or lack of bleeding with debridement of the ulcer should immediately raise concern for underlying arterial insufficiency. Other signs suggesting arterial insufficiency include pallor with elevation, fissures (particularly at the heel) and absent hair growth. Although poor skin condition and hyperkeratosis may not always be good indicators of arterial disease, they should be noted, as they may help confirm initial clinical impressions.

The pulse examination, including the status of the foot pulses, is the single most important component of the physical exam, since *ischemia is always presumed to be present in the absence of a palpable pulse.*

Although not difficult, an accurate pulse examination of the lower extremities is an acquired skill, and time should be devoted to practicing and perfecting the technique. The femoral pulse is palpated midway between the superior iliac spine and the pubic tubercle, just below the inguinal ligament. The popliteal pulse should be palpated with both hands and with the knee flexed no more than 15 degrees. Palpation of the foot pulses requires a knowledge of the usual location of the native arteries. The dorsalis pedis artery is located between the first and second metatarsal bones, just lateral to the extensor hallucis longus tendon, and its pulse is palpated by the pads of the fingers as the hand is partially wrapped around the foot. If the pulse cannot be palpated, the fingers may be moved a few millimeters in each direction, as the artery may have an occasional slight aberrant course. A common mistake is to place a single finger at one location on the dorsum of the foot. The posterior tibial artery is typically located in the hollow curve just behind the medial malleolus, approximately halfway between the malleolus and the Achilles tendon. The examiner's hand should be contralateral to the examined foot (i.e., the right hand should be used to palpate the left foot and vice versa), so as to allow the hand curvature to follow the ankle.

A variety of noninvasive arterial tests may be ordered in an effort to quantify the degree of ischemia. However, in the presence of diabetes, *all* of these tests have significant limitations. Although Doppler-derived pressures have proven to be reliable in localizing the degree and level of arterial occlusive disease in nondiabetic patients, their use is limited in the presence of diabetes. Medial arterial calcinosis occurs frequently in diabetic patients and is characterized by a *nonobstructive* calcification of the vessel wall at the media layer; its presence can result in noncompressible arteries with artifactually high segmental systolic pressures and ankle-brachial indices. Medial calcification should be suspected whenever the ankle pressure greatly exceeds arm pressure or when the Doppler signal at the ankle cannot be obliterated with greater than 250 mm Hg pressure. Lower levels of calcification in the toe vessels supports the use of toe systolic pressures as a more reliable indicator of arterial flow to the foot. However, the use of toe pressures is often limited by the proximity of the foot ulcer to the cuff site, the size of the cuff itself, and other extrinsic variables.

Segmental Doppler wave forms and pulsed volume recordings are unaffected by medial calcification. A normal Doppler waveform is triphasic; with proximal obstruction, the waveform becomes monophasic. Pulse volume recordings rely on plethysmographic recordings of the change in volume that occurs with each pulsation. A sharp upstoke, narrow peak, and dicrotic notch characterize a normal recording. With increasing levels of arterial insufficiency, the waveform loses the dicrotic notch, followed by loss of amplitude and blunting of the waveform. Since neither of these tests rely on obliterating flow within a vessel (unlike Doppler-derived pressures), they may prove useful in the diabetic patient with suspected arterial insufficiency. However, significant limitations exist in their use and caution should be exercised when interpreting their results. Evaluation of these waveforms is primarily qualitative and not quantitative. A flat forefoot tracing is a convincing demonstration of ischemia, but it is difficult to make clinical decisions based on the magnitude of the waveform. Similarly, severity of arterial insufficiency cannot be accurately interpreted, since no reliable quantitative scoring exists. In addition, the quality of the waveforms is affected by peripheral edema, cuff size, and motion artifact. Finally, the presence of ulceration, especially at the forefoot level, often precludes accurate cuff placement.

Regional transcutaneous oximetry ($TcPO_2$) measurements are also unaffected by medial calcinosis, and recent studies have noted its reliability in predicting healing of ulcers and amputation levels. Limitations, including a lack of equipment standardization, user variability, and a large "gray area" of values, preclude its applicability. Furthermore, $TcPO_2$ measurements are higher in diabetic patients with foot ulcers when compared to the nondiabetic population, which further limits the ability of this test to predict ischemia.

The limitations of noninvasive vascular testing in diabetic patients with foot ulceration emphasize the continued importance of a thorough bedside evaluation and clinical judgment. To reiterate, the status of the foot pulse is the most important aspect of the physical exam and occlusive disease is present if the foot pulses are not palpable. Because restoration of pulsatile flow maximizes the chances of healing in the diabetic foot, nonpalpable foot pulses are an indication for contrast arteriography in the clinical setting of tissue loss, poor healing, or gangrene, even if neuropathy may have been the antecedent cause of skin breakdown or ulceration. The arteriogram is obtained to determine and plan the type of arterial reconstruction which will result in restoration of the foot pulse.

Concern about contrast-induced renal dysfunction in the presence of diabetes should not mitigate against the performance of a high-quality arteriogram of the entire distal circulation. Several prospective studies have documented that the incidence of contrast-induced nephropathy is not higher in the diabetic patient without preexisting renal disease, particularly with the judicious use of hydration and renal protective agents. Alternatively, magnetic resonance angiography, carbon dioxide angiography, and duplex scanning may be used, either in conjunction with or in place of contrast arteriography.

Whatever preoperative imaging modality is chosen prior to arterial reconstruction, it is mandatory that consideration be given to the pattern of lower-extremity vascular disease in patients with diabetes, and that the complete infrapopliteal circulation be incorporated, including the foot vessels. Because the foot vessels are often spared by the atherosclerotic occlusive process, even when the tibial arteries are occluded, it is essential that arteriograms not be terminated at the midtibial level.

PRINCIPLES OF ARTERIAL RECONSTRUCTION IN THE DIABETIC FOOT

Restoration of the foot pulse is a fundamental goal of revascularization in the diabetic foot. Although bypass to the popliteal or tibio-peroneal arteries may restore foot pulses, the characteristic pattern of occlusive disease in the diabetic patient usually requires more distal bypass grafting. Specifically, autogenous vein grafting to the dorsalis pedis, distal posterior tibial, and plantar arteries incorporates knowledge of this anatomic pattern and will result in the maximal pulsatile blood flow that is required for healing. Experience with the dorsalis pedis bypass graft has demonstrated technical feasibility and excellent short-term and long-term patency. More importantly, 5-year limb salvage rates of approximately 85% have been reported. Fundamental to its success is meticulous technique and its appropriate use. The principal indication for the pedal graft is when there is no other vessel that has continuity with the foot, particularly in cases with tissue loss, and is unnecessary when a more proximal bypass will restore foot pulses. Autogenous vein is the preferred conduit for all lower-extremity bypass operations, and, in our opinion, should always be used for the pedal bypass grafts. The distal location of the dorsalis pedis artery theoretically necessitates a long venous conduit, which is often not attainable. However, by using the popliteal or distal superficial femoral artery as an inflow site, a shorter length of vein may be used, with excellent long-term patency. This is particularly true in the diabetic patient, again due to the pattern of atherosclerotic disease.

Active infection in the foot is commonly encountered in the complicated ischemic diabetic foot. However, it is not a contraindication to lower-extremity revascularization, as long as the infectious process is controlled and located remotely from the proposed incisions. Adequate control implies absence of sepsis and resolution of cellulitis, lymphangitis, and edema, especially in areas of proposed incisions required to expose the distal artery or saphenous vein.

Despite the technical success of lower-extremity bypass in patients with diabetes, there continue to be concerns about long-term patient function and survival. However, recent studies have clearly demonstrated equivalent long-term survival and limb salvage in patients with and without diabetes.

Following successful revascularization, secondary procedures may be performed for both limb *and* foot salvage. Chronic ulcerations may be treated by ulcer excision, arthroplasty, or hemiphalangectomy. In the patient with extensive tissue loss, both local flaps and free flaps may be used. Due to the architecture of the diabetic foot, underlying bony structural abnormalities are often the cause of ulceration and may be corrected by metatarsal head resection or osteotomy. Heel ulcers may be treated by partial calcanectomy and local (e.g., flexor tendon) or even free flap coverage.

CONCLUSION

The patient with diabetes and peripheral vascular disease represents a uniquely complex pathophysiology involving microcirculatory and macrovascular disease. Because much of the disability and morbidity of diabetes are caused directly by these vascular changes, an understanding of diabetic vascular disease is critical for reducing the overall morbidity and mortality of diabetes.

ADDITIONAL READINGS

Akbari CM, LoGerfo FW. Diabetes and peripheral vascular disease. *J Vasc Surg* 1999;30:373.

Akbari CM, Pomposelli FB Jr, Gibbons GW, et al: Diabetes mellitus: A risk factor for cartoid endarterectomy? *J Vasc Surg* 1997;25:1070.

Akbari CM, Pomposelli FB Jr, Gibbons GW, et al: Lower extremity revascularization in diabetes: Late observations. *Arch Surg* 2000;135:452.

LoGerfo FW, Coffman JD: Vascular and microvascular disease of the foot in diabetes. *N Engl J Med* 1984;311:1615.

Veves A, Akbari CM, Primavera J, et al: Endothelial dysfunction and the expression of endothelial nitric oxide synthetase in diabetic neuropathy, vascular disease, and foot ulceration. *Diabetes* 1997;47:457.

For a more detailed discussion of this topic and a bibliography, please see Porte *et al: Ellenberg & Rifkin's Diabetes Mellitus,* 6th ed., Chapter 50.

28 | The Diabetic Foot
William C. Coleman

INTRODUCTION

The history of caring for the feet of persons with diabetes is fraught with frustration for medical professionals, family members, and patients. During the last decade of the twentieth century there was a continuing refinement of interventional techniques to improve vascular flow to the lower extremities of persons with diabetes. And, new topical medications and dressings were introduced to improve the management of foot wounds. However, during this same period of time, there was a disappointing 22% increase in the total number of amputations performed in diabetic patients. By the end of the 1990s the annual number of lower-extremity amputations in the diabetic population had risen to over 67,000, with most performed on patients who receive Medicare benefits.

Despite this sobering trend, successful amputation prevention practices have been repeatedly confirmed by several groups, with up to a 68% reduction in amputations over a 2-year period. In Spain, 318 diabetic patients with neuropathy were followed by Calle-Pascual and associates for 3–6 years for their compliance with participation in an education and foot monitoring program. Participants who complied with all aspects of the program had a 13 times lower risk of developing a first ulcer and 44 times lower risk of amputation, as compared to noncompliant patients.

Successful programs have utilized multidisciplinary foot care teams, including foot specialists and/or specialized education techniques on foot care directed by a knowledgeable, influential leader. Regular preventive visits were scheduled to help the patients monitor their feet and to reinforce the need for constant protective behavior. Key to the success of the programs that are able to significantly reduce the numbers of lower-extremity amputations is their ability to manage the ramifications of lower-extremity sensory loss.

SENSORIMOTOR POLYNEUROPATHY

In the context of foot management, it is sensory neuropathy that increases the likelihood that the patient will develop a serious foot wound. Mantey and associates found that foot ulcers most frequently recurred in patients with the poorest glycemic control and the most profound distal neuropathy. Peripheral vascular disease rarely increases the chance of injury occurring, but an injury to a limb with severe arterial occlusive disease increases the possibility of limb loss.

Peripheral, symmetric, lower-extremity sensorimotor polyneuropathy affects approximately 50% of all persons who have had diabetes for more than 15 years. A foot may be vulnerable to damage long before gross sensory loss is noted. The diabetic patient with neuropathy often fails to notice pain associated with foot injury, or other telltale signs and symptoms such as swelling and infection.

The physician or therapist must identify the degree of sensory loss that puts a person at risk. This involves a quantitative test of sensation, which should be repeated at least annually for every person with diabetes. A test commonly used to identify feet that need protection and areas of the foot at most risk utilizes monofilament nylon fibers of varied diameters, which are calibrated to bend when different forces are applied to the ends of the fibers. Three monofilaments are recommended for the testing of diabetic feet: (1) the 1-g fiber (Semmes-Weinstein), which can be felt by normal feet and identifies the early onset of sensory neuropathy at a stage when special care may not be necessary; (2) the 10-g fiber to identify the areas that need to be protected; and (3) a 75-g fiber to identify areas that have lost all protective sensation. Clearly, the 10-g fiber is the important one. Busy diabetic clinics may benefit from frequent tests with one fiber, rather than less frequent full mapping of sensation.

RISK CATEGORIZATION

Several studies were conducted during the last decade to identify factors that contribute to the morbidity of the diabetic foot. In a prospective study of 749 patients, Boyko and coworkers found that diabetic foot ulcers develop as the result of neuropathy, diminished vascular perfusion, foot deformity, higher pressures under the foot, severity of diabetes, and co-morbid complications from diabetes. Persons with diabetes and neuropathy are 1.7 times more likely to develop foot ulceration. Those with foot deformity (limited great toe motion, bunion, or toe deformity) are 12.1 times more likely to experience a foot ulcer. If an individual diabetic patients has already had an amputation of a lower extremity, the risk of ulceration on the opposite limb increases to 36.4 times normal. By being aware of these data, the clinician can begin to categorize patients according to their risk of developing foot injury (Table 28-1).

CALLUSES

When subjected to repeated pressure, skin thickens to form callus tissue. Callus strengthens the skin's ability to withstand pressure. Callus of a moderate thickness is protective, whereas it can act as a foreign body if it is too thick. At that point, when pressure is again applied to the area, the callus can contribute to damage in deeper tissues. Plantar callus has been shown to be highly predictive of eventual foot ulceration.

WOUNDS OF THE FOOT

A foot may be damaged by external forces in one or more of three ways: (1) An unrelenting, low pressure, as from a tight shoe, may cause ischemic necrosis or a pressure sore. Its pathology is similar to that of a decubitus ulcer. (2) A much higher pressure may cause direct mechanical damage, as when a foot lands heavily on a sharp stone, broken glass, or a thumbtack, and the skin is broken or penetrated. (3) Constantly repeated moderate pressure with every step may result in inflammation at high-pressure points, followed by blister or ulcer formation. The pathology is not ischemic necrosis, because the blood supply is not continuously blocked, but is more consistent with inflammatory enzymatic autolysis. We have termed these three pathogenic factors *ischemia, mechanical damage,* and *inflammatory autolysis.*

TABLE 28-1 Classification of Diabetes Patients According to Risk of Developing Foot Injury

Category of risk for foot injury	Patient characteristics	Education needs	Monitoring of feet
0	All patients with diabetes	Co-morbidities of diabetes related to poor glycemic control Signs that suggest damage to the vasculature or nerves Need for properly fitting, conservative footwear	Once-a-year evaluation by a health care professional for signs of lower-extremity neuropathy or extremity arterial occlusive disease A quantitative test of sensation conducted at least annually Assessment of properly fitting shoes by a competent professional Toenails and calluses should be maintained by a trained medical professional Feet should be medically evaluated at least once every 6 months
1	Diabetes and peripheral neuropathy	Need for daily visual foot inspection Sensation in feet cannot be trusted as an indication of the presence or severity of foot wound Contact physician for assistance with wound care	
2	Diabetes, neuropathy, and foot deformity	Strict adherence to the use of proper footwear at all times Custom footwear or shoe inserts are often needed Any lesion should be treated immediately	See a foot specialist every 3 months for nail and callus care Feet should be examined for changes in shape or mobility
3	Diabetes and neuropathic feet	Must always wear prescription footwear to lower weight-bearing stress at previous site(s) of ulcer Walking without shoes or with nonprescribed footwear poses a threat to the foot	Visit a foot clinic every 1–2 months Footwear needs to be examined at every visit for proper fit and function

431

Ischemic Pressure Ulceration

A neuropathic foot is vulnerable to injury from unrelenting pressure. Sustained external pressure that is greater than capillary or local arteriolar blood pressure will occlude vessels wherever the tissues are compressed between the shoe and an underlying bony structure.

Localized necrosis of the skin of the foot may occur with pressures as low as 1 pound per square inch (psi). This level of pressure, often painless, can be exceeded with tight shoes (Fig. 28-1). With this in mind, a diabetic patient should wear a new shoe for only 2–3 hours on the first day. When it is removed, the patient should look carefully for any area of redness and feel for any localized warmth. If the skin becomes flushed after only 2 hours, there is reasonable chance that it might become severely damaged if that shoe were worn for 8–10 hours. A leather shoe may be moistened (using a 50% water/50% isopropyl alcohol solution) and stretched on a special last, and may then be worn again for only short periods until it is "broken in." People with diabetes should be advised to wear only leather shoes, because vinyl and other plastic uppers do not adapt to the shape of the foot to relieve localized pressure.

Although it may seem logical to encourage persons with diabetes to purchase loose shoes, this should actually be avoided. The danger from friction is as great or greater than that from ischemia. Friction blisters or ulcers may occur behind the heel or around the rim of the shoe as the foot moves in the vertical axis due to the loose fit. These blisters and ulcers are prevented by ensuring that the heel is snug and well shaped, and that the lacing or strap over the dorsum reaches far enough up and back over the instep to hold the shoe firmly onto the foot.

Direct Mechanical Damage

Approximately 1000 times more force per unit area is required to damage skin directly than it does to damage it via ischemia (Fig. 28-2). Direct damage to the sole of the foot might occur if the whole weight of a 144-lb person

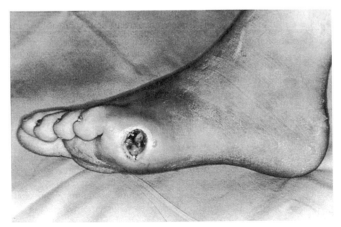

FIG. 28-1   Pressure necrosis at the lateral border of an insensitive foot due to the wearing of a tight shoe all day.

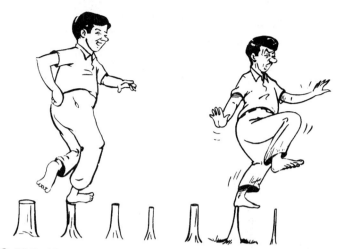

FIG. 28-2   His weight remains the same, but the area of the stump on which he stands is smaller. Under the foot, damage is caused more readily by narrowing the area of support than by increasing force.

were to rest on an area of ⅑ of a square inch (e.g., stiletto heels). Thus, it is unlikely that a person wearing shoes could ever suffer direct damage from any external force unless a small, sharp object were under the foot inside the shoe. And, because insensate feet are sometimes damaged by walking in stocking feet or barefoot on sharp objects, diabetics should never walk without footware. Other practical advice includes always wearing shoes with soles thick enough to prevent a thumbtack from penetrating to the foot and always to shake out the shoes before putting them on.

Along with direct damage from very high forces, direct damage from heat, cold, or corrosive chemicals should be considered. All persons with peripheral neuropathy need to be alert to such danger and to maintain a margin of safety. Such individuals require extra socks when skiing, protective footwear in chemical plants, and special awareness of hot floors in automobiles and trucks. They should be wary of fires or car heaters, and they must never rest their feet on steam pipes or use electric heaters in close proximity to warm their feet on frigid days.

Inflammatory Autolysis

Inflammatory autolysis is by far the most common cause of ulceration in the diabetic foot. The pressures that cause it range from 20 to 70 psi and are quite similar to the pressures that are ordinarily tolerated by normal individuals who go jogging or walking briskly in firm-soled shoes. Such pressures do not harm normal or diabetic feet unless:

1. They are frequently repeated on a daily basis on the same areas of the foot.
2. The tissues are already inflamed as a result of excessive mechanical stress.
3. The tissues are structurally abnormal as a result of previous ulceration and scarring.

The typical diabetic foot ulceration is postulated to begin as a callus on the surface of the skin. Due to repeated impacts to this callus as a result of walking, breakdown occurs between the callus and the deeper tissue. This breakdown comes as the result of the accumulation of inflammatory cells. These cells release enzymes that lyse underlying tissues, resulting in a pocket of accumulated fluid. Because the foot is insensate, the patient may continue to walk. The inflammation and associated tissue damage becomes exacerbated by hydraulic fluid pressure as the result of stresses on the pocket. This eventually results in the formation of a blister adjacent to the callus or a break in the skin. The hole in the skin will be smaller than the deeper pocket. For the inexperienced clinician, this could result in an underestimation of the extent of damage. When a blister rather than an open wound is found, and the foot is neuropathic, the clinician should appreciate that the real damage is deep to the callus rather than under the blister.

WALKING MANAGEMENT

The fact that persons with diabetes do not appear to limp or change their gait (as would normally occur) in the early stages of traumatic inflammation may allow them to continue until they develop necrosis, a blister, or ulceration. Every person who has insensitive feet needs to be educated about the dangers of repetitive, moderate stress to the feet and the need for extra foot protection to compensate for the reduction in sensation. Preulcerative changes (i.e., blisters, petechiae, erythema, and increased skin temperature) can alert patients and clinicians at a stage when the foot can be better protected to prevent further damage.

Patients need to know that they will be able to walk further if they reduce localized high-pressure areas on the sole. A study by Edmonds and colleagues demonstrated the value of proper footwear in the prevention of recurrent ulceration in a population of patients with diabetes. They found an 83% recurrence of ulceration in patients who reverted to wearing their regular shoes, while only 26% who wore only their prescribed footwear experienced recurrence. Likewise, Uccioli and Italian associates selected a group of diabetic neuropathic patients and randomly assigned them to either wear their own footwear or footwear with custom-molded inserts in extra-depth shoes for a year. Of those who wore nonprescription footwear, 58.3% developed foot ulcers within a year, in contrast to just 27.7% of those who were wearing the custom-molded inserts in extra-depth shoes.

At the point while walking when the "swing" foot is moving forward in preparation for the next step, the heel leaves the ground, and the entire body weight rests on the forefoot and toes, and the pressure is at the peak. The heel and midfoot bear no weight, and there may be only a few square inches to carry the body's weight. Under these conditions, pressures under the metatarsal heads or toes may rise to 40, 50, or even 60 psi. It is these levels of pressure that will result in inflammation and ulceration if they are repeated too frequently.

THE DAILY FOOT EXAMINATION

The person with diabetes is advised to check his or her feet every night before bed. Localized redness, heat, and callus formation are all good indications of stress. If any of them is progressive, it means that the patient is walking too much or wearing the wrong kind of shoe. Small areas of increased surface temperature that are still present the next morning represent inflammation.

If a person with diabetes finds a wound during the daily examination, he or she must promptly communicate its presence to the physician, nurse practitioner, or foot care team. Serious problems associated with the diabetic foot occur after the skin is broken and a wound or ulcer forms. In a survey of causal factors that resulted in lower-extremity amputation in diabetic patients, Reiber and associates showed that 84% had foot ulceration as the initial pathology. While it is important to prevent the wound or ulcer, it is absolutely essential to concentrate on the care and healing of the foot after it is wounded. Much of the reputation for nonhealing wounds on the feet of persons with diabetes has emerged because such wounds have gone undetected or are allowed to progress with each step for months or even years.

ACUTE CARE

The care giver must feel the skin around the ulcer. If it is warm and erythematous, the prognosis for healing is good. If it is cool, bluish, or dusky, the limb needs careful evaluation for vascular competence, and it may be a candidate for revascularization, angioplasty, or possible amputation. All necrotic tissue and callus should be debrided from the wound site by a trained specialist.

All foot wounds should be probed with a sterile instrument such as a nasal sinus probe to reveal any sinus tracts. The presence of a tract is often masked by granulation or necrotic tissue. Gentle insertion of the sinus probe in several parts of the wound from various angles will reveal the presence of the tract. Grayson and colleagues found in a study of 75 patients that simply probing for osteomyelitis had a specificity of 85% and a sensitivity of 66%. The predictive value of probing for osteomyelitis was 89% when bone was felt. However, if bone is not felt, osteomyelitis cannot be ruled out. Probing compares very favorably in sensitivity and specificity to radiographic and radionuclide studies. If the opening of the wound on the foot is narrow in proportion to its depth, it should be opened. Nonviable tissue may be removed and the wound lightly packed.

A new ulcer or infection may require immediate bedrest and antibiotics. In the past, many contended that all persons with foot infections and diabetes must be hospitalized. However, a prospective study by Lipsky and colleagues found that diabetic patients with non-limb-threatening infections can be successfully managed on an outpatient basis. If outpatient management is selected, the principles of controlling pressure and motion must be addressed. Patients with foot infections or severe peripheral vascular disease can be managed with posterior splints or other special protective devices as described by Hampton and Birke.

When the acute phase has subsided (with alleviation of fever and swelling), the foot may be treated by providing a protective plaster cast for ambulation.

Total contact casting remains the most reliable method for treatment, with chronic ulcers (present for months to years) predictably healed within 8 weeks when weight-bearing relief is provided by these specialized devices. Location and size of the ulcer correlate with the time it takes to close these wounds. Longer healing times have been attributed to severe vascular compromise or poor patient compliance. Forefoot ulcers healed in 30 days, and more posterior plantar ulcers took an average of 63 days to close.

The safe criteria for treatment in a plaster cast are: (1) only feet with adequate blood supply (warm around the wound) should be casted; (2) wait until the infection is localized and systemic symptoms have subsided (e.g., fever, tender inguinal lymphadenopathy); (3) make sure the wound is wide open so there is no danger of skin closing over, leaving a deep pocket of infection; and (4) close contact with the patient; remove the cast if any new or recurrent symptoms are noted.

The first cast is usually removed and casting reapplied after 7 days because the limb always shrinks from loss of edema as soon as it is immobilized. If there is obvious swelling at the time the cast was first applied, it should be changed even sooner, because a loose cast is liable to produce friction blisters. The second cast can often be left on for 2 weeks without significant loosening. A "window" should also never be left in a cast. The edges of the window cause shear stress on the tissues that bulge through.

MANAGEMENT OF NEWLY HEALED ULCERS

When an ulcer has finally epithelialized, it is not necessary to keep the patient in bed or in a cast. However, the foot is not yet completely healed, and walking has to be carefully graded, as the scar has not consolidated and the tissues are still friable. When a healed ulcer breaks down again, it usually occurs in the first month after healing. This has often been attributed to a recurrence of infection, but the actual explanation is commonly the shear stress from walking. A predictable result is that the newly formed tissues are torn, with a hematoma forming under the new skin. The damage is repeated with continued walking until the wound breaks down once again.

Several simple rules should be followed to minimize such recurrence of foot ulcers:

1. The patient must understand the problem; otherwise he or she will make no real attempt to curtail activity.
2. Shear stress occurs maximally with fast walking, quick starts and stops, and when making long strides. It also occurs with extension of the toes at the metatarsophalangeal joint when the foot bends at the ball of the foot in the propulsive phase of gait.
3. For the first few weeks after an ulcer heals, the patient should walk as little as possible, slowly and with short steps, preferably with a rigid-soled shoe.
4. Friction between the skin of the sole and the insole of the shoe must be minimized. The inner layer of the insole should be slick and slippery (leather or nylon, rather than rubber or polyethylene foam products). Talcum powder, silicone, or a double layer of socks helps to minimize the extent to which the skin of the foot sticks to the shoe.

SURGICAL INTERVENTION

Elective surgery on the diabetic foot is mainly directed at the prevention of localized pressure and shear. If for any reason it is difficult to avoid high stress to a single aspect of the foot, even with well-fitted shoes, then a foot surgeon should be consulted. Clawed toes or hammer toes may be straightened to avoid stress on the tip of the toe or on the dorsal aspect of the interphalangeal joint. Bunions and hallux valgus may need correction.

If one metatarsal head is prominent on the sole and is shown to be under undue stress during walking in a well-fitted shoe, it may be useful to do an osteotomy at its neck to allow the head to move into alignment with the other metatarsals. Less often, a metatarsal may be shortened to bring it into line with other, already shortened metatarsals. Rarely should a metatarsal be removed. Although it allows the ulcer under it to heal, its removal decreases available weight-bearing surface and increases the stress under the remaining metatarsals, creating new concerns.

Sometimes a foot may have an intrinsic imbalance, such as a foot drop or inversion. If such an imbalance or deformity can be corrected surgically by tendon transfer or by an osteotomy, it may avoid the need for custom-made shoes or braces on a permanent basis.

NEUROPATHIC FRACTURES

The definition of a "Charcot's" fracture has evolved over time. Jean Martin Charcot described arthropathy that developed without known cause in patients with tabes dorsalis or other neuropathies. The term *Charcot's fracture* (or *Charcot foot*) is now used to describe a fracture in the presence of neuropathy. It should also be extended to include cases in which the tarsus collapses due to ligamentous failure, but no fracture can be identified radiographically.

The key to success in the treatment of neuropathic joint deformity is early diagnosis. The most constant sign of early joint damage is a patch of localized heat, often on the medial aspect of the midfoot. At that stage the X-ray may show early fragmentation of the navicular, the medial cuneiform, or the head of the talus.

When confronted with a red, warm, swollen foot on a diabetic patient, and no open wound can be found, in addition to cellulites, the clinician should consider that a Charcot's fracture may be present. Even if radiologic studies fail to show the presence of a fracture, if the surface skin temperature remains hot, the foot must be immobilized and weight bearing should be supported until the temperature returns to normal.

CONCLUSION

The vast majority of lower-extremity amputations can be avoided. To accomplish this on a national scale, the medical community must embrace changes in its current approach to this epidemic. The physician must learn to appreciate the unique environment in which neuropathic injuries occur. A multidisciplinary team is needed to successfully manage diabetic foot problems. Injury prevention through education, appropriate footwear, and regularly scheduled clinic visits should be at the heart of such a program. Members of this team should have a knowledge of psychology, social intervention, patient education, footwear and orthoses, biomechanics of the lower extremity, neuropathic wound and fracture care, and diabetes management. Professionals who accept the challenges of helping patients with diabetes should be willing and able to provide treatment and rehabilitation on an ongoing basis, often for many years.

ADDITIONAL READINGS

Boulton AJ: Pressure and the diabetic foot: clinical science and offloading techniques. *Amer J Surg* 2004;187:17S.

Brem H, Sheehan P, Boulton AJ: Protocol for treatment of diabetic foot ulcers. *Amer J Surg* 2004;187:1S.

Frykberg RG: Diabetic foot ulcerations: management and adjunctive therapy. *Clin Podiatr Med Surg* 2003;20:709.

Jeffcoate WJ, Harding KG: Diabetic foot ulcers. *Lancet* 2003;361:1545.

Zgonis T, Jolly GP, Buren BJ, et al: Diabetic foot infections and antibiotic therapy. *Clin Podiatr Med Surg* 2003;20:655.

For a more detailed discussion of this topic and a bibliography, please see Porte *et al: Ellenberg & Rifkin's Diabetes Mellitus,* 6th ed., Chapter 51.

29 | Diabetes and the Skin
Jennifer Bub   John Olerud

The skin is affected in one way or another in essentially 100% of diabetic patients. Dysregulation of glucose, insulin, and lipids leads directly to physical signs in the skin of patients with diabetes. In this chapter, we review conditions that appear to be linked directly to the endocrine, vascular, neurologic, and immunologic impairment seen in diabetes mellitus (DM). These conditions include ulcers, acanthosis nigricans, diabetic thick skin, cutaneous infections, and cutaneous xanthomas. A number of other clinical conditions associated with diabetes will be reviewed, although the pathobiology of the disorders remains unclear. These include necrobiosis lipoidica, granuloma annulare, diabetic dermopathy, bullosis diabeticorum, and acquired perforating dermatosis. Complications of insulin injection are reviewed as well, because of its importance in the management of diabetic patients.

DIABETIC ULCERS

Without question, the most important skin lesions in diabetic patients are lower-extremity ulcers. Approximately 15% of people with DM will develop at least one foot ulcer during their lifetime, and 15–24% of diabetic patients with foot ulcers will eventually undergo amputation. It is estimated that the vast majority (up to 85%) of lower-extremity amputations are preventable; still, rates of amputation continue to rise. Underuse of recommended preventive care practices among patients with DM is a major contributor.

Reiber *et al* found neuropathy, minor foot trauma, and foot deformity to be the most common causes of lower-extremity ulceration. Edema, ischemia, and callus formation were also important. Three factors important in all lower-extremity ulcerations, regardless of etiology, include venous insufficiency, stasis dermatitis, and infection. For the diabetic patient, skin conditions such as necrobiosis lipoidica and bullosis diabeticorum can also eventuate in ulceration.

Vasculopathy is a major factor in the pathogenesis of diabetic ulcers. Transcutaneous oxygen ($TcPO_2$), and carbon dioxide ($TcPCO_2$) pressure monitoring allows for quantification of the degree of peripheral vascular disease and has been shown to correlate with risk of amputation. Levels below 20 mm Hg result in a 16-fold excess risk of amputation. The degree of vasculopathy is also strongly associated with failure of diabetic ulcers to heal.

Sensory neuropathy also plays a major role in diabetic ulcers and lower-extremity amputation. Diabetic patients who lack vibratory sensation have been shown to have a 15.5-fold excess risk of amputation compared to those with intact vibratory sense. Unperceived trauma from friction blisters and ingrown toenails, and diminished influences of neuropeptides on skin immunity and tissue repair all play a role in the pathogenesis. Of importance, ulcers heal very slowly in diabetic patients with neuropathy. One study showed that only 31% of 349 patients with diabetic neuropathic foot ulcers receiving standard treatment healed in 20 weeks. Frequent clinical examination and the use of a 5.07 Semmes-Weinstein filament are imperative to identify patients at risk for foot ulceration.

Management of lower-extremity ulcers requires modification of contributing factors. These include stasis dermatitis, peripheral edema, infection, and mechanical trauma. Stasis dermatitis should be treated with topical steroids on the skin adjacent to the ulcers. Control of peripheral edema may be accomplished by bedrest, leg elevation, sodium restriction, or appropriately used diuretics. Unna boots, Ace wraps, compression stockings, and even contact casting for weight off-loading may be useful if severe arterial insufficiency does not preclude these interventions. Edema was associated with amputations in 58% of diabetic patients undergoing amputation in one series. Diagnosis and treatment of underlying local soft tissue infection is important. Osteomyelitis occurs in approximately 15% of diabetic lower-extremity ulcers, and should be suspected in deep or chronically draining ulcers, particularly if bone is exposed. Mechanical protection for neuropathic extremities is another key element in therapy of diabetic ulcers (see Chap. 28).

Trials of growth-promoting factors and skin equivalents have been under investigation to enhance diabetic ulcer healing. Adjunctive use of these new topical technologies show "modest benefit" if used with adequate off-loading, debridement, and control of infection. Arterial reconstruction for critical limb ischemia (severe diabetic ulceration and gangrene) should be considered. The use of multidisciplinary diabetic foot units, and specialized ulcer care teams in outpatient departments, has produced impressive results in the prevention and management of lower-extremity ulcers as well as the prevention of amputations.

Without question, the most important ulcer interventions by physicians and other health care professionals are in the area of prevention. These interventions can be summarized as follows:

1. Implement formal outpatient education that includes teaching daily foot inspection, particularly for neuropathic patients.
2. Advise careful selection of footwear that is not rigid or constricting in design or requires a break-in period. Ill-fitting shoes or socks were the most common reasons for foot ulcers in a study of 314 diabetic patients with ulcers. Issuing sports shoes to a group of diabetic patients as an experimental variable resulted in a measurable reduction of calluses.
3. Advise patients to inspect shoes for foreign bodies before putting them on, and to avoid walking barefoot.
4. Seek early health care attention for calluses, blisters, ingrown toenails, dermatitis, or athlete's foot.
5. Personally inspect the feet of diabetic patients at each visit.
6. Advise patients with a history of ulceration that they are at high risk for reulceration (34% at 1 year, 61% at 3 years, and 70% at 5 years). Redouble education and prevention efforts in this group. Life-long surveillance is required.

ACANTHOSIS NIGRICANS

Clinical/Epidemiology

Acanthosis nigricans (AN) presents as "dirty" black or gray-brown, velvety, warty, thickened skin in the flexural areas, including the back and sides of the neck, the axillae, and the anogenital region (Fig. 29-1). The neck is the most consistently affected area. AN is common in the general population, and most cases are associated with obesity, insulin resistance, and hyperin-

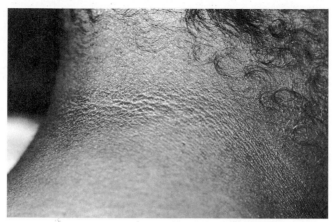

FIG. 29-1   Acanthosis nigricans on the neck of an African-American woman with T2DM.

sulinemia. In certain studies, AN is present in approximately three-fourths of obese adults, and two-thirds of primary school children weighing 200% of ideal body weight (IBW). Overall, AN was present in 7.1% of unselected primary school children, with a significantly higher prevalence among African-American and Hispanic children compared to those of European descent. Rates of AN are also very high in certain Native American subpopulations in which the development of type 2 diabetes mellitus (T2DM) is strikingly common. A prospective longitudinal study found AN to be an independent risk factor for development of T2DM. Since AN is strongly correlated with hyperinsulinemia, and hyperinsulinemia has been demonstrated to be an independent risk factor for the development of ischemic heart disease, some investigators have recommended that AN be used as an inexpensive surrogate marker for hyperinsulinemia to identify children and adolescents with a future risk of T2DM and ischemic cardiovascular disease.

Pathogenesis

In conditions of insulin resistance and hyperinsulinemia, excess binding of insulin to insulin-like growth factor (IGF-1) receptors has been proposed as a mechanism for AN as well as for androgen excess. High concentrations of insulin stimulate DNA synthesis and cell proliferation *in vitro* through the IGF-1 receptor in fibroblasts, and perhaps keratinocytes. Ovarian cells capable of steroidogenesis also possess IGF-1 receptors. Molecular biology has been used to identify a number of specific mutations in the insulin receptor gene in patients with AN and type A insulin resistance. These patients have both severe insulin resistance and hyperandrogenemia.

Treatment

Treatment for AN is generally ineffective. Resolution may occur with weight loss in obese patients. Treatment of hyperinsulinemic diabetic and nondiabetic patients with metformin was found to result in a decrease in AN. Topical retinoids and ammonium lactate have shown varied success. Discontinuation of certain drugs reported to cause AN, such as nicotinic acid and diethyl-stilbestrol, usually results in skin clearance. Although earlier authors have emphasized a relationship between AN and malignancy, the high frequency of AN in the general population and its lack of specificity for malignancy suggest that when history and physical examination are negative, an extensive cancer workup is unlikely to be productive.

DIABETIC THICK SKIN

Several specific syndromes are associated with localized thickening of the skin in DM and are discussed below.

Scleroderma-Like Syndrome and Limited Joint Mobility

Clinical/Epidemiology

Scleroderma-like syndrome (SLS) is typically described in children and young adults with type 1 diabetes mellitus (T1DM) in the context of the "diabetic hand syndrome," limited joint mobility (LJM), or "cheiroarthropathy." Skin and joint findings usually coexist in most cases, although each may exist independently. Clinical findings include cutaneous thickening and induration of the dorsal fingers associated with painless loss of interphalangeal joint mobility. Involvement proximal to the metacarpophalangeal joints may occur in patients with long-term diabetes, and larger joints of the elbow, knee, and foot may be affected. LJM is thought to result from deposition of connective tissue in the periarticular soft tissues around the joint capsule rather than from a true arthropathy. LJM may be demonstrated by the "prayer sign" (Fig. 29-2), which shows an inability to flatten the palmer surface with fingers spread apart.

Approximately 50% of adolescent patients with T1DM for more than 5 years are affected. SLS and LJM are common in T2DM as well. Longitudinal control of diabetes as measured by HbA_{1c} is strongly associated with the presence or absence of LJM. Most important, LJM is strongly correlated with microvascular disease, and retinopathy appears to be most closely associated.

Pathogenesis

The pathogenesis of SLS and LJM is not fully understood. Nonenzymatic glycosylation (NEG) of connective tissue and attenuated hyaluronic acid deposition in the dermis may be involved.

Treatment

Intensive insulin therapy may be beneficial in the prevention and treatment of LJM and SLS. Small studies have shown that tight glycemic control results in decreased skin thickness and delayed onset of LJM. Treatment of LJM with sorbinil, an aldose reductase inhibitor, was effective over a 10-year period in 2 patients. Physical therapy to preserve range of motion should be considered as well.

Scleredema

Clinical/Epidemiology

Scleredema of diabetes, or scleredema diabeticorum (SD), is characterized as firm, "woody," nonpitting edema of the skin, symmetrically distributed over

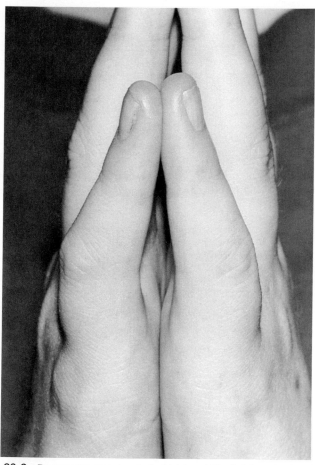

FIG. 29-2   Prayer sign showing limited joint mobility (LJM) and scleroderma-like syndrome (SLS) skin changes. This young woman with T1DM also has severe diabetic retinopathy and nephropathy.

the posterior neck, upper back, and shoulders. Occasionally, the skin thickness can be so severe as to limit complete range of motion of the neck and shoulders (Fig. 29-3). However, SD is usually asymptomatic and may go unnoticed by the patient. This condition is present in 2.5–14% of diabetic patients, depending on the study.

SD may be seen in both T1DM and T2DM, but is much more common in type 2 disease, and is associated with obesity. Other forms of scleredema include the classical scleredema adultorum of Buschke, which occurs after a febrile illness, and idiopathic scleredema adultorum. Clinically, these types of scleredema are similar to SD, but facial involvement is more common and, unlike SD, they may resolve spontaneously within 2 years. Monoclonal gammopathy and multiple myeloma have been reported with scleredema. SD does not appear to correlate with retinopathy, nephropathy, or neuropathy.

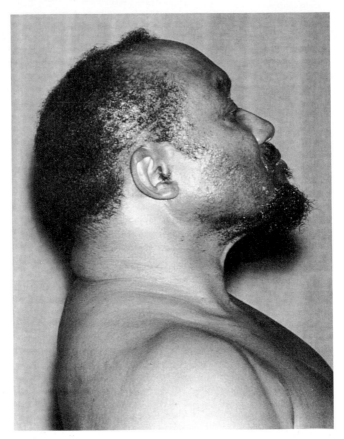

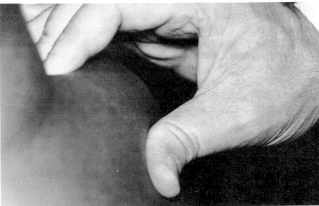

FIG. 29-3   *(Top)* A man with adult-onset DM with sclerodem diabeticorum so severe that it restricts his efforts at neck extension. *(Bottom)* A close-up view of the remarkable thickening of skin on his neck.

Pathogenesis

Although the pathogenesis is unclear, on histopathology, SD is characterized by remarkable thickening of the dermis and increased mucin (acid mucopolysaccharide) deposition. One study showed enhanced synthesis of extracellular macromolecules in cultured fibroblasts incubated with serum from patients with scleredema and paraproteinemia. Unfortunately, most of the studies have focused on paraproteinemia-associated scleredema and involved a small numbers of cases.

Treatment

No current established therapy exists for SD, and it usually persists chronically. Case reports regarding the use of electron-beam radiation, penicillin, cyclosporine, bath photochemotherapy (psoralen plus ultraviolet A light treatment, PUVA), and prostaglandin E_1 have recently been referenced.

CUTANEOUS INFECTIONS

The true association between DM and cutaneous infections is not known; however, infection clearly makes diabetes more difficult to manage and, conversely, hyperglycemia and ketoacidosis diminish chemotaxis, phagocytosis, and bactericidal ability of white blood cells. Few population-based studies have looked at the prevalence of cutaneous infections in DM. Still, we will discuss some of the cutaneous infections that appear to be over represented, occur with greater severity, or are associated with worse adverse outcomes in diabetic patients.

Bacterial Infections

Streptococcal Infections

Population-based studies have shown diabetes to be a risk factor for invasive group B streptococcal infection in adults. Skin and soft tissues were the most common local sites of infection. Approximately 30% of the patients had DM, and the overall case mortality rate was 21–32%. Diabetes is also associated with a 3.7-fold increased relative risk of invasive group A streptococcal infections.

Malignant External Otitis

Malignant external otitis (MEO) is a life-threatening pyogenic infection of the external ear canal with the potential for intracranial extension. *Pseudomonas aeruginosa* is often the causative organism. Usually seen in older diabetic patients, MEO presents with facial swelling, unrelenting pain, hearing loss, purulent discharge, and granulation tissue in the ear canal. The onset may be indolent, and the diagnosis is often delayed. The majority of patients who develop MEO have DM. Preceding aural irrigation with tap water has been implicated. The mortality rate is cited as 20–40% despite appropriate antibiotics.

Necrotizing Fasciitis

Necrotizing fasciitis (NF) is a potentially lethal infection seen postoperatively, following minor trauma, and occasionally at injection sites. Synergistic infection involving two or more organisms is the rule; however, monomicrobial NF does occur, most commonly with streptococcal species. Polymicrobial infections result most often from facultative gram-negative organisms such as *Escherichia coli,* and anaerobes such as *Bacteroides,* peptostreptococci, and *Clostridium* species. The perineum, trunk, abdomen, and upper extremities are most commonly involved. Toxicity is often out of proportion to signs. Skin findings include redness, induration, cyanosis, and necrosis with overlying bullae. Approximately 10–60% of patients with necrotizing soft tissue infection have diabetes. Mortality rates of 21–80% have been reported. The most important aspect of treatment is early aggressive surgical debridement.

Staphylococcal Infections

The prevalence of staphylococcal infections in diabetic patients has been a source of controversy. Recent reviewers agree that available data do not permit an estimation of the proportional risk of staphylococcal infection in patients with DM, but that an increased rate of staphylococcal carriage may be found in certain subsets of patients.

Erythrasma

Erythrasma is an infection of intertriginous skin with *Corynebacterium minutissimum.* The organism produces a porphyrin pigment that results in characteristic coral red fluorescence when a Wood's lamp is shined on the skin. The infection is of little medical consequence but has been observed in up to 61% of diabetic patients. Erythrasma may be treated with topical or oral erythromycin.

Fungal and Yeast Infections

Candidal Infections

Candida albicans causes angular cheilitis, glossitis, vulvovaginitis, balanitis, finger web space infection, and paronychia in diabetic patients. *Candida* infection appears to be more common in patients with poorly controlled diabetes. Clinical evidence of candidal paronychia was observed in 9.6% of 250 diabetic women, compared with only 3.4% of 500 nondiabetic women. Treatment includes oral or topical antifungals. In the case of paronychia, prolonged wetness should be avoided (e.g., wear cotton gloves under rubber gloves when working in water). Treatment with drying agents is beneficial, e.g., 15% sulfacetamide in 50% ethanol (3–4 drops four times per day and each time the hands get wet).

Dermatophyte Infections

The prevalence of toenail onychomycosis appears to be increased in patients with diabetes. Treatment of tinea pedis and onychomycosis in diabetic patients is important because the infection may provide a portal of entry for subsequent bacterial infections. Topical antifungals usually suffice to control fungal infection on skin adjacent to affected nails, but oral agents are needed to clear the onychomycosis.

Rhinocerebral Mucormycosis

Rhinocerebral mucormycosis (RCM) is a destructive nasal mucosa and sinus infection caused by Zygomycetes (*Mucor* and *Rhizopus* species). RCM usually presents as facial or ocular pain and nasal stuffiness with or without discharge. Later manifestations may include proptosis, necrotic lesions on the palate or nasal turbinate, ophthalmoplegia, and vision loss. Approximately 75–80% of RCM occurs in diabetic patients with uncontrolled disease. Amphotericin B and surgical debridement are the treatments of choice. Mortality rates for RCM have been reported to be 15–34%.

ERUPTIVE XANTHOMAS

Clinical/Epidemiology

Eruptive xanthomas appear as asymptomatic to mildly pruritic 1- to 4-mm reddish-yellow papules on the buttocks and extensor surfaces of the arms and legs. They are a cutaneous manifestation of severe hypertriglyceridemia, and may be the first indication of diabetes. Complications of severe, untreated hypertriglyceridemia include abdominal pain, pancreatitis, hepatosplenomegaly, lipemia retinalis, hypoxemia, abnormal hemoglobin oxygen affinity, decreased pulmonary diffusing capacities, and psychologic changes.

Pathogenesis

Diabetes is the most common cause of acquired hypertriglyceridemia (see Chap. 24). In uncontrolled diabetes, the activity of lipoprotein lipase, the enzyme that normally clears triglyceride-rich chylomicrons, is decreased. In addition, insulin is necessary for normal clearance of plasma lipoproteins. In eruptive xanthomas, plasma lipoproteins enter the skin and are phagocytosed by macrophages that appear as foam-laden cells on histopathology.

Treatment

Hypertriglyceridemia responds rapidly to diet and insulin therapy, and the eruptive xanthomas usually resolve completely in 6–8 weeks.

NECROBIOSIS LIPOIDICA

Clinical/Epidemiology

Many investigators prefer the term *necrobiosis lipoidica* (NL) to the previously used *necrobiosis lipoidica diabeticorum,* because NL can occur in patients without diabetes. Clinically, NL presents as one or more asymptomatic, oval, sharply marginated, reddish-brown plaques over the anterior lower legs (bilateral 75% of the time) on young (mean age, 30 years) diabetic women (3:1 female:male ratio). The plaques often slowly enlarge, with central development of yellowish glazed-porcelain sheen and prominent telangiectasias (Fig. 29-4). The active margins remain erythematous and slightly elevated. Ulceration occurs in about one-third of diabetic patients with NL, and spontaneous remission is relatively rare (19%). Other sites can be involved, but NL only rarely spares the legs (2% of the time).

Between 11% and 66% of patients with NL have DM. However, most patients with diabetes do not have NL (less than 1%).

Pathogenesis

NL is characterized by altered extracellular matrix and degenerative changes in collagen and elastic fibers. The exact pathogenesis of NL remains unknown. Proposed mechanisms include heredity, microangiopathy, increased produc-

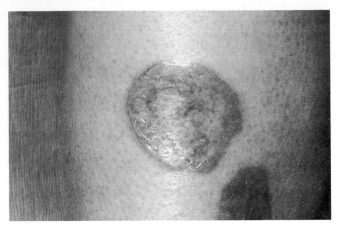

FIG. 29-4   Plaques of necrobiosis lipoidica. The lesion has a typical glazed-porcelain sheen and yellowish hue with prominent telangiectasia.

tion of fibronectin by endothelial cells, increased factor VIII-related antigen, abnormal platelet function and prostaglandin synthesis, accelerated collagen aging, and immune-mediated vasculopathy. Expression of metalloproteinases has been noted in early lesions, suggesting that collagenolysis may play an early role. Poor glycemic control does not appear to be a factor in NL.

Treatment

Treatment of NL is difficult. In early, inflammatory lesions, high-potency topical steroids may be useful. Likewise, injection of triamcinolone in perilesional skin has been used with success; however, care should be exercised with local steroid use because ulceration may occur. Oral treatments include short-term use of systemic steroids, and pentoxifylline. Experience with dipyridamole and aspirin has been disappointing. Cover-up products such as Dermablend or Covermark may be useful cosmetically. Protective padding is advised for ulcer protection during high-risk activities, and a nightlight is useful to prevent inadvertent trauma at night. Cyclosporine has been reported for the treatment of persistently ulcerated NL. For very large or recalcitrant ulcers in NL, excision down to fascia with split-thickness skin grafting may be necessary.

GRANULOMA ANNULARE

Clinical/Epidemiology

Granuloma annulare (GA) is a benign, self-limited condition characterized by annular plaques usually seen over the dorsal hands, feet, or ankles. The plaques often consist of a ring of red to violaceous papules with clearing or flattening in the center. Other presentations include solitary or generalized papules. Rarely, subcutaneous nodules or perforating lesions may occur. About 15% of patients have more than 10 lesions, and 7–10% have generalized lesions. Localized GA occurs at a younger age (two-thirds before age 30) and usually clears within 2 years, whereas generalized GA occurs in an older population (mean age of onset is 52 years) and rarely clears spontaneously.

Although most patients with GA have no underlying disorder, an association with DM is supported in the literature. Approximately 10–20% of patients with GA have DM. Patients with generalized GA are more likely to have diabetes than those with localized lesions.

Pathogenesis

The pathogenesis of GA remains unknown. Like NL, GA is characterized by altered extracellular matrix and degenerative changes in collagen and elastic fibers in the dermis. Expression of metaloproteases was also noted in lesions of GA.

Treatment

GA is usually an asymptomatic, self-limited process. Treatment with high-potency topical steroids or steroid injection may be effective for localized lesions. Generalized GA may be more pruritic and persistent, and is more cosmetically disabling. Encouraging results for generalized GA have been reported with PUVA. Limited success has been reported with systemic corticosteroids, chloroquine, potassium iodide, sulfones, niacinamide, and chlorpropamide. A careful history and physical examination should be done with the question of diabetes in mind. It can be argued that a fasting blood sugar should be obtained in older patients with generalized GA.

DIABETIC DERMOPATHY

Clinical/Epidemiology

Diabetic dermopathy is the term used to describe the small (2–10-mm), rounded, brownish, atrophic lesions over the pretibial surface of the legs in diabetic patients (Fig. 29-5). Prevalence of atrophic shin spots ascertained from diabetic patients in outpatient clinics has ranged from 24% to 65% for males and from 4% to 39% for females. The prevalence in nondiabetic control groups was between 1.6% and 20% depending on the chosen control group population (i.e., healthy versus patients in an endocrine clinic). A population-based study in Sweden found shin spots in 33% of patients with T1DM and in 39% of patients with T2DM, compared with 2% of a control group comprised of 100 healthy people, mainly hospital personnel aged 15–50 years.

Pathogenesis

The pathogenesis of the condition is unknown. It is likely that the lesions are related to repetitive, minor, antecedent trauma, even though most patients are unaware of associated trauma and the lesions are asymptomatic. Arguments in favor of trauma are supported by the location on the shins and the increased prevalence in men. In the most recent study of 173 patients with DM (69 with atrophic shin spots), a strong statistical relationship with retinopathy, nephropathy, and neuropathy was reported.

Treatment

No treatment is necessary, since the lesions of diabetic dermopathy are without symptoms or direct morbidity. Attempts to avoid trauma to the shins may be appropriate.

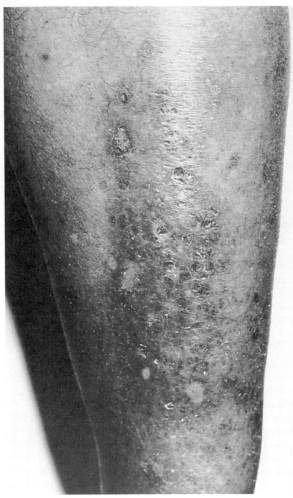

FIG. 29-5   Atrophic "shin spots" or diabetic dermopathy on the legs of a diabetic man.

BULLOSIS DIABETICORUM

Clinical/Epidemiology

The abrupt onset of bullae on the extremities has been reported as a rare condition associated with diabetes. The lesions of bullosis diabeticorum (BD) are usually on the toes, feet, and distal lower extremities, but may be observed on the fingers, hands, and forearms. They are unrelated to any apparent trauma or infection and heal without scarring in 2–5 weeks unless they become infected. The condition may resolve spontaneously or recur over a number of years.

Pathogenesis

The pathogenesis is unknown. Patients with BD do not have an antecedent history of trauma. The histopathology shows an inconsistent level of separation varying from intraepidermal to subepidermal. Direct immunofluorescence is usually negative, and no immunopathologic features are consistently found. Increased skin fragility has been implicated.

Treatment

Treatment consists of supportive wound care. It is of utmost importance that other blistering disorders of the skin be considered in the diagnostic workup. The differential diagnosis includes bullous impetigo, bullous pemphigoid, pemphigus vulgaris, epidermolysis bullosa acquisita, porphyria cutanea tarda (PCT), bullous erythema multiforme (e.g., due to drugs), and insect-bite reaction. Distinguishing BD from other blistering conditions is important because treatment of the latter may involve the use of systemic steroids or immunosuppressive therapy, which confers significant risk of toxicity to diabetic patients.

ACQUIRED PERFORATING DERMATOSIS

Clinical/Epidemiology

Acquired perforating dermatosis (APD) has been reported in association with diabetes and renal failure. A variety of terms used for this group of conditions include Kyrle's disease, reactive perforating collagenosis (RPC), perforating folliculitis, and elastosis perforans serpiginosa (EPS). Because histology may vary from location to location on the same patient and the pathogenesis is unclear, it appears more logical to consider these conditions together rather than to emphasize differences.

Clinically, APD presents as pruritic, keratotic, papules and nodules located on the extremities, trunk and, to a lesser extent, the face. The lesions are often perifollicular. In one series, 16 of 22 patients (72%) with RPC had diabetes, and 10 were on dialysis. Many had systemic complications of diabetes. These observations are supportive of the association of APD with DM and chronic renal failure, and suggest that APD may be more common than previously appreciated.

Pathogenesis

APD is characterized by transepidermal elimination of what appears to be altered collagen. The pathogenesis is unclear, but has been postulated to involve deposition of "uremic substances," such as uric acid or hydroxyapatite. The deposition is thought to elicit an inflammatory response and foreign-body reaction resulting in transepidermal elimination of dermal constituents. Local trauma and chronic rubbing may also play a role.

Treatment

Treatment with glycemic control, ultraviolet light, retinoic acid, or topical steroids is at times effective.

INSULIN INJECTION COMPLICATIONS

Intensive insulin therapy with multiple daily insulin injections or external insulin pumps has become the norm (see Chap. 19). Although the possibility of increased skin complications exists with intensive insulin therapy, the incidence of complications has actually decreased with the more recent use of purified pork and bovine insulin as well as with human insulin (HI). Possible complications of insulin injection are discussed below.

Lipoatrophy

Insulin induced lipoatrophy has been attributed to local immune complex formation and complement fixation with release of lysosomal enzymes in response to a presumed antigenic component of the less purified insulins. The current use of highly purified insulin results in significantly less lipoatrophy than with earlier preparations (0–2.5% versus 16%, respectively). Still, lipoatrophy from injection of intermediate- and long-acting HI has been reported.

Lipohypertrophy

Lipohypertrophy is thought to occur because of a local anabolic effect of insulin that promotes fat and protein synthesis. Approximately 20–30% of patients may develop localized fat hypertrophy. Unlike lipoatrophy, the frequency of lipohypertrophy has not decreased with the use of highly purified insulin and HI. The problem can usually be alleviated by rotation of injection sites. Insulin absorption can be delayed or inconsistent in the hypertrophic areas, so patients should be discouraged from using the sites for injection.

Allergic Reactions

Local and systemic allergic reactions have been reported with insulin injections. Local reactions are by far the most common. Etiologic factors include contaminating proteins, zinc, protamine, and insulin itself (including HI). Clinically, local reactions usually present as a wheal and flare within 30 minutes of injection. Most are IgE-mediated. Local reactions to insulin are often transient and of no major significance.

Systemic allergic reactions, though rare, are potentially life-threatening. They include urticaria, angioedema, anaphylaxis, and the Arthus reaction. Although highly purified insulin and HI are less immunogenic, allergic reactions are still observed. Intradermal testing may be used to find an insulin preparation to which the patient does not react. Desensitization techniques are useful for generalized insulin allergies. Systemic steroids and antihistamines are occasionally required.

Nonimmunologic Cutaneous Reactions

Nonimmunologic reactions include infections (e.g., *S. aureus, S. epidermidis,* and *M. chelonei*), zinc granulomas, sterile abscesses, silicon oil granulomas from disposable syringes, keloid formation, and pigmentation that can resemble acanthosis nigricans.

Continuous Subcutaneous Insulin Infusion (CSII)

Skin complications are the most common reason for discontinuation of CSII. Complications include inflammation, infection, subcutaneous nodule formation, and scarring. *S. epidermidis* and *S. aureus* are among the bacteria that can be cultured from CSSI catheters. In one study, pyogenic skin inflammation was described in 48% of 50 patients treated with CSII, compared with 6% of the insulin-injecting patients and 3% of healthy volunteers. Recommendations regarding skin care with CSII include needle change every 48 hours, no catheter reuse, hand washing before insertion of needles, antiseptic preparation of needle insertion sites, and sterile covering of the needles.

ADDITIONAL READINGS

American Diabetes Association. Consensus Development Conference on Diabetic Foot Wound Care: 7–8 April, 1999, Boston, Massachusetts. *Diabetes Care*.1999;22:1354.

Bub JL, Olerud JE. Diabetes mellitus. In: Freedberg IM, Eisen AZ, Wolff K, et al, eds. *Fitzpatrick's Dermatology in General Medicine,* 6th ed. New York: McGraw-Hill; 2003:1651.

The Diabetes Control and Complications Trial Research Group. The effect of intensive treatment of diabetes on the development and progression of long-term complications in insulin-dependent diabetes mellitus. N Engl J Med. 1993;329:977.

Joshi N, Caputo Gm, Weitekamp MR, Karchmer AW. Infections in patients with diabetes mellitus. *N Engl J Med.* 1999;341:1906.

Reiber GE, Vileikyte L, Boyko EJ, et al. Causal pathways for incident lower-extremity ulcers in patients with diabetes from two settings. *Diabetes Care.* 1999;22:157.

For a more detailed discussion of this topic and a bibliography, please see Porte *et al: Ellenberg & Rifkin's Diabetes Mellitus,* 6th ed., Chapter 53.

New Treatments for
Diabetes Mellitus:
Outlook for the Future

Lester B. Salans

INTRODUCTION

The importance of achieving and maintaining normal or near-normal blood glucose levels ("tight" glucose control) in individuals with diabetes mellitus is well established. In the great majority of diabetic patients, however, glycemic levels necessary to completely control the disease and to eliminate chronic complications are not achieved. As a result, the disease progressively worsens over time and complications develop. New therapeutic tools can achieve tight glucose control and treatment of diabetes has improved, but the intensive regimens required are neither practical nor feasible for many patients. Even under circumstances where best current treatment is optimally applied by highly motivated patients, tight control of blood glucose reduces but does not entirely eliminate disease progression and complications. Clearly, there is a need for still better treatments *and* better treatment approaches.

This chapter will review some of the major shortcomings of current treatment for type 1 diabetes mellitus (T1DM) and type 2 diabetes mellitus (T2DM), and some of the pharmacologic agents and technologies under investigation and in development for the treatment of diabetes and its complications in the future.

T1DM: TREATMENT SHORTCOMINGS

Intensive Treatment Regimens Are Difficult for Patient Compliance

Achievement of levels of blood glucose necessary to prevent or control disease progression and diabetic complications requires strict therapeutic regimens that are neither practical nor feasible for many patients and their families. Intensive therapy requires multiple daily injections of insulin and frequent monitoring of blood glucose. Adherence to stringent dietary practices coupled with the necessity to coordinate food intake, physical activity, and insulin administration is difficult, especially for children and adolescents.

Intensive Therapy Regimens Cause Frequent Episodes of Hypoglycemia

Current therapeutic regimens that achieve normal or near-normal glycemia cause frequent episodes of hypoglycemia. Hypoglycemia and the accompanying counterregulatory hormone response produced by iatrogenic hypoglycemia are often the major limiting factor in achieving tight glucose control. Frequent hypoglycemia causes hypoglycemic unawareness. Avoidance of frequent hypoglycemia restores hypoglycemia awareness.

Insulin Is Not Delivered Physiologically

Delivery of insulin by subcutaneous injection does not adequately imitate physiologic control of blood glucose achieved by normal pancreatic β-cells, which continuously adjust insulin secretion according to the prevailing blood glucose. Subcutaneous administration by injection delivers insulin to the peripheral circulation rather than portally, the physiologic route, thereby bypassing its first-pass effect to rapidly decrease hepatic glucose output. As another consequence of bypassing first-pass hepatic extraction, insulin is delivered to the peripheral tissues in pharmacologic doses, causing chronic exposure to excessive levels of insulin, especially in the fasting or basal state. Chronic hyperinsulinemia impairs insulin action and may increase the risk of diabetic complications.

While providing excessive amounts of insulin during basal or fasting conditions, current practice often does not provide insulin in sufficient amounts or with the appropriate timing and pharmacokinetics to control mealtime and postprandial glucose levels. As a result, mealtime and postprandial blood glucose excursions are excessive.

Complications Begin at Blood Glucose and HbA$_{1c}$ Levels below Current Therapeutic Targets, and Treatments Begin after Complications Exist

The pathophysiologic processes responsible for development of complications, and the risk for micro- and macrovascular disease, begin at levels below the current treatment targets of fasting glucose of ≤ 7 mM/L and HbA$_{1c}$ of <7%. Furthermore, the complications of diabetes often begin before their clinical diagnosis, and specific treatments are begun after complications are well advanced, perhaps at a point when intervention can have only limited effect.

Optimal Glycemic Therapy Requires Costly Multidisciplinary Resources

The integrated, multidisciplinary resources required for intensive therapy, e.g., dietitians, nurse educators, etc., are often not available. Intensive diabetes treatment is costly, beyond the capability of families with limited financial resources, and is inadequately reimbursed.

CHANGES IN THERAPEUTIC APPROACHES FOR T1DM

New Prevention Approaches

Genes

The prevention, cure, and effective treatment of T1DM diabetes may ultimately come from genetic research establishing the genes conferring disease susceptibility, and identifying the mechanisms by which they produce their effects. In spite of enormous progress and promise, gene-based therapy for this polygenic disease is unlikely to be accomplished soon.

Immune System

Primary prevention clinical trials are underway to assess whether immune modulation can prevent T1DM in individuals at high risk. Several approaches for preventing autoimmune β-cell destruction are being pursued, including antigen-, cytokine-, and monoclonal antibody-based interventions. However, applicability of results of trials in high-risk relatives to the general population, in which 90% of new cases of T1DM occur, is uncertain, and broad population-based trials will be necessary.

Environment

Prevention of T1DM might be achieved by blocking environmental factors that activate or interact with T1DM diabetes susceptibility genes. Unfortunately, the offending environmental factors, whether infectious, toxins, dietary, or otherwise, have yet to be identified with certainty.

New Treatment Options

Noninjectable Routes of Insulin Administration

Inhaled insulin: Administration of insulin by pulmonary route is currently in Phase III clinical testing (see Chap. 9), and may be available for treatment in the near future. Issues of reproducible absorption, inhalation technology, powder versus liquid formulations, and, most important, long-term pulmonary safety, remain to be resolved. Given its short duration of action, inhaled insulin will have to be administered in combination with long- and/or intermediate-acting insulin to meet basal requirements and achieve 24-hour glycemic control.

Oral, nasal, and transdermal routes of insulin administration: Proteolytic degradation and poor absorption have made efforts to produce an orally bioavailable insulin difficult. Efforts to develop modified insulins that can be administered orally and absorbed reproducibly through the buccal or intestinal mucosa without loss of biologic activity, and technologies for controlled release of insulin with predictable oral bioavailability and activity using polymer encapsulation and osmotic release are ongoing, and progress is being made. Nasal and transdermal delivery by iontophoresis are being investigated. All of these approaches have encountered significant hurdles and are far from clinical application.

New Injectable Insulin Formulations

Rapid-onset, short-acting insulin: Rapid-onset, short-acting lispro insulin, insulin aspart, and glulisine insulin have enabled better control of mealtime glucose and improved overall glycemic control when used in combination with long-acting insulin in many people with T1DM. Other rapid-acting insulins are in development.

Long-acting insulin: Insulin glargine and insulin detemir are newer long-acting insulin analogs that are now available for clinical use. These insulin formulations provide relatively constant levels of basal insulin over 24-hours, and, in many patients, achieve better control of fasting glucose and HbA$_{1c}$ levels with less nocturnal hypoglycemia than NPH (Neutral Protamine Hagedorn) insulin. When used in combination with premeal short-acting insulin, they can enable significantly better overall 24-hour glucose control.

Hepatoselective insulin analogs: A novel hepatoselective insulin analog, N$^{\alpha\beta1}$L-thyroxyl-insulin (B1-T4-Ins), is currently in early development. It or subsequent analogs have the potential to provide more physiologic insulin action than current insulin preparations.

Pancreatic Islet Transplantation

The use of islet allographs and novel combinations of immunosuppressive agents in type 1 diabetes has recently shown promise, and multicenter trials are underway. However, this highly visible approach has significant hurdles to overcome before successful clinical application. A major hurdle is the lack of sufficient numbers of donor islets to meet the needs for successful islet transplantation. Pluripotential stem cells, and genetically engineered somatic cell lines, may provide a source of cells, and may enable successful transplantation *without* requirement for life-long immune suppression to prevent rejection and autoimmune destruction of transplanted cells. Xenographic transplanted pig islets must overcome concerns about possible transmission of infectious porcine microorganisms.

The "Artificial Pancreas"

An implantable "artificial pancreas" that provides continuous, on-line measurement of blood glucose, activating a mechanical device (pump) to deliver insulin directly to the liver, would permit a more physiologic and readily applicable replacement of insulin (see Chap. 9). Progress is being made, but an acceptable device is unlikely to become available in the near future.

Implantable Insulin Pumps

Delivery systems that are implantable, able to be regulated with great precision, and have more safety features are being developed and may be available in the not-too-distant future for treatment of T1DM (see Chap. 9). Insulin pumps should be used only by well-trained health care personnel, and after thorough training of patients and their families.

Noninvasive Glucose Sensors

Significant progress is being made in developing accurate and sensitive, noninvasive glucose sensors for continuous measurement of blood glucose, displaying, downloading, and storing real-time blood glucose levels at suitable intervals, and containing reliable hypoglycemia alert alarm systems. These will greatly enhance glucose control and reduce risk of hypoglycemia and hypoglycemia unawareness (see Chap. 9).

Control of Mealtime and Postprandial Glucose Levels

Achievement of normal or near-normal glycemia requires control not only of fasting glucose, but also of mealtime and postmeal blood glucose. Treatment of T1DM will therefore increasingly utilize premeal administration of fast-onset, short-acting insulins such as lispro, aspart, glulisine, and possibly inhaled insulin. An analog of amylin, pramlintide, when administered before meals and used as an adjunct to insulin, is reported to reduce postprandial glucose, improve HbA_{1c}, reduce body weight, and decrease insulin dose in both T1DM and T2DM, and may soon be available as an adjunct to insulin therapy. The requirement for parental administration, and inability to mix it with insulin in the same syringe, may limit its clinical use.

Treatments to Induce Remission and Ameliorate Autoimmune β-Cell Destruction

Several antigen-based approaches utilizing antigens postulated to play a role in the autoimmune destruction of β-cells in T1DM, including fragments of the insulin B chain, GAD_{64}, and heat-shock proteins, are in clinical trials.

Other immune targets are also being evaluated in animal and human T1DM. Studies in animal models of diabetes such as the NOD mouse demonstrate that several of these approaches can prevent development of insulitis and T1DM, but the relevance of these results to prevention of human T1DM must await the outcomes of ongoing and future controlled human clinical trials.

Initial clinical studies of a humanized anti-CD-3 monoclonal antibody have recently reported efficacy in inducing remission or slowing rate of progression in newly diagnosed type 1 diabetic patients with sufficient remaining β-cell function.

Methods to Stimulate β-Cell Regeneration and Growth, and Inhibit β-Cell Apoptosis

Advances in β-cell biology could lead eventually to development of methods to stimulate β-cell regeneration in patients with diabetes. Factors such as GLP-1, exendin-4, IGF-1, nitric oxide, and certain β-cell transcription factors, e.g., pancreas duodenum homeobox-containing transcription factor 1 (PDX-1), have been shown to possess stimulatory activity for islet cell growth in laboratory animals, but their specificity is unknown. This approach may also be useful in T2DM. In T1DM it will have to be coupled with immune suppression to prevent autoimmune destruction of newly formed β-cells; it may therefore be more feasible initially in patients with T2DM.

T2DM: TREATMENT SHORTCOMINGS

Limitations of Existing Oral Hypoglycemic Agents

Current oral agents, at least as utilized by most physicians, are limited in their ability to achieve normal or near-normal glycemia in most type 2 diabetic patients. Significant side effects such as hypoglycemia, gastrointestinal dysfunction, fluid retention, edema, liver failure, and lactic acidosis compromise proper dosing and limit patient compliance. Both more effective and safer drugs, as well as better use of existing agents, are required, as discussed below.

Therapy May Be Initiated Too Late

Treatment of T2DM is usually begun after the disease has progressed significantly, perhaps to the point where intervention can have only limited effect. Numerous studies, most recently the UK Prospective Diabetes Study (UKPDS), have established that the complications of diabetes often begin before clinical diagnosis of the disease, and before the development of fasting hyperglycemia and elevated HbA_{1c}. Epidemiologic evidence from the UKPDS indicates that increase risk for micro- and macrovascular disease begins at HbA_{1c} levels of 6.5% or lower. The progressive loss of β-cell function observed in the UKPDS may also reflect initiation of treatment too late in the disease, rather than inevitable loss of function.

Both underlying defects of T2DM, insulin resistance and defective insulin secretion, exist before fasting hyperglycemia occurs, HbA_{1c} becomes elevated, diagnosis of diabetes is made, and therapy is initiated. Both of these defects predict subsequent development of overt disease and may be risk factors for complications; both defects may therefore be targets for earlier therapeutic intervention. Weight loss is perhaps the best of example of reducing insulin resistance to prevent or improve T2DM (see Chap. 6); on the other hand, restoration of acute/early-phase insulin secretion also improves glucose tolerance in T2DM. Loss of acute-phase insulin secretion is often the earliest clinically detectable abnormality of T2DM, commonly lost at fasting glucose levels between 6.1 and 6.5 mmol/L, yet treatment usually does not begin until the diabetes is diagnosed by fasting hyperglycemia. Clearly, T2DM needs to be treated earlier, even before development of fasting hyperglycemia of 7 mmol/L and HbA_{1c} of 7%. As discussed under T1DM earlier, detection and treatment of the complications is also required for improved outcomes in T2DM.

Therapy Is Too Narrowly Focused

Although insulin resistance and defective insulin secretion exist early in the course of the disease, current treatment approaches usually address only one of these two abnormalities. Treatment is likely to be more effective if both defects are addressed—the earlier the better. This requires the use of two oral hypoglycemic drugs with different mechanisms of action, one acting on insulin action, the other on insulin secretion, or insulin.

Additionally, current therapy is often focused solely on managing fasting hyperglycemia and on targeting this endpoint as a measure of adequate glycemic control. Mealtime and postprandial glycemia are often ignored, yet they contribute much to overall 24-hour hyperglycemia, worsen the underlying defects of insulin secretion and action, and may increase risk of complications. Current treatment targets focus on fasting plasma glucose levels and give scant attention to the importance of reducing postprandial hyperglycemia.

Therapy Is Insufficiently Aggressive

Blood glucose levels are often allowed to remain too high for too long because patients are asymptomatic, or for fear of inducing hypoglycemia. Combination therapy with oral agents and addition of, or switching to, insulin is too often delayed until the disease is well advanced and glycemic control has deteriorated substantially.

CHANGES IN THERAPEUTIC APPROACHES FOR T2DM

Prevention

Overweight and Obesity

The most obvious means of preventing a large percentage of T2DM is to prevent obesity. Indeed, clinical studies demonstrate that lifestyle intervention including diet, reduced dietary fat intake, weight loss, and exercise can significantly improve glucose tolerance in individuals at high risk for T2DM. However, societal attitudes, lifestyles, and nutrition tend to increase body weight and reduce physical activity, and preventing obesity or reducing body weight has proven difficult to achieve and to maintain over time. Unless these lifestyle issues can be addressed more effectively other interventions, primarily pharmacologic, will be required.

Genes

Prevention of T2DM may ultimately come from identification of the genes responsible for this disease, *and* discovery of how they function to cause abnormalities of insulin secretion and action. In spite of great progress and promise, gene-based therapy for this polygenic disease is unlikely to occur soon.

New Treatment Options

Because current treatment is often too late, too little, and too narrowly focused, a major shift in the approach to the treatment of T2DM is required.

Earlier Diagnosis and Treatment

T2DM and its complications need to be treated earlier. Increased efforts to detect and treat asymptomatic patients with fasting hyperglycemia, elevated HbA_{1c}, and postprandial hyperglycemia must become standard medical practice. The recent downward revision of the fasting plasma glucose levels diagnostic of diabetes, i.e., ≥ 7 mmol/L (126 mg/dL), and treatment target levels to $HbA_{1c} \leq 7\%$, will enable earlier diagnosis and treatment, but these levels may still not be low enough. The risk of complications begins at even lower levels of fasting glucose and HbA_{1c}. Perhaps treatment should begin even before development of fasting hyperglycemia as defined by current criteria (≥ 7.0 mmol/L), and the therapeutic target for HbA_{1c} of 7% should be lowered to considerably less than 7%. Further downward revision of the current criteria may be necessary. The results of the National Institutes of Health-sponsored Diabetes Prevention Program (DPP) support this view, demonstrating that in prediabetic patients at high risk for developing T2DM (patients with impaired glucose tolerance), treatment intervention to improve glucose control can significantly reduce progression to overt clinical diabetes. Lower diagnostic criteria will enable earlier diagnosis and treatment of abnormalities that contribute to disease progression and complications, with the likelihood of more effective outcomes.

The establishment of categories of impaired glucose tolerance (IGT) and impaired fasting glucose (IFG) provides another opportunity for a major shift in the management of T2DM by potentially enabling earlier intervention. The DPP indicates that treatment during IGT, either with an effective program of diet and exercise or with the oral hypoglycemic drug metformin, can decrease the rate of progression of IGT to frank T2DM. Thus, in all likelihood, future therapy may be directed toward treating individuals with what is currently categorized as IGT with lifestyle-change programs (diet, weight control, and exercise), or with oral hypoglycemic agents capable of overcoming insulin resistance and/or restoring acute insulin secretion and lowering postprandial blood glucose. Drugs with proven safety and very low risk of hypoglycemia will have to be utilized. At this time, in the view of this author, lifestyle modification, including better nutrition, weight loss, and maintenance of normal body weight, and an appropriate program of physical activity, appears to be safer than currently available oral hypoglycemic agents for long-term use for early intervention in patients with IGT.

Future therapy may also be directed toward treatment of patients with impaired fasting glycemia (IFG). As currently defined, IFG identifies a different group of at-risk patients in the population than does IGT, with perhaps as little as 30–50% overlap with IGT. Thus, if IFG were utilized to determine treatment intervention, large numbers of patients with IGT would go undetected. Since IGT is known to be a significant risk factor for development of cardiovascular disease, detection and treatment of IFG *alone,* without detection and treatment of IGT, would appear to be an undesirable strategy for early detection of risk and early intervention. For this reason, it has been suggested that the fasting glucose level diagnostic of IFG be lowered to ≤ 6 mmol/L (108 mg/dL) in order to define individuals more similar to those with IGT with regard to risk of cardiovascular disease, and that oral glucose tolerance testing continue in high-risk patients.

Control of Mealtime and Postprandial Blood Glucose

Therapy of T2DM in the future should focus not only on controlling fasting blood glucose and HbA_{1c}, but also on control of mealtime and postmeal glucose levels. In some type 2 diabetic patients, reduction of postprandial glucose levels has been shown to contribute to lowering HbA_{1c} at least as much as reduction of fasting glucose. In the future, mealtime and postprandial hyperglycemia may be treated before *fasting hyperglycemia occurs* (i.e., before fasting glucose reaches 7 mmol/L or 126 mg/dL). For example, patients with elevated postprandial glucose levels but normal fasting glucose may be treated with proven-safe oral hypoglycemic agents capable of stimulating early insulin secretion and lowering postmeal hyperglycemia. Screening of patients at high risk for developing T2DM with oral glucose tolerance tests, although cumbersome, is desirable. Appropriate targets for postprandial glucose levels will have to be established. Current epidemiologic data on increased cardiovascular risk suggest that a 2-hour postprandial plasma glucose of 11 mmol/L is too high. A level of less than 8.9 mmol/L (160 mg/dL) may be more appropriate.

Combination Therapy

It is unlikely that a single oral agent will successfully control 24-hour blood glucose levels for very long in most patients with T2DM. Some have therefore proposed that combinations of two or more drugs (see Chaps. 10 and 12) that target *both* underlying defects of T2DM, impaired insulin secretion and action, and *both* fasting and postprandial hyperglycemia, should begin early in the course of the disease, perhaps at time of diagnosis, in order to achieve better overall glycemic control, and perhaps more successfully modify the disease process. Earlier addition or switch to insulin may be required in certain patients in order to control blood glucose more aggressively.

New Orally Active Drugs to Stimulate Insulin Action and Overcome Insulin Resistance

Numerous targets exist for drugs to decrease insulin resistance, enhance insulin action, and increase glucose disposal, principally insulin signaling proteins (see Chap. 5). Although defects have been demonstrated at several molecular sites in the insulin signaling pathway, which one (or ones), if any, accounts for the insulin-resistant state in human T2DM is not known. Therefore, which might be a viable target for new drugs to overcome insulin resistance remains conjectural. Given the high likelihood that there is a heterogeneity of defects responsible for insulin resistance in T2DM, that the relative contribution of each defect varies among T2DM patients, and that insulin resistance may be the result of additive effects of several interacting genetic and environmental factors on several insulin signaling proteins, a single drug to prevent or correct all forms of insulin resistance in type 2 populations is unlikely. Rather, multiple drugs targeted to different signaling molecules, together with lifestyle interventions, may have to be utilized.

Insulin mimetics, potentiators, and sensitizers: Molecules are being developed to act at the insulin receptor or at one or more postreceptor signaling event to either mimic, potentiate, or sensitize cells to insulin action in order to overcome insulin resistance and promote glucose disposal. Among those currently in development are molecules mimicking insulin action through phosphorylation of the tyrosine kinase domain of the insulin receptor, inhibitors of protein tyrosine phosphatase, especially PTP-1B, and stimulators of insulin receptor substrate 1 (IRS-1), second messenger systems such as phosphatidylinositol-3-phosphate kinase (PI-3 kinase), glucose transport, and other downstream signaling proteins.

PPARγ activators: Drugs acting through the nuclear receptor peroxisome proliferator-activated receptor complex (PPAR) increase insulin sensitivity, decrease insulin resistance, and increase glucose disposal, thereby lowering blood glucose (see Chap. 12). The two drugs currently clinically available, rosiglitazone and pioglitazone, acting through the PPARγ component of the nuclear complex, have significant but modest hypoglycemic efficacy but can be associated with significant weight gain, fluid retention, edema, and increased risk for congestive heart failure, side effects that may limit their long-term usefulness. They are most helpful when used in combination with other oral agents or insulin. Thiazoladinedione (TZD) and non-TZD agents with greater efficacy and safety are being sought. Several agents, acting either through PPARγ or as dual PPARα–PPARγ agonists, are in clinical trials, the latter appearing to have greater benefits on plasma lipids. Whether they possess meaningful efficacy and safety advantages remains to be demonstrated. The reported anti-inflammatory effects of the TZDs are intriguing with respect to their potential influence on accelerated atherosclerosis in diabetes.

β₃-Adrenergic receptor agonists: β₃-Adrenergic receptor agonists, which increase insulin-stimulated glucose disposal and improve glucose tolerance in laboratory animals and humans, have been hampered by having modest hypoglycemic efficacy, insufficient selectivity, limited bioavailability, and significant sides effects in humans.

Inhibition of hepatic gluconeogenesis and hepatic glucose output: Inhibitors of gluconeogenic enzymes such as PEPCK and F1-6 bisphosphonate have been associated with serious hypoglycemia. Progress toward developing safer agents is being made. New avenues of research are being pursued, such as overexpression of the bifunctional hepatic enzyme 6-phosphofructo-2-kinase/fructose-2-6-bisphosphonate, thereby decreasing gluconeogenesis and increasing glycolysis.

Stimulation of glycogen synthesis: The demonstration that reduced levels of hepatic glycogen contribute to increased hepatic glucose production in T2DM has led to efforts to seek drugs that increase the capacity of the liver for glycogenesis. Focus has been on molecules that enhance the activity of glycogen synthase, hepatic glucokinase, and subunits of hepatic protein phosphatase-1 (PTP-1) in order to enhance glucose disposal and glycogen storage in diabetic patients, thereby lowering blood glucose.

Growth hormone and insulin-like growth factor-1 (IGF-1): Fragments of growth hormone (e.g., hGH 6-13) have been shown to increase insulin action and improve glucose tolerance in laboratory animals. Several analogs are in preclinical development. IGF-1 stimulates insulin action in rodents and humans, and has been explored for treatment of T2DM. However, IGF-1 has been associated with significant side effects, which appear to be reduced by combination with its binding protein, IGF-BP3.

Glucagon inhibition: Inhibitors of pancreatic glucagon secretion, e.g., GLP-1, somatostatin, exendin-4, and of glucagon action in the liver (e.g., glucagon receptor antagonists), have been shown to reduce blood glucose in laboratory animals. These agents are discussed in more detail in this chapter under "Glucagon-like-peptide-1."

Obesity-Related Approaches

The most obvious target for increasing insulin action in T2DM and returning blood glucose to normal or near-normal levels is reduction of excess adiposity. Indeed, several clinical studies demonstrate that lifestyle intervention can significantly improve glucose tolerance in individuals at high risk for T2DM. Although recent progress in basic research progress has been great (see Chap. 6), many years will probably be required to develop effective drugs to prevent obesity or achieve and *maintain* weight loss. It is unlikely that a drug targeted to a single mechanism (e.g., leptin, PPY), a neuroendocrine peptide or receptor, or an uncoupling protein, will be successful given the redundancy and complexity of the process regulating eating behavior, energy homeostasis, and the adipose tissue mass. Rather, a combination of agents targeted to different sites in this process is likely to be required.

New Drugs to Stimulate Insulin Secretion

Nonsulfonylurea insulin secretagogues: A new class of nonsulfonylurea insulin secretagogues is now available for reducing mealtime and postprandial hyperglycemia in T2DM. Two drugs from this class are available: repaglinide, a benzoic acid derivative, and nateglinide, an amino acid derivative. A third agent, KAD 1229, currently in development, has only limited clinical experience at this time.

The major value of these nonsulfonylurea insulin secretagogues appears to be their stimulation of early insulin secretion after a meal and control of mealtime and postprandial glucose. They stimulate insulin secretion with very rapid onset and short duration of action, thereby reducing excessive mealtime and postprandial glucose excursions that adversely affect overall glycemia, and they do so with minimal elevation of plasma insulin levels and exposure of tissues to hyperinsulinemia. These drugs offer the opportunity, in certain subsets of type 2 patients, to achieve better overall glycemic control and lower HbA_{1c} levels than can be achieved with current sulfonylyureas that primarily target fasting glucose. They appear to be most useful when used in combination with drugs that enhance insulin action and control fasting glucose, e.g., metformin or $PPAR\gamma$ agonists. Combination with sulfonylureas appears to have no added benefit. As monotherapy, these drugs should be limited to treatment of patients with T2DM with mild hyperglycemia (≤ 7.5 mMol/L [≤ 135 mg/d]), either early in the course of their disease or elderly T2DM patients in whom meal-related hyperglycemia is the most pronounced glycemic abnormality. For T2DM patients with more severe degrees of hyperglycemia, monotherapy with these agents is insufficient. To date, drugs of this class appear to be well tolerated and safe. If this remains the case over the long term, and the risk of hypoglycemia is low, these drugs may have a role in treatment of IGT.

Glucagon-like peptide-1 (GLP-1): Several GLP-1 agonists and drugs that raise plasma levels of GLP-1 are being developed as a new approach for improving glycemic control. Because of its extremely short half-life, native GLP-1 itself is unsuitable as a therapeutic agent. Modified GLP-1 molecules with longer half-lives, requiring only once- or twice-daily injection, are currently undergoing clinical trials and may soon be available. Nevertheless, these peptides must be administered parenterally on a daily basis, and thus their practicality for the treatment of T2DM may be limited.

Exendin-4, a 39-amino acid peptide isolated from saliva of the Gila monster, has a 53% sequence homology to GLP-1. A synthetic exendin-4 molecule, Exenatide, when injected subcutaneously twice daily to patients with T2DM already being treated with oral hypoglycemic agents, stimulates insulin secretion, reduces glucagon secretion, enhances insulin action, slows gastric emptying, and reduces plasma glucose and HbA_{1c}. If ongoing clinical trials demonstrate adequate safety and efficacy, this drug may soon be available for T2DM. Since this peptide, like the modified GLP-1 analogs, must be administered parenterally on a daily basis, its widespread clinical application may be limited. A long-acting formulation that will not require daily injection is being developed, which could have large-scale clinical application and be of considerable value.

Orally bioavailable inhibitors of DPP-IV, the enzyme that degrades GLP-1, are currently in clinical development. These agents raise and maintain increased GLP-1 levels, increase insulin secretion and insulin action, inhibit glucagon secretion, reduce plasma glucose levels, and improve glucose tolerance in T2DM humans and animal models. Clinical trials are in progress, and if efficacy and safety (DPP-IV inhibits several key regulatory peptides) are demonstrated, this could be an attractive drug for treatment of T2DM. These drugs will be used in combination with other hypoglycemic agents.

β-Cell glucokinase: Efforts to restore or enhance β-cell sensitivity to glucose-stimulated insulin secretion by stimulation of β-cell-specific glucokinase activity are currently under investigation. Even if a defect in glucokinase does not exist in the great majority of type 2 diabetics, increased β-cell sensitivity to glucose should be useful.

COMPLICATIONS OF DIABETES

Therapies for Prevention and Treatment

Methods for Earlier Detection of Complications

Earlier detection of the complications of diabetes might enable earlier intervention, thus prevention or slowing the rate of progression. Among tools currently under study are the use of magnetic resonance imaging (MRI) to detect early retinopathy, measurement of methylglyoxal and other α-dicarbonyl glucose derivatives to detect early diabetic nephropathy, cardiovascular autonomic function, and cardiovascular PET scanning.

Tissue-Specific Therapies

Identification of potential molecular and biochemical mechanisms by which hyperglycemia causes tissue damage gives rise to potential new therapeutic interventions targeted directly to diabetic complications. Many of these approaches are directed toward hyperglycemia-induced alterations in vascular endothelial cells. A few of them are discussed below.

Inhibitors of AGE and AGE-RAGE interactions: A second generation of inhibitors of advanced glycation end-product (AGE) formation and cross-link inhibitors is being developed after the first-generation molecule encountered safety and efficacy problems. Inhibition of the AGE-RAGE (receptors for AGE) interaction by blocking RAGE on endothelial, vascular smooth muscle, neural, mesangial, immune, and inflammatory cells shows promise in laboratory animals. Soluble RAGE (sRAGE) is reported to be effective against microvascular disease in animals, and may provide a basis for developing a small, oral inhibitor of human AGE-RAGE interaction or AGE receptors.

Inhibition of protein kinase C (PKC): PKC is believed to play an important role in the development of the vascular, neurologic, and possibly renal complications of diabetes. At least one inhibitor of PKC is currently in Phase III clinical studies for treatment of diabetic retinopathy and neuropathy. Initial clinical results have been disappointing, but may reflect faulty study design rather than lack of drug efficacy.

Inhibitors of the renin–angiotensin system: Blockade with angiotensin-converting enzymes or angiotensin II receptor inhibitors, alone or in combination, has been shown to improve microalbuminuria and retinopathy in human T1DM and T2DM, and is being increasingly used for diabetic nephropathy.

Inhibitors of aldose reductase and sorbitol formation: Inhibitors of aldose reductase have been developed by several companies for treatment of diabetic neuropathy. Most appear to have limited efficacy and unacceptable toxicity.

Inhibition of angiogenic growth factors to decrease the formation of new blood vessels in diabetic retinopathy: A major focus of current drug discovery and development is inhibitors of vascular endothelial growth factor (VEGF) for the treatment of diabetic retinopathy. Other targets receiving attention for micro- and macrovascular disease include IGF-1, growth hormone, TGF-β, bFGF, other growth factors, integrins and endothelin.

Stimulation of angiogenic growth and other factors: Stimulation of angiogenesis to increase formation of new blood vessels for treatment of coronary and peripheral vascular disease, and to treat neuropathy, is also under study. Gene therapy approaches to stimulate growth of new blood vessels are currently under investigation. Drugs that stimulate VEGF are also being sought for this indication, but these will have to be highly tissue-specific and selective, because systemic effects could adversely affect retinopathy by stimulating new retinal vessel growth.

Antioxidants: A variety of antioxidant drugs and natural substances such as vitamin E, β-carotene, α-lipoic acid, γ-linolenic acid, and inhibitors of superoxide dismutase, catalase, and the hexosamine pathway are being tested in laboratory animals in an attempt to decrease oxidative stress and reactive oxygen species in cells and tissues of the body, a pathologic process thought by some to contribute to development of diabetic complications.

ADDITIONAL READINGS

Ahren B, Gomis R, Mills A, et al: The DPP-4 inhibitor LAF237, improves glycemic control in patients with type 2 diabetes (T2DM) inadequately treated with metformin. *Diabetes* 2004;53(suppl 2):A354.

Bruttomesso D, Pianta A, Mari A, et al: Restoration of early rise in plasma insulin levels improves glucose tolerance of type 2 diabetic patients. *Diabetes* 1999;48:99.

Buse J, Henry R, Han J, et al: Effect of Exenatide(exendin-4) on glycemic control and safety over 30 weeks in sulfonylurea-treated patients with type 2 diabetes. *Diabetes* 2004;53(suppl 2):A352.

Diabetes Prevention Program Research Group: Reduction in the incidence of type 2 diabetes with lifestyle intervention or metformin. *N Engl J Med* 2002;346:393.

Lando H: The new "designer" insulins. *Clin Diabetes* 2000;4:154.

Skyler, J; For the Exubera Phase II Study Group: Sustained long-term efficacy and safety of inhaled insulin during 4 years of continuous therapy. *Diabetes* 2004;53(suppl 2):A486.

For a more detailed discussion of this topic and a bibliography, please see Porte *et al: Ellenberg & Rifkin's Diabetes Mellitus,* 6th ed., Chapter 57.

Index

Page numbers followed by *f* refer to figures; those followed by *t* refer to tables.